NURSING

THE REFLECTIVE APPROACH TO ADULT NURSING

Second Edition

Ann Faulkner

Honorary Professor in Communication Studies,
University of Sheffield, UK and freelance
consultant, author and lecturer, Educational
Consultant to Trent Palliative Care Centre

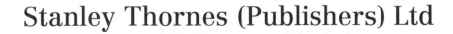

Stanley Thornes (Publishers) Ltd

First edition published in 1985 by Baillière Tindall
Second edition published in 1996 by Chapman & Hall

Reprinted in 2000 by:
Stanley Thornes (Publishers) Ltd
Delta Place
27 Bath Road
CHELTENHAM
Glos.
GL53 7TH
United Kingdom

00 01 02 03 04 / 10 9 8 7 6 5 4 3 2 1

A catalogue record for this book is available from the British Library.

ISBN 0 7487 5834 8

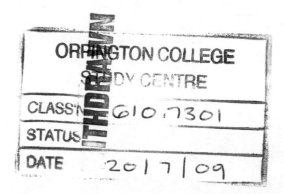
Typeset by Best-set Typesetter Ltd, Hong Kong
Printed and bound in Italy by G. Canale & C.S.p.A., Borgaro, T.se, Turin

NURSING

I would like to dedicate this book
to 'Grannie' and Ellen,
who knew but were not told, and
to Peter
who turns black and white into technicolour

Contents

Preface to the Second Edition, ix

Preface to the First Edition, xi

Acknowledgements, xiii

PART ONE: INTRODUCTION, 1

1   An overview of patient-centred nursing, 3
2   The individual in his normal environment, 20

PART TWO: ASSESSMENT, 65

3   The patient on admission, 67
4   Assessment of the patient's needs, 83
5   The disease process, 105
6   Defining nursing problems, 131

PART THREE: PLANS FOR CARE, 145

7   Care plans, 147
8   Maintaining records, 175

PART FOUR: PROBLEMS AND PLANS FOR CARE, 193

9   Towards diagnosis, 195
10   Planning care: medical interventions, 243
11   Planning care: surgical interventions, 353
12   The elderly patient, 422
13   The dying patient, 460

PART FIVE: EVALUATION AND DISCHARGE, 493

14   Measuring outcomes, 495
15   The patient on discharge, 513

PART SIX: CARE IN THE COMMUNITY, 541

16   Life after hospital, 543
17   Community services, 558
18   The changing role of the nurse, 579

      Index, 611

Preface to the Second Edition

In the 10 years since the first edition of *Nursing: A Creative Approach*, much has changed in health care. The NHS reforms are currently being implemented with much greater emphasis on community and social care. Nursing itself has changed. The implementation of Project 2000 has brought proper student status to nurses and a need for nursing to link more closely with higher education. The new deal for junior doctors has enhanced the role of the nurse and widened considerably her scope of practice.

In some areas of health care, tremendous strides have been made. These include much more sophisticated investigative procedures and certainly one area where there has been vast improvement and refinement has been in surgical procedures, with many hospitals having around 60% of their surgery on a day care basis. The development of laparoscopic and laser techniques has helped to make this possible.

Reading the preface to the first edition, I find the one area where the situation has not changed has been in terms of patient needs. Now, more than ever, individualized care is an imperative. As a result, in writing the second edition, I have retained the mode of writing from the patient's perspective rather than from a medical systems approach, which militates against the identification of the psychosocial problems of both the patient and his relatives.

The aim of the book has not changed. Nurses need skills to identify patients' deficits and needs from the individuals' perspective of their disease so that creative and coherent care may be planned within the framework of the process of nursing. As before, I have included some basic physiology, but the intention remains to leave this area to those who have written specialist texts in order that I could concentrate on the patient's understanding of and reactions to his illness.

Many of the patient vignettes that were in the original edition have remained because they illustrate particular nursing situations. Some new vignettes have been added and, as before, each one comes from a real case study and reflects both my own nursing experience and that of the many students with whom I have worked, both at basic and post-basic level. The importance of the vignettes remains rooted in individuals' reactions to their current situation rather than the diseases from which they have suffered.

Part Four of the book has been divided as before to meet the needs of general nurses for specialized knowledge. This includes nursing patients who require medical intervention and those who require surgical intervention. It also covers care of the elderly and the dying. Other specialties such as psychiatry, paediatrics and learning disabilities have again been left to experts in those fields. In the specialized chapters, common specific diseases have been used to illustrate patients' deficits and needs. In this edition, AIDS has also been addressed. Further reading offers more in-depth knowledge on the areas covered.

In 1996, 11 years after the first edition, there are many more signs that nursing is developing along a problem identification path which can be applied to any individual rather than a stereotyped approach to disease on the part of the nurses. To this end, a new approach in this book is the addition of exercises that are designed to encourage discussion and debate but, more importantly, to encourage reflective practice.

The book has been updated throughout and changes made where necessary. My belief about what nursing is and should be, which underpins this book, has not changed at all.

Ann Faulkner

Preface to the First Edition

For many general nurses, a patient is someone who appears on a hospital ward with a specific disease which will require medical treatment and nursing care. Little is known of the person who is the patient in terms of his background, his responsibilities and his beliefs, and less on how he feels in a new and stressful role.

Individualized care can only be given if something is known of the patient as a person. I have attempted to write this textbook from the patient's perspective rather than from a medical systems approach, which may militate against the psychosocial problems of the patient and his relatives. If it could be said that I have used a model for this book, it is a model of nursing as a function which responds to an individual's reactions to deficits in his normal life pattern. This concept is incorporated in the nursing process by assessment of reaction to deficits, which is followed by planning, implementation and evaluation of care as a dynamic, continuous process.

In the 1984 Winifred Raphael lecture, Dr Wilson-Barnett suggested that the key functions of nursing included understanding illness and treatment from the patient's viewpoint and situation, the provision of continuous psychological care and the provision of comfort for the patient. This book is about these key functions.

The aim of the book is to teach nurses to identify patients' deficits and needs from the individual's perspective of his disease, so that creative and coherent care may be planned within the framework of the nursing process. Although it has been necessary to include some physiology, it has not been my intention to diminish the importance of this subject by scant coverage. Rather, I have left this area to those who have written the specialist texts, in order that I could concentrate on the patient's understanding of, and reactions to, his illness.

Patient vignettes have been used to illustrate nursing situations where possible, and some of these appear in several chapters to form threads throughout the text. Each vignette comes from a real case study and of necessity they reflect my own nursing and personal experience.

The importance of the vignettes is in the individual's reactions rather than the diseases from which he has suffered.

Part Four of the book has been divided to meet the needs of general nurses for specialized knowledge. This includes nursing patients on a medical ward, a surgical ward and a ward for the elderly. Other specialties, such as psychiatry, paediatrics and mental handicap, have again been left to experts in those fields. In the specialized chapters, common specific diseases have been used to illustrate patients' deficits and needs. It is hoped that this will lead to the development of a problem-identification approach to nursing care which can be applied to any individual, rather than a stereotyped approach to disease, on the part of the nurses. There is some overlap between diseases but each disease or operation may be consequently referred to separately.

I hope that this will be a book which the general nurse will use throughout her training alongside the specialist texts recommended in the 'Further reading' at the end of each chapter. I have enjoyed writing a 'different' book and trust that students, and perhaps their tutors, will enjoy reading it. To facilitate ease of reading I have throughout the book used 'she' for a nurse and 'he' for a patient except where a disease is only applicable to the female gender. There is no bias intended towards either sex.

Ann Faulkner

Acknowledgements

The second edition of this book has been made possible by three people, one of whom I have not met. My daughter, Sarah, a Senior Nurse, brought me a paper from the *Nursing Standard* 1993 written by Paul Morbath, who had surveyed books which were considered necessary for nurses studying on Project 2000. Of the 109 titles received, seven were out of print, including *Nursing: A Creative Approach*, which was considered both essential and background reading by respondents. The first edition of this book was published by Baillière Tindall and I worked very closely during that time with Rosemary Morris who was the Nursing Editor. In the meantime Rosemary had moved to Chapman & Hall and she was the third person in the equation, having enough faith in the book to persuade Chapman & Hall to publish the second edition. Many thanks to Sarah, Rosemary and to Paul Morbath.

There are almost too many people to thank for their help with this second edition. Christine Ingleton, a colleague at Trent Palliative Care Centre, took the first edition to senior colleagues in the Sheffield College of Nursing and brought back a precis of their beliefs of how the book should be updated. Her husband gave me much help on Project 2000. Steve Page at Seacroft Hospital in Leeds kindly agreed to allow me to use the documentation work that the Practice Development Unit and staff across the hospital have developed. There are many others too numerous to mention, colleagues and friends who have encouraged me in what was quite a large endeavour in bringing the book up to date, while maintaining its practical approach. The manuscript for the first edition was typed by Joyce Fernandez, who has sadly since died of cancer. I would like to thank Barbara Grimbley for her work on this second edition, typing the changes and retyping the revised changes, all with great good humour.

I will not be the first author who likens writing a book to producing a baby. In writing this second edition, I have been privileged to have Rosemary Morris once again as the midwife, Sarah, a constant source of love and support, and Peter, who is always there with both loving and practical support.

PART ONE
INTRODUCTION

1

An Overview of the Nursing Process and the Holistic Approach to Nursing

CHAPTER SUMMARY

The traditional model of nursing, 3
Why examine the traditional
model? 3
How does the medical model
work? 5
Task-oriented care, 6
The interrelated role of doctor and
nurse, 7

The patient as a person, 8
Patient versus disease, 8
On being a person, 9

The person and roles, 10
Nurse–patient interaction, 11

Nursing as a process, 12
Assessment, 14
Planning, 15
Implementation, 16
Evaluation, 17

Summary, 18

References, 18

Further reading, 19

The traditional model of nursing

Why examine the traditional model?

Since 1977, when the General Nursing Council adopted the nursing process as the preferred vehicle for nursing care, there has been a need to rethink the long-held values inherent in the 'traditional' model of nursing. Nurses have been heard to say that the nursing process is 'what we have always done', truly believing that any change is in documentation. Such beliefs call for clear definitions of both approaches to nursing so that distinctions may be drawn between them.

Most people have a clear idea of what a nurse is. Sometimes this idea is very simple as with the young girl dressed in apron and cap who knows that being a nurse means putting a bandage on her doll or giving a pill to the cat. Many adults share this view of the nurse as one who does things to or for the patient. Others may see her as one who helps the doctor and carries out his orders while others may see her as a professional in her own right. Nurses themselves do not always agree on their role and from time to time the nursing journals will debate the issue of whether or not nurses are professionals.

The 'new deal' for junior doctors (NHS Management Executive 1991) has refuelled the debate. The reduction in junior doctors' hours has led to nurses picking up such tasks as venepuncture, taking a patient's history, refer- ring a patient for investigation and writing discharge let- ters (Cole 1994). Some nurses see this as the opportunity to develop their role into that of a 'practitioner', that is an autonomous professional with an expanded range of skills. Others claim that the nurses are merely being given tasks that doctors do not wish to carry out.

This expansion of the nurse's role which has been a direct response to the change in junior doctors' hours is supported by the UKCC (1992). The debate has been brought into the public arena by the case of a nurse who carried out an appendicectomy under the direction of a surgeon. She was subsequently accused of operating on a patient, thereby putting him at risk, acting unprofession- ally and neglecting her role as patient's advocate (Day 1995).

If there is some discrepancy in individual perceptions of what a nurse is, there is even more on what nursing is. There has been increasing emphasis and interest in 'mod- els' of nursing. Table 1.1 shows the basis of six of these models (Pearson and Vaughan 1991).

The traditional model does not suggest such complex- ity in nursing that at least 14 different theories could have been generated (Kim and Moritz 1982). Rather it suggests the more simple approach of doing things to or for a patient with a certain diagnosis, which have been pre- scribed by the doctor. Of course it is not quite so simple. The nurse is expected to observe and report on the pa- tient's condition and on his reaction to treatment. And although this traditional, medical model may give the im- pression of a nurse subservient to a doctor, the doctor is often dependent upon the nurse for information about the patient.

One thing which the medical model implies is 'owner- ship' of the patient by the consultant. This is an important concept when examining the nursing process and may account for the reservations some doctors are said to feel

Author of model	Rationale
Roper *et al.* (1980) *(Activities of Living)*	Care is based on activities of daily living in good health
Orem (1980) *(Self Care)*	This model is based on self-care as far as the individual is able
Roy (1976) *(Adaptation)*	The underpinning of this model is based on adaptation to change
Neuman (1980) *(Health Care Systems)*	This is also an adaptation model but is related to the stress inherent in illness
Peplau (1980) *(Developmental)*	Although labelled a 'developmental' model, this approach depends heavily on effective interaction
King (1971) *(Interaction)*	This is also an interactive approach to care, using the concepts of interaction and its relationship to individual perceptions

Table 1.1 Rationale for six models of nursing.

towards this approach to nursing. This concept of 'ownership' implies both responsibility and accountability on the part of the medical profession and may suggest that the nurse does not have a decision-making role. This is very different from the notion that care of patients is an ongoing process.

How does the medical model work?

In the medical model, both doctor and nurse are working towards the successful treatment of a disease. This depends on an accurate diagnosis on the part of the doctor, who takes a history from the patient and gives him a physical examination. Various tests and examinations, such as X-rays, may be carried out to assist in an accurate diagnosis. The nurse's role at this diagnostic stage may include observation of temperature, pulse and respiration (TPR), monitoring of blood pressure (BP) and fluid balance, and testing of urine. It may also include the collection of specimens such as urine and faeces for laboratory examination.

With the changing role of the nurse, it may be in future that the patient may be assessed, X-rays ordered and blood taken before the doctor first sees the patient. This will depend on how ill the patient is on arrival.

Once a diagnosis has been made, the doctor may prescribe medical treatment and/or decide that surgical intervention is necessary. The nurse may carry out medical treatment in the form of administering medications, or she may co-ordinate care given by other health professionals such as physiotherapists and dietitians. When surgical intervention is necessary, the nurse's role includes preparation of the patient for surgery, and post-operative care.

In the above situations, whether medical or surgical, the nurse's actions are largely dictated by the medical profession. The nurse is not and cannot be an autonomous decision maker since all decisions on patient care are made by the medical profession, and these decisions are tied to the patient's medical diagnosis. In fact it was not uncommon to hear patients referred to as 'the appendicectomy in the third bed' or 'last night's suicide', before the advent of the nursing process.

Another effect of the traditional model appears to be the making of value judgements about patients. The 'alcoholic' or the 'attempted suicide' may be seen as of little worth compared to the 'gallbladder' or the 'carcinoma of uterus' because their illnesses are thought of as self-inflicted. Of course the nursing process is not a panacea for all ills. Even if a patient is seen as a person with problems rather than as a disease, it may be easier to be tolerant with the physically ill than with those who cannot cope but who still need help with their problems.

Task-oriented care

'Task-oriented care' means that each nurse on a ward takes responsibility for certain tasks, performing them for all patients for whom they have been prescribed. Sharing of the workload in this way is organized by the Ward Sister or Staff Nurse and junior nurses may be linked with more senior nurses so that they can learn how to complete a particular task. Under this system, patients will be cared for by a number of nurses. One may come to attend to pressure areas, another to take temperature, pulse and respiration, while yet another will administer drugs. Patients may not always be aware of the distinctions and may ask the 'wrong' nurse for a bedpan or a drink only to be told, 'Sorry, I am on dressings, dear. Ask Nurse Green.'

If the nurse is concerned with only a part of the patient's care, it becomes difficult for her to build a relationship with the patient or to see him as an individual. It is also difficult for the patient to see enough of any one nurse in order to find someone he can confide in. Both care and patient are fragmented. Such a situation puts the Ward Sister and Staff Nurse in a powerful position since they are the co-ordinators of care and, hopefully, have an overall picture of the patient and his progress.

It could be argued that task allocation militates against individualized nursing care. Further, it may reduce the chances of nurses and doctors working as equal members of a team since it is only the person in charge of the ward who has enough information to liaise with the doctors, and much of that information is second hand.

The interrelated role of doctor and nurse

If nursing is something different and more complex than doing things to or for the patient, and carrying out doctors' orders, what is the relationship between doctor and nurse? A distinction which will be used throughout this book is that the primary role of the doctor is to diagnose and treat a patient's disease while the nurse is more

Fig. 1.1 The interrelated roles of the health care team, showing some of the health professionals involved.

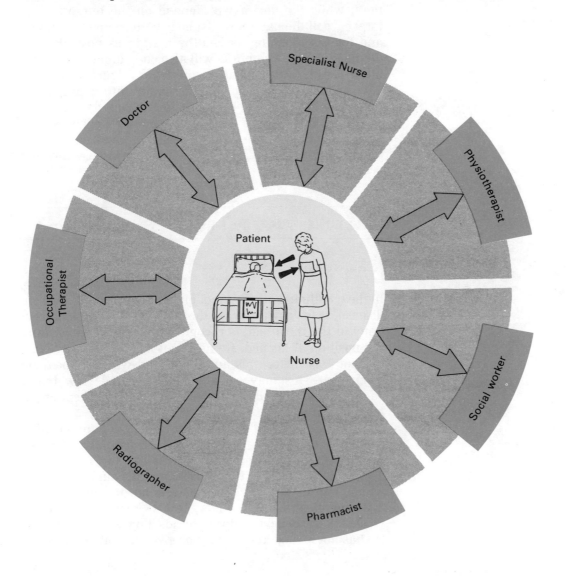

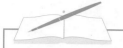

Choose two 'models' of nursing. Identify common themes in both models. Which elements, unique to a particular model, give it strength and credibility?

concerned with the patient's reaction to that disease. This is of course an oversimplification. The nurse cannot ignore the patient's disease, and she will be involved in carrying out treatment prescribed by the doctor. (Similarly, the doctor should note patients' reactions to illness.) However, the nurse will have the added dimension of caring for the whole person and making nursing decisions about his care.

Such an interpretation of the nurse's role moves away from the concept of the nurse being subservient to the doctor. Both can be seen as health professionals with something unique to offer the patient and they should be truly interdependent along with other members of the health care team. The nurse will depend on the doctor for accurate diagnosis and appropriate treatment of the patient, while the doctor will depend on the nurse for the total care of the patient whilst he is undergoing treatment, and for his reaching as healthy a state as possible or a dignified death. The nurse will also co-ordinate care from other health professionals in the team (Figure 1.1).

The above ideas do not fit readily into a pattern of task-oriented, fragmented care but rather demand that the nurse looks after a few patients in all respects. Such a move, inherent in the nursing process, gives each nurse an autonomy which carries with it both responsibility and accountability.

The patient as a person

Patient versus disease

In the traditional medical model, where the emphasis is on disease, it is easy to forget the patient. 'The appendicectomy in the third bed' is recognized by his diagnosis and the position of his bed. He need not have a name or face, did not exist before his admission and will disappear on discharge. This may seem an exaggerated view but it could adequately describe the patient's perception of hospitalization.

It is not only in nursing that such dehumanization occurs. Some people suggest that one cannot be a good nurse without knowing what it feels like to be a patient. This may be true, but there are examples outside nursing which help us to realize how it feels not to exist. A ticket collector on the train shouts 'Tickets please' in a bored voice, takes the ticket, clips it, hands it back and moves on. He has not looked at your face or given any indication that you are anything but a hand holding a ticket. The nurse who silently takes the patient's temperature and moves on with the inquiry 'Have you had your bowels open?' is showing the same lack of awareness of another person as the ticket collector who says 'Change at Crewe' before moving on.

On the train it does not matter; the impersonal contact is short-lived and the passenger is free. But in hospital each nurse may behave in a similar manner and the patient's sense of not existing as a person will be intensified. If each patient is nursed as an individual, depersonalization is far less likely to occur. It is often suggested in nursing literature that nurses put barriers up between themselves and the patient. If the patient becomes a person rather than a disease, the nurse will need to take down those barriers. This will make her more vulnerable to emotional stress. This should not put nurses against the notion of entering their patient's world, provided they are given emotional support from peers and senior staff.

On being a person

What is it that makes each of us an individual person? Psychologists talk of individuals having a 'self-image'. This image of each person as a unique individual depends partly on other people reinforcing such beliefs. It may also be influenced by the environment and the clothes which are worn by the individual. If you believe yourself to be a witty personality, you will need others to laugh at your jokes. If they do not laugh, you may have to change your view of yourself. Similarly, if you feel yourself to be smartly dressed, you will need the appropriate clothes plus the assurance from others that you are smartly dressed. This assurance will not necessarily be verbal but it needs to be there in some form to reinforce your image of yourself.

It can be seen that the patient in hospital is at an immediate disadvantage in that he is out of his own environment and has had to leave behind the trappings of his own individuality. He may no longer have reinforcement of his self-image since many of the elements of that image have been left at the ward door. This may cause problems even to the friends and relatives of the patient. They may come to visit their friend, George, bon viveur, caustic and witty, only to find a middle-aged man in Paisley pyjamas, meekly eating processed cheese. They sit stiffly, unable to think of much to say and, when they leave, the nurse may be faced with an unexplained outburst from a patient who

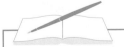

Think of the last time you met a total stranger. How did you feel? Identify the factors that affected your feelings. How can these observations help you to make a new patient feel comfortable with you?

is miserably wondering if life will ever be the same again.

Self-image is not simply a visual image but embraces all aspects of 'me as a person', including intellect. It could be said that the nurse does not test the patient's intellect if he is not involved in the discussions on his care and treatment.

The person and roles

What is it that affects a person so that when he is admitted to hospital or is ill at home, he no longer behaves in the same way as he had previously? Just as the environment and other people reinforce an individual's view of himself, so they also put constraints upon him by their expectations of his behaviour.

Psychologists and sociologists talk of role theory, suggesting that each individual has several roles. Think of the nurse. She may have a role as a student nurse but may also have roles as Mrs Smith's daughter, Miss Jones's niece, and Matthew's wife. Would her husband recognize the quietly efficient nurse? Or would her aunt, who has been heard to call her a 'sweet girl', recognize Matthew's sexually attractive wife?

It is not that people deliberately behave differently in each role, so much as that the circumstances of each role demand something different from them. What is appropriate in one situation may be totally inappropriate in another. What remains in each role is the central image of 'me as a person'. Each role reveals a different facet of 'me'.

Some roles carry certain expectations from society. A policeman, for example, is expected to be honest, a vicar to be righteous and a nurse to be kind and thoughtful. One has only to read newspapers or watch television to observe these views reinforced, or the horror prevailing when someone breaks the rules of any role. If the police are called to break up a noisy party, the local paper may carry the headline 'Neighbours complain of noisy party'. If the party were held by a nurse, it can be said that she is being neither kind nor thoughtful. The headlines might then read 'Noisy party in nurse's flat'. It can be seen that the expectations of some roles spill over into 'off duty' time for that role.

Most people have ideas about the role of the patient. Words used may include 'grateful', 'quiet', 'acquiescent' and 'compliant'. The patient may feel that he must conform to this role or suffer retribution. Stockwell (1972) in her work on the unpopular patient showed that the popular patient is the one who is cheerful, quiet and unde-manding. If the patient is to remain an individual, the popular concept of 'the patient' may need to be amended, both by the patient and by those who care for him. It should be possible to admit a patient to hospital without requiring him to leave his personality, intellect and image at the ward door.

Nurse–patient interaction

If both the nurse and the patient have a concept of what is a patient's role, this will affect their interactions with each other. Roles fall into two main categories, one in which the role is chosen (achieved), i.e. the role of nurse or wife, and one in which the role is imposed (ascribed), i.e. the role of an ill person, so it can be seen that the role of patient will not necessarily be adopted willingly and indeed may conflict with other roles of the individual.

In this situation, it can be appreciated that the nurse often lacks information about the real person who has been admitted or whom she is visiting at home. The patient may be in conflict with his own self-image and react in a number of ways.

Imagine John Hollings. His self-image includes ideas that he is clever and charming, articulate and reasonably attractive. He fills the roles of husband, father, college lecturer, risqué friend and church official. He is admitted to hospital, barely conscious, with a subarachnoid haemorrhage. He cannot speak clearly or focus properly. No one reinforces his self-image, nurses talk to him as if he were a child and, as his condition improves, his temper worsens. A nurse might describe him as 'difficult and demanding', when neither adjective describes the real person.

'Interaction' suggests the involvement of more than one person. If the nurse does not see the real individual in a patient, it might be true to say that the patient's view of the nurse may also be inaccurate. To a certain extent any barriers put up by the patient could be due to frustration caused by the effects of a 'sick' role. Even the pyjamas may not be his own if an individual is used to sleeping naked. Jourard, as long ago as 1960, suggested that the nurse puts up barriers to her real self. He described the 'bedside manner' being used to distance the nurse from the patient. Uniform was seen to be an aid to this distancing.

If both patient and nurse are putting up barriers, then it is very unlikely that meaningful interaction will occur between them. If the nurse wishes to form a relationship with the patient so that meaningful interaction may take place, then both she and the patient must 'disclose' to each other. Such an approach calls for a change in the role of both nurse and patient.

'Disclosure' implies that an individual will allow others to know something of himself. In other words, something is given. This does not necessarily fit the traditional role of the nurse, who may feel she has a right to disclosures from the patient without having to give anything in return. Indeed she may have the idea that she needs to remain aloof in order to maintain authority over the patient.

An argument could be made that it is not necessary to get to know patients. Interaction will not mend a broken leg. Returning to the example of the ticket collector, his lack of attention does not really alter a traveller's journey in any way. However, interaction between patients and those who care for them does seem to affect the outcome.

Many researchers have shown links between the information given to patients, the recovery rate, and the need for analgesics. Others have suggested that stress can affect outcomes for patients. To obtain and give information, and to reduce stress, it is necessary to interact successfully with the patient (Faulkner 1992).

The nurse and the patient are both individuals. If they allow that individuality to show through the constraints of their respective roles, there may be gains in terms of improved interactions. There may also be losses, in that they will both be vulnerable, the nurse to the patient's pain from which she had previously distanced herself, and the patient to the nurse as a human rather than an idealized object.

Nursing as a process

Nursing is often described as a process in which problems are identified and solved. This may be rather misleading since it assumes that all problems have a solution. This may be so in physical terms if one accepts death as a solution in some cases. It is far less likely to be true in psychological terms, however, and with these cases the nurse may identify problems which she cannot solve. If a patient's marriage has broken up, for example, the nurse who identifies the problem may be able to help the patient to come to terms with reality, or may refer him to someone else. What she cannot expect to do is to re-unite the couple.

The traditional model of nursing would not necessarily have concerned itself with emotional problems if the patient was being treated for a physical disease. It is thought, however, that there may be a link between stress and disease (Cooper 1983), and certainly, if the patient is to be nursed as an individual, it would be foolish to ignore those problems which could well be affecting the patient's will or ability to recover.

The nursing process was introduced as a method of nursing that concerns itself with an individual's physical, social and psychological reactions to disease, and which takes into account that the patient is a member of society with his own stresses within that society, which may affect his reaction to disease.

Early authors, e.g. Kratz (1979) and McFarlane and Castledine (1982), divided the process into four main stages, as follows:

1 Assessment
2 Planning
3 Implementation
4 Evaluation

It is useful to make such a division for purposes of explanation, if nursing is to be accepted as a process, but this should be seen as dynamic and continuous if, as a patient's physical and emotional state changes, there will be a need for reassessment with resulting adjustments to other stages (Figure 1.2).

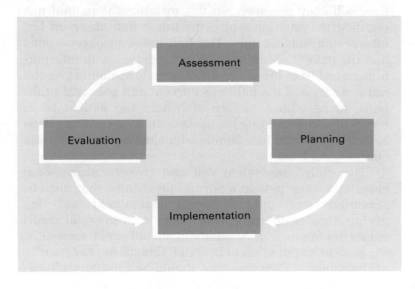

Fig. 1.2 The dynamic nature of the nursing process.

Assessment

Assessment is the first and possibly most crucial interaction with the patient after he has been admitted and settled into the ward. It involves taking a nursing history. For this history to accurately reflect the patient's current problems, the nurse needs to communicate effectively. She also needs to be able to conduct an interview which will facilitate trust in the patient so that he is able to disclose his concerns without fear or embarrassment (Faulkner 1992).

It is inevitable that a nursing history will have areas of overlap with a medical history taken by the doctor. Some information may therefore be taken from the patient's notes and then checked for accuracy, e.g. name, address, and other demographic data. Details of the patient's illness, however, should be obtained directly from the patient – not to check up on the doctor but rather to elicit the patient's perception of his present state.

Assessment is more than a nursing history. It also includes observational assessment of the patient, both subjective and objective. An objective observation, for example measuring a patient's temperature, may help to identify physical problems. More subjective observations may help to identify psychological and social problems. It may be that the nurse will observe that the patient seems frightened. If she says to him, 'You seem a little scared' she may elicit what the fear is and the underlying problem or, indeed, she may find that the patient laughs and says, 'Oh no, I am not scared but I am worried about how long they will keep me here'. In this instance the patient has clarified the emotion which the nurse had observed but interpreted inaccurately. The link between observations and the patient's view of his state, together with information gained from the assessment interview, should give the nurse an idea of the patient's current and potential problems, along with a picture of 'where the patient is' in terms of understanding his disease and the resulting deficiencies in normal functioning which have given rise to his current problems.

Hopefully, assessment will also give the nurse some clues about the patient's normal lifestyle so that her observations can be put into context for that individual. This is considerably different from the more traditional medical model of nursing. Assessment should occur soon after the patient's admission to hospital, though not necessarily at the same time. Assessment should be continuous, however, and observations made on admission may be incorporated into the nursing history, which may be taken on another day.

Planning

Accurate assessment of a patient's physical, social and psychological state should help a nurse to identify problems, both actual and potential, and to make some decisions on the care that is needed from the health care team, as opposed to that which the patient is able to continue doing for himself. In the traditional model of nursing, the patient was often seen to be dependent on health carers. With a more patient-centred approach, each individual remains as independent as possible, given the constraints of each particular hospital.

Although the aim of planning care is to meet an individual's needs, there are of necessity some constraints which cannot be ignored. A patient may have problems concerned with nutrition, for example. The nurse may be able to plan appropriate action over content and size of meals but would normally find it very difficult to deviate from hospital meal times.

Planning must take reality into account while attempting to meet each patient's needs. Without planning, care could be delivered on a hit-and-miss basis which might result in too much or too little attention being paid to an individual. Inevitably, when problems are identified, some will be more pressing than others and will need to take priority when care is planned. Such ordering of priorities can happen only if care is carefully planned with a particular patient in mind. The most pressing problems may be physical or psychological, for although a patient who is anxious may seem to have more important physical problems, alleviating the psychological stress may bring a reduction in physical symptoms.

Once priorities have been established, goals need to be set which are agreed with the patient. Such goals set out proposed outcomes which must be realistic, specific and measurable. There is little point in setting goals that cannot be achieved since this could engender a feeling of failure in both nurse and patient. Rather, goals should be set that can be reached in a reasonable time. Other, more ambitious, goals can then build on past success.

When goals have been set, appropriate actions can be planned. Some authors use the term 'nursing actions'. This appears to imply that nursing care is being 'done to' the patient, and it is worth remembering that planning care also involves the patient. Some actions that are planned may be actions the nurse is going to take in providing care. Others may be taken by the patient as he co-operates in the plans for his care. Whichever applies, in planning care the appropriate actions for dealing with a patient's problems will be selected in order that goals can be realized.

When the necessary action has been agreed, a record needs to be made for each patient that is readily understood by all those who care for him. This record is called a 'care plan'. Care plans are discussed in Part Three of this book and it will be seen that they need constant updating as the patient is reassessed and his problems change. Planning is an important step in nursing since, once problems are identified, planning sets out a logical method of care which is geared as far as possible to the needs of the individual. Just as poor assessment will lead to poor planning, poor planning may lead to inappropriate care being given to the patient.

Implementation

'Implementation' is a rather grand word for actually caring for the patient. All the work that goes into assessment and planning will come to nought if the quality of nursing care is poor.

For the standard of nursing care to be high, the nurse needs to understand what she is doing and to have the necessary skills to carry out care, whether it be physical or emotional.

The concept that the nurse needs to understand what she is doing is an important one since it brings into question how much she needs to know about a patient's diagnosis. If it is argued that nursing is different from medicine, it might be possible to suggest that nursing could be carried out without knowledge of a patient's diagnosis. That this is a fallacy should be immediately obvious by thinking of any nursing action. It is not possible to attend *safely* to a patient if there is no understanding of the relationship between a nursing action and the action of disease upon the patient.

An example of this is nutrition. Disease may have an effect on the absorption of different foods or upon their action. Planning to meet a patient's nutritional needs without this knowledge could be very difficult indeed and in some cases, for example the diabetic patient, actually dangerous. Similar examples can be found for other nursing actions. Nurses therefore need a good knowledge base of disease and its treatment if they are to give a high standard of nursing care.

Knowledge is also necessary of the nursing actions themselves. For example, it is relatively easy to test urine, fill in a chart or indeed to ask open questions. Such basic skills could easily be taught to young children. Yet nursing is not an easy but a highly skilled activity because it requires knowledge to make sense of the information received, whether the information comes from observations or from the patient. It also requires knowledge in terms of subsequent actions for the patient.

As with knowledge, so with skills. Many nursing actions could possibly be carried out by the unskilled, but a skilled nurse is required to deliver a high level of nursing care, not only in sophisticated nursing actions but also in basic care. In implementing care, the nurse is a member of a multidisciplinary team of which no member can give care in isolation. As far as the patient is concerned, the nurse is the most constant member of that team. As such she will not only implement nursing plans but will co-ordinate care with other team members and will often liaise between them and the patient. A notable example of this may be in the nurse's role of communicating information to the patient on medical and paramedical plans and actions. It should be remembered that nursing care involves both care planned by the nurse and treatment prescribed by the doctor.

Evaluation

The evaluation component of the nursing process is an attempt to measure outcomes of practice. As such it is a dynamic process, rather than something performed at the end of a patient's stay in hospital. If, for example, a patient is admitted to the ward and is found to have a pressure sore, certain nursing actions will be planned after the sore has been assessed. Evaluation in this instance will determine if the action taken has caused the pressure sore to improve after an agreed period of time. If not, then the sore may need to be reassessed and perhaps different actions planned. It can be seen that the care will be periodically evaluated until, hopefully, healing has occurred.

Similarly with psychological problems. The patient who is anxious on admission to hospital may be seen to need information to help him understand the care prescribed. The effect of this nursing action will need to be evaluated, and, if the patient remains anxious, reassessment of the cause of the anxiety may be required and questions asked, perhaps about the quality and appropriateness of the information given to the patient.

It will be seen that assessment and evaluation are closely tied, in that assessment elicits problems which lead to care being planned. By measuring care (evaluation) we return to assessment and so to more plans for care, which need re-evaluation. Stages of this process will overlap but care cannot be evaluated until it has been planned and given. The inference in evaluation is that all care can be measured. We can in fact measure care by asking if goals set for patient care have been met. This is yet another reason for setting realistic goals in a 'build-on' fashion. An example can be given by returning to the patient with a pressure sore. He may be in hospital for two weeks. Goals may therefore be set for stages of healing so that evaluation, and reassessment if necessary, can occur at intervals.

The important point about evaluation is that it encourages nurses to question the care given to patients and to make any necessary adjustment. It does not mean changing action every day but it does require that the nurse is able to make judgements and decisions about patient care and is able to set realistic, measurable goals for her patient's recovery from physical, social and psychological problems.

Summary

This chapter has examined the traditional method of nursing in which the nurse's role was largely concerned with carrying out care prescribed by the doctor and based on medical problems. A case has been made for nursing the patient as an individual rather than as a disease with the resultant change in both the nurse's role and that of the patient.

An overview of nursing as a process has been given along with a description of the demands made upon the nurse when using this approach to patient care. It will be seen that the process requires the nurse to be a thinking person with a dynamic attitude to patient care. It also requires the nurse to make decisions and to take responsibility for such decisions.

Each stage of the process has been briefly described and examples given of the interrelatedness of the stages.

References

Cole, A. (1994) A problem shared. *Nursing Times*, *90*(47), 16.
Cooper, D. L. (Ed.) (1983) *Stress research. Issues for the eighties.* Chichester: Wiley.

Day, M. (1995) Drama in the theatre. *Nursing Times*, *91*(4), 14–15.

Faulkner, A. (1992) *Effective interaction with patients*. Edinburgh: Churchill Livingstone.

Jourard, S. M. (1960) The bedside manner. *American Journal of Nursing*, *60*(1), 63–66.

Kim, M. & Moritz, D. (1982) *Classification of nursing diagnosis*. New York: McGraw-Hill.

King, I. M. (1971) *Towards a theory for nursing*. New York: John Wiley.

Kratz, C. (Ed.) (1979) *The nursing process*. London: Baillière Tindall.

McFarlane, J. & Castledine, G. (1982) *A guide to the practice of nursing using the nursing process*. London: Mosby.

Neuman, B. (1980) The Betty Neuman health care system model: a total approach to patients' problems. In Rheil, J. & Roy, C. (Eds.) *Conceptual models for nursing practice*. New York: Appleton Century Crofts.

NHS Management Executive (1991) *Junior doctors. The new deal*. London: NHS Management Executive.

Orem, D. (1980) *Nursing: concepts of practice*, 2nd ed. New York: McGraw-Hill.

Pearson, A. & Vaughan, B. (1991) *Nursing models for practice*. London: Butterworth Heinemann.

Peplau, H. E. (1980) The psychiatric nurse: accountable? to whom? for what? *Perspectives in Psychiatric Care*, *18*(3), 128–134.

Roper, N., Logan, W. & Tierney, A. (1980) *The elements of nursing*. Edinburgh: Churchill Livingstone.

Roy, C. (1976) *Introduction to nursing: an adaptation model*. New Jersey: Prentice Hall.

Stockwell, F. (1972) *The unpopular patient*. London: Rcn.

UKCC (1992) *The scope of professional practice*. London: United Kingdom Central Council for Nursing, Midwifery and Health Visiting.

Further reading

Alfaro, R. (1989) *Applying nursing diagnosis and nursing process: A step by step guide*, 2nd ed. Philadelphia.

Giles, S. (1993) Passing the buck. *Nursing Times*, *89*(28), 42–43.

Moyse, G. (1994) Growing pains. *Nursing Standard*, *8*(25), 53.

Pickersgill, F. (1993) A 'new deal' for nurses too? *Nursing Standard*, *7*(35), 21–22.

Salvage, J. & Kershaw, B. (1990) *Models for nursing*, *2*. London: Scutari Press.

Vestal Allen, C. (1991) *Comprehending the nursing process: a workbook approach*. Michigan: Appleton and Lange.

Walsh, M. (1991) *Nursing models in clinical practice*. London: Baillière Tindall.

2

The Individual in His Normal Environment

CHAPTER SUMMARY

Concepts of health, 20
The National Health Service, 21
The Social Services, 22
The Health Education Authority, 22
The individual's responsibility for health, 23

The physiology of physical health, 25
Intake of oxygen and food, 25
Transport to and from the cells, 30
Elimination of waste products, 32
Body control systems, 34
The body's framework, 41

The psychology of mental health, 45
Personality, 45
Stress, 46
Perception, 47
Attitudes, 48

Interaction, 49
Sexuality, 50
Communication, 50
The psychological individual, 52
Spirituality, 53

Sociological aspects of health, 54
Social class, 54
Status, 55
The family, 56
The community, 57

Culture, 60

Summary, 62

References, 62

Further reading, 63

Concepts of health

Health is something that is taken for granted by many individuals until they become ill, yet health does not just happen. In the Third World, for example, there is considerable ill-health due to famine, overcrowding, ignorance and poverty. Ironically, in the Western culture, ill-health is often caused by affluence and ignorance.

The World Health Organization (WHO) has a definition of health that is useful, although it is not the only one available. The WHO definition states: 'Health is a state of complete physical, mental and social well-being and not merely the absence of disease or infirmity.'

In the United Kingdom the government takes responsibility for health in a number of ways that fit in with the following elements of the WHO constitution:

'The enjoyment of the highest attainable standard of health is one of the fundamental rights of every human being without distinction of race, religion, political belief, economic or social condition.

The health of all people is fundamental to the attainment of peace and security and is dependent upon the fullest co-operation of individuals and States.

The achievement of any State in the promotion and protection of health is of value to all.

Health development of the child is of basic importance; the ability to live harmoniously in a changing total environment is essential to such development.

The extension to all people of the benefits of medical, psychological and related knowledge is essential to the fullest attainment of health.

Informed opinion and active co-operation on the part of the public are of the utmost importance in the improvement of the health of the people.

Governments have a responsibility for the health of their peoples which can be fulfilled only by the provision of adequate health and social measures.'

The National Health Service

One way in which the government takes responsibility for health in the United Kingdom is by the provision of the National Health Service (NHS); which came into being in 1948. All employed people make contributions to the NHS and as a result free hospitalization can be offered to all who require it, as can consultations with General Practitioners (GPs) and care in the community. Standard charges are made for such items as drugs, spectacles and false teeth, but those in need and special cases such as patients suffering from diabetes are exempt from some or all of these charges.

Within the NHS there is provision for monitoring the health of young children by the Health Visitor (Chapter 17) and educating other groups for health. Programmes of immunization and vaccination have eradicated smallpox and virtually eradicated other diseases such as diphtheria and tuberculosis in the United Kingdom. Other NHS services that promote health include family planning services, education for prospective parents, well-women clinics and other health promotion and maintenance clinics of a wide variety. These services are increasingly available at GP practices. Those GPs who are fundholders, and manage their own budget, get some financial reward for making such health promotional services available.

In recent years, other major changes have occurred in the NHS. There has been a shift to general management to improve efficiency and cost-effectiveness since 1984 with the result that a clear management hierarchy has arisen. Secondly, since 1991 there has been a gradual introduction of an internal market initiative with emphasis on the dynamics of a purchaser/provider system. This is likely to have far-reaching effects on the whole of health care.

In 1992, the government introduced the Patient's Charter which outlines improvements to the NHS and promises a service that:

- always puts the patient first, providing services that meet clearly defined national and local standards, in ways responsive to people's views and needs. The Patient's Charter is a central part of achieving this objective by seeking to ensure everywhere the high standards of the best;
- provides services that produce clear, measurable benefits to people's health, with more emphasis than in the past on health promotion and prevention. The consultative document *Health of the Nation*, which can be obtained from local libraries, suggests explicit targets for improvements in health for the first time in Britain;
- is highly efficient, representing really good value for money, achieved through better management following the implementation of the proposals in the White Papers *Working for Patients* and *Caring for People*;
- respects and values the immense resource of skill and dedication which is to be found amongst those who work for and with the National Health Service.

The Social Services

The Social Services also contribute to health in a number of ways, such as the provision of income to the aged and unemployed, benefits to help parents with the expenses of child rearing and supplementary benefits to those in need. This means that, in theory, no one should be unhealthy as a result of having insufficient money to purchase the necessities of life. The Social Services also offer support and emotional care to families in need along with members of the primary health care team (Chapter 17). With the reforms in the NHS, Social Services have also taken greater responsibility for care of the elderly. This includes providing some funding for elderly placements in nursing homes.

The Health Education Authority

The Health Education Council (now the Health Education Authority, HEA) was set up in 1968 by the government as an independent public body supported by the Department of Health and Social Security (DHSS). Its remit is to plan and promote health education at a national level in England, Wales and Northern Ireland. The Scottish Health Education Group (SHEG) performs a similar function in Scotland.

The HEA, in its educative programme, lays emphasis on those factors in Western life which are known to be a risk to health, such as smoking, over-indulgence of alcohol, inappropriate nutrition and sexual ignorance.

The smoking programme, for example, has included a mass campaign for children and has used a well-known comic character, Superman, as the anti-smoking hero. Television programmes have been aimed at teenagers to help them see smoking as an antisocial habit, and at parents and adults. Hints on how to give up smoking are also available to adults.

Besides other campaigns, through schools and the media, to help people appreciate the dangers of alcohol abuse and an unhealthy diet, the HEA is also concerned with promoting other aspects of healthy living, such as care of the teeth and a responsible attitude to sexual behaviour. Other special educational programmes include preparation for parenthood, prevention of coronary heart disease and cancer education.

The HEA links with health education units which are provided within the NHS. These units are open to the public and to health professionals and carry HEA-produced posters and leaflets. These units also produce their own material to suit local needs. Much of this work is linked with other agencies. The 1993/4 annual report states that HEA has '. . . worked in partnership with many different organisations during the year in alliances aimed at achieving THE HEALTH OF THE NATION targets for coronary heart disease and stroke'. Highlights of the year included a physical activity task force, a nutrition task force and projects in community care. There are also ongoing educational programmes on HIV and AIDS.

The individual's responsibility for health

Although the government takes overall responsibility for the nation's health, individuals remain relatively free to make their own choices. This is not as simple as the foregoing would suggest, for in a consumer society much is advertised and available which could be detrimental to health. Cigarettes, for example, are freely advertised on hoardings and in glossy magazines, but government legislation bans such advertisements on commercial television and insists on a government health warning on both cigarette packets and advertisements.

A similar picture emerges with alcohol. The government has passed legislation to ban those drivers who are found to have over a certain level of alcohol in their blood, and the HEA warns of the dangers to health of too much alcohol, but alcohol is advertised as a desirable aspect of a successful lifestyle.

The general public still gets mixed messages about harmful elements in lifestyle. The tobacco companies, for example, are still allowed to sponsor televised sports, so sports fans will see advertisements for cigarettes on the hoardings as they watch their favourite programmes. Cigarettes are still used in some TV dramas but much less than in old films, showing that cigarette smoking is less socially acceptable than it used to be. Similarly with alcohol, the drink driving campaigns show that this is now socially undesireable to a level that anyone who drinks and drives is portrayed as a potential killer. Nevertheless, in television and films alcohol is still seen to be part of everyday life.

Given such mixed messages, it is often difficult for individuals to make informed choices. Health education aims to assist in the difficult task of helping individuals to make informed choices for themselves and for the younger generation for whom they are responsible.

Information alone will not necessarily change behaviour, particularly in youngsters who are finding their own way in the world and often see their parents and teachers as old-fashioned 'fuddy-duddies'.

Young people often experiment with drugs, little realizing that this could lead to addiction and that by not using clean needles they run the risk of becoming HIV positive and thus developing AIDS. Again, health education programmes aim to help young people understand the risks, and the government sponsors educational programmes and include needle exchange schemes.

One educational programme, 'Populace in the 80's', explores the above point. This is the 'Look after Yourself' programme initiated by the HEA, in which people met regularly with trained tutors to learn about healthy living. Interest grew as individuals heard about it from their friends and subsequently decided to join one of the groups.

Choice, in the absence of motivation and information, may be made on the basis of an individual's life experiences. Smoking, for example, can be rationalized as safe if an elderly relative appears to be a healthy smoker, while diet can be dismissed as a cause of overweight by a member of a 'big' family who sees his problems as genetic.

In some individuals, choice may be absent through an inability to read. Healthy people do not necessarily come into contact with health professionals who could talk to them about smoking and other dangerous practices. They are left to depend on their own life experiences and whatever they hear on the radio or television.

The choices open to individuals in the past have been largely concerned with physical health. There is, however, a growing awareness of the need to promote mental health, especially in times of life crisis. The HEA funded research into pre-retirement education since retirement is known to be a time of mental and physical adjustment.

Occasionally, the government does not leave choice to the individual on matters of safety and health. Two examples of this are the legislation on drinking and driving and the mandatory wearing of seat belts by the driver and all passengers of a car.

The physiology of physical health

For an individual to remain physically healthy he requires an adequate intake of oxygen, food and fluid. Oxygen is needed for the metabolic breakdown of food constituents ('cellular respiration') to provide energy and to allow the functioning and replacement of cells throughout the body. He needs to excrete waste products from the body and to maintain a constant temperature, fluid balance and pH (acid–base balance) since enzymes vital for all metabolic processes work in an aqueous medium at optimal temperature and pH. Figure 2.1 shows how the various metabolic activities interact in health.

Intake of oxygen and food

Oxygen

Oxygen constitutes about 20% of atmospheric air, which is inhaled via the nose, where any particles are trapped and the air is warmed before passing into the bronchial tree (Figure 2.2). The main bronchi subdivide many times, producing smaller and smaller airways, culminating in the terminal bronchioles and alveoli where gases are exchanged (Figure 2.3).

An adult normally breathes about 20 times a minute and draws in about half a litre of air with each inspiration. Of this, about 150 ml plays no part in gaseous exchange

Fig. 2.1 Metabolic activities in the body.

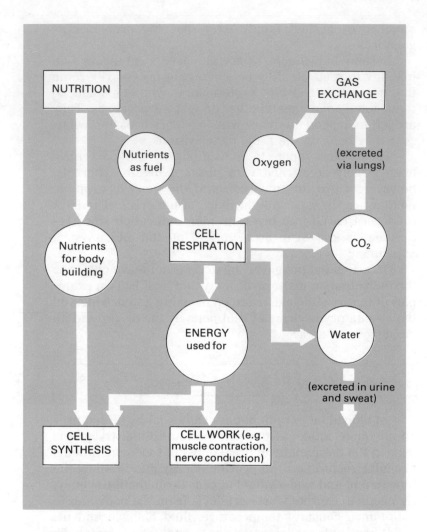

and only acts to fill what is termed the 'dead space' between the nose and the terminal bronchioles. The remaining 350 ml of air is available for oxygen consumption by the body. The terminal bronchioles and alveoli are lined with a very thin membrane which is surrounded by a network of thin-walled capillaries (Figure 2.3). Gases can pass between the air in the alveoli and the blood in the capillaries and it is here that oxygen in inspired air crosses into the blood. The blood is then returned to the heart for circulation around the body.

Food
Food intake is essential if cells are to receive nutrients for energy production. Foods can be either solid or liquid and their intake is largely under the voluntary control of the individual, although the ultimate control of appetite and satiety lies in the hypothalamus in the brain.

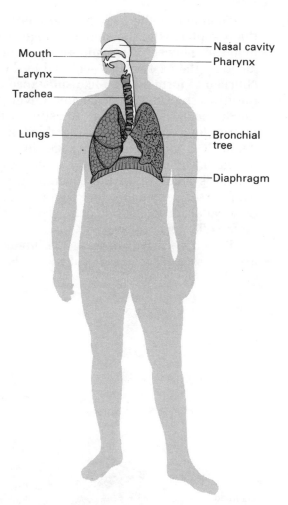

Fig. 2.2 The respiratory system.

Mouth

Nasal cavity

Pharynx

Larynx

Trachea

Lungs

Bronchial tree

Diaphragm

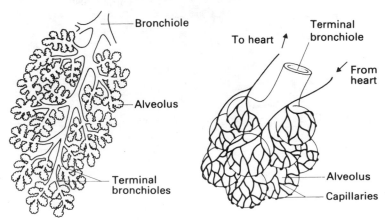

Bronchiole

Alveolus

Terminal bronchioles

To heart

Terminal bronchiole

From heart

Alveolus

Capillaries

Fig. 2.3 The terminal airways in cross-section (*left*) and showing the sites of gaseous exchange (*right*).

Food enters the body by the mouth and passes down the oesophagus to the stomach (Figure 2.4), where it remains for between 30 minutes and five hours. Bacteria are killed by the gastric acid secreted in the stomach, food is churned to form a paste-like substance called chyme and the process of digestion begins. Chyme is released from the stomach into the small intestine, which is about five metres long and includes the duodenum, jejunum and ileum. It is the main site of digestion. Food is then propelled through the one and a half metres of large intestine (which is made up of the caecum, appendix, ascending, transverse, descending and sigmoid colons), rectum and anal canal. Propulsion is achieved by a wave-like movement called peristalsis.

Proteins, carbohydrates, fats, minerals and vitamins are all essential in the diet if health is to be maintained (Table 2.1).

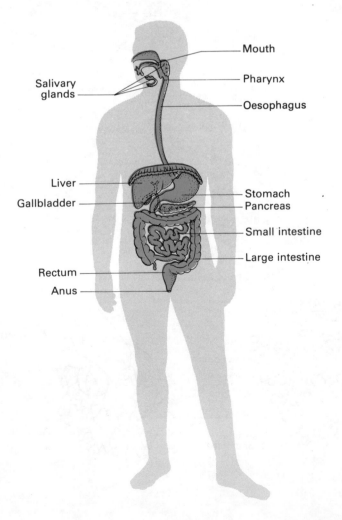

Fig. 2.4 The digestive system.

Dietary constituent	Broken down by (to)	Produced in	Absorbed from	Used for
Protein	Pepsin (peptides) Trypsin, chymotrypsin, carboxypeptidase	Stomach Pancreas	Small intestine	Growth and repair of tissues Transamination to other proteins, e.g. plasma protein Energy production Excess stored as fat
Carbohydrate	Amylase (maltose)	Pancreas	Small intestine	Oxidized to produce cellular energy
	Maltase (glucose)	Small intestine		Excess stored as glycogen (short-term)
	Sucrase (glucose and fructose)	Small intestine		Excess converted to fat and stored in adipose tissue (long-term)
	Lactase (glucose and lactose)	Small intestine		
Fat	Bile salts (emulsified fat)	Liver (stored in gallbladder)	Small intestine	Cellular energy
	Lipase (glycerol and fatty acids)	Pancreas		Synthesis of cholesterol, bile salts and steroid hormones Excess stored in adipose tissue

Table 2.1 Digestion of major dietary constituents.

Protein is found in foods such as meat, fish, cheese and soya beans. Some amino acids, the 'building blocks' of proteins, can be manufactured by the body but others cannot and it is essential that these are taken in the diet. Proteins are used for the growth and repair of tissues throughout the body and, indirectly, are broken down to produce energy.

Protein digestion begins in the stomach where the enzyme pepsin is produced; it acts to break the long protein chains into smaller polypeptides. This process is not essential and humans can survive with no stomach. In the duodenum, enzymes secreted from the pancreas continue the digestion of protein – trypsin, chymotrypsin and carboxypeptidase break down the chains until the constituent amino acids are released. Pancreatic enzymes are essential for protein digestion and the pancreas is thus essential for life. The amino acids are absorbed into the bloodstream from the intestine and carried to tissues throughout the body. Some of them undergo transamination in the liver – that is, they are used to make other proteins, such as plasma proteins. Any amino acids in excess of the body's requirements are deaminated in the liver to produce glucose which cells can use to provide energy.

Carbohydrates are found as starches and sugars and are the staple constituents of all traditional diets – flours and cereals such as wheat and rice, fruit and vegetables. They tend to be cheap, filling and readily available. Simple carbohydrates are the principal source of energy for the cells and are broken down (oxidized) by them. The liver and muscles can store carbohydrates as glycogen to act as a short-term energy store. Excess carbohydrates are converted to fat and stored in the adipose tissue beneath the skin where they form a more long-term energy store.

Carbohydrate digestion commences in the duodenum, where amylase from the pancreas is released and breaks it down to maltose. Other enzymes produced in the duodenum break the maltose down to the simple sugars glucose (80%), fructose and lactose (20%). These are absorbed into the blood for use by cells throughout the body.

Fats are found in animal products such as butter, cream, meat and fish (saturated fats) and can be made from plants such as sunflowers and corn (unsaturated fats). The cells oxidize fats to produce heat and energy and any surplus is stored in adipose tissue, where excess deposition can lead to overweight.

Fat digestion also begins in the duodenum, where bile secreted from the liver emulsifies the fat and allows it to break into minute particles. Lipase from the pancreas breaks down the globules to glycerol and fatty acids, which are absorbed by blood. Fatty acids are further broken down in the liver to a form that can be used by the cells.

Minerals are found as salts in food and many of them have important functions in the body. Sodium is needed to ensure the working of most cells in the body, iron is necessary for the production of red blood cells (erythrocytes), iodine is essential for thyroid function, and calcium is important for bone formation and for muscle and nerve function. Chlorine, cobalt, copper, fluoride, magnesium, potassium, sulphur and zinc are other minerals necessary for the maintenance of health.

Vitamins are found in small amounts in many foods and may be divided into those that are fat-soluble, including vitamins A, D, E and K, and those that are water-soluble, B and C. Vitamin A is essential for normal vision, the B vitamins for metabolism of proteins and carbohydrates, C for growth of cells, especially in bone, and K for blood clotting.

Transport to and from the cells

Oxygen and nutrients from food are absorbed into the blood and carried to tissues throughout the body in the circulatory system, which comprises the heart, blood vessels and lymphatic system. They are then transferred via the extracellular fluid, which surrounds the cells, into the cells themselves, where they can be used (Figure 2.5). All of these processes occur in water-based fluid and so water is essential to life. About 60% of body weight is water (about 40 litres) and, of this, two-thirds is found in the cells. All food contains some water and liquids are drunk to make up the total needed by the body. Average fluid intake is about 2600 ml per day, which is in excess of the body's requirements. Intake is largely under the control of the individual who may drink in response to physiological thirst, social expectation, or purely for pleasure.

The heart is a muscular organ with four chambers, the left and right atria and left and right ventricles. Cardiac muscle does not need nervous stimulation in order to beat; it beats at rest at about 70 beats per minute and acts as a pump to circulate blood around the body. About 70 ml is pumped with each beat. The heart can increase both its rate and the volume pumped per beat (stroke volume) in response to the body's needs – output can be increased sevenfold if necessary. Blood from the right side of the heart is pumped, via the pulmonary circulation, to the lungs and back, and from the left side to the rest of the body via the systemic circulation. Blood pressure must remain constant if tissue perfusion is to be maintained.

The blood vessels contain about five litres of blood of which 70% is in the veins. This entire volume is pumped around the body once a minute at rest. The vessels form an extensive network to convey blood to all the tissues (Figure 2.6). The arteries are large vessels which carry blood under pressure from the heart to all parts of the body and dampen out its pulsatile flow. If an artery is occluded, the tissue which it supplies will die. The main arteries subdi-

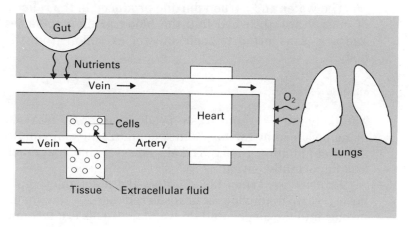

Fig. 2.5 Transfer of oxygen and nutrients to the cells.

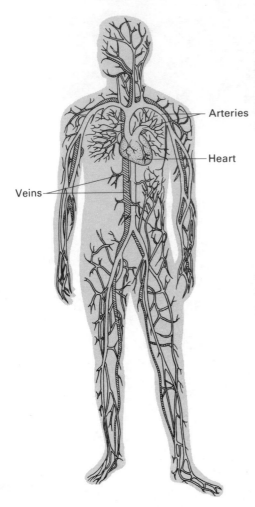

Fig. 2.6 The cardiovascular system.

vide until blood reaches the small arterioles which control blood flow and maintain a constant blood pressure by dilating and constricting. If they are not functioning properly, pain will result. Blood flows into the capillaries, which have thin walls, unlike the great vessels. The walls are permeable and it is here that gases, nutrients and waste products pass between the blood and the cells. Blood pressure forces oxygen and nutrients out of the capillaries at the arteriolar end and the osmotic pressure of plasma proteins sucks in fluid containing carbon dioxide and waste products at the venular end. Plasma proteins and red blood cells do not cross the capillary membrane because they are too large. Malfunction of capillaries, for example after a bee sting, will result in localized swelling (oedema). From the capillaries, blood is pushed into the venules and then veins, which return it to the heart. Veins, particularly in the legs, contain valves which act to break up the long columns of blood and to prevent the blood flowing backwards with gravity. Veins contain most of the body's blood and, if it is not returned to the heart efficiently, fainting occurs.

The lymphatic system consists of lymph, lymphatic vessels, lymph nodes and nodules, thymus and tonsils (Figure 2.7). It removes excess fluid from the tissues and absorbs digested fat for transport to the liver. Localized oedema will result if lymphatic drainage is absent or blocked.

Oxygen is needed for the complex chemical process of cellular respiration in which the nutrients transported to the cells are broken down. Energy is released during this process and water and carbon dioxide are produced. This energy is in the form of high-energy compounds such as adenosine triphosphate (ATP), which can subsequently provide the energy needed for cellular activities such as muscle movement, growth and replication of cells.

The water and carbon dioxide produced in the release of energy are absorbed into the blood at the capillaries and are transported to their sites of excretion from the body.

Elimination of waste products

The body must excrete waste products in order to avoid being poisoned by the toxins they contain. The main methods of elimination are expired air, faeces, urine and, much less importantly, sweat.

Expired air: When blood enters the pulmonary capillaries, carbon dioxide is transferred across the membranes into the alveoli and then exhaled. This is a fast and

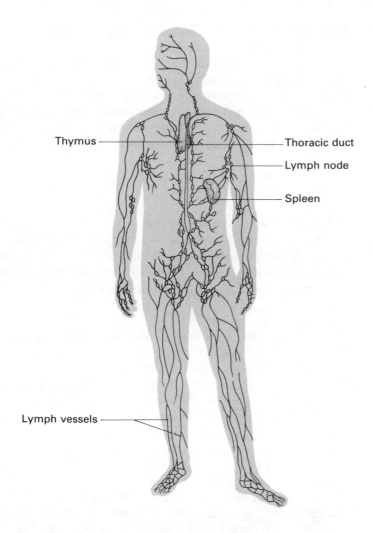

Fig. 2.7 The lymphatic system.

Thymus

Thoracic duct

Lymph node

Spleen

Lymph vessels

efficient method of eliminating carbon dioxide from the body.

Faeces: Food that has not been absorbed from the small intestine continues through the large intestine, where it is mixed with bacteria, sloughed off cells from the gut wall and bile pigments, which give faeces their characteristic colour. Water is absorbed from the large intestine, leaving solid faeces. Dietary fibre is important as it is not digested and gives bulk to help form the stools.

When the rectum fills, the individual feels the need to defecate but can usually suppress the reflex until time and place are appropriate. Diarrhoea results if water is not properly absorbed from the gut.

Urine: At rest about 1250 ml of blood per minute pass through the kidneys, where water is filtered out. Water that is in excess of the body's requirements is passed as urine. Urine also contains urea (a waste product of protein breakdown), sodium, creatinine (from worn-out muscle cells), potassium, bicarbonate and other mineral salts. When the bladder is full, the urge to urinate is felt, but can be controlled under normal conditions. Approximately 1.5 litres of urine are voided per day by an adult.

Sweat: The two to five million sweat glands throughout the body excrete water, sodium and urea in small quantities. Loss via the sweat glands can be significant in hot climates.

Body control systems

Cells and tissues do not function in isolation and the body has two important methods of ensuring the smooth running of all bodily functions and maintaining homeostasis – hormonal and nervous. The two systems often work very closely together but can function independently.

The endocrine system

Hormones are produced by the ductless, endocrine glands and are carried in the bloodstream to their target organs, which may be some distance from the production site. Hormone production is dictated by the body's needs and control is slower and more long-term than that of the nervous system. Endocrine glands include the hypothalamus, pituitary, thyroid, four parathyroids, two adrenal glands, the pancreas, two gonads (testes or ovaries) and the placenta during pregnancy. Figure 2.8 indicates their location in the body.

The **hypothalamus** provides the link between the endocrine and nervous systems and produces several relasing hormones which regulate the secretion of specific hormones from the anterior pituitary.

The **pituitary** gland has an anterior and a posterior part which function separately. The posterior part produces antidiuretic hormone (ADH), which causes water retention by the kidney, and oxytocin, which is important in uterine contraction and lactation in the female. The anterior pituitary produces a number of hormones which act on other endocrine glands (the target organs), which in turn release hormones of their own (Figure 2.9). Production is governed by the amount of a hormone circulating in the blood by a 'negative feedback' system. For example, if thyroid hormone levels in the blood are low, the hypothalamus will stimulate the anterior pituitary to produce thyroid-stimulating hormone (TSH), which will act on the thyroid gland to stimulate release of thyroid hormones into the circulation. When levels return to normal, the production circuit will be switched off.

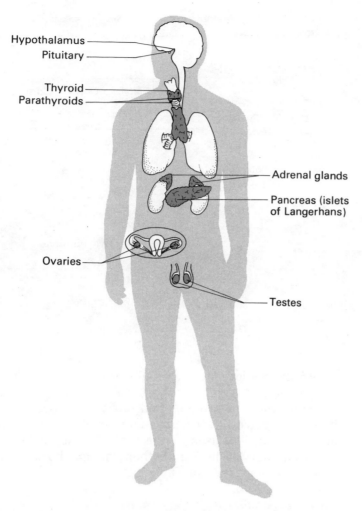

Fig. 2.8 The endocrine system.

Hypothalamus
Pituitary
Thyroid
Parathyroids
Adrenal glands
Pancreas (islets of Langerhans)
Ovaries
Testes

The **adrenal** gland also has two separately functioning parts, the cortex and the medulla. The cortex produces steroids which control sugar metabolism, salt and water balance and growth of the sex organs; the medulla produces adrenaline and noradrenaline which help the body to cope with stress. Adrenaline is poured into the circulation in situations where an individual needs to respond by 'fight or flight'.

Thyroid hormones contain iodine, which must be taken in the diet, and control the body's metabolic rate, that is, the amount of energy used by the tissues.

The **pancreas** produces two hormones from cells in the islets of Langerhans which work together to control blood sugar levels. Insulin, from the beta cells, is produced in response to raised blood glucose levels and acts to lower them by allowing glucose to enter the cells and be used; glucagon, from the alpha cells, is produced in re-

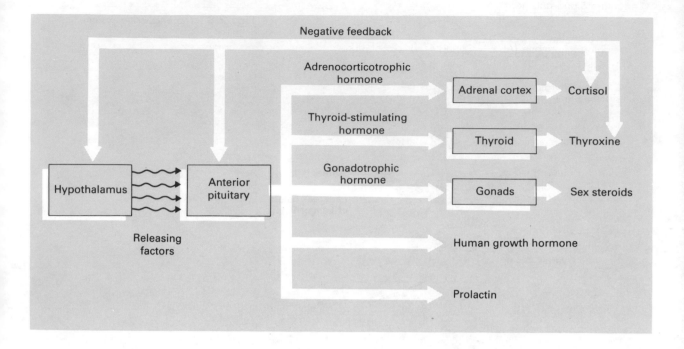

Fig. 2.9 The influence of the anterior pituitary gland on other endocrine glands.

sponse to low levels of blood glucose and raises them by mobilizing glycogen stored in the liver and by increasing the conversion of proteins and fats to glucose. It is vital that blood glucose levels are maintained because it is the only food nutrient used by the brain for metabolism.

A summary of these and other principal hormones and their actions is given in Table 2.2.

The nervous system

Nervous control is provided by the nervous system, which provides the body's links with the outside world and, with the endocrine system, maintains homeostasis within the body. The two major divisions of the nervous system are the central nervous system (CNS), comprising the brain and spinal cord, and the peripheral system, which includes the sensory receptors and nerves to and from the CNS. The CNS is protected by bone and three layers of membrane and is bathed in the cerebrospinal fluid. The brain is the major control centre of the body, with different areas responsible for functions such as speech, posture, personality, appetite and memory. Brain cells must receive a constant supply of glucose and oxygen in order to function.

The peripheral nervous system is subdivided for convenience into the somatic and autonomic systems. The somatic division receives messages via sensory nerves about the external environment and returns messages via

Table 2.2 Principal endocrine hormones and their actions

Endocrine gland and hormone	Acts on (target)	Actions
Posterior pituitary		
Antidiuretic hormone (ADH)	Distal tubules of kidney	Stimulates conservation of water by reabsorption
Oxytocin	Uterus and mammary glands	Stimulates uterine contraction and ejection of milk into ducts
Anterior pituitary		
Adrenocorticotrophic hormone (ACTH)	Adrenal cortex	Formation and secretion of adrenal cortex hormones (see below)
Thyroid-stimulating hormone (TSH)	Thyroid gland	Formation and secretion of thyroid hormones (see below)
Gonadotrophic hormones (follicle-stimulating hormone and luteinizing hormone)	Gonads	Stimulates gonad hormone production (see below)
Human growth hormone (HGH)	General	Stimulates growth – promotes protein synthesis, raises blood glucose level, mobilizes fat
Prolactin	Mammary glands	Stimulates milk secretion
Thyroid		
Thyroxine (T_4) and tri-iodothyronine (T_3)	General	Control metabolic rate, mobilize fat, affect metabolism of carbohydrates essential to normal development
Calcitonin	Bone	Lowers blood calcium level by inhibiting breakdown of bone
Adrenal cortex		
Aldosterone	Kidney tubules	Maintains sodium balance
Cortisol	General	Promotes synthesis of glucose in liver to raise blood glucose, mobilizes fat
Adrenal medulla		
Adrenaline and noradrenaline	General	Helps body to cope with stress, e.g. by increasing heart rate, metabolic rate, rerouting blood, increasing blood sugar
Parathyroids		
Parathyroid hormone	Bone, gut, kidneys	Increases blood calcium level
Pancreas		
Insulin	General	Lowers blood sugar by allowing glucose to enter the cells for use, stimulates fat storage and protein synthesis
Glucagon	Adipose tissue, liver	Increases blood glucose by stimulating fat breakdown and glucose production in the liver
Testes		
Testosterone	General	Maturation of reproductive organs of male, development of secondary sexual characteristics in male, bone growth and fusion of epiphyses
Ovaries		
Oestrogen	General	Preparation of endometrium for pregnancy and maintenance during pregnancy
Progesterone	Uterus, breasts	Maturation of female reproductive organs, development of secondary sexual characteristics in female, thickening of endometrium, development of breast lobules and areolae
Placenta		
Production of oestrogen and progesterone is taken over from ovaries at about the twelfth week of pregnancy		

motor nerves to adjust the position of skeletal muscles; it is under voluntary control by the individual. The autonomic system is responsible for ensuring a steady state within the body's internal environment by regulating such things as temperature and heart rate. It works automatically without voluntary control.

Stimuli are carried from the peripheral to the central nervous system where decisions are made or reflex actions triggered. Messages are then returned via the peripheral system to the appropriate muscles and glands which carry out the order.

Maintaining homeostasis

If homeostasis is to be maintained, temperature, fluid levels and pH must remain constant and nutrients must always be available.

Temperature at the core of the body is kept at about 37°C, whatever the external temperature, by the control centre in the hypothalamus. It receives messages from heat receptors in the skin and is sensitive to the temperature of the arterial blood surrounding it. The hypothalamus is 'set', rather like a thermostat, at around 37°C, and initiates mechanisms to ensure that body temperature remains constant. To some extent the individual can influence his own temperature by the clothes he wears, the food he eats, and the temperature of the environment in which he chooses to spend his time.

If the temperature at the hypothalamus falls below 37°C, thyroid hormones are excreted to increase the metabolic rate and more food is metabolized in the liver to produce heat. Nerves are stimulated to contract capillaries in the skin so that heat is conserved. If the core temperature continues to fall, shivering begins; the muscles contract and this produces heat. Once temperature is returned to normal, these mechanisms are switched off.

If the temperature rises above 37°C, the hypothalamus initiates dilatation of the capillaries in the skin so that more body heat is carried to the surface where it is radiated off. Nerves also stimulate the sweat glands, perspiration increases and heat is lost by evaporation. Again the mechanisms are switched off once homeostasis is achieved.

Respiration is under voluntary control to a point but usually it is impossible to stop breathing until death occurs since the respiratory centre in the medulla of the brain will intervene to ensure that breathing is resumed. Receptors in the carotid arteries are sensitive to low levels of oxygen in the blood and send messages to the respiratory centre, which in turn stimulates the respiratory muscles. The rate and depth of breathing are increased and in consequence more oxygen is absorbed into the blood. Other receptors, in the brain, sense any rise in blood levels of carbon dioxide and inform the respiratory centre, which increases the breathing rate so that more carbon dioxide is exhaled. It is important that carbon dioxide is not allowed to build up because it is an acid and enzymes will only function at the correct pH.

Fluid balance is achieved in the distal tubules of the kidneys, which can reabsorb water or excrete it into the urinary system for elimination as urine. The process is under the control of ADH from the posterior pituitary gland. Receptors in the brain sense the osmotic pressure of the blood (an indication of its dilution). When this is higher than normal, indicating that the blood is too concentrated, the receptors inform the hypothalamus which stimulates the posterior pituitary to release ADH. ADH acts on the distal tubules to increase the volume of water reabsorbed into the blood, i.e. antidiuresis. If osmotic pressure is below normal because the blood is too

Fig. 2.10 Diagrammatic representation of homeostasis.

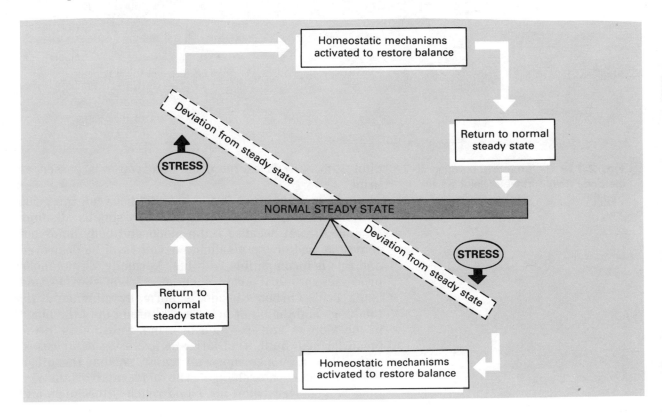

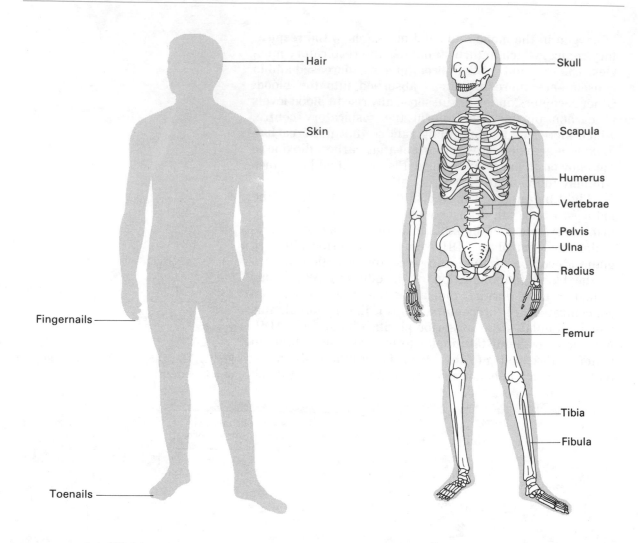

Fig. 2.11 The protective covering of the body (*left*) and the skeletal system (*right*).

dilute, no ADH is excreted and the water is passed as urine.

Acid–base balance is the balance between the acids and alkalis in the blood – it is normally slightly alkaline. Balance is vital because if the blood and body fluids become too acid or too alkaline, enzymes will be destroyed and this is incompatible with life. Normally all metabolic processes produce acids such as carbon dioxide and lactic acid. Carbon dioxide is normally eliminated via the lungs and the other acids are filtered out of the blood in the kidneys and excreted in urine. Substances in the blood termed 'buffers' absorb any excess acids or bases, rather like a sponge mops up water, so that the pH of the blood does not change. The acids and alkalis can then be removed when the blood reaches the lungs and kidneys.

Figure 2.10 summarizes diagrammatically how

homeostatic mechanisms act to maintain a steady state in body functions.

The body's framework

All the tissues of the body are held together and in shape by other tissue systems, the skeleton, the muscles and the skin, which must also function efficiently if physical health is to be maintained.

The **skeleton** is made up of bones connected together by joints (many of which are movable), cartilage, ligaments and tendons (Figure 2.11). It allows movement and acts as support and protection for many parts of the body. Bones also store calcium and phosphorus and manufacture blood cells.

There are nearly six hundred **muscles** in the human body, some of which are indicated in Figure 2.12. Voluntary muscles such as the biceps and quadriceps need nervous stimulation before they can be moved. Cardiac muscle and smooth muscle are involuntary and work automatically without the need of nerves to stimulate them. Examples of smooth muscle are that in the blood vessels, where it helps to maintain blood pressure, and that in the gut, where it acts to propel food along.

The **protective covering** layer includes skin, hair, nails and sweat glands. It protects the body from injury and infection and is an important organ for controlling temperature. It prevents water entry and loss and has a sensory function; pain, temperature and pressure are all sensed in the skin. It can be a useful health indicator since heat, colour and hydration all vary with an individual's physical state.

This section has introduced the systems of the body. Figures 2.13 to 2.18 are designed to show how they are sited anatomically in relation to one another. Surface structures have been progressively removed to show the deeper structures.

It has been necessary, for the sake of clarity, to talk of body systems and functions as though they work independently of one another; this is clearly not the case. Even a seemingly simple action such as respiration involves several of the body systems – circulating blood carries carbon dioxide (a product of cellular respiration) to receptors in the brain, which alert the nervous system to influence the muscles of respiration. The human body is an extraordinarily complex machine of many interdependent parts, which must all function in conjunction with one another to maintain physical health.

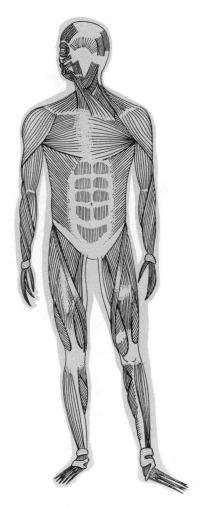

Fig. 2.12 The muscular system.

Fig. 2.13 Anterior view: skin and muscle removed.

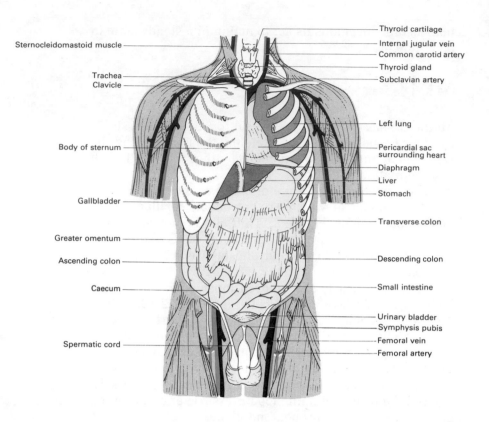

Sternocleidomastoid muscle

Trachea
Clavicle

Body of sternum

Gallbladder

Greater omentum

Ascending colon

Caecum

Spermatic cord

Thyroid cartilage
Internal jugular vein
Common carotid artery
Thyroid gland
Subclavian artery

Left lung
Pericardial sac surrounding heart
Diaphragm
Liver
Stomach

Transverse colon

Descending colon

Small intestine

Urinary bladder
Symphysis pubis
Femoral vein
Femoral artery

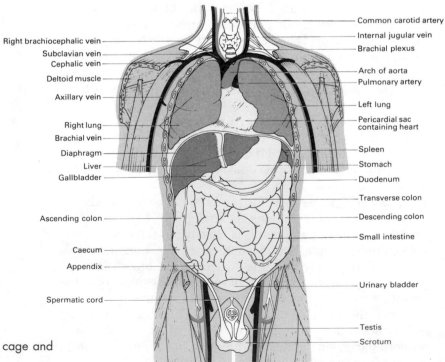

Right brachiocephalic vein
Subclavian vein
Cephalic vein
Deltoid muscle
Axillary vein

Right lung
Brachial vein
Diaphragm
Liver
Gallbladder

Ascending colon

Caecum

Appendix

Spermatic cord

Common carotid artery
Internal jugular vein
Brachial plexus

Arch of aorta
Pulmonary artery

Left lung
Pericardial sac containing heart

Spleen
Stomach
Duodenum

Transverse colon

Descending colon

Small intestine

Urinary bladder

Testis
Scrotum

Fig. 2.14 Anterior view: rib cage and greater omentum removed.

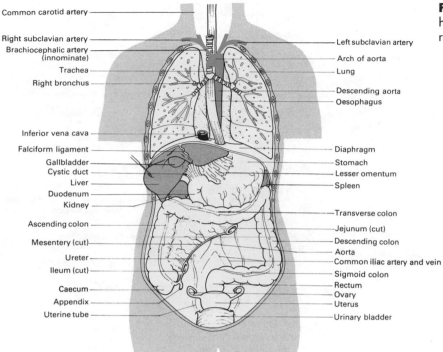

Common carotid artery

Right subclavian artery
Brachiocephalic artery
(innominate)
Trachea
Right bronchus

Inferior vena cava

Falciform ligament
Gallbladder
Cystic duct
Liver
Duodenum
Kidney

Ascending colon

Mesentery (cut)

Ureter
Ileum (cut)

Caecum

Appendix
Uterine tube

Left subclavian artery

Arch of aorta

Lung

Descending aorta
Oesophagus

Diaphragm
Stomach
Lesser omentum
Spleen

Transverse colon

Jejunum (cut)
Descending colon
Aorta
Common iliac artery and vein
Sigmoid colon
Rectum
Ovary
Uterus
Urinary bladder

Fig. 2.15 Anterior view:
heart and small intestine
removed. Lungs in section.

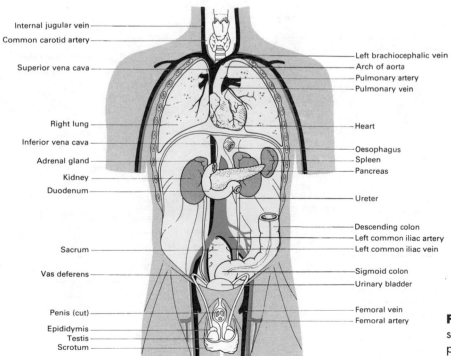

Internal jugular vein
Common carotid artery

Superior vena cava

Right lung

Inferior vena cava

Adrenal gland

Kidney
Duodenum

Sacrum

Vas deferens

Penis (cut)

Epididymis
Testis
Scrotum

Left brachiocephalic vein
Arch of aorta
Pulmonary artery
Pulmonary vein

Heart

Oesophagus
Spleen
Pancreas

Ureter

Descending colon
Left common iliac artery
Left common iliac vein

Sigmoid colon
Urinary bladder

Femoral vein
Femoral artery

Fig. 2.16 Anterior view:
stomach, small intestine and
part of large intestine
removed.

Fig. 2.17 Anterior view: all viscera removed.

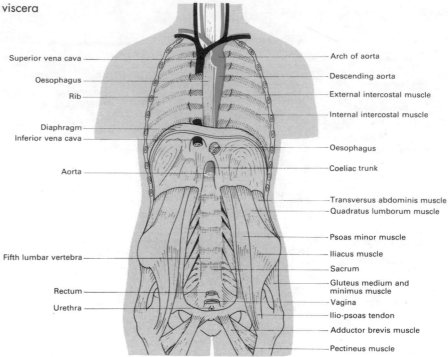

Superior vena cava
Oesophagus
Rib
Diaphragm
Inferior vena cava
Aorta
Fifth lumbar vertebra
Rectum
Urethra

Arch of aorta
Descending aorta
External intercostal muscle
Internal intercostal muscle
Oesophagus
Coeliac trunk
Transversus abdominis muscle
Quadratus lumborum muscle
Psoas minor muscle
Iliacus muscle
Sacrum
Gluteus medium and minimus muscle
Vagina
Ilio-psoas tendon
Adductor brevis muscle
Pectineus muscle

Fig. 2.18 Posterior view: muscles removed.

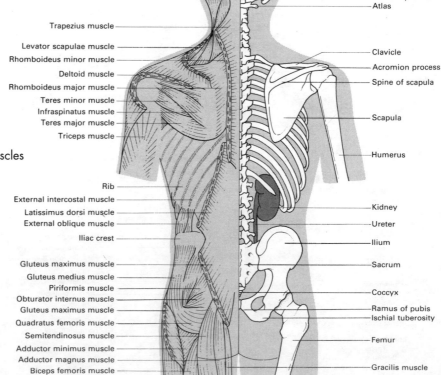

Trapezius muscle
Levator scapulae muscle
Rhomboideus minor muscle
Deltoid muscle
Rhomboideus major muscle
Teres minor muscle
Infraspinatus muscle
Teres major muscle
Triceps muscle

Rib
External intercostal muscle
Latissimus dorsi muscle
External oblique muscle
Iliac crest
Gluteus maximus muscle
Gluteus medius muscle
Piriformis muscle
Obturator internus muscle
Gluteus maximus muscle
Quadratus femoris muscle
Semitendinosus muscle
Adductor minimus muscle
Adductor magnus muscle
Biceps femoris muscle

Mastoid process
Atlas
Clavicle
Acromion process
Spine of scapula
Scapula
Humerus
Kidney
Ureter
Ilium
Sacrum
Coccyx
Ramus of pubis
Ischial tuberosity
Femur
Gracilis muscle

The psychology of mental health

The human individual is much more than a physiological machine. His brain does not exist to control bodily needs alone, but also gives him the power to think, learn, feel and express emotion. The study of man's mental processes is called psychology. Nurses require an understanding of psychology to allow them to assess mental health in their patients.

Personality

Although the physiological functioning of each human follows a well-defined pattern, each one may be seen to be a unique individual in his own right. The difference may be described in terms of personality, though this is of course an oversimplification. Personality has been studied by psychologists for many years and a number of theories to explain differences in personality have emerged.

Early theories, such as that of Freud, can be described as 'conflict models', and portray each individual developing his personality in terms of compromise. More recent theorists, such as Rogers and Maslow, use a 'fulfilment' model, in which personality develops as the individual attempts to actualize his full potential.

The Rogerian view is that each individual is influenced by his view of himself as a person. Where Freud might talk of man having basic self-centred instincts, e.g. survival and reproduction, Rogers proposes an inherent potential to maintain and enhance life, which in enhancing an individual's view of himself will also lead to his valuing and respecting other people. In Rogers' view, suspicion and competitive feelings about others come from misunderstanding rather than from selfishness.

For an individual to actualize his potential, he has two basic requirements – the need for positive regard from others and the need for positive regard of self. Both are seen to be learned needs which lead to the development of a self-concept. In other words, the view of oneself as a person will be influenced by feedback from other significant individuals.

It can be seen that if the inherent potential is to be reached, social influences, such as positive feedback about self-concepts, are necessary. Rogers explains this in terms of 'conditions of worth'. In effect this is saying that society gives an individual values by the simple method of approval and disapproval, and suggests that if potential is not approved, actualization may not occur.

Disapproval can be seen to lead to feelings of guilt, which can be lessened by defence mechanisms. In Rogers' view such defence lessens the chance of self-actualization and can have a crippling effect on personality development. If, however, individuals are held in positive regard by the significant people in their lives, they are likely in turn to regard others positively.

Theories such as those of Rogers and Maslow (Chapter 4) are useful in that they explain human behaviour in terms of needs, many of which are met by others. This view of individuals as dependent upon each other suggests the possibility of vulnerability and stress, particularly if others undermine the self-concept or self-image which has been developed. Mental health may be affected if the need for a positive regard of self is not met.

Stress

Stress may be described as an individual's reaction to a challenging situation. The body has a mechanism which responds to stress by preparing for 'fight or flight'. This is under the control of the autonomic nervous system, which triggers the secretion of adrenaline from the adrenal medulla and at the myoneural junctions in a challenging situation.

Adrenaline in the blood causes peripheral blood vessels to constrict so that blood is diverted to muscles ready for action. The circulatory increase to muscles and brain, along with an increase in glucose from the liver, all prepare the body to face the challenge or run away.

This reaction would be appropriate if stress were always in the form of physical danger, but much stress in modern life is to do with interaction with others or with distressing happenings. A further complication is that what is seen by one individual as a stressful situation might not upset another at all. Similarly, what is seen as stressful can vary because of its relationship with other factors in life.

Mary Wong found much of life stressful. She became angry and upset if her family were late for meals and was known to cry if a cake was burnt. Her son later died in tragic circumstances abroad. A few days after this the bedroom ceiling was brought down by snow. In normal circumstances this would have caused Mary tremendous stress, but in relation to her son's death it caused no anger or panic at all.

Meichenbaum (1983) describes stress as 'a byproduct of the transaction between the individual and the environment'. Modern living is seen to be stressful in day-to-day problems such as the burnt cake, in lifestyle problems in terms of job, relationships and social expectations, and in life crises such as the death of someone who is much loved.

Stress is a fact of life and indeed a certain level of stress is seen to be necessary, for if too much is inhibiting, in that it engenders the fight or flight feelings of panic, anger and alarm, too little may prevent an individual from maximum achievement.

The normal healthy individual is usually able to cope with those situations which he perceives as stressful, either by consciously regulating his emotional responses or by changing the situation which is causing the stress. These and other coping strategies allow an individual to maintain mental health while living in a stressful society. Alternative strategies such as smoking and taking alcohol or drugs may be used to reduce stress but do not deal with the underlying problems.

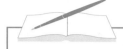

Think of a recent occasion when a problem caused you to feel stressed or anxious. How did you cope with the problem? With hindsight, what would you have done differently?

Perception

Perception can be described as the way the individual views the world, using his eyes and other senses such as touch, taste and smell.

Each individual attempts to make sense of his world. This means that in each new situation, past experiences will be used to classify and explain that situation. In Mary Wong's case, for example, the potential stress of the fallen ceiling was measured against the enormous stress of the loss of her son. The thoughts which led to the perception of the ceiling damage may not have been conscious but it seems reasonable to assume that, had her son not died, the ceiling would have been viewed as an all-time tragedy.

Perception is more to do with knowledge stored in the brain than with what is actually seen. Looking out of the window, the house at the end of the road appears smaller than the pot plant on the window sill, yet their real sizes have been learned, as is the principle that items in the distance look smaller than they actually are.

The brain interprets the senses in perception of depth, width, distance and colour. Similarly with the perception of events. Individuals see what they want to see or what they expect to see. For instance, an experiment in which a film was shown of police dealing with a riot elicited very different reports from the police and public who watched it. The police described the violence of the rioters towards the police, while the public described the police as assaulting the rioters.

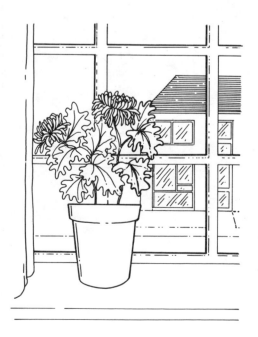

The above example shows how individuals pick out of a situation that part which is pertinent to themselves. This selectivity in perception means that no two individuals will interpret a situation in the same way, and that almost all situations are open to misinterpretation. If an individual is under stress, he is more likely to have errors in perception, which can affect normal healthy functioning.

Attitudes

Attitudes are derived from perceptions of the world and the way in which an individual deals with its stresses. As such, an attitude may be described as a belief held about some aspect of life such as politics, religion or sexuality. Once an attitude is formed it may be resistant to change.

Mr North had a very negative attitude to his neighbour, whom he described as useless because he neglected his garden and changed jobs frequently. When Mr North was told that the neighbour was in fact in poor health and unable to do heavy work he did not change his attitude but rationalized that the neighbour was unable to 'pull himself together'. This distortion of fact allowed Mr North to maintain his original attitude towards his neighbour rather than admit that he had held an inaccurate belief.

Individuals tend to be drawn to others who hold similar attitudes. Liking someone who holds different attitudes may lead to 'cognitive dissonance' originally described by Festinger in 1957. This dissonance is thought to be caused by the difficulty of accepting opposing views in an otherwise likeable person. Festinger suggested that an individual will work to reduce dissonance either by changing his own views or by deciding that he does not like his friend after all. An alternative is to rationalize in order to explain a friend's divergent views.

Finding that attitudes match those of a friend can strengthen friendship since each individual is positive towards the other's beliefs no matter how trivial. This is illustrated by the story of Matthew, who, in telling his mother about the girl he planned to marry, explained, 'I knew we were going to like each other as soon as I realized that we both hated macaroni cheese'.

Extreme attitudes are called prejudice. Examples of this are racial prejudice, where a negative attitude to a whole race is made on the basis of colour, or prejudice towards a whole group on the basis of the behaviour of a few. Few people are without any prejudice, though the mentally healthy person accepts that he is occasionally prejudiced and that some of his attitudes would not bear close scrutiny. Awareness of self helps an individual to understand others, and to become tolerant of human frailty.

Interaction

Interaction with others and the environment is necessary for mental health since it has been shown that sensory deprivation can produce psychiatric states (Davis *et al.* 1960). Isolation is not quite the same as total sensory deprivation but it may lead to delusions, abnormal behaviour (e.g. talking to oneself) and loss of interest in life. Humans are undoubtedly social. They are reared in a social group and learn to look for confirmation of self-image from significant people around them. The newborn infant learns first to look to his mother for love and affection and later to friends and peers (Klein 1987).

Friends are chosen usually because of common interests and attitudes, and, as a child develops, friends may replace parents as confidants and mentors, as each reinforces the other's view of self as a worthwhile person. In adolescence, the need for love and affection from peers or a special same-sex friend may be succeeded by the need for friendship with the opposite sex as well as interaction with peers.

Interaction with others fulfils a basic need. The loving sexual relationship can be the ultimate in close relationships since it fulfils the need both for friendship and esteem and for sexual expression. It may also lead to production of the next generation. Society has an expectation that the normal behaviour of adults is to marry and reproduce. This can be hard on individuals who do not wish to express their sexuality physically and on those who do not wish to or cannot reproduce.

Interaction, then, may be with family and friends and may include one particularly significant person of the same or opposite sex. Other interactions may occur with strangers such as a waiter in a restaurant, with colleagues at school or at work, or with like-minded people in a club or an association. The important element is the individual's choice to develop any relationship or bring it to a close. Dissonance will occur only if the individuals do not agree on the level of relationship desired. To have friendly overtures rebuffed may be damaging to an individual's self-image.

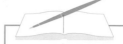

Do this with a colleague who knows you quite well (you can both participate):

1 Each note three positive aspects about the other.
2 Each note one aspect of the other that does not fit the overall 'picture' of the persona.

Did you agree with each other?
If not, how did you feel?
How did you deal with these feelings?
Did you discuss your reactions with anyone?

Sexuality

Sexuality and the need to reproduce were seen by Freud as a basic driving force which explained many of man's actions. This view is less popular today but most people would agree about the strength of the force of sexuality. Part of an individual's self-image is concerned with his sexual attractiveness to another, no matter at how low or high a level. Unfortunately much that is written about sexuality does not include the concept of love. The two are not necessarily synonymous since a man can pay a prostitute if all he wants is a sexual encounter. A loving sexual relationship concerns a level of regard and respect and a level of self-disclosure totally lacking in a purely sexual exchange. As Kaplan (1978) suggests, 'Love involves shedding the carapace upon which we depend to protect us from pain and it renders us so vulnerable to the other. And yet, to get in touch with feelings of mutual love can profoundly change the quality of life from black and white to technicolour . . .'

Although romantic novels describe 'love at first sight', it is more likely that love develops as a relationship progresses. When a couple are sexually attracted there is a natural urge to express sexual feelings. Men are still seen to take the lead in heterosexual relationships, but this may be changing as women strive for equality. Certainly there is an increase in couples who live together for a period before getting married to make sure that they are suited to each other and some couples live together permanently in same-sex relationships with all the commitment of marriage.

Sexual expression within a loving relationship can be incredibly binding to both partners. Should one of the partners subsequently reject the other for any reason, considerable stress may develop which, in some instances, can seriously affect mental health. It is also true that if a relationship is close and confiding, the partners are more able to cope with stressful situations (Maguire 1984). Sexuality without love fulfils a biological need, while sexuality with love fulfils both biological and psychological needs.

Communication

In order to interact with others, an individual needs to learn to communicate. Language has to be learned, and most children have a wide vocabulary, grammar and syntax by the time they are five years old. In the early days of interaction between mother and child, there is considerable non-verbal communication such as smiling and touching to show pleasure, and frowning and distancing to show displeasure. Even when language is learned, non-verbal behaviour remains an integral part of the communication system.

Verbal communication

Language is a vital part of verbal communication, although what is said is almost always interpreted in the context of the non-verbal behaviour which accompanies the message, and also by the expectations of the individual giving the message. For example, information is likely to be taken more seriously from someone who is trusted and respected than from someone the receiver is suspicious of. It can be seen from this that interpretation of language depends not only on the individual transmitting the message but on the perceptions and attitudes of the receiver.

Lindgren (1973) cites studies to suggest that the kind of language used by an individual will indicate his identity in terms of culture and status. Lindgren also suggests that language will be used differently by an individual according to the status of the person with whom he is interacting.

It can be seen that to use the same language does not necessarily mean that what is said by one individual will be understood by another, and even written messages may be misunderstood. In the early days of supermarkets, the trolley bays used to have signs above saying 'Please take one'. Many people interpreted this to mean that they could actually keep the trolley rather than use it within the supermarket.

Many words in the English language are ambiguous in that their meaning expresses a personal value. The word 'good' is an example of this in that it infers judgement of what is good. If, for example, a child is noisy and active his mother might describe him as 'good' on a quiet day, while the mother of a normally quiet child might only describe him as 'good' if he performs a special service for her. Past experiences are colouring the meaning of the word so that its use is subjective and not necessarily understood in the same way by others.

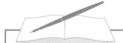

Identify six ambiguous words. List the different meanings attributed to each word. How can we be sure we undertand the real meaning of a particular message? (See Chapter 4.)

Non-verbal communication

If language can be misunderstood through misinterpretation of the words used, there can be further room for error from the non-verbal communication which surrounds it.

People who are used to interacting with each other learn to 'read' each other's non-verbal messages and will usually have a common meaning for words.

The tone and manner in which language is used can give information about the verbal message. For example, the message 'I have some news for you' can be given many meanings by non-verbal cues. If it is said in a serious voice it could be imagined that the news is bad, an excited voice could imply good news, while a hesitant voice with poor eye contact could mean that there was some doubt about the way the news will be received. Non-verbal behaviours such as eye contact, posture, gestures and the clothes we wear (Argyle 1972) can all affect communication. Examples are given in Chapter 4.

The need to communicate

Although communication is a complex process, individuals exhibit a need to communicate from birth. The need to have others communicate positively with them can be seen in mothers who are anxious for their baby's first smile. There is comfort and support in positive interaction and communication between people, and a potential for stress if the majority of communication is negative.

There are, however, wide discrepancies between individuals' needs. Eysenck (1970) used a scale to describe individuals on a continuum from introversion to extroversion (Figure 2.19). Although we may describe people as extroverts and see them as gregarious, or introverts who tend to be loners, most people fall somewhere between these two extremes. What is important is that each individual is content with the level of interaction and communication available to him.

Many healthy people in society feel cut off from communication more by circumstances than desire – for example, the young mother who is constrained by her children, or the elderly person who is constrained by the thought that society has abandoned her and that her family, who live far away, do not need her.

The psychological individual

Each individual develops a personality that contributes to his uniqueness. Psychologists such as Freud see this personality developing from selfish instincts whereas others, such as Rogers, talk of inherent unselfish potential.

To develop and maintain a healthy self-image, positive regard for self and positive regard for others is required. Negative feedback may cause stress, as may life events both large and small. The psychologically healthy

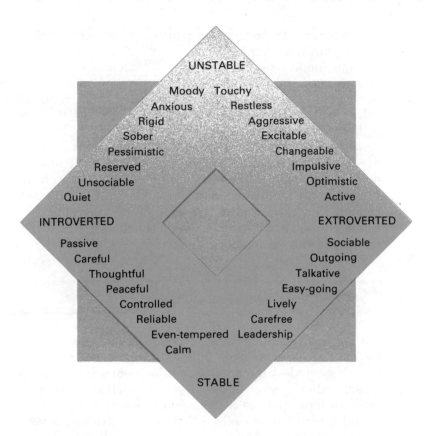

Fig. 2.19 Eysenck's introversion–extraversion scale.

UNSTABLE

Moody Touchy
Anxious   Restless
Rigid   Aggressive
Sober   Excitable
Pessimistic   Changeable
Reserved   Impulsive
Unsociable   Optimistic
Quiet   Active

INTROVERTED   EXTROVERTED

Passive   Sociable
Careful   Outgoing
Thoughtful   Talkative
Peaceful   Easy-going
Controlled   Lively
Reliable   Carefree
Even-tempered Leadership
Calm

STABLE

individual develops mechanisms to cope with normal stress.

Perception will affect attitudes to life as each individual makes sense of his environment, using past experiences to interpret the present. Chosen interactions will be with other individuals with similar attitudes. From the safety of the family group, the individual will widen his circle of peers, friends and loved ones. A partner may be chosen for a loving relationship which may or may not be sexual. The ability to communicate effectively is necessary for the building of relationships and the fulfilment of needs. This includes verbal and non-verbal communication, which combine to produce a composite message.

It can be seen that, psychologically, man is a complex individual who from his genetic pattern, environmental influences and interaction with others becomes totally unique.

Spirituality

Part of the uniqueness of each individual is spirituality. Too often this is interpreted as religion (Stoter 1991) and therefore any spiritual distress is seen as peripheral to

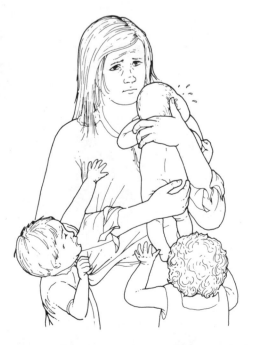

nursing care. In fact, spirituality **may** include religious beliefs, but not necessarily.

Spirituality may be seen as the 'essence' of an individual and is inextricably tied to a view of oneself as a person. Most people do not consciously concern themselves with their beliefs until some crisis leads them to rethink who and what they are.

Illness is just such a crisis, particularly if it is interpreted as a punishment, as is often the case if the disease does not appear to make much sense. In a search for meaning, the individual may have his views of himself shaken. This can result in strong emotions emerging such as anger, guilt and blame. If religious beliefs are involved, then faith may be temporarily shaken.

Sociological aspects of health

Both physiology and psychology study the individual – how he develops, reacts and functions in his environment. Sociology studies the society of which each individual is a part, either by studying small groups such as families, or large groups such as a community. Because each individual interrelates to others, often in a structured way, and because he is often constrained by his place in society, it can be said that sociological factors may affect health.

Social class

The idea of social class is unpalatable to many people since it evokes connotations of status and privilege. However, at regular intervals a census is held in the United Kingdom in which each household has to give particulars about its members and the amenities of the home in which they live. From this, statistics are developed about society, and its members are divided into five social classes according to the occupation of the head of the household. Table 2.3 shows the classification into classes according to occupation.

Many would argue that this classification is old-fashioned and no longer pertinent. However, differences do exist and can have an effect on patterns of illness and on health care (Bond and Bond 1993). For example, social class 1 members used to have most earning power, but today many semi-skilled jobs, such as working on oil rigs, carry enormous salaries because of the danger and hardship involved. Similarly, many nurses are now graduates

Social class	Occupation (examples)
1	Graduate professionals e.g. doctors, university professors
2	Professionals e.g. teachers, nurses
3	Skilled (white collar workers) e.g. clerks
4	Semi-skilled (blue collar workers) e.g. postmen
5	Unskilled e.g. labourers

Table 2.3 The social classes.

and would see themselves as of similar status to doctors. Finally, in a society where women wish for equality, judging their social status by their husband's occupation can seem to be insulting.

Perhaps a more realistic classification in terms of health is that of marketing, where groups are identified according to their media consumption. This includes which newspapers and consumables are bought, and which TV programmes are watched. Such classification can give some information on whether healthy foods are bought as opposed to those seen to be less healthy, and can tell whether consumption of alcohol and cigarettes is going up or down, but it actually tells us very little about the health of the nation.

Status

On paper, status may be linked to social class. In society, other attributes may be added to social class to determine status. These may include the sort of house a person lives in, the number of cars, a person's standing in society in terms of privilege and club membership, and other tangible signs of success.

Attempts have been made to break down the barriers in society caused by class and status. Early in this century a man called Webb built an estate of private houses in Purley, Surrey. The idea was to provide houses at all prices so that there would be a social mix of people. Today, only the rich can afford to buy houses on the Webb estate, no matter how small. Money has been used to control the status of house owners.

A similar example of 'like to like' organization is that of Cutteslowe Park in Oxford, where an illegal wall was built across the road to divide private houses from a council estate (Collison 1963). Examples such as these suggest that society tends to resist attempts to destroy groups formed according to class or status. Whether this need for division applies to all groups, or more to the privileged groups, is unclear.

The family

Whatever an individual's class or status, the family is the basic unit in society. It used to be common for families to be **extended**, in that when a young couple married, they would settle with or near parents and other relatives (Figure 2.20). Grannies might live no more than a street away, and thus would influence the new marriage group in terms of running the home and rearing the children. Such a family (and many still exist) can be very supportive

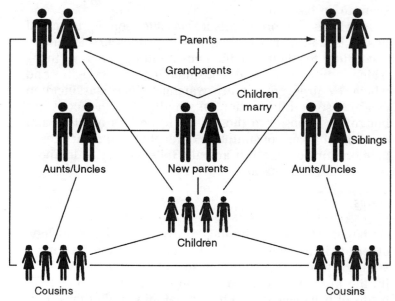

Extended family. All live in close proximity

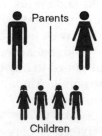

Nuclear family. Other relatives live at a distance

Fig. 2.20 The extended family (*above*) and nuclear family (*below*).

to its members, since an inexperienced bride may be helped by parents who will later be cared for by their children when they get old. Children growing up in such families have a loving network of carers when they are needed.

Education and mobility of employment have led to an increase in the number of **nuclear** families, in which the basic unit is the parents and their children, often living hundreds of miles away from their relatives. When the first child arrives, the mother often feels very isolated if she has given up employment and does not know her neighbours well. Social outlets may be curbed by the ties of a child and the marriage may suffer as the husband sees his wife totally absorbed in the child.

It can be seen that individuals within a family will be affected by its structure. In the extended family a young couple may live with parents for some time. Whether or not a couple both work may depend on the co-operation of their parents in caring for a child during working hours. Gulfs are unlikely to occur in the extended family because each new generation is continuously socialized by the past.

The nuclear family has the chance to set new traditions, far away from the influence of parents. It may be then that a 'generation gap' occurs, which means that family reunions for holidays and celebrations can be difficult if the various generations are not tolerant of each other's views. In such a situation the elderly are not likely to settle happily into a son's or daughter's home in old age.

The family gives a child its first experience of co-operation between a small group of people. The nature of the relationships within the family and the level of responsibility expected of each member will give each individual the values with which he will operate in the community.

The community

If the family is the basic unit of society, groups of families may be seen as a community. A community is a geographical area where there is a level of sharing and interdependence among the families within it. A village is commonly given as a good example of a community, while a town could be seen to be composed of a number of communities. Both village and town will say something of the families and communities within them.

Chester, for example, is a town serving a number of fairly affluent communities and is noted for its jewellers and antique shops, whereas nearby Wrexham developed to provide the needs of first a mining area and later an industrial area. This is reflected in shops which are geared to practical needs. Similar comparisons may be made between Oxford and Swindon.

Communities share meeting places such as schools, churches, pubs and clubs. They often have local magazines and papers, and, if the community is a close one, they share informal information networks. Members of a community are free to have as much or as little contact with other members as they wish, but there is often an assumption that individual members will 'pull together' for the good of the community.

In villages where the extended family survives, there is a sense of loyalty and belonging to the community which is not seen in commuter communities with a rapid turnover of residents. There may be a sense of isolation for people who live in an area where neighbours are out at work all day and little social interaction is possible to an extent that mental health is at risk.

The working community

Family members and other people who live in a community may work within or outside that community. The local vicar, postman, farmworker or shopkeeper may spend both his working and social life within the same community. Others may work away, often travelling some distance from home to a different type of community.

Industrial organizations, educational establishments, prisons and hospitals may be described as 'working communities' where individuals use their work as the common factor among them. Sociologists use the concept of roles to describe different behaviour in different circumstances, and people who work outside their own community can be seen to have different working and social roles, which may be less clearly defined for someone working within his own community.

For example, the university lecturer who is authoritarian with his students may appear to bear little relationship to the darts player full of bonhomie in the 'local' at the weekend, whereas the local milkman is expected to behave in the same way to the villagers whether he is delivering milk or playing darts.

Working may impose a strain on health, both mental and physical, if there is role strain. It may be that the image an individual feels is expected at work may be difficult to maintain. There may be a risk of job loss if goals are not met or mistakes are made.

Unemployment and redundancy have been a problem

in recent years with devastating effects on many in society. For most people employment not only provides the money for supporting a home and family but also provides the classification of class and status for self and family. The individual who loses his job may feel that he has also lost his status in the community. Because of the strong work ethic which still exists, he may feel it degrading to accept unemployment benefits from the state. Self-image may be affected, as may relationships within the family.

The social community
Individuals do not necessarily socialize within their own community, but there are opportunities to do so. In Christian Communities the church is one organization which offers socialization, not only in religious services, but in social groups such as the Mothers' Union, the Pathfinder Clubs and other activities.

Most communities, and the individuals within the community, have religious beliefs. These beliefs are not the same for all religions, but they do appear to have common elements. One of these elements is that individuals within the community meet together to reiterate their beliefs. Another is that each belief, be it Christian or not, involves a superior, powerful being, God or deities.

Many people, at both an individual and a community level, gain strength from the thought that they can depend on their belief for comfort, safety and support. Further, such belief usually offers the promise of a better life after death. It can be seen that this element of community interaction offers both religious and social interaction. People's involvement in the community aspects of religion varies: for some, their involvement with the church is an integral part of their lives, while others may not feel the need to make their belief, or lack of it, public.

Local community activities may also arise in response to specific conditions in an area. For example, some villages have societies for the preservation of footpaths. Such groups have both a social and a community function in that the members act as watchdogs in their area so that they can bring pressure to bear on those who seek to obstruct or close local pathways. Other examples of this type of group are tree preservation societies, and groups such as rotary clubs which fulfil both a social and a charitable role.

In any of the above activities, whether an individual attends a place of worship, or belongs to a club or a society, his commitment to the community is likely to increase as the result of his involvement with others in his area.

Health risks in the community

The family and the community may be seen to be a supportive network for the individual in his social, home and working life. However, it must be remembered that these networks are not always ideal.

All families do not have ideal accommodation. In some depressed areas housing is poor and families overcrowded so that strains are put upon relationships. This may result in violence within the family, particularly towards women (Bart 1993), and in health problems for children (Wyke and Hewison 1991). Although this could happen at all levels of society, it is more likely to occur when conditions are poor and money is limited.

Some families may have outside or shared lavatories and no more than a cold water tap available indoors. Physical health and cleanliness become more difficult in such circumstances, and those who try to keep standards up in such conditions may become very disillusioned.

Social Services' provision should mean that there is no poverty in the United Kingdom. However, secondary poverty, where families cannot manage their money, may lead to malnutrition and other symptoms of deprivation which are detrimental to mental and physical health.

Finally, lifestyle may affect health in that individuals tend to accept group norms in society even if they are harmful. Thus groups of youngsters may experiment with drugs in order to be acceptable to peers, while others misuse alcohol at clubs and pubs to remain 'part of the community'. One of the problems of health education is in motivating an individual to change behaviour which is acceptable to family, friends and colleagues.

It can be seen that society provides a supportive network for an individual but that this network may also have negative effects on physical and psychological well-being.

Culture

'Culture' is a word used to describe those aspects of a society which make it unique. This includes the arts, technology, eating habits, beliefs and customs of a society.

Since the Second World War, the United Kingdom has changed from an almost exclusively white population to a multiracial one with immigrants from all over the world. Many come into the country expecting a better life than they had experienced previously, and are often disappointed when they are unable to find work or accommodation in the area of their choice.

Immigrants tend to live in separate areas from others. This may not be from choice but from discrimination in that, if black families move into an area, white families may move out. Often there is quite strong prejudice against immigrants, which may be based on ignorance of their culture.

Because of its multiracial society, the United Kingdom has many subcultures, which can be seen in specialist restaurants, clothes shops and food shops in an area. Just as integration was seen to be resisted between classes, so it is between races living in the same country.

This may change as third-generation children grow up. Their first language may be English so they will not have the problems of being understood that many immigrants experience. Similarly they may take a more Westernized view of life although this may cause its own tensions. This process is helped by the fact that white children now grow up with black friends, and religious education in state schools very often involves all religions represented by the pupils. Major religious festivals are celebrated in the cultures represented in the school and children are encouraged to understand the different cultures within UK society.

A major problem lies in the poorer areas of the country where there may be more people of ethnic minorities and fewer facilities than in richer areas. It can then be seen that white families get preferential treatment to that of ethnic minority families.

It may be difficult for members of a different culture to maintain health. For many, the climate is cold and unfriendly and the food strange. There may also be problems of poverty and overcrowding. The HEA produces booklets in many languages to help parents from different cultures with nutrition and health, but little attention is given to the integration of immigrants into society.

Because of hostility and prejudice towards other cultures in society, the government introduced the Race Relations Act. This means that if a job is advertised, employers are not allowed to exclude people from that job on the basis of their race or colour. The problem with legislation of this sort is that it is very difficult to enforce. Prejudice cannot be written out of existence by the law, and it is difficult to prove that an individual was unsuccessful in obtaining work because of his race.

A better understanding of the cultural patterns of immigrants might reduce prejudice. The other view is that many immigrants are resentful of their host country and feel 'let down' when they find that their standard of life has not improved to the level of their expectations. They are unwilling to give up their own cultural patterns and this is understandable. Culture and belief are part of each individual's heritage.

Summary

This chapter has examined the individual in his normal environment. It can be seen that health is often a matter of choice, although there may be a conflict of choices between healthy behaviour and socially accepted behaviour.

Physiologically and psychologically, the individual has needs which, if not met, will affect his health. Many of the physical needs are met automatically, such as breathing, while others can be controlled by the individual, such as nutrition. Psychological needs may be met by others in terms of approval and confirmation of self-image.

The need for others has led to a discussion of the construction of society and its supportive role in the life of the individual. Society may also have a negative effect on an individual. This may be seen in racial prejudice and discrimination, where there is a lack of understanding of others' cultures.

References

Argyle, M. (1972) *The psychology of interpersonal behaviour*. Harmondsworth, London: Penguin.

Bart, P. (1993) *Violence against women: bloody footprints*. London: Sage Publications.

Bond, J. & Bond, S. (1993) *Sociology and health care: an introduction for nurses and other health care professionals*. Edinburgh: Churchill Livingstone.

Collison, P. (1963) *The Cutteslowe walls*. London: Faber and Faber.

Davis, J. M., McCourt, W. F. & Solomon, P. (1960) The effect of visual stimulation on hallucinations and other mental experiences during sensory deprivation. *American Journal of Psychiatry*, **116**, 889–892.

Eysenck, H. J. (Ed.) (1970) *Readings in extraversion–introversion. Theoretical and methodological issues*. London: Staples Press.

Festinger, L. (1957) A theory of cognitive dissonance. In

Lindgren, H. (Ed.) (1973) *An introduction to social psychology*. New York: J. Wiley.

Kaplan, H. S. (1978) *The new sex therapy*. Harmondsworth, London: Penguin.

Klein, J. (1987) *Our need for others and its roots in infancy*. London: Tavistock.

Lindgren, H. (1973) *An introduction to social psychology*. New York: J. Wiley.

Maguire, P. (1984) Psychological reactions to breast cancer and its treatment. In Bonadonna, G. (Ed.) *Breast cancer: diagnosis and treatment*. London: J. Wiley.

Meichenbaum, D. (1983) *Coping with stress*. Amsterdam: Multimedia Publications.

Stoter, D. (1991) Spiritual care. In Penson, J. & Fisher, R. (Eds.) *Palliative care for people with cancer*. London: Edward Arnold.

Wyke, S. & Hewison, J. (1991) *Child health matters*. Milton Keynes: Open University Press.

Further reading

Abraham, C. (1992) *Social psychology for nurses*. London: Edward Arnold.

Altschul, A. (1991) *Psychology for nurses: nurses' aids series*. London: Baillière Tindall.

Birch, A. (1994) *Individual differences*. London: Macmillan Press.

Blaxter, M. (1990) *Health and lifestyles*. London: Routledge.

Cannon, C. (1992) *Changing families, changing welfare*. Harvester.

Goffman, E. (1959) *Presentation of self in everyday life*. Harmondsworth: Penguin.

Green, J. (1975) *Introduction to human physiology*, 4th edn. Oxford: Oxford University Press.

Ham, C. (1991) *The new National Health Service: organisation and management*. Oxford: Radcliffe Medical Press.

Haynes, N. (1994) *Foundations of psychology*. London: Routledge.

Holiday, I. (1992) *The NHS transformed*. Manchester: Baseline Books.

Jacobson, B., Smith, A. & Whitehead, M. (1991) *The nation's health: a strategy for the 1990s*. London: King's Fund.

MacKinnon, P. (1993) *Oxford textbook of functional anatomy: musculoskeletal*. Oxford: Oxford University Press.

Niven, N. (1994) *Health psychology: introduction for nurses*. Edinburgh: Churchill Livingstone.

Paton, C. (1992) *Competition and planning in the NHS*. London: Chapman & Hall.

Riddle, J. (1985) *Anatomy and physiology applied to nursing*. Edinburgh: Churchill Livingstone.

Wilson, K. (1990) *Ross and Wilson anatomy and physiology: in health and illness*. Edinburgh: Churchill Livingstone.

PART TWO
ASSESSMENT

3

The Patient on Admission

CHAPTER SUMMARY

Physical signs of disease, 67
The need for help, 68

Notice of admission, 69

The concept of stress on admission, 70
The nurse's role, 70
The need for information, 71

The ward environment, 71
Ward structure, 71
Noise and smell, 72
Ward personnel, 73
Other staff, 74

Admitting a patient, 75

Waiting, 76
Introductions, 76
Orientation to the ward, 76
Pattern of the day, 77
Patient concerns, 77
Documentation, 78
Adaptation to a new environment, 79

The relatives, 80
The need for reassurance, 81

Summary, 81

References, 81

Further reading, 82

Physical signs of disease

In Chapter 2, people were considered as healthy individuals within an environment familiar to them. It would be simplistic to assume that no illness enters this normal life, as most people suffer from occasional aches and pains or have coughs or a cold. How these common disorders are dealt with will depend on the individual. Some people, for example, will treat a cold quite seriously, staying at home and maybe taking some medication, while others will stoically go on with their lives as normal, stating that they will not be beaten by a simple cold. It could be argued that the person who stays at home is being neurotic or that the person who ignores the cold is a risk to other, unaffected people. What is important, though, is that there is a level of unhealthiness which each individual will consider as a cause for concern, and this will vary considerably from person to person.

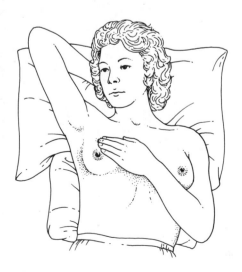

The need for help

Although an individual may not worry about the common cold, other symptoms, which are less common, will alert the average healthy person. An occasional headache may not seem important, but constant headaches with accompanying symptoms such as dizziness and loss of focus may send an individual to the doctor for advice. This is so for most pain – be it headache, indigestion, backache or 'muscle' pains – the individual will consult the doctor or seek other help (Figure 3.1) when the level can no longer be explained in normal terms for that person. It is reasonable to believe that the patient seeking advice in these circumstances will be concerned for his health to some degree.

Other physical signs may so frighten a patient that he or she feels bound to consult he doctor.

John Hughes was very proud of the fact that he 'never had a day's illness' and had little time for doctors. At 50 he began to have bouts of 'thumping' in his chest together with a feeling of 'tightness'. He ignored his wife's pleas to visit the doctor until he had an attack while driving his car one day, when he had to pull over to the slow lane to recover.

While fear of a particular sign or symptom may send a patient to the doctor, it may well keep him or her away.

Ingrid Olson found a lump in her breast many months before she approached her doctor. She was terrified of cancer and felt that if she ignored the lump it might go away.

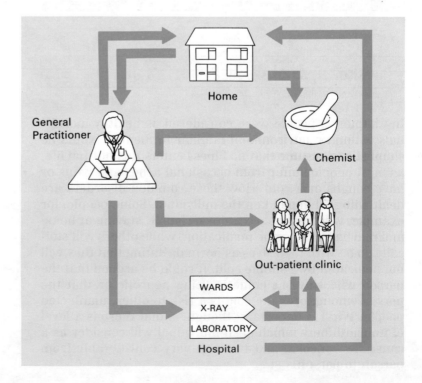

Fig. 3.1 Possibilities for action in illness.

The General Practitioner (GP) may be able to deal with many of the ailments which otherwise healthy individuals present to him in surgery. For example, Mr Hughes was sent for an ECG (electrocardiogram), where the tracing showed some irregularity of heart beat which could be treated at home with medication. Other patients may need to be admitted to hospital for investigations and treatment or operation.

Notice of admission

Of the patients that the GP believes need hospital care, some will have to go on a waiting list. Usually such patients are considered non-urgent, though they may be feeling uncomfortable or restricted in some way.

Mr Zolman had noticed that he was not walking as easily as before, and suffered pains in his leg. The GP diagnosed arthritis and the possible need for a replacement hip joint. It is usual to have to wait for such an operation. It can be argued that the disease will not affect Mr Zolman's general health and that his pain can be controlled, though he may not understand why he has to wait for an operation.

Ingrid Olson, however, would normally be admitted very quickly since a lump in the breast **may** be cancer, and without treatment it could spread. She could be admitted within a week of seeing her GP.

The Patient's Charter (updated 1995) sets down limits for how long a patient has to wait to see a Consultant, and how long he has to wait for an operation.

Most hospitals send information to patients prior to their admission to hospital. Usually such information is in the form of a small booklet. It may list things to bring into hospital, visiting times, details of bus routes, and other items of information necessary for the patient's stay.

When admitting a patient it is worth asking if such information has been received. Some patients are admitted as emergencies, straight from home, the surgery, or an accident. They may be too ill to care about visiting times, but their relatives will need information and may not think to ask for it. A supply of such booklets on the ward is useful since such information given verbally may not be remembered.

There will be local standards for the admission procedure. These may include the concept of a 'named nurse', i.e. a nurse who will take responsibility for the patient and his care during his stay, although other members of the

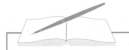

Ask your librarian for a copy of your Health Authority's Local Charter Standards. How long would a patient in your area have to wait for a first out-patient's appointment? What other local standards do **you** think are important?

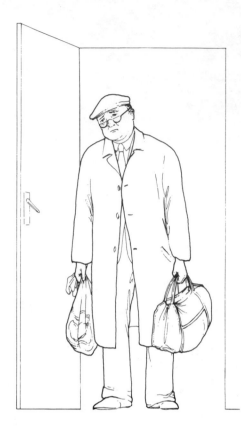

team will also be involved. Such procedures are aimed at helping the patient to adapt to the new environment with the minimum of added stress.

The concept of stress on admission

It has already been shown that normal body mechanisms prepare an individual for 'fight or flight' in the face of threat or danger. It is also true that many people are threatened by the unknown. This is not too difficult to believe. One only has to think back to a new experience – say starting a first job, flying in an aeroplane for the first time or going to one's first disco – to remember that, even though the event could be foreseen as pleasurable, it also brought anxiety. This anxiety may take many forms but usually it is a concern over the ability to cope with the situation. How much more stressful is admission to hospital, which is not normally seen as a pleasurable experience, can readily be appreciated.

Patients on admission are already experiencing physical signs or symptoms of disease. Depending on their knowledge, experience and personality, they may be in some fear for their health and future. Additionally, coming into hospital may be a totally new experience compounded by the inevitable restrictions of normal life.

The nurse's role

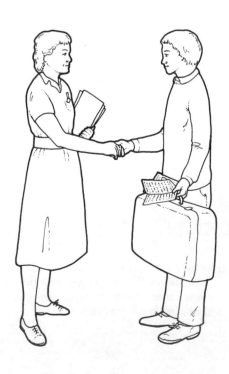

The nurse is part of the patient's new experience and her interactions with him on admission are most important. At the point when the patient actually arrives on the ward the need is for social interaction, i.e. greetings and an introduction, yet often patients complain that they are taken to a bed and left there without greeting or explanation. Such casual treatment is almost bound to raise anxiety levels in the patient.

It is not always possible to deal with all the fears and worries of a patient on admission. It will not be known until after investigation if Ingrid Olson's lump is cancer; nor can we foretell the cause of many other physical signs and symptoms. For this reason many patients are not given a diagnosis and may be very anxious about the outcome of the investigations or operation. What the nurse can do is to be calm and friendly while appreciating that anxiety does exist.

As long ago as 1978, Wilson-Barnett suggested that for most patients stress is highest in the first 24 hours after admission. An interesting book (Cooper 1983) takes a wider view of stress and disease, and makes some links with personality. However, for many patients the stress of admission may be compounded by fears and worries about diagnosis, treatment and the resultant uncertainty. How quickly the patient adapts to the hospital environment can be largely in the hands of the nurse, through her attitude, her accurate assessment of the patient's initial needs, and her ability to meet those needs.

The need for information

Stress and anxiety reduce concentration, so that much of what is said to the patient in his first few hours in hospital may need to be repeated later. It has been argued that information should be kept to a minimum during the first day or so in hospital, but the patient may ask questions which the nurse can answer. This willingness to meet the patient's need for knowledge could reduce his anxiety and is therefore worthwhile even if he does forget and ask the same questions again later.

Individuals do not always show that they are anxious, nor do they necessarily tell anyone about it. Some patients may be very quiet and withdrawn, while others may appear to be aggressive. Learning to assess patients' reactions accurately should help to reduce their anxiety and will increase their faith in the nurse as a professional, which in turn will allow them to cope better in the new situation.

The ward environment

Nurses soon become familiar with the hospital and may forget their first impressions of the hospital ward, but for the patient arriving for admission the ward may seem both frightening and confusing.

Ward structure

In older hospitals the wards are often large and open. These are called Nightingale wards. The beds are arranged down each side of the ward with perhaps a table or desk in the middle. Seeing such a ward for the first time, it will almost certainly look enormous and not very friendly. What are those machines beside some of the beds? Why is that old man groaning and being ignored? What's going on behind those closed curtains? The patient will be bombarded with new impressions, many of which will add to his anxieties.

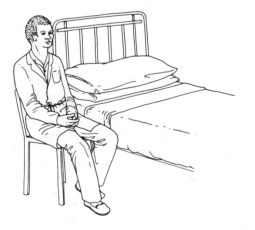

More modern wards are divided into smaller rooms or open bays. Here there are perhaps four patients in a group. There is less of an overall impression of vastness and illness in such settings, thought it is more difficult for the nurses to observe the patients. All wards are likely to have at least one single room and this is usually reserved for a patient who is very ill or who is in need of special care.

Most wards have a day-room for patients where the atmosphere is less clinical than the main ward. There are other rooms such as bathroom, shower and toilet, sluice, clinical room, kitchen and Sister's office. It may take a new patient a considerable time to find his way around and to learn where he may and may not go.

Noise and smell

Added to the confusion of the ward layout for a new patient are the strange smells and level of noise. The smell on a ward is quite unique and will obviously affect individuals differently. Some may find it pleasant, picking up the antiseptic 'cleanness' of the smell, while others may find it rather overpowering with its essence of illness and people, overriding the sharp clean smells of the clinical room. The important thing is that the new patient will almost certainly be aware of the hospital smell and may take some time to adjust. Similarly, some adjustment is needed to the noise. A lay person may have an impression of hospitals as quiet hushed places and may therefore be rather surprised at the noise of rattling trollies, clanging lift gates, crunching bedpan machines and the general buzz in an average ward.

The patient is admitted in a confusion of impressions of space, smell, people and noise. He is taken to a bed and may sit there, looking around and trying to make sense of his surroundings. Again, this will be different for each person. When confronted with something new, individuals look to their past knowledge and experience to make sense of the unknown. Such a mechanism is very useful because it saves time but it can also lead to misconceptions.

The new patient sitting waiting to be admitted may not have enough knowledge to make accurate sense of his surroundings and may see what is going on around him as far more frightening than it really is. He may see several people in white coats standing round a bed. Is the patient seriously ill? Why are there so many of them? Why are they not talking to the patient? It will be a day or two

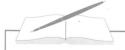

Choose a patient with whom you feel comfortable. Ask him/her to tell you what he/she particularly remembers about being admitted. What was most helpful? What caused most concern?

Discuss your findings with a colleague and plan how differently you will handle future admissions.

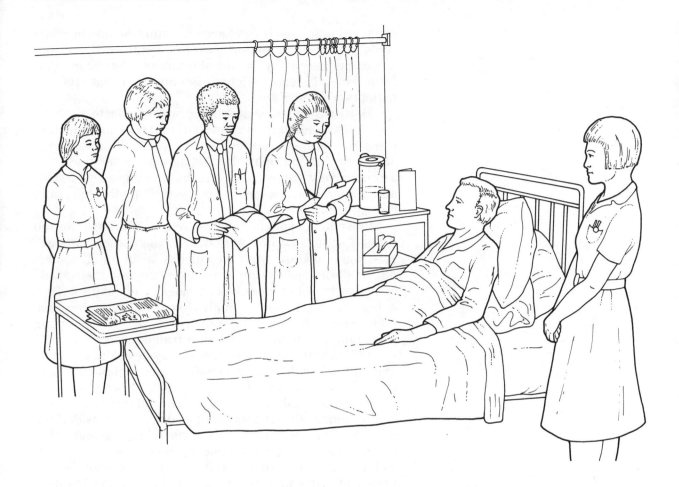

before the patient realizes that what he has seen is part of a normal ward round.

The nurse cannot explain all the strangeness at once but sensitive assessment of the patient's level of awareness will help him make sense of his new surroundings as quickly as possible.

Ward personnel

In the previous section there has been an assumption that new patients may be very naive in their knowledge of hospitals. Television programmes may give a romantic view or go to the extreme of overdramatization of events in hospital wards or emergency departments. There are also romantic novels woven around nurses and hospitals, but neither of these will help the patient with his new impressions on admission and may hinder him in identifying ward personnel. Most people, for example, 'know' that the ward manager is in charge and that people in white coats are doctors, but in fact the reality can be very confusing, especially in the absence of a standard uniform. For this reason alone it is important that staff tell patients who they are.

Many personnel wear white coats, e.g. doctors, physiotherapists, dietitians, pharmacists and laboratory technicians. Obviously the patient will not meet all these people at once, but he may be helped if he is told that a protective white coat is worn by many grades of staff, and if personnel wear badges giving their name and designation.

In some hospitals, nurses wear different-coloured dresses or suits according to their grade and patients will soon come to know what the colours mean. In other hospitals, all the nurses' uniforms are white and their grade is shown by different-coloured belts or epaulettes. To a new patient, a nurse is simply that, and it may be some time before he can differentiate between a nursing assisstant, a student nurse and a trained nurse.

This means that junior nurses may be asked for information that would be more appropriately obtained from a trained member of staff.

If a patient asks a junior nurse for information it does not, of course, always mean that he does not know that the nurse is a learner. As long ago as 1961, Maghee found that patients often feel more able to relate to junior staff, feeling that both patients and nurses are under the authority of Sister and the Doctor. If this relationship does exist between junior nurses and their patients, it is important that trust also exists. This requires honesty on the part of the nurse when she cannot help the patient, and a commitment to keep promises to fetch a more senior member of staff. It is very easy, on the way to find a senior colleague, to become diverted and forget the promise to the patient. The patient, waiting and anxious, may believe that no one cares about him or his problems.

Other staff

Apart from doctors and nurses, whom the patient will expect to see, there are numerous other staff in hospital who will visit the ward. Lelean (1973) reported no fewer than 33 categories of personnel visiting a ward in a four-hour period. These included technicians, clerks, maintenance staff, porters, teachers, chaplains and senior nursing staff. (This still relevant study, with others carried out during the period, has become a classic and forms part of a series published by Scutari Press.) Lelean's study focused on interruptions of the Sister's work, but from the patient's point of view these people represent quite a confusion, especially since many will be dressed in a similar way. The patient's main concern will be the personnel with whom he is expected to interact.

A n example of a patient's confusion is that of Miss Reilly. She had been a patient before, so she knew a little about the organization of staff. Each morning, a rather aloof woman dressed in tweeds and twinset came into her room and asked how she was. Miss Reilly treated this as a social enquiry but was puzzled about the woman's identity. Since the daily enquiry was always accompanied by a searching look around the room, Miss Reilly decided that her visitor was the domestic supervisor. In fact she was a senior nursing manager. Had Miss Reilly known her identity she may have felt able to discuss her problems, since Sister was off sick and she felt she needed to talk to a senior person.

Often the ancillary staff seem most friendly to patients and as a result gain more of their confidence. This can be a cause for concern, since the understanding cleaner, however friendly, may give the patient information that is either false or inappropriate. This in turn may lead to patients confiding, to the cleaner, important information that is more relevant to nursing and medical staff. If nursing and medical staff can meet the needs of patients for information, anxiety will be considerably reduced.

The nurse can help the patient to become accustomed to the many different personnel on the ward. When a porter arrives to take a patient to X-ray he may ask for Mrs Smith. It is much more pleasant for the patient if the nurse accompanies the porter to the bed and explains his presence, than if the nurse points out the patient and leaves the porter to make his own introductions.

It could be argued that most patients are able to ask personnel who they are and why they are there. In fact it is well documented that patients do not ask questions, and it therefore falls to the nurse to help the patient make sense of all the many people who will be concerned in his care and treatment.

Admitting a patient

The main aim in admitting a patient should be to meet his need to settle into his new environment as soon as possible. This may seem to conflict with the nurse's need to gain some information about the patient and his current problems. In fact the patient may be too anxious for a full assessment, and it is probably best to take the essential details only on admission. When the patient has settled into his new surroundings, he will be more able to disclose his problems, his fears and his worries (Faulkner 1992).

Waiting

It is not always possible to admit a patient as soon as he arrives. Some wards have waiting rooms or areas. If the patient has arrived with a relative it is better to leave them both in the waiting room than to separate them and sit the patient by his bed. In such a situation anxiety levels may be raised in both the patient and his relative. In a study of childhood cancer (Faulkner *et al.* 1995), one small boy vividly describes being put on a bed while his mother was taken outside: 'I were right afraid'. This could have been avoided.

It may help the patient to know how long the wait will be. He can then discuss whether it is worth the relative waiting, since she may have other appointments such as collecting children from school. A relative who is short of time may feel unable to explain this or leave in case she is thought uncaring. The perceptive nurse will give the relative an opportunity to leave without guilt.

Introductions

The nurse who greets the patient on admission is likely to be remembered by him and soon becomes a familiar face among the many strangers. When the nurse takes the patient to his bed, it may help to introduce the patients on either side. There are now three people known to the patient and to whom he can relate. This helps in his orientation to the ward, and may help him to relax as he begins to understand his new environment.

Orientation to the ward

If the patient is able to walk, he should have the geography of the ward shown to him. Initially he needs to know the whereabouts of the bathrooms and lavatories, the dayrooms, the Ward Manager's office and/or the nurse's station. In his own bed area he needs to know which is his locker, where the bell is to call a nurse, and how to use the headphones if a radio is provided.

Many of the rules of a new environment are not explicit and need to be learned. In the main, such rules are in operation for the good of the majority and as such may irk a newcomer. For example, some hospitals are now completely non-smoking, though they may have designated smoking areas. If a nurse explains this rule she has an opportunity at an early stage to discuss the patient's smoking habits. This may be the start of an opportunity for health education. The fact that smoking in the ward is a fire risk is unlikely to help a patient change his habits for the good of his general health.

Pattern of the day

Although the new patient will need to learn the pattern of the hospital day, his immediate need on admission is to know what will happen **next**. Given that anxiety on admission affects the patient's ability to absorb information, it is very helpful if the nurse checks that the patient has had the booklet giving meal times and other aspects of the ward day, and then concentrates on the next happening. This will need to be consistent with the patient's beliefs about his admission.

When Ingrid Olson was admitted to hospital it was with the belief that she would come in at 10 a.m., have her breast biopsy in the afternoon and go home the following day.

On admission, Ingrid was told by the nurse that lunch would be along in just half an hour. She began to worry because she had expected to starve before her operation. When she tried to explain to the nurse she was cut off: 'Now, don't start worrying. You will feel better after a meal'. It would have been more useful if the nurse had tried to establish what Ingrid believed she had been told about her biopsy.

Patient concerns

On admission the patient may have some concerns about the hospital which are not explained in the booklet. As long as there is adequate opportunity to air these concerns, they are best dealt with as they arise. To attempt to cover all the queries which might possibly arise will put the nurse in the position of giving more information than an individual patient can absorb.

Of major concern may be the patient's illness and treatment. It may be that the patient has a clear understanding of his disease and what will happen to him. In this case he may simply ask for confirmation from the nurse of the length of stay, day of operation, types of investigation or possible outcomes.

If the patient is unsure of what will happen, he may ask for more information. Again, the nurse should deal with what will happen next. If the patient knows that his investigations will start tomorrow he will be reassured that the hospital staff are efficient. The patient who is in hospital for two days before anything happens seldom understands the necessity for inactivity and may need help in understanding the need for bedrest.

Documentation

Although the nurse should help the patient to settle into his new environment as a primary aim, she needs to collect some data from him on admission and deal with some practical matters.

The patient's notes usually arrive on the ward with the patient and will contain his home address, telephone number and name of next of kin. Although the nurse may take these details from the notes for her nursing history, she does need to confirm with the patient that the information is accurate.

Names are very important at any age. Many people have names which they never use in everyday life and therefore do not react to. It is always worth asking patients what they like to be called. It may be that some patients feel more comfortable on first or pet name terms; others may prefer to be addressed more formally. It is the patient's preference which counts. Old people especially can get very upset when called 'Gran' or 'Grandad', 'lovey' or 'pet'.

It is usual on admission to put a nameband on the wrist of each patient, bearing full forenames, surname and hospital number. Many patients do not like being labelled in this way. Such patients may accept the indignity if the reasons are explained to them in terms of concern for their protection and accurate treatment.

Other practical matters that a nurse has to deal with are clothes, safe storage of jewellery and money, and initial standard investigations such as urinalysis. Patients are more likely to be co-operative if they understand the reasons behind the actions. The nurse, however, needs to be sensitive to her patients' reactions.

Sarah Burns had worn a fine gold chain around her neck for years, 24 hours a day. She was asked to give it to the nurse for safe keeping until after her operation. Sarah understood that jewellery was not allowed in theatre, but after her operation it was almost the first thing she asked for. To the nurses, it was a trivial request and as such forgotten. To Sarah, it was a part of her; she felt naked without it and was therefore upset to have her request ignored.

It is difficult for an individual to maintain his identity in hospital when he is wearing anonymous nightclothes. A nurse can recognize the patient's dependence on small personal items like Sarah's chain and go far in reassuring the patient of his worth as a unique person.

Adaptation to a new environment

If the ward is considered as a social system (Menzies, 1970) it will be found to have unique facets with which the individual has to deal. The patients, for instance, may have only their illnesses in common and may differ markedly in other respects.

Although some individuals choose to take advantage of private treatment, the ward caters for all social and cultural groups. Normally society tends to be divided so that people mix with their own class for most of the time. This applies to work, social life and the places where people live. In hospital the class barriers are removed and adaptation to the new environment may include meeting

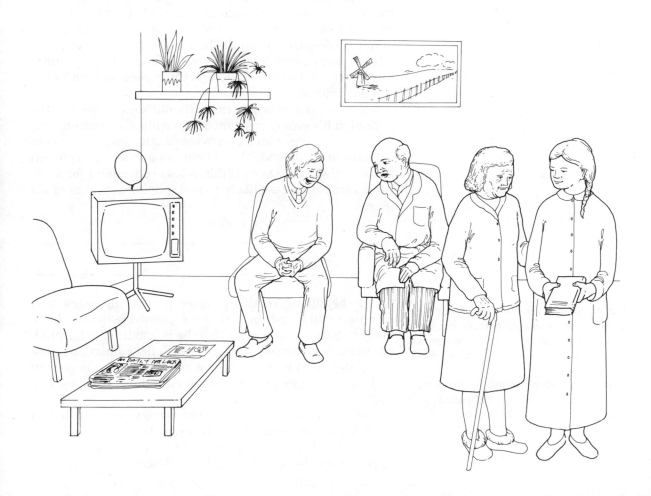

people very different from those with whom the patient normally interacts (Bond and Bond 1993).

It is usually thought a good idea to encourage patients to socialize with each other in the day-room and particularly at mealtimes. But insisting that all patients who can should sit at a common mealtable can be very stressful for patients, since eating is a social act for most people. Think of going to a restaurant with a friend – most people would rather wait for a table for two than share with strangers. Patients are individuals who should be able to choose either to join other patients in the day-room or to eat alone by their beds.

The timing of meals in hospital is often different from the patient's normal pattern of eating. There is logic in serving meals at a set time, but the time may require adjustment on the patient's part. If the last meal of the day is over at six p.m., the patient who normally eats much later may be hungry at bedtime and unable to sleep.

It can be seen that for someone who has been healthy previously, there is considerable adjustment necessary in the first few days in hospital in terms of both the social and the working life the ward. Added to this is an adjustment of personal space – even the bed and locker are not inviolate territory since time in or out of bed is largely under the control of the ward staff, and the contents of the locker are not private.

Nursing is a process which should seek to involve the patient in his own care (Hunt 1990) while the environment of the ward gives him a relatively passive role in terms of organizing his lifestyle. The nurse can encourage a patient in his individuality even if this is less convenient for staff. In this way he is less likely to feel a helpless victim of his illness.

The relatives

At the beginning of this chapter it was suggested that when an individual has concerns about his health, he is likely to become stressed. When he is admitted to hospital, the nurse is concerned primarily with his admission to the ward. Relatives may be at least as stressed as the patient and may require help and understanding from nursing staff.

To a busy nurse, relatives may seem selfish, but in fact their behaviour is due to a preoccupation with their own family, which gives them a different perception, rather than to their being selfish. This is demonstrated by rela-

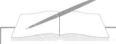

Work with a colleague. Each of you should ask a patient's relative if he/she will spare you 20 minutes for a short interview. Ask the relative for his/her perceptions of the patient's current illness. What are the relative's major concerns?

Compare notes with your colleague. Are there any common areas of concern? How different are the relative's perceptions from (a) the patient's view and (b) reality? Share ideas of how you might address problems that you have identified.

tives telephoning the ward and asking 'How is Dad?' or 'Has Mabel had her operation?' Their concern for their own relative eliminates the other patients on the ward to such a degree that they are often surprised that the nurse answering the telephone needs to be given Dad's name.

The need for reassurance

The relative needs reassurance that the patient will be well cared for and will get better. The nurse is not always able to reassure relatives on all points, particularly when diagnosis is in doubt. What the nurse can give to the relative is the assurance that everything possible will be done for the patient and that the nurse will be approachable and as helpful as possible.

Practical information can often be reassuring to relatives. Knowing when it is convenient to telephone the ward, what one is allowed to bring to patients, and whether children may visit will all help the relative to see how she fits in to the hospital routine. Initial stress may affect the absorption of this information, so it may need to be repeated at a subsequent visit, or written down.

Summary

In this chapter the transition from healthy independence to hospital admission has been considered, along with the many problems which may initially beset the patient and his relatives.

The nurse's role requires that she can perceive the situation from the patient's point of view, assess his individual needs, and help him to adjust to the new situation with the minimum of stress.

Relatives need to be treated with sensitivity and an awareness that they too may be under considerable stress.

References

Bond, J. & Bond, S. (1993) *Sociology and health care: an introduction for nurses and other health care professionals*, 2nd edn. Edinburgh: Churchill Livingstone.

Cooper, C. L. (Ed.) (1983) *Stress research. Issues for the eighties.* Chichester: John Wiley & Sons.

Faulkner, A. (1992) *Effective interaction with patients.* Edinburgh: Churchill Livingstone.

Faulkner, A., Peace, G. & O'Keeffe, C. (1995) *When a child has cancer*. London: Chapman & Hall.

Hunt, J. (1990) *Nursing care plans: the nursing process at work*. London: Scutari.

Lelean, S. (1973) *Ready for report, Nurse?* London: Rcn.

Maghee, A. (1961) *The patient's attitude to nursing care*. London: Livingstone Press.

Menzies, I. (1970) *Social systems as a defence against anxiety*. London: Tavistock Press.

Wilson-Barnett, J. (1978) *Stress in hospital*. Edinburgh: Churchill Livingstone.

Further reading

Altschul, A. (1972) *Patient–nurse interaction*. Edinburgh: Churchill Livingstone.

Franklin, B. L. (1974) *Patient anxiety on admission to hospital*. London: Rcn.

Mitchell, J. (1984) *What is to be done about illness and health?* Harmondsworth, London: Penguin.

Sinclair, H. & Fawcett, J. (1991) *Altschul's psychology for nurses*. London: Baillière Tindall.

Taylor, S., Field, D. & James, N. (1993) *Sociology of health and health care: an introduction for nurses*. Edinburgh: Blackwell Scientific Publications.

Winefield, H. & Peay, M. (1980) *Behavioural science in medicine*. Beaconsfield: Allen & Unwin.

4

Assessment of the Patient's Needs

CHAPTER SUMMARY

The concept of need, 83
Levels of need, 84
Physiological needs, 84
Safety needs, 85
Psychological needs, 86

Communication, 87
Verbal communication, 88
Non-verbal communication, 90

Interviewing skills, 94
Questioning techniques, 94
Cues, 97
Reflection, 97

Silence, 98
Educated guesses, 98
Clarification and encouraging precision, 99
Reassurance, 100
Control, 100
Summarizing, 101
Closing an interview, 102
Assessment forms, 102

Summary, 103

References, 103

Further reading, 104

The concept of need

When considering 'need' in relation to the process of nursing, there is the suggestion of a deficit of some sort. These deficits may be small or large, physical, social or psychological. A patient may present a number of deficits at the same time and the nurse may have to decide, on a priority basis, what action to take for the patient initially. Such decisions should represent the patient's priorities where possible, though occasionally a physiological need may seem more pressing to the health professional than to the patient.

Maslow (1954), an American psychologist, used the concept of need as part of his explanation of personality development. He suggested that man has a tendency to satisfy needs to ensure physical and psychological survival, and further suggested that these needs may be seen in a hierarchical order (Figure 4.1). The basic physical needs, i.e. air, food and warmth, are seen as fundamental because, if they are not met, there will be no motivation to

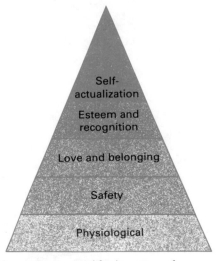

Fig. 4.1 A simplified version of Maslow's hierarchy of needs.

meet higher-order needs. Maslow's theory is not dissimilar to that of Rogers, which was discussed in Chapter 2, for both theorists are interested in how each individual reaches his full potential.

Levels of need

What is useful for nursing in Malsow's (1954) theory is the idea of different **levels** of need. In extreme cases where there are deficits in basic needs, we do not need to have this spelt out. At other levels there may be difficulties in assessing needs accurately.

Martha Jones, aged 22, was admitted for a simple operation on her foot. She was quiet and withdrawn with both staff and other patients, in spite of their reassurance and encouragement about her forthcoming operation. In fact, Martha Jones was pregnant but had not admitted this to anyone and was concerned about the effect of the anaesthetic on her baby.

The above case illustrates that we cannot make assumptions about needs until we know all the facts. In Miss Jones's case, her boyfriend had been killed in an accident, and she was desperate to keep his baby. One of her problems was that she did not have the courage to confide in anyone. Her physiological and safety needs were not in question, but she had lost her fiancé, was frightened for her baby, and had lost her self-esteem because of an imagined rejection by her family once they knew the facts.

Nurses cannot always meet assessed needs themselves, though sometimes meeting the need to confide will be helpful to the patient. The relationship between physical and mental health is not yet properly understood but there is a belief among some researchers (e.g. Fox 1983; Kasl 1983) that distress can affect physical health.

When Maslow developed his concept of man's drive to meet physical and psychological needs, his model was based on a normal individual with motivation to achieve his own potential. A patient coming into hospital usually has deficits which he cannot correct himself. It is these deficits with which the doctors and nurses concern themselves.

Physiological needs

Physiological needs may be affected by disease or physical malfunction of some part of the body. The individual can then be described as having a problem because he can no longer cope alone. For example, disease of the lungs will affect the ability to take in an adequate amount of oxygen.

Physiological needs can also be affected by social factors, e.g. an inadequate income may lead to malnutrition and hypothermia. This should not happen in a country with adequate Social Services but unfortunately some people, especially the elderly, do not know their rights, and some, through inadequate education, may not manage their income too well.

Physiological needs may also be affected by psychological factors. An example of this is anorexia nervosa, a condition most common in teenage girls where the need for food is not met because of an underlying, stressful condition, or occasionally because of an attempt to be slimmer.

In a situation where there is a physiological deficit which the patient cannot correct himself, plans have to be made to meet the individual's need in the light of the reason for the deficit and the physical condition of the patient.

Safety needs

Safety needs may be affected by physical disorders. In everyday life the senses are used to avoid danger, e.g. fire can be seen and heat felt; obstructions can be seen and so avoided. Further, memory ensures safety in normal circumstances, so that, for example, a kettle which is put on a stove to heat will be removed when it boils.

Miss Prince was 82 years old and lived by herself. She was fiercely independent and not prepared to admit that she could not see too well or that she had lapses of memory. She managed quite well in her own home because she knew where everything was, and so could manoeuvre her way through the house with no bother. She would occasionally forget to eat and had no electricity because she had not paid the bill.

A niece decided that Miss Prince was not safe and took her to her own home. As a result of being in a strange place, Miss Prince fell several times because she could not see the obstructions, burnt out two kettles because she had forgotten about putting them on the stove, and was finally admitted to hospital with a badly burnt hand, having fallen against the fire.

Patients in hospital cannot always meet their own needs for safety. The unconscious patient is a clear example of this, as is the confused patient who may need cot sides on his bed to stop him from falling out. Such cases show the responsibility of the nurse to ensure the safety of every patient. Each patient should be assessed individually so that proposed interventions may be agreed with the patient and/or relevant family members. Often patients feel overprotected when they are not given responsibility for their own safety, even though they could cope perfectly well.

Psychological needs

The effects of hospitalization on patients in terms of stress and loss of identity were discussed in Chapter 3. Physical disease may also lead to an increase in the psychological need for love and belonging, esteem and recognition. Some diseases, such as cancer or AIDS, may be seen to carry a stigma so that the patient feels somehow unclean and unacceptable to society. Such a patient may suffer a tremendous sense of emotional isolation. Similar feelings may be experienced with skin diseases. The patient's feelings may not reflect the way his family and friends really feel, but it is his own perceptions which are important when a nurse is trying to assess his needs.

Because of the loss of identity which may be associated with admission to hospital, the patient may lose his self-esteem. His normal means of sustaining self-esteem are in the past, replaced by the role of a patient. If the patient is frightened and anxious, his self-image may suffer another blow as he tries to remember his positive real life image.

Being admitted to hospital removes responsibility, not only for oneself but also for one's dependants. In fact there may be a role reversal that the patient finds difficult to cope with. It is almost impossible to feel a person of worth in such circumstances. Injury to self-esteem may lead to aggressive behaviour towards loved ones, causing further loss to feelings of worth. A nurse who can find the cause of such aggression may be able to help both the patient and his relatives to understand the situation and so help to meet the needs for psychological well-being.

Psychological deficits may also be caused by traumatic surgery. Ingrid Olson had to have her breast removed because she had cancer. She had been under stress for some time before admission and was worried that the cancer might spread and, more immediately, that the surgery would affect her husband's love for her. Because she saw herself as a freak she no longer felt a person of worth or someone lovable. In such a situation, the nurse may not be able to restore the patient's confidence since she cannot know if the husband's love has been affected. What she can do is accept the patient's concerns, emphasize the positive side of aftercare, and herself treat the patient as a worthwhile individual.

Some patients may believe that illness is a punishment that they have deserved. This can lead to feelings of guilt if the illness causes them to give up responsibility for their families temporarily.

Psychological problems are often more difficult to assess than physical problems, but a proper assessment of the patient should include physical, social and psychological needs. Psychological problems may also be more difficult to resolve than physical ones. Indeed some of them may not have a solution. The reader may wonder if there is any point knowing about these. In fact, just talking about the problem may help the patient and enable the nurse to initiate referral to an appropriate agency. Knowledge of such problems may also explain otherwise puzzling behaviour in a patient.

Communication

Communication is an integral part of patient care and is particularly important in the assessment of the patient. Communication is also part of what may be described as 'life skills' which any individual needs in order to function in society. For this reason it is often argued that such skills are innate and do not need to be learned. Even if this were true, communication in nursing is different from normal social interaction for a number of reasons.

It is accepted that patients are often under stress while they are in hospital. This alone would have the result of disturbing their normal pattern of communication and would involve the nurse in needing to make more effort than usual in order to interact with the patient. If the fears and worries held by many patients are added to this situation, particularly if they are not verbalized, it can be seen that social interactive skills alone are insufficient for nursing care.

In fact, research shows us that nurses do not communicate well with patients. Both Faulkner (1980) and Macleod Clark (1982) found that nurses generally do not meet their patients' needs for communication. However, Faulkner and Maguire (1984; 1994) have shown that if health professionals are taught communication skills, not only are they better able to assess their patients but the patients benefit in terms of being less stressed. Faulkner and Maguire (1984) concentrated on patients following mastectomy, but their later work generalized to health professionals involved in both cancer and palliative care.

Verbal communication

Verbal communication is largely concerned with the words we use, though other elements, such as tone of voice, will help to convey meaning. If English is the common language used, there should theoretically be few problems of understanding between nurse and patient. Reality is somewhat different from theory and much ambiguity can exist in communication in hospitals.

Jargon

It is usual for a profession to have its own 'language' or 'jargon'. This means that a nurse will build up a repertoire of terms and shorthand which other nurses will understand but which patients may not. The problem arises when this professional language becomes so familiar that one forgets it is not understood by everyone. If Sister says, 'Nurse, ask Mr Smith to let you know when he wants to PU so that you can get an MSU – Oh! and while you are there warn him about the i.v. drips', you will probably have to translate before Mr Smith understands enough to co-operate.

This professional language may also result in patients being ignorant of the reason for their admission.

J anet Curtis had been suffering from heavy periods. Her doctor told her that she had fibroids and would need a hysterectomy. Mrs Curtis thought that a 'hysterectomy' meant the removal of the fibroids, and it was not until after her operation, when she asked how soon she could become pregnant, that she learned that a hysterectomy meant removal of the womb.

Meaning

In Mrs Curtis' case, her misunderstanding is not surprising given that the technical term 'hysterectomy' could not be described as an everyday word. It might be used in the doctor's pages of women's magazines but even here there is often an assumption that its meaning is well known.

A more subtle problem of meaning may arise with everyday words which have a distinct meaning for the communicator but a different meaning for others. Such words may be very important in assessment terms. For example, a patient may describe himself as 'depressed'.

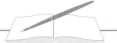

Think of the word 'normal'. It may mean different things to different people. To test this, ask a group of friends if they eat a normal breakfast. Then ask each one what they **actually** eat for breakfast. How could you rephrase the question to get a more meaningful answer? See p. 95 on open questions.

This could mean anything from being 'fed up' to clinical depression and needs to be clarified. Questions asked by nurses should avoid words which do not have clear meanings, such as 'social', 'enough', 'adequate', 'often' and 'frequent'. There are many others.

In assessment of the patient it is important that words mean the same to each speaker and that doubtful words are either omitted or clarified.

Social class

It has been suggested that the way we use language is affected by our social class (Bernstein 1959), working class people having a more restricted vocabulary than middle class people and a more restricted way of using language. This means that a nurse (whom one would expect to have a wide vocabulary) might confuse a patient if she does not keep her explanations simple. If a careful assessment is made of the patient's language pattern it should be possible to meet his need for information without talking down to him.

Mistakes may be made at the other end of the scale, in that it is easy to imagine that a patient with a wide vocabulary needs less explanation, or that a well-spoken patient has a wide vocabulary. Each patient needs an individual assessment without the nurse making prior assumptions.

Culture

There is an increasing number of patients whose first language is not English. It can be very distressing for a patient who wishes to communicate not to have enough command of the language to be able to do so. The nurse needs to be very sensitive to such distress. Inability to speak the language can easily be associated with low intelligence, yet how many of us could give a clear history of our symptoms if we were taken ill abroad in a place where English is not spoken? Many hospitals have interpreters available, but there is still a need to remember that patients who speak little English may feel very isolated.

Sowsan was an Arab patient on a gynaecological ward. She spoke little English and was described by the staff as 'sulky and withdrawn'. Staff Nurse Forbes had been in Abu Dhabi for two years nursing Arabs in an American hospital. One day, while making Sowsan's bed, Staff Nurse Forbes said a few halting sentences in Arabic. The transformation in Sowsan was immediate — here at last was someone who could communicate with her, if only on a simple level.

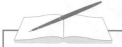

Join with a few colleagues. One of you should attempt to give a message to the others without using words. The rest of the group should attempt to interpret the message. How successful was the exercise? What misinterpretations were made?

Non-verbal communication

Verbal communication requires words, which can be recorded, evaluated and measured to determine if the exchange has fulfilled its intended function (Faulkner 1992; Argent *et al.* 1994).

Non-verbal behaviour is equally important, if not more important, than words for if there is a mismatch between the verbal and non-verbal message, the non-verbal message is most likely to be believed.

Mr Abraham was admitted to hospital for investigations. Nurse Brown could see that he was very frightened and told him, 'I am always available if you want to discuss things'.

As Mr Abraham saw Nurse Brown moving swiftly up and down the ward, he perceived that she was far too busy to spend time with him in spite of her reassuring words.

Non-verbal behaviour is well described by Argyle (1988) and must form part of assessment. However, such body language is very open to misinterpretation so no assumptions should be made until the behaviour observed has been clarified.

If we return to Mr Abraham, Nurse Brown noticed that he was very quiet and withdrawn and stopped by his bed to speak to him:

Nurse Brown You seem very quiet – I guess it all seems pretty overpowering?

Mr Abraham It isn't that, nurse. I've got loads of questions buzzing around my head but you are all so busy

Nurse Brown Not too busy for you

Mr Abraham Well, you never stop. I don't want to be a nuisance

In the above exchange, both nurse and patient had made assumptions about the other's non-verbal behaviour that needed to be clarified with words. What is important is that non-verbal messages are being sent and interpreted all the time that two or more people are together, and they can portray a wide variety of emotions, many of which can be reassuring to the patient. These include warmth, empathy and the willingness to give time. The risk is that other, less helpful, messages may be given including busyness, impatience and censure.

Clothes

In normal society, clothes are a strong non-verbal way for an individual to say something about himself, and society has certain expectations about dress. Students, for example, are expected to wear jeans and sweaters while businessmen are expected to wear suits. At a party, clothes are often an indicator of a person's status and subtle differences may be drawn between the wearer of a well-cut, well-brushed suit and the wearer of an old and shiny one.

For both the hospital patient and the nurse, the part of personality and status afforded by clothes is absent in that patients normally wear nightclothes and nurses wear a uniform. This approach denotes status for all within the hospital system but tells us little about individuals. What does happen in this situation may be seen as a loss of status for the patient and an authority (uniform) status for the nurse. In some areas of care, e.g. psychiatry, rehabilitation and care of the elderly, this problem is recognized and patients are encouraged to dress in their own clothes.

In normal society, meeting someone in nightclothes might well cause embarrassment and a loss of dignity to both parties. Hospital patients may take time to adjust to meeting people while dressed in night attire. This might be one possible explanation for why quite positive, articulate people become quiet, submissive patients.

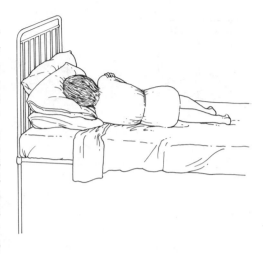

Posture

Posture is a strong non-verbal indicator of an individual's personality and the way he is feeling. By observing patients we can assess their posture for clues into areas we may need to explore. For instance, the patient who turns his face to the wall may be described as 'withdrawn' but needs to be assessed to discover the cause of the withdrawal. It may be that he is unhappy and does not want the other patients to see. Or it may be that something is worrying him which causes him to withdraw into his own thoughts. Posture will give the clue but the real reason for a patient's withdrawal needs sensitive assessment.

Similarly the patient will be assessing the nurse's posture. The nurse who stands by the bed, hands on hips, is unlikely to do more than frighten the nervous patient and anger the others. For the patient to be able to trust the nurse, he needs to feel that she is friendly and concerned for him. Sitting at the same level as the patient gives a feeling of friendliness and equality. This should help the patient to relax with the nurse. Even sitting postures communicate how friendly or formal we are feeling, by whether we are leaning forward or sitting upright, how

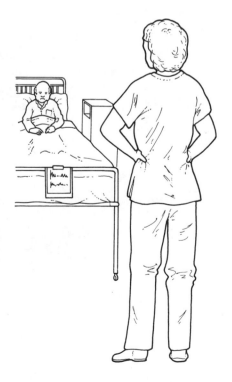

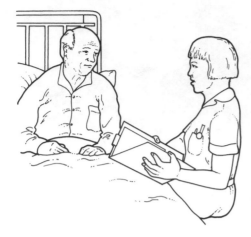

far apart we sit and at what angle our chair is to the person with whom we are communicating.

Eye contact

People tend to be judged on whether or not they make eye contact. 'He is shifty, not to be trusted' is a common assumption about someone who will not look another person in the eye. In fact there are many reasons why individuals avoid eye contact. They may be shy, embarrassed or merely trying to preserve their personal space.

In interacting with patients, eye contact is important since it indicates that the nurse is attending, that she is interested and that she is someone to be trusted. If a nurse is alone on the ward it may be that several patients need attention at the same time. A patient will be very aware of any divided interest from non-verbal behaviour, especially the eyes. Most patients understand the nurse who says 'I am alone at the moment and worried about Mr Smith, who is restless. I can see you need to talk and I will come back later when I can give you my full attention.' Of the important points here, actually going back later will show the patient that his concerns matter to the nursing staff.

Sometimes patients ask questions that may embarrass the nurse. Perhaps she knows the answer but does not feel free to divulge it, or perhaps she is unsure of the answer. The patient will make his own interpretation on lack of eye contact and may draw conclusions which are worrying or inaccurate.

Observation

Just as the patient will be trying to make sense of a nurse's non-verbal behaviour, the nurse may also observe a patient's responses to an attempted interaction. The patient's posture, facial expression and hands may all give clues to how he is reacting to being in hospital. Sometimes, however, the patient's non-verbal behaviour may conflict with what he is actually feeling.

Joe Timms had been brought into hospital because his daughter could no longer manage the old man at home. Mr Timms felt that he was in disgrace but that it was not his fault. He was angry with his daughter but felt that, if he showed it, she would refuse to have him home again. The nurse assessed him as a 'quiet, sad man'. His non-verbal behaviour was meek and still. His hands did not clench or twist as they might have in stress or anger. His eyes seemed expressionless. He said little, and did not smile. Had his assessment included his feelings about his admission, some of his underlying anger may have surfaced. In fact it finally came out in aggressive behaviour towards the nurses. Only then were his psychological problems identified.

Observation can also help with physical assessment. When bathing a patient, the skin may be observed for rashes, sores or non-accidental injury. Poor circulation may be observed in the feel and colour of the extremities. Signs of undernourishment may also be observed, as may disorders in the state of nails and hair. All these observations are non-verbal communication of the physical state of the patient's health. Again the face is important. Are the eyes clear and bright, or dull with maybe a yellowish tinge to the whites? Is the patient dark under the eyes? Are his lips cracked and sore?

Sometimes the patient's disease will explain the signs observed, but sometimes they may point to a need for further investigation.

Molly Witherington was a day patient, in for a simple procedure. A nurse noticed that she visited the toilet very frequently and so asked for a specimen of urine. This was found to contain glucose, further investigations showing Mrs Witherington to be diabetic. This condition was discovered and stabilized early as a result of the nurse making sense of observations of a patient's non-verbal behaviour.

Touch

Touch is an important area of non-verbal communication and is particularly important in nursing, where many of the socially acceptable rules on touch are overridden. For example, British people tend to be restrained in their use of touch (Argyle 1972), using just hand touching in interactions with the majority of people outside their family circle. Close proximity and touch may be interpreted as aggressive or sexual according to the situation and the people involved.

Nurses are often involved in intimate contact with patients that might cause embarrassment to some individuals. Bathing, attention to pressure areas and help when a patient requires a bedpan or bottle, all need to be dealt with in a sensitive way. If assessment suggests that there are problems, steps may be taken to explore the area and make any possible adjustments. For example, a male patient may feel more comfortable if he is bathed by a male nurse.

Touch can be used to express empathy and to convey comfort. Some authors (e.g. Krieger 1979) suggest that touch can be therapeutic and have healing qualities. Perhaps the most important aspect of touch is that both nurse and patient should feel comfortable about its use. Assessment may help a nurse decide if touch would be helpful or acceptable to a patient. Some might argue that touch

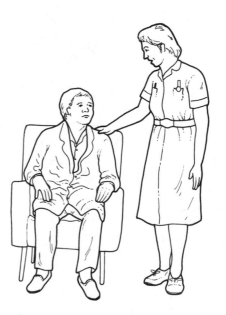

should always be spontaneous, but if a patient 'flinches' or misinterprets the touch, the result may be embarrassment or unhappiness on both sides. The maxim 'if it feels right, do it' is very applicable to touch.

Interviewing skills

If a nurse develops her communication and observational skills, she should be able to take a meaningful history from each patient and be able to assess him in terms of any deficits in his understanding of his present problems or disease. To make such an assessment, she will need to use her communication skills to develop a successful interviewing technique.

The aim of an assessment interview is to monitor the patient's physical, social and psychological state so that appropriate nursing care may be planned or referral made to other agencies. It is therefore important that the interview takes place in the best possible environment. The patient needs to feel safe with the nurse if she is to gain his trust, and privacy should be arranged if at all possible. This may pose problems on a busy ward where there is no interview room. If the assessment takes place by the patient's bed, drawing the curtains at least gives an illusion of privacy. It may also be the case that, even when a separate room is available, the patient feels more comfortable by his own bed than in a strange place. In either event, the nurse needs to sit where she has good eye contact and is on a similar level to the patient. If the nurse 'stands over' the patient, he may be very intimidated and unable to articulate his concerns.

One question which often arises in a discussion of 'good' interviewing techniques is whether the interviewer should write things down. Probably the most satisfactory method is for the nurse to make brief notes, and then write the full history as soon as possible after the interview. In this way, major points are noted but maximum attention is paid to the patient. Ideally, each nurse will develop her own style which is acceptable to her patients while allowing her to document interviews accurately.

Questioning techniques

Because the assessment is designed to monitor how the patient feels and what he understands, the patient should do most of the talking. For this to occur, the nurse needs

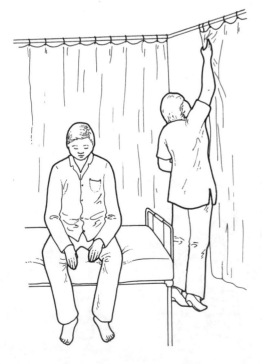

to develop questioning skills appropriate to the information required.

Closed questions

Closed questions are those which restrict the answer to yes/no or to some fact. They can be used when the nurse is checking information which she may have gained from the patient's notes. For example:

Nurse   Hello. Are you Mary Brown?
Patient Yes
Nurse   Is this address right? 46 Yew Tree Drive?
Patient Yes
Nurse   How old are you?
Patient 46

Such questions may be inappropriate. In the above example, the first questions were asked about stated facts so there was no misunderstanding about the patient's answers. Similarly, the question 'how old are you?' has only one meaning, though there may be some cultural differences in how age is assessed. In that case, asking for the year of birth would be an improvement, though a closed question would still be appropriate. Where closed questions are **not** appropriate is where assumptions are made that may mean different things to the two people involved. For example:

Nurse   Is this your first baby?
Patient Yes
Nurse   Have you been here before?
Patient Yes
Nurse   Why were you admitted?
Patient I had a miscarriage

Open questions

Open questions allow a patient to express how he feels, and will give the nurse an insight into aspects of the patient's problems which she may not have considered. For example:

Nurse   How do you feel about being admitted here?
Patient Well, I am worried about leaving the children at home
Nurse   Why are you worried?
Patient Oh, I suppose it is silly – I think my husband has a girlfriend and I am afraid he will neglect the children

In this situation, the patient is disclosing a personal worry. The questioning technique has allowed this, plus the fact that the nurse did not make assumptions. Had she done so, the interaction might have gone very differently:

Nurse How do you feel about being admitted here?

Patient Well, I am worried about leaving the children at home

Nurse You mothers are all the same. I expect they will survive

Patient (trying to explain) Well . . . it is more than that

Nurse Do them good. Tell me what you understand about your illness

In the above example, the nurse understands about asking open questions, but is making incorrect assumptions and not properly exploring the patient's feelings.

Open questions do not lead the patient in any way. They simply give someone a chance to talk freely on a topic. They may also be used to prompt a patient. For example:

Patient I hope they get things right here. Better than last time

Nurse Tell me what happened then?

Patient Happened! I'll tell you what happened . . .

Leading questions

Questions are called 'leading' when they put the idea of a response into the listener's head. This may cause difficulties in a nurse–patient interaction and can lead to misunderstandings as the patient tries to live up to the nurse's expectations. For example:

Nurse You are feeling better today aren't you?

Patient Mm

Nurse And I am sure you would like to have a bath

Patient Mm

Nurse Good. I will go and get the trolley

In the above situation, the patient may have been feeling unwell but even so responded to the nurse's expectations. If the nurse's enquiries had been open she could have made a better assessment of her patient. For example:

Nurse How are you feeling today?

Patient Not too good really

Nurse Tell me about it

Patient Oh! headachy; hot and sticky

Nurse I will get you something for the headache. Do you think a bath would help?

Patient Well, it might freshen me up

In this exchange, the patient is choosing to have the bath and will feel that he is an active participant in decisions made about his care.

Cues

Even with open questions, a patient may not feel free to disclose all his concerns. He may, however, mention worries in an oblique way – that is, he may give cues. A rule of thumb is that if a cue is given several times, the patient is hoping for a chance to air a real concern. Research suggests that nurses are not good at picking up cues, but this may be more a reluctance to deal with difficult matters than an inability to spot the cues. Consider the following conversation.

Nurse How do you feel about your operation?
Patient Oh! I know a hysterectomy is necessary. There may not be any more babies but I will still be a woman
Nurse Did you want more babies?
Patient Not me
Nurse Well. You will be home in about three weeks
Patient I suppose I will feel normal again
Nurse It will be several weeks before you can do everything you could, but see how you go
Patient Well it is not just me
Nurse No, you can rope the family in to help you

In that conversation, there were obvious cues which the nurse could have picked up on about the patient's concern for her femininity and the involvement of (possibly) her husband. If the nurse had explored these she might have assessed personal concerns as well as the patient's feelings about the operation itself.

Cues are usually given about areas on which it is not normally acceptable to talk. Taboo subjects such as dying, fear and sex are often tentatively mentioned in the form of cues. One way to pick up cues is to use a reflective technique.

Reflection

Reflection simply means repeating the last few words a patient has said. This prompts a patient without leading him. It also gives him the chance to shrug off the subject if he regrets raising it. If we look again at the hysterectomy patient, a different picture emerges if just one cue is picked up:

Nurse Did you want more babies?
Patient Not me
Nurse Not you?
Patient No, it is my husband. He thinks if it's all gone and I cannot have babies, I will not be a proper

wife to him anymore. But I won't go frigid – will I?

Here the patient feels safe enough to air her fears. The reflective technique also gives the freedom not to discuss fears:

Patient I reckon I won't get over this
Nurse Not get over it?
Patient Oh, take no notice of me, nurse. I'm feeling low today

In this situation, the patient has retracted, but the nurse is alerted to the concern and will be ready to talk about it when the patient feels ready.

Silence

Good questioning technique will only work if the patient is given time to think through before answering. Using silence effectively should result in a more accurate assessment. Silence can seem to be oppressive and then the nurse, having asked a question and not gained an answer, can be tempted to fill the space with another question or with a suggested answer.

The effective interviewer learns to wait at the end of a question, and also at the end of an answer to make sure it is the end of the answer. This is particularly true if the subject is one where the individual finds difficulty in verbalizing his thoughts. If such an individual seems 'stuck' then just a word may be enough to prompt the patient to continue.

Educated guesses

Often, as a patient is describing his present situation, a nurse gets a strong indication that the patient has feelings that are not being articulated. It is always worth testing this out by making an educated guess (sometimes called an understanding hypothesis). The patient will usually do one of the following:

1 confirm
2 confirm and elaborate
3 deny
4 deny and correct

When Mr Abraham shared his concerns with Nurse Brown, she gained the strong feeling that he was more upset than he admitted:

> *Nurse Brown* Mr Abraham, I get the feeling that you are far more upset about your admission than you say.
>
> *Mr Abraham* Yes . . . well . . .
>
> *Nurse Brown* Well?
>
> *Mr Abraham* It's work, you see. They are planning redundancies and if I'm seen to be ill, I may be for the chop. And how would we manage then?

In the above exchange, Nurse Brown's educated guess was correct and Mr Abraham was able to elaborate.

Such guesses tell a patient that the nurse is concentrating on his problems. If the guess is wrong, most patients will give the actual problem.

> *Nurse Atkin* Martha, I get the feeling that you are far more worried about the operation on your foot than you say.
>
> *Martha Jones* No.
>
> *Nurse Atkin* No?
>
> *Martha Jones* Oh Nurse. I am worried, but not about my foot [starts crying]. I'm . . . I'm . . . pregnant.

In the above exchange, the patient corrected the guess and was able to disclose her most pressing problem.

Clarification and encouraging precision

It was seen on page 89 that clarification is necessary to avoid ambiguity in the meaning of words. This links with the need to encourage precision when assessing a patient. This sounds quite hard but in fact will be interpreted as interest by the patient.

When Martha Jones felt able to share her worries with the nurse, she was quite vague. Nurse Atkin asked for clear, precise information and Martha later told a close friend, 'I felt that she really cared about me, wanted to know dates and just what had happened – even asked me just what I meant when I said I couldn't tell me Da for fear of what he'd do. Funny though, it sort of dropped into place then – and I knew it would be OK.'

Questions such as 'can you tell me what you mean by that?' or 'when exactly did it happen?' will lead to an accurate account of the patient's history and concerns and help the patient to articulate facts and events.

Reassurance

It would be rare in an assessment if the patient did not have some concerns which needed answers. Such questions should be answered if possible or referred if the nurse feels unable to deal with them. It is tempting to want to reassure the patient about his worries and sometimes this is possible. Difficulties arise if it is not possible to reassure the patient or if the nurse has not properly assessed the real area of concern.

It is never worth giving false reassurance to a patient. Sooner or later the truth will emerge and then the nurse will not be trusted. A patient may be worried that a procedure will hurt. If it will, then an explanation should be given in simple terms. For example:

Patient I am a terrible coward when it comes to pain
Nurse Well, I cannot say that it won't hurt but you will be given an injection (local anaesthetic) beforehand which should help, and pain-killers afterwards if you need them

Sometimes a patient will ask for impossible reassurance. The patient after mastectomy who fears that her husband may stop loving her, or the patient with cancer who fears he may die, are both in need of reassurance, but it is unlikely that either would respect the nurse who gave false reassurance. With such patients, their main need may be to talk through their fears. Such situations are difficult for nurses as it is very hard to say things like, 'I do not know how your husband will feel about you. Can you talk to him?' or 'Things are not too good at the moment. Do you want to talk about it?'

Other difficulties arise when the nurse makes assumptions about the patient's fears. This can result in reassurance being given in the wrong area. It is common, for example, for nurses to assume that patients with a diagnosis of cancer fear death. It may be that an individual is more concerned with the way of dying rather than death itself. Similarly, it is easy to assume that patients undergoing surgery may worry about their operation while they may, in fact, be more concerned with loss of income or other social factors related to the operation.

Control

In interviewing, it is important that the nurse is able to control what is happening, both to elicit necessary information about the patient and also to ensure that the interview is not too time-consuming. This may seem a hard approach but, in reality, no nurse has unlimited time available for one patient.

Most people do not object to a nurse who says, 'Hello, I've come to ask you a few things about yourself so that we can give you the proper care you need. It will take about 20 minutes, but if you feel you need to talk more after that, I'll arrange to come back later.' This approach sets the scene for the sort of interaction, but also shows the patient that the nurse is interested in him as a person, to the point that she will make further time available if necessary.

If setting the scene in this way helps to control time, it also helps to control content. The patient knows that the nurse has not come to discuss the weather, but to take a serious account of how things are for the patient. It is often thought that for the nurse to put the patient at ease, the interview should start with social chit-chat. This is not the case. It is the nurse's manner which is important in helping the patient to relax. In fact, a very anxious patient may well be irritated by social questions when what he really needs is someone with whom he can discuss his problems. If social material is used in an interview, it is called 'neutral' material, and may even be used by a nurse in an attempt to avoid more serious matters.

Of course some patients like to talk, and can be very difficult to keep to the point. In such a situation it is probably best to interrupt with 'Of course I would like to hear more about that, but I wonder if we can return to . . .' or something similar. Such interruptions do not generally upset patients if they are made firmly and with humour.

Summarizing

From time to time in an assessment, a small summary should be given to the patient. This has two functions:

1 It gives the patient the feeling that he has been heard and his problems identified
2 It gives the nurse the chance to check out that she has identified concerns from the patient's perspective

Towards the end of the interview a final summary should be given and a 'screening' question asked:

Nurse Atkin Well Martha, it seems that you have several problems. You seem to be in balance about the operation itself, but are worried about the effect of the anaesthetic on your baby. There are problems to do with your boyfriend's death and about your parents in terms of support. Before we begin to plan the way forward, I wonder if you have other problems?

Martha Nothing serious. The main worry is my baby.

Occasionally, screening may elicit further problems. A decision then has to be made on whether to address them straight away or whether to make another time for further assessment.

Closing an interview

An assessment interview may be quite demanding on a patient in that it asks him not only to give information about himself, but also to examine his feelings about his illness. He may disclose information to the nurse which he would not normally divulge to a stranger.

It is up to the nurse to leave the patient as little upset as possible and to bring the interview to a close in a sensitive way. Not all patients will get upset, but if one should then often sitting quietly for a few minutes will help him regain his composure. The skills of non-verbal communication will be more important than worrying the patient with words.

Before leaving a patient, the nurse should thank him for answering her questions and ask if he feels that there is anything else he would like to say. If important issues crop up at the end of an interview and there is not the time to discuss them further, a future time should be set aside.

Assessment forms

It can be seen that the assessment interview is important in monitoring an individual's social, psychological and physical reaction to his illness in order that plans may be made to give him the care that will meet his individual needs. An accurate record of the assessment should be made so that other members of staff can build up a picture of the patient without repeating questions that have already been asked. The assessment form needs to be regularly updated as goals are met and further concerns identified. Records will vary from hospital to hospital. The important point is that information is clear and concise.

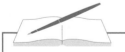

List the important elements of assessment and compare with the form used in your hospital. How could the form be improved? Discuss with a tutor, or your Nurse Manager, the possibility of making amendments to the assessment form.

Summary

In this chapter the concept of need has been explored alongside the sorts of deficiencies which can occur when a person is no longer in perfect health.

It has been shown how important it is that the nurse should develop her communication skills so that she may accurately assess her patients' needs. Finally, the elements of an assessment interview have been considered.

References

Argent, J., Faulkner, A. & O'Keeffe, C. (1994) The development and modification of a rating scale for measuring the communication skills of health workers in palliative care. *Medical Education*, *28*, 559–565.

Argyle, M. (1972) *The psychology of interpersonal behaviour*. Harmondsworth, London: Penguin.

Argyle, M. (1988) *Bodily communication*, 2nd edn. London: Methuen.

Bernstein, B. A. (1959) A public language: some sociological implications of a linguistic form. *British Journal of Sociology*, *10*, 311–326.

Faulkner, A. (1980) *The student nurse's role in giving information to patients*. Unpublished M. Litt. Thesis, Aberdeen University.

Faulkner, A. (1992) The evaluation of training programmes for communication skills in palliative care. *Journal of Cancer Care*, *1*, 75–78,

Faulkner, A. & Maguire, P. (1984) Teaching assessment skills. In Faulkner, A. (Ed.) *Communication*. Edinburgh: Churchill Livingstone.

Faulkner, A. & Maguire, P. (1994) *Talking to cancer patients and their relatives*, pp. 169–184. Oxford: Oxford University Press.

Fox, B. H. (1983) Current theory of psychogenic effects on cancer incidence and prognosis. *Journal of Psychosocial Oncology*, *1*(1), 17–32.

Kasl, S. (1983) Pursuing the link between stressful life experiences and disease: a time for reappraisal. In Cooper, C. (Ed.) *Stress research. Issues for the eighties*, pp. 79–103. Chichester: John Wiley & Sons.

Krieger, D. (1979) *The therapeutic touch*. Englewood Cliffs, N. J.: Prentice-Hall.

Macleod Clark, J. (1982) *Nurse–patient verbal interaction: an analysis of recorded conversations from selected surgical wards*. Unpublished Ph.D. Thesis, University of London.

Maslow, A. H. (1954) *Motivation and personality*. New York: Harper.

Further reading

Adler, R. B., Rosenfeld, L. B. & Towne, N. (1980) *Interplay*, 2nd edn. London: Holt, Rinehart, Winston.

Bullmer, K. (1975) *The art of empathy*. New York: Human Sciences Press.

Collins, M. (1983) *Communication in health care*, 2nd edn. London: C. V. Mosby.

Faulkner, A. (1992) *Effective interaction with patients*. Edinburgh: Churchill Livingstone.

Helman, C. (1985) *Culture, health and illness*. Bristol: Wright & Sons.

Maslow A. H. (1969) A Theory of metermotivation: The biological rooting of the value of life. *Humanities*, *4*, 301–343.

Rambo, B. T. (1983) *Adaptation nursing: assessment and intervention*. Philadelphia: W. B. Saunders.

Tyler, P. Taptich, B. & Bernocchi-Losey, D. (1991) *Nursing process and nursing diagnosis*. Philadephia: W. B. Saunders.

5

The Disease Process

CHAPTER SUMMARY

The person rather than the pathology, 105
Understanding pathology, 106
The nursing focus, 106

The deficits produced by disease, 107
Oxygen, 108
Food, 110
Fluid, 112
Rest, 114
Exercise and daily functioning, 116
Psychological factors, 116
Social factors, 117

Recognizing deficits in individuals, 118
Temperature, 118
Pulse, 124
Respiration, 125
The place of TPR in recognizing deficits produced by disease, 127
Other measures of an individual's functioning, 127

Summary, 129

References, 129

Further reading, 130

The person rather than the pathology

In recent years, as the move has been made towards more individualized nursing care, the 'medical model' has been denigrated as being against the patient's interests. Certainly to talk of 'admitting an appendix' or 'bathing a tonsil' dehumanizes patients by turning them into diseases or operations and should be avoided, but this by no means suggests that medical diagnosis is of no interest to nurses.

It has been shown in previous chapters that a knowledge of the biological and behavioural sciences is necessary to understand how individuals function, both as independent people and as part of society. Such knowledge gives an overview of sciences from which we may make some assumptions about any particular individual.

For example, studies in psychology suggest that man is a social animal. Such knowledge is useful to nursing in that opportunities can be arranged for patients to interact with each other by the provision of day-rooms and facilities for communal eating and television watching. If it is forgotten that patients are individual people, there may be a tendency to expect them all to go into the day-room, and insist that all who are able to will eat together. In Chapter 3 it was suggested that this is not the way to treat patients.

What is required is that facilities for socializing are offered, but individuals may choose how sociable they wish to be. Nursing is then using psychology creatively to help understand people rather than dictate how they should behave.

Understanding pathology

Because patients in hospital are usually there through some deficit of body functioning, it can be seen that a knowledge of pathology is as vital as a knowledge of human biology, sociology and psychology. Such knowledge does not necessarily reduce the patient to a disease any more than a knowledge of social psychology would reduce an individual to a rigid norm of behaviour. What a knowledge of pathology can contribute to nursing is an understanding of disease and dysfunction which will alert nurses to immediate and potential problems in a particular patient.

There has been much debate on whether nursing may call itself a profession in that it borrows from other disciplines rather than having a unique body of knowledge. What can be seen to be unique in nursing is the creative way in which nurses take eclectically from other disciplines in order to help patients achieve their health potential.

So it is with pathology. Nurses should not be seen as mini-doctors concerned with medical diagnosis, nor yet should the process of nursing be seen as a threat to the unique function of the doctor. What is important is the emphasis on pathology, which will be very different for the doctor and for the nurse.

The nursing focus

The nurse is concerned with each individual's reactions to his disease or dysfunction, so she needs to know not only her patient's diagnosis but also the effects of a particular diagnosis on an individual's normal functioning. She needs to realize which particular deficits a given disease may produce and how these can affect an individual socially, psychologically and physically.

With this emphasis, the disease process becomes a vital piece of knowledge in the total make-up of the patient, rather than a label to obliterate the individual. An example of this is diabetes mellitus, a disease where there is a deficiency of insulin secreted by the pancreas. The doctor will diagnose the disease and prescribe one of three possible regimens – diet alone, diet and tablets, or diet and insulin – depending on the type of diabetes, the age of the patient and other relevant factors.

Since the nurse is concerned with the patient's reaction to his diagnosis she will be concerned with assessing his ability to understand and cope with the prescribed regimen and with helping him with problems that may arise as a result of the diagnosis. She will also have a teaching role to perform. By thinking of this patient as 'a diabetic' it is possible that the nurse will apply a rigid regimen of no sugar, rigid adherence to meal times, pre-meal urinalysis and other inhibiting measures. By seeing this patient as an individual there is a much better chance of helping him to cope in a way that fits in with his normal lifestyle. He may, for example, find that a teaspoonful of sugar on his cornflakes gets over the problem of being expected to eat more carbohydrate than he is used to at breakfast time.

There are many ways of coping sensibly with diabetes. The nurse will not be able to help her patient if she does not have a knowledge of pathology. Ignorance leads to poor assessment and often to rigid behaviour on the part of the nurse.

The diabetic diagnosis is just one example of how the individual is the focus of the nurse's attention, rather than his disease, but in which a knowledge of the disease is crucial to planning effective nursing care. This patient-centred approach requires more knowledge than the medical-model approach since it deals in principles rather than prescribed rules, which can be applied without understanding.

By talking of the person rather than the pathology, the pathology is put into the context of the total person. For each deficit there will be standard problems that can be foreseen, but each of these problems will be affected by the individual who has them. There will also be non-standard problems that may be explained in other than pathological terms. A nursing assessment that does not make assumptions should elicit the needs of the individual, not simply the symptoms of his disease.

The deficits produced by disease

The deficits produced by disease fulfil a useful function in that they alert an individual, or his family, to the fact that something is amiss, and this will generally lead to action being taken and a diagnosis being made. Deficits may occur in any part of the body and may affect an individual's functioning physically, socially and/or psychologically. It will depend on the particular deficit whether it shows itself early in the disease process or not. Some organs, e.g. the kidneys and liver, are larger than needed to maintain an individual in perfect health. Unfortunately this means that malfunctioning of these organs may be quite advanced before the person feels the effect of deficits. At the other end of the spectrum, deficiencies in the temperature control of the body become apparent very quickly.

In Chapter 2, normal physiological function was considered. Now, the effects of disease on those functions, and the subsequent effects on the individual as he becomes aware that all is not well with his body, will be considered. Physiologically, an individual needs an adequate supply of oxygen, food and water to survive, along with the ability to excrete waste products from his body. He also needs rest and exercise. An old adage suggests that one can live three minutes without air, three days without water and three weeks without food. In reality, most individuals are not called upon to test this, but disease may affect the ability to take these vital substances into the body and so cause deficits. Such deficits will give rise to symptoms which may, sooner or later, affect a person's ability to lead a normal life. Nurses are concerned with the effect of these symptoms on an individual, and with planning care to reduce or eliminate the resulting problems.

Oxygen

For an adequate supply of oxygen to the body, the respiratory tract needs to be clear and functioning, and the oxygen-carrying capacity of the blood should be normal. The muscles of respiration need to be unaffected by disease and the respiratory centre needs to be functioning as a control over the system.

Disease may affect the area of lung tissue available for the exchange of oxygen and carbon dioxide. One such disease is carcinoma of the lungs, where proliferating malignant cells invade normal tissue (Figure 5.1). Another is pneumonia, where the alveoli fill with fluid (Figure 5.2). Disease may also affect the respiratory tract, so narrowing the respiratory passages. The common cold, obstructive tumours, bronchitis and asthma are examples of diseases that affect oxygen uptake and carbon dioxide excretion by restricting normal breathing. Cardiovascular disease, or diseases of the blood, may reduce the oxygen-carrying capacity of the blood, so reducing the exchange of oxygen and carbon dioxide in the alveoli.

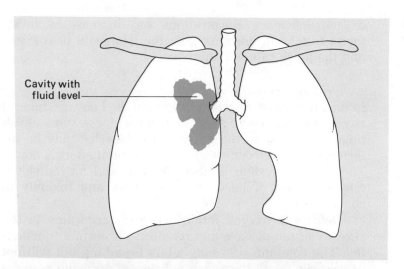

Fig. 5.1 Diagram showing carcinoma of the lung.

Cavity with fluid level

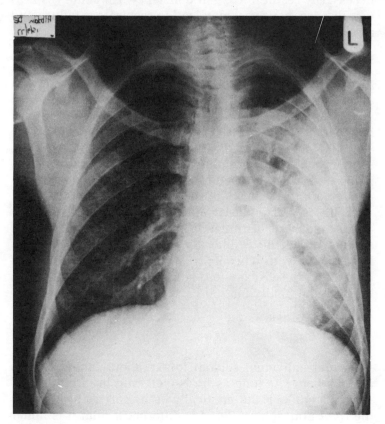

Fig. 5.2 X-ray showing pneumonia. From Swash and Mason (1984) with kind permission of the authors.

Breathing

If disease causes a reduced intake of oxygen and an accompanying deficiency in the removal of carbon dioxide, breathing will be affected. If there is infection present, other symptoms such as a cough, with or without sputum, may be present. The whole body will respond to the oxygen deficiency. Respirations may increase in an attempt to take in more oxygen, the heart will beat faster and the pulse rate will increase.

General effects

In the absence of sufficient oxygen to the body, peripheral circulation may be affected, causing coldness and a bluish tinge (cyanosis) to the extremities. Muscles may be affected, causing tiredness and exhaustion if effort is made. The nervous system is also affected, and an individual may complain of headaches, dizziness and inability to concentrate.

Deficits in oxygen intake will vary according to the severity of the disease and its effect on normal functioning. The common cold may affect breathing but will not necessarily result in oxygen deficiency. An acute respiratory disease, however, may lead to respiratory failure and a resulting acute oxygen deficiency.

Individual reactions

An individual's reaction to oxygen deficiency will vary according to a number of factors, not least his knowledge of what is happening. If the causative disease is infectious, body temperature may be raised and the patient may feel very ill. Most people know that oxygen is essential for life, so any problems in breathing may cause the individual to panic and become fearful and anxious, to a degree depending on the severity of the symptoms.

This is particularly obvious in acute respiratory disease such as asthma. When the individual has an asthma attack he is literally fighting for every breath. In patients with chronic respiratory disease such as bronchitis, the disease may affect the individual's whole lifestyle and ability for self-care.

Food

A normal individual seldom thinks about taking oxygen into his body. As long as he is well, and breathing naturally, his intake is automatically at the correct level, given the right atmosphere. Food is different in that it is under individual control. Eating fulfils a physical, social and psychological function, yet disease may be caused by poor nutrition or by overindulgence. There are situations, however, where an adequate diet may be followed, but where disease of the organs associated with digestion may cause deficits in an individual.

Digestive tract

Disease may affect any part of the digestive tract and its associated organs (Figure 5.3). Diseased teeth can make eating a painful process, as can swelling of the oesophagus and the resulting difficulty in swallowing (dysphagia). Ulceration of the stomach not only affects the digestive process but again causes pain and discomfort, which is likely to result in a reduced diet as eating is no longer seen as a pleasurable act.

Disease and infections of the intestines are likely to cause food to pass through the body without its nutrients being absorbed. Parasites in the intestine may also affect the absorption of nutrients. The effect is similar to that of an insufficient diet, in that the individual will lose weight.

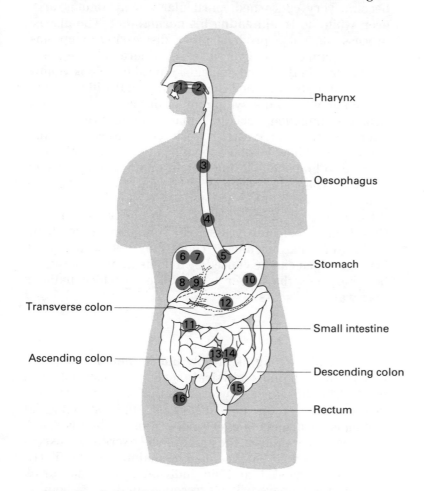

1. Stomatitis 2. Tonsillitis 3. Oesophageal stricture 4. Oesophagitis
5. Hiatus hernia 6. Cirrhosis 7. Hepatitis 8. Cholelithiasis
9. Cholecystitis 10. Gastric ulcer 11. Duodenal ulcer
12. Pancreatitis 13. Malabsorption syndrome
14. Crohn's disease (most common in small bowel) 15. Ulcerative colitis
16. Appendicitis 17. Carcinoma can occur from mouth to anus

Fig. 5.3 Sites of disease in the digestive tract.

Organs associated with digestion

Disease of the liver may affect the absorption of fat. If fat has been taken as part of the individual's diet, it will be excreted in fatty, bulky faeces. A diseased liver may also be unable to detoxicate drugs such as alcohol, so causing a build up of toxins. If the pancreas does not secrete enough insulin, carbohydrate cannot be used by the body and is excreted as glucose in the urine.

Individual reactions

The above are just a few of the deficits produced by diseases affecting the intake of food, but the symptoms which can be produced, e.g. pain, loss of weight, loss of energy and abnormal excretion, may cause a patient to become very concerned, particularly if symptoms arise even while he is still eating his normal diet. The disease process may also produce other distressing symptoms, such as jaundice in liver disease, where bile pigments accumulate in the blood and cause the skin to look yellow.

It cannot be assumed that an individual will react in a particular way to the symptoms of diseases which cause deficits in nutrition. Socially, females are admired for slim figures, yet in the Western world there is considerable overeating. It may be that a female patient may initially be pleased to find she is losing weight and may only become worried when she becomes tired and listless. Another patient may explain his symptoms in terms of his lifestyle, 'Of course I am losing weight. I am always on the go.' Others may feel embarrassed to complain of (to them) trivial items like tiredness. There may not be the panic feelings which can be caused by deficits in oxygen uptake, but there may be longer term concerns which patients may want to discuss.

Fluid

Drinking, like eating, is largely under the control of the individual and fulfils physical, social and psychological needs. The difference, however, is that if an individual is healthy and overeats, the excess food will be stored as fat and cause problems of overweight. If more fluid is drunk than the body requires, the kidneys will excrete the excess liquid so that fluid balance may be maintained. Similarly, if thirst is ignored and an individual does not drink enough, the kidneys will act to retain fluid in the body so that balance is maintained.

If disease affects the kidneys, fluid balance may be disturbed with the result that an individual holds too much fluid in his body. If through disease, e.g. heart failure or dehydration, fluid is retained, there will be a build up of toxins in the blood, the most damaging being urea.

Diseases outside the urinary tract, such as diabetes, can affect fluid balance, for as the kidneys discard the excess sugar in the blood, water is also removed (Figure 5.4).

Urine excretion

Although disease of the kidneys may affect the amount of urine produced, disease of the bladder and urethra may prevent the excretion of normal urine. If the prostate gland is enlarged, or a tumour grows in the bladder, urine may be retained (Figure 5.5). Pressure on the bladder from outside, as in pregnancy when the uterus is enlarged, may also cause retention (Figure 5.6).

Alternatively, disease may cause incontinence of urine, as when a patient is unconscious or when there is damage to the spinal cord.

If the bladder is inflamed, as in cystitis, urine may be passed more frequently than usual although the overall volume may not increase. Increased volume (polyuria), as in diabetes, will also cause frequency of micturition.

Diseases such as enlargement of the prostate gland

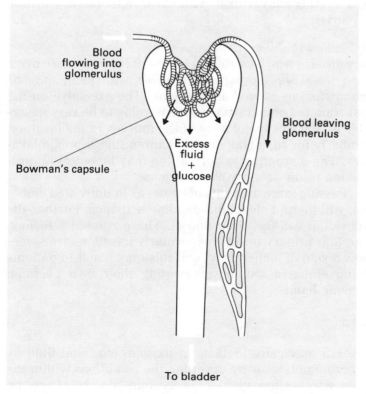

Fig. 5.4 Excess fluid loss from blood with high level of glucose.

Fig. 5.5 Enlarged prostate gland blocking urinary output.

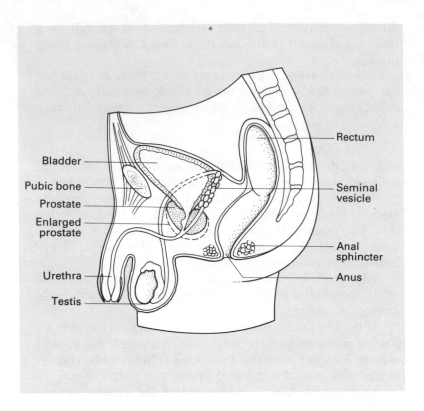

and cystitis may cause painful or difficult micturition (dysuria).

Effects on the individual
Any disease which causes an individual to pass more urine than usual, or more frequently, or with pain, may be embarrassing as well as worrying. The executive on the fast train to London with cystitis is going to be very miserable as she will spend most of the journey in the lavatory. Similarly for the shopper who cannot find a public lavatory. The disruption to normal life may be out of all proportion to the severity of the disease.

Passing large amounts of urine, as in untreated diabetes, will disrupt sleep and daytime activities. Further the individual will feel tired and ill. There is often a feeling, too, that urinary upsets, particularly infection, are somehow a sign of 'being dirty' and this may result in patients being embarrassed, or overstating their own personal hygiene habits.

Rest

Disease may cause deficits in oxygen, food and fluid by affecting uptake or by upsetting the conditions within the body which allow uptake. There may also be effects on

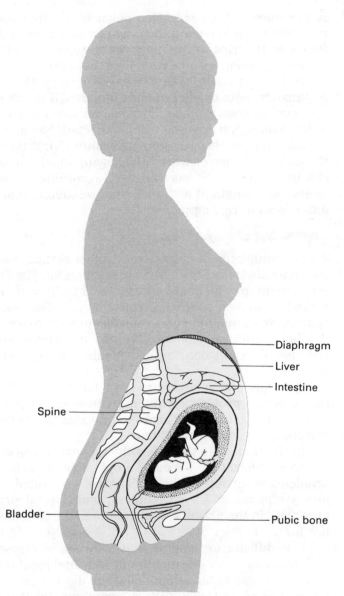

Fig. 5.6 Pregnancy blocking urinary output.

Diaphragm
Liver
Intestine
Spine
Bladder
Pubic bone

excretory functions which are allied to disease. As symptoms of disease occur, a patient may panic, worry, be embarrassed or frightened. These feelings, along with his symptoms, may soon begin to disrupt his usual living pattern.

Anxiety may affect patterns of rest in a number of ways. It may be that an individual cannot get off to sleep at night, falls asleep but then wakes up in the small hours, or wakes very early in the morning and cannot get back to sleep. Worries may seem much worse at night, so anxiety grows as the problem goes round and round without an obvious solution. Symptoms of disease may also affect rest patterns. For example, polyuria or frequency of micturition will have a patient awake many times during the night for trips to the toilet, while pain or breathlessness can prevent or interrupt sleep patterns.

It does not matter what the cause of sleep disturbance is – anxiety, pain or altered body function, if things do not improve the result will be the same: an individual's ability to function in the daytime will be affected. Sleep, albeit a variable amount, is necessary for healthy living. If disease, through symptoms or worry about symptoms, causes deficits in sleep, the effects will vary according to the frequency and length of disturbance in relation to individual differences in resting patterns.

Exercise and daily functioning

Just as symptoms of disease may affect resting patterns, they may also affect normal daily functioning. The breathless patient may be unable to run for a train, walk uphill, make love to their partner or ride a bicycle. Someone who is tired from malnutrition may be unable to complete the housework, be too tired to go to employment or, because of exhaustion, become unable to cope with the family.

Pain may be so severe that an individual is loath to move, while problems with diarrhoea or urinary frequency may cause such problems outside the home that travelling becomes a nightmare.

In situations like this a healthy balance of work, exercise and relaxation becomes impossible to achieve. If problems of anxiety and sleeplessness are added to this, new symptoms of frayed tempers, tears and depression may arise in the absence of diagnosis and treatment (Figure 5.7).

It is difficult to imagine that a nurse, in assessing a patient, could take a sympathetic and intelligent interest in his reactions to his symptoms if she did not understand the pathology underlying those symptoms. Further, such knowledge will enhance her teaching ability so that she can involve the patient in understanding his problems and co-operating in his care.

Psychological factors

Some symptoms may have a psychological rather than a physical explanation. It will be apparent, for example, that sleep may be as readily disturbed by anxiety as by pain. Anxiety may also affect breathing patterns. A psychological need to be slim may lead to deficits in nutrition or indeed to self-induced vomiting. The same need may lead to the effects of taking diuretics unnecessarily.

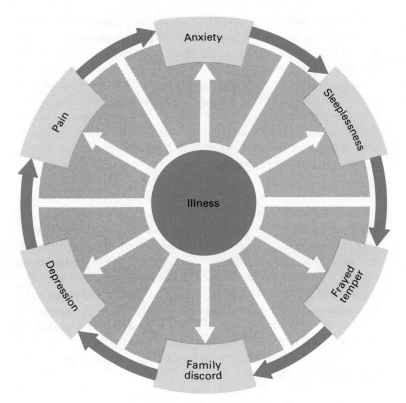

Fig. 5.7 Effects of illness on daily functioning.

In such cases, a differential diagnosis will need to be made by the doctor. Sometimes this will be a simple matter. At others, the doctor may be helped by a nurse's careful assessment of the patient.

Social factors

Social factors may also lead to deficits in an adequate uptake of oxygen, food and fluid, and in sleep and exercise. People who are unemployed or pensioners may not have enough money for basic needs and luxuries. Since spending money is a matter of choice, it may often be spent unwisely in terms of maintaining physical health.

Food

Granny Woodruffe (as she asked others to call her) lived by herself on a state pension. Her children lived some distance away though they visited regularly. Granny paid her bills, including six small life insurances, and bought food with what was left. Her diet was inadequate because other things were more important to her, such as the regular visits of the insurance men and the savings she wished to leave her children.

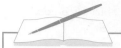

Join with one or two colleagues to note your food and fluid intake over 24 hours. Check against the information given by the Department of Health (1991). How do you compare in terms of a balanced diet? How different was your intake from that of your colleagues?

Similar deficits in nutrition may be caused in families on the dole, where money is spent on alcohol in an attempt to escape the misery of unemployment, or simply by spending the money on unsuitable 'junk' foods which may be high in fat and carbohydrate but low in protein. Many individuals do not understand the elements of a balanced diet, despite educational initiatives such as those from the Health Education Council (1983), now the Health Education Authority, which makes leaflets readily available in several different languages.

Fluid

Occasionally, a symptom of disease may cause a deficit because of its social implications. For example, many elderly people suffer from mild incontinence of urine. Even if incontinence pants are worn, the symptom is embarrassing for a number of reasons. There may be a leakage, the individual imagines that he smells offensive, clothes may be stained. A common though totally inappropriate response to this upsetting condition is for the patient to drastically reduce his fluid intake. Thus he adds dehydration to his problems with resultant concentrated urine and continued incontinence.

Oxygen

Polluted air may affect oxygen uptake. This is a national social problem which the UK Government approaches through legislation such as the Clean Air Acts of 1956 and 1968.

Recognizing deficits in individuals

It will be seen from the previous section that social, psychological and physical factors are interrelated in a healthy individual becoming affected by disease and its accompanying symptoms. It is this interrelatedness which is important in assessment and which should prevent assumptions being made on symptoms alone.

Recognizing deficits requires careful observation of the patient, both on admission and subsequently. Careful documentation of what has been observed should be part of every nursing assessment.

Temperature

Acute diseases, particularly infections, may result in a rise in normal body temperature. Such a condition is called pyrexia. Psychological upset such as fear or anger can also cause slight pyrexia. Similarly, hot social conditions may produce a rise in temperature. A lowered body temperature is called hypothermia. This condition is most commonly seen in elderly people in the winter and may be caused by cold, damp accommodation, poor diet, inadequate clothing and too little exercise. Newborn babies are also susceptible to this condition.

It is usual to take a patient's temperature on admission to hospital and at intervals during his stay. The intervals will depend on the condition of the patient. Pyrexial patients may have their temperature taken four-hourly, while patients with chronic diseases may have only a weekly check taken. Taking a temperature once is of little use, particularly since there is a range of normality. Taking the temperature of an ill patient at regular intervals will give a pattern of recording and will show when a return to normal is achieved and maintained (Figure 5.8).

Taking a temperature

Body temperatures are most commonly measured using a glass thermometer (Figure 5.9), orally, anally or under the axilla. The glass thermometer has mercury within it which expands with the heat of the body to give a reading between 35°C and 43.5°C. Patients thought to be suffering from hypothermia need to have their temperature taken with a special thermometer which starts to register at 21°C.

Disposable thermometers are also available. These are sealed strips, and therefore sterile until the seal is removed; they contain heat-sensitive chemicals in dots in the tip (Figure 5.10).

Electronic thermometers, some with a digital display, are also available but can be expensive. They are, however, time saving since they register the body temperature in seconds rather than minutes, and are extremely accurate.

Time

The accuracy of temperature taking with a glass thermometer is largely in the hands of the nurse. It is not an uncommon sight to see a nurse on a ward attempt to take several patients' temperatures at the same time. If she is using an oral thermometer, she will put one under the tongue of each of, say, six patients. She may then go back to the first patient and read the thermometer, which may have been in for one or two minutes. It will be some time before the last patient has had the thermometer removed,

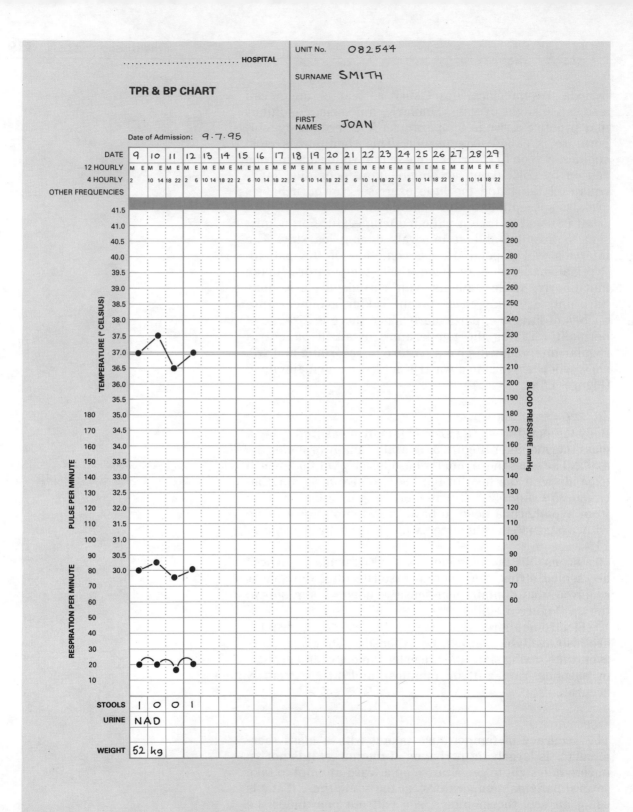

Fig. 5.8 The TPR & BP chart.

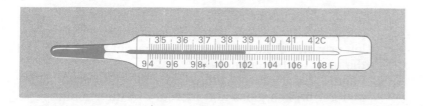

5.9 A glass thermometer.

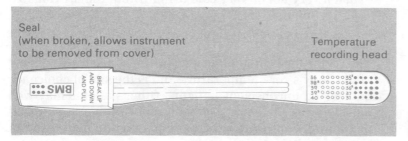

Seal
(when broken, allows instrument
to be removed from cover)

Temperature
recording head

Fig. 5.10 A disposable
thermometer.

say nine or ten minutes. Extreme variations may occur if
the last patient on this occasion is the first patient next
time. For an accurate recording, the thermometer should
be left *in situ* for the correct length of time, and for the
same length of time at each recording.

Oral site – minimum of two minutes
Axillary site – minimum of five minutes
Anal site – minimum of one minute

The thermometer

It is preferable for each patient to have an individual
thermometer, kept in a container by his bed. This will
prevent infection being carried from one patient to another (cross-infection), which can happen if one thermometer is used by several patients.

A thermometer should be clinically clean but need
not be sterile. Before use, the nurse should check that
the mercury has been shaken to the bottom of the thermometer. Doing this is a knack, and is achieved by
holding the thermometer halfway along between thumb
and forefinger and giving a sharp flick of the wrist.

After use, the mercury should again be shaken to the
bottom of the thermometer, the thermometer wiped clean
and replaced in its container.

Oral site

Although the oral site is popular for recording body
temperature (Figure 5.11) because it is seen to be most
sensitive to changes in temperature, it has several
drawbacks.

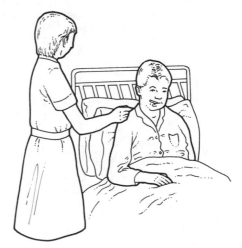

Fig. 5.11 Taking a temperature at the
oral site.

1 Some areas under the tongue will record a lower temperature than others. Siting is important, either at the left or right of the junction of the floor of the mouth and the base of the tongue.
2 Children or confused adults may bite the thermometer and get broken glass and mercury in their mouths.
3 Temperature reading will be affected if the patient has had a very hot or very cold drink within the previous 10 or 15 minutes.

Rectal site

The rectal site is thought to give the most accurate reading of the body's core temperature and is the site of choice for babies and unconscious patients. Other patients may well object to this site being used and find it embarrassing and degrading. Concern for the patient's dignity may result in other sites being used.

Axillary site

This site does not have embarrassing connotations and may be used for any patient when the oral site is contraindicated. The thermometer needs to be held securely under the axilla and not allowed to slip (Figure 5.12). This site is probably the least reliable of the three available.

No matter which site is chosen, some general rules apply. Firstly, a patient's temperature should not be taken if he has had a bath in the last hour, or has recently been exercising, as both may affect the recordings. Secondly, taking a temperature is a nursing task which should be explained to the patient. Faulkner (1980) found that nurses may take a patient's temperature without any verbal interaction between them. It may be that both patient and nurse understand the procedure, but still the impersonal approach tends to dehumanize a patient.

Observations of temperature

Although measuring body temperature may give an accurate objective measure to record, it may also increase a patient's feeling of illness and, for this reason alone, questions may be asked about routine temperature taking. It is possible, by careful observation, to note signs of abnormal body temperature and for a nurse to make a decision about the necessity to record with a thermometer.

Pyrexia

A high temperature affects body processes and the first complaint may be that the patient feels 'unwell' with headache, tiredness and loss of appetite. He may also complain of feeling 'shivery'. This 'shivery' feeling is due

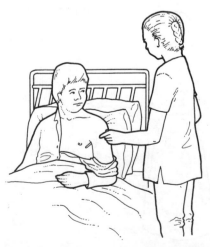

Fig. 5.12 Taking a temperature at the axillary site.

to vasoconstriction as the body adjusts to the higher temperature.

These symptoms should alert the nurse to check the patient's temperature immediately. If the nurse misses this 'onset' period, observations will show the established features of pyrexia. The patient will look hot and flushed and sweaty. This is due to vasodilatation and considerable fluid loss may occur through the skin, causing reduced urinary output and possible dehydration.

The patient will try to cool down by removing bed-clothes. He will complain of thirst, headache and possibly disorientation. He will not wish to eat, and if the pyrexia persists may lose weight and become lethargic.

Unless pyrexia is marked, the nurse may miss the symptoms if she is not observant, and this may be a good reason for taking a temperature on admission. It will not necessarily give baseline data but it will show abnormality in an objective way.

Hypothermia

In hypothermia, the temperature is below the normal range. Observation may lead a nurse to suspect that the patient is hypothermic. This is important, since a normal thermometer does not record very low temperature. The patient will be cold to the touch and will look very pale and waxen. The patient's only complaint may be extreme tiredness and drowsiness, but in fact the metabolic rate is slowed down so that pulse rate will be slow, breathing will be slow and shallow and blood pressure will be low. The patient may become drowsy, which will cause the metabolic rate to decrease again and coma may result.

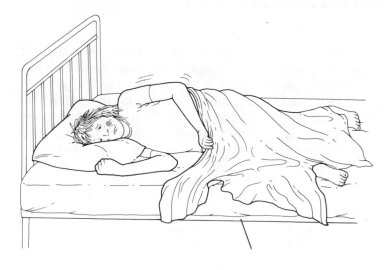

Table 5.1 Observations suggesting pyrexia or hypothermia

Pyrexia	Hypothermia
Patient looks and feels hot	Patient looks and feels cold
Obvious sweating	Shivering
Pulse rate ↑	Pulse rate ↓
Respirations ↑	Respirations ↓
Thirst	Blood pressure ↓
Urine ↓	Extreme tiredness
No appetite (anorexia)	Drowsiness – coma
Headache	
Disorientation	

Table 5.1 shows the observations that will indicate the possibility of pyrexia or hypothermia to a nurse.

Pulse

An individual's pulse rate reflects the heart beat and may be seen as an indicator of disease and its progress, although other factors can also have an effect, e.g. emotion is likely to increase pulse rate, as is exercise. It was seen earlier that pyrexia is accompanied by an increased pulse rate. Other causes are attributable to particular diseases such as thyrotoxicosis and some other diseases of the heart. Haemorrhage may also result in an increased pulse rate. The term 'tachycardia' is used to describe an increased heart rate.

A slow pulse rate is associated with advancing age but can also occur in disease. It was seen that the pulse rate is slow in hypothermia. It can also be slow if brain disease is present, in jaundice, heart disease, myxoedema and some forms of poisoning. The term 'bradycardia' is used to describe a decreased heart rate.

Taking a pulse
It is usual to take a patient's pulse rate at the time of taking temperature and respiration measurements. The radial artery in the wrist is the most common pulse to examine (Figures 5.13 and 5.14), though the pulse rate may also be felt in the carotid artery in the neck and in the temporal artery, slightly forward and above the ear.

The nurse should note not only the rate of the pulse but its rhythm and volume, and should feel it for a full minute, using a watch with a second hand.

Rate
The nurse should place two fingers lightly on the radial artery just above the wrist (Figure 5.14), and start count-

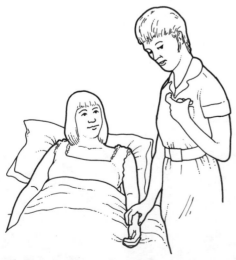

Fig. 5.13 The nurse taking a pulse.

ing when she feels the pulse. Too much pressure will slow the flow of blood through the artery and will be uncomfortable for the patient. The number of pulses per minute should be recorded on the temperature chart (Figure 5.8).

Rhythm

The rhythm of the heart and therefore the pulse, which is normally regular, may become irregular in disease. When counting the pulse rate, the nurse should note the rhythm. Are there 'gaps' and then a quickening of rate? This is called 'extrasystole' and is present in some heart conditions, though it may have little significance alone.

A pulse which is completely irregular in all respects can be said to be 'fibrillating' and may be due to diseases such as thyrotoxicosis and some heart conditions. If any irregularities of pulse rhythm are felt they should be noted on the chart, and a senior member of staff should be informed.

Volume

The volume of the pulse may vary in disease. It may be weak and difficult to feel when disease of the heart is present and the circulation is poor. A 'full' feeling pulse may occur when infection is present with a resulting pyrexia.

Because emotion and exercise affect the pulse rate, it should be taken when the patient is at rest, except of course when a measure is required of the effect of exercise on the pulse rate. The patient should understand what is happening and why it is happening. Obviously if the nurse is concentrating on the feel of the pulse and looking at her watch, she will not be able to interact with the patient until after the measurement is recorded. She should be careful not to walk away wordlessly.

Respiration

Respirations are a further indication of the deficits produced by disease. They should be observed by the nurse for a full minute and the rate recorded on the temperature chart. Respirations are normally observed while temperature and pulse are recorded, the three measurements being linked as 'TPR' (temperature, pulse and respiration). It is preferable if the patient is unaware that breathing is being observed, since the rate of respiration can be controlled and varied by an individual.

Rate, rhythm, sound and ease of breathing should be observed. If the patient has a cough this should also be noted.

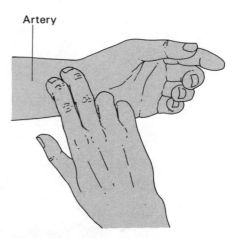

Artery

Fig. 5.14 The nurse's fingers on the radial artery.

Rate

Deficiencies in the oxygen supply will result in an **increased** respiration rate as the body tries to take in more oxygen. A **decreased** respiration rate is associated with a depressed respiratory centre which may be due to disease or poisoning.

Rhythm

In a normal individual, there is an equal rhythm between respirations. If an individual has chest pain he may consciously breathe less deeply than usual, so affecting rhythm, in an effort to ease his pain. Alternatively, the patient in coma has a deeper, slower rhythm than normal.

Patients who are critically ill may have a peculiar rhythm called Cheyne–Stokes breathing, a cyclic pattern of a gradually increasing rate and depth of respirations which peak and then are followed by a period of apnoea (absence of respirations).

Sound

Normal breathing is relatively quiet but deficits in the respiratory system may cause distinctive alterations in sound, e.g. patients with asthma may make wheezing, whistling sounds, while unconscious patients may make loud snoring noises. Even the common cold can affect the sound of breathing.

Difficulty in breathing (dyspnoea)

One does not usually think of breathing unless the respiratory system is affected by disease when difficulty may be experienced. The dyspnoeic patient is aware that his breathing is not normal and becomes distressed as he experiences discomfort. Dyspnoea may be due to physical disease or psychological distress.

Cough

Coughing is a reflex action which interrupts normal breathing. Most people cough occasionally, in a smokey atmosphere or if a drink 'goes down the wrong way'. A cough can also be associated with disease that affects breathing.

A cough may be 'dry' and 'hard' as in a heavy smoker, or moist and productive when there is an infection. It may be associated with breathlessness in cardiac failure, and may cause the patient considerable distress.

There may also be a pattern in the coughing in that it is more apparent on waking, or is associated with exertion or smoking.

The place of temperature, pulse and respiration in recognizing deficits produced by disease

Measurements of temperature, pulse and respiration are probably the most common observations carried out by nurses. Variations from normal will give indications that disease is present but will not, on their own, indicate which disease is causing deficits. For example, pyrexia may suggest that an infection is causing deficits such as fluid loss, but laboratory tests of blood and urine may be necessary to establish which infection is present. The nurse, however, in her assessment will note the fluid-related deficits so that her care plan can meet the resulting physical needs.

Other measures of an individual's functioning

Temperature, pulse and respiration are just one set of measurements which may be taken from an individual and have been considered here since few patients do not require these observations. Other objective measurements of a patient's functioning may be taken by a nurse, such as blood pressure (BP) and urinalysis. These will be considered in Part Four, when specific diseases are discussed and their relevance more clearly seen. Less objective measures of an individual's functioning can be equally important in recognizing deficits and may be achieved by observation and by questioning the patient.

Weight

A patient may be weighed on admission and it is possible, by consulting a 'weight for height' chart, to make assumptions about that patient's approximation to the ideal weight. This in itself gives little information about the individual since he may always have been over- or underweight. By talking to the patient and asking if there has been any **change** in weight recently, we can assess whether or not the patient's weight should be a cause for concern. It may be that an individual is overweight because of his lifestyle and therefore may benefit from health education, but if the patient reports change then there may be an underlying disease process causing deficits.

If a patient reports that change has occurred in his weight, questions to elicit if there have been changes in eating habits, exercise or sleep patterns will all help to build a picture of the patient's health which is related to what is normal for him.

Skin

Skin may be observed for indications of disease. It has been seen that the look and feel of skin can indicate pyrexia and hypothermia. For example, in Caucasians, the skin may be pale or flushed, it may also be blue in some circulatory disorders or yellow in liver disease. Again, what is normal for the individual is important in establishing if there has been change. Some people, for example, have naturally dark or fair skin or a ruddy complexion.

Skin may also be observed for blemishes and for signs of injury. Occasionally there may be signs of non-accidental injuries which should be reported, for although these may not indicate the presence of disease, they may be a clue to social problems which need attention.

Observations such as these may be made unobtrusively while helping a patient prepare for bed or whilst bathing him. Pertinent open questions should give the patient the opportunity of putting the observations into perspective.

Expression

All individuals are liable to a gamut of emotions, e.g. from happy to sad, optimistic to pessimistic, angry to pleased. Personality has a part to play in reaction to situations along with an individual's attitude to life.

The nurse often sees a patient for the first time when he is feeling unwell, worried and apprehensive and this may make it difficult for her to assess if change has taken place in his emotional state. Expression can register current feelings but, since it is non-verbal, it may be misconstrued.

If a nurse is to assess how the patient is feeling, she should ask him. She may use the perceived expression as an opener, e.g. 'You look worried Mr Smith . . .', so giving him a chance to confirm or deny. Certainly reactions should not be assumed from non-verbal communication.

A patient's emotional state may change as a result of disease, e.g. brain tumour, or as a reaction to disease. Pain, for example, may turn a sunny-natured person into a very anxious one. It is sometimes thought that pain may be assessed from expression, but careful assessment needs to be made to ascertain the level, site and cause of pain (Raiman 1988). Expression and body posture are indicators which can be observed, but the patient needs the chance to express the nature of the pain in order that appropriate treatment can be given.

Mobility

Observation will give considerable information about an individual's mobility but again needs to be linked to the concept of normality for each individual. Elderly people, for example, may seem less mobile in hospital because of unfamiliar floor surfaces and a ward layout which is strange to them. There may be wide open spaces and nothing to hold on to to steady themselves.

General observations

Any observation will give some information but, to be useful, the information generally needs to be put into the context of what is normal for the patient.

If the patient reports that his present state is different from that which he perceives to be normal, it may be that the change is an indication of deficits produced by disease or by social or psychological factors.

If the patient's present state in any area, e.g. weight, is normal for him, it may still cause concern by its implications for health. This aspect of observations could be seen to be linked with potential deficits for the patient.

In this section, various aspects of a patient's functioning have been taken separately for ease of explanation. In reality, while making her observations, the skilled nurse will be building a picture of the whole person and eliciting those areas of his functioning which are a cause for immediate or potential concern.

Summary

In this chapter the relevance of the medical diagnosis has been discussed in relation to nursing. Some of the deficits produced by disease have been explored along with their possible effects on individuals.

Recognizing deficits produced by disease requires skilled objective and subjective observation, put into the context of what is normal for each individual.

Specific diseases and appropriate observations will be discussed in Part Four.

References

Department of Health (1991) *Dietary reference values for food energy and nutrients for the United Kingdom*. Report on health and social subjects No. 41. London: HMSO.

Faulkner, A. (1980) *The student nurse's role in giving information to patients*. Unpublished M. Litt. Thesis, Aberdeen University.

Health Education Council (1983) *Discussion paper on guidelines for nutritional education in Britain*. Report of the National Advisory Council. London: Health Education Council.

Raiman, J. (1988) Pain and its management. In Wilson Barnett, J. & Raiman, J. (Eds.) *Nursing issues and research in terminal care*. Chichester: John Wiley.

Swash, M. & Mason, S. (1984) *Hutchison's clinical methods*, 18th edn. London: Baillière Tindall.

Further reading

Bates, B. (1979) *A guide to physical examination*. Philadelphia: J. B. Lippincott.

Beland, I. L. & Passos, J. Y. (1981) Clinical nursing: patho-physiological and psycho-social approaches, 4th edn. London: Macmillan.

Block, C., Nolan, J. & Dempsey, M. (1981) *Health assessment for professional nursing*. New York: Appleton-Century-Crofts.

Gibson, R. S. (1990) *Principles of nutritional assessment*. Oxford: Oxford University Press.

Hinchliff, S. & Montague, L. (1988) *Physiology for nursing practice*. London: Baillière Tindall.

McCaffery, M. & Beebe, A. (1989) *Pain: clinical manual for nursing practice*. St Louis: C. V. Mosby.

Muirhead, N. & Catto, G. R. (1986) *Aids to fluid and electrolyte imbalance*. Edinburgh: Churchill Livingstone.

Rickards, R. (1980) *Understanding medical terms*. Edinburgh: Churchill Livingstone.

Riddle, J. T. (1985) *Anatomy and physiology applied to nursing*, 6th edn. Edinburgh: Churchill Livingstone.

Thompson, R. (1980) *An introduction to physical signs*. Oxford: Blackwell Scientific.

Tighe, J. R. & Davies, D. R. (1984) *Pathology*, 4th edn. London: Baillière Tindall.

6

Defining Nursing Problems

CHAPTER SUMMARY

Patient's problems versus nurse's problems, 131
Patient's problems, 131
Patient's lifestyle, 132
Nurse's problems, 133
Defining problems, 134

Problem anticipation, 135
Anticipating physical problems, 135
Anticipating psychological problems, 136
Anticipating social problems, 138

The dangers of anticipation, 138

Formulating aims for care, 139
Problems with possible solutions, 140
Problems which may be alleviated, 141
Problems where there is no solution, 141

Summary, 142

References, 143

Further reading, 143

Patient's problems versus nurse's problems

One major criticism of the nursing process is that it generates so much paperwork that it is difficult to gain a quick summary of the patient's problems. For example, a nurse who was writing out a patient's history once identified 57 problems. Some of these were concerned with the patient's long-standing disagreements with the local council, some were to do with his lifestyle and a few were linked with the deficits produced by his current illness.

It is possible to argue, of course, that personal feuds and lifestyle may have a direct bearing on a patient's well-being but, in order to plan care, priorities must be set and a distinction made between a problem which is agreed between patient and nurse, a problem in either the nurse's view or the patient's, and a problem not directly concerned with current illness but which may need attention or referral to an appropriate agency.

Patient's problems

Assessment of the patient should elicit the most pressing physical, social and psychological problems. Some of these may be expected. For example, the patient with respiratory disease may complain of problems in breathing, while the patient newly diagnosed as diabetic may have problems in understanding the need for his new regimen. Other problems may be more specific to a particular individual, and it is here particularly that a difference may arise in the perception of what is a problem or what is the priority of that problem.

When Mrs Witherington (Chapter 4) was found to have diabetes, her major problem was that she had come into hospital as a day patient and expected to go home that evening. She had had several previous stays in hospital with the result that her small daughter was showing signs of insecurity. Mrs Witherington had promised that on this occasion she would be home before Sarah's bedtime. To the medical and nursing staff, the patient's problem was that her diabetes had not been stabilized and she therefore needed immediate treatment. The nurses and doctors were persuaded to accept the patient's priority on problems and she went home for two days to arrange her domestic life so that she could come back to be stabilized with a peaceful mind. The registrar, however, commented in the case notes that Mrs Witherington was an 'uncooperative' patient.

This difference in perception can often affect realistic assessment of the patient's problems. In the above case the welfare of an individual's daughter, the trust between mother and child, and the diabetes were all problems. To the nurse, before she understood the psychological aspects of the case, the diabetes was the major problem, but to the patient the keeping of her promise was paramount and she was able to argue that since the diagnosis was made by chance, another day or so without insulin would not make much difference.

All patients are not so articulate and it is often up to the nurse to make sure that problems identified are agreed by the patient. If not, the patient's perspective needs to be gained if co-operation is to be achieved.

Patient's lifestyle

Often it seems obvious to the nurse that aspects of a patient's lifestyle are problems in that they may affect his chance of recovery. Smoking, for example, is known to be associated with a number of diseases, while being overweight can also cause problems. If, however, smoking is a normal part of a patient's lifestyle, and he can list elderly relatives who smoke and are healthy, he may not agree that smoking is a problem for him. Similarly with weight: many people are not prepared to believe that their weight is associated with inappropriate eating habits.

With these and other lifestyle-related problems, it is easy to set goals in hospital which will apparently 'solve' them. Many consultants will not operate on or treat patients who do not stop smoking while they are in hospital, and many overweight patients are put on a diet. In fact such regimens may not have any long-term benefits for the patient. Faulkner and Ward (1983) for example, when looking at the teaching function of the nurse, found that those patients who had stopped smoking in hospital intended to start again as soon as they were discharged. It appeared that they had not accepted that smoking was a problem for them, but for the hospital.

In areas such as this, the nurse, because of her knowledge of disease processes, identifies problems which may not be agreed by the patient. In such instances the problems will need to be defined in educative rather than prescriptive terms, and the nurse may have to accept that the patient may not necessarily be interested in being educated.

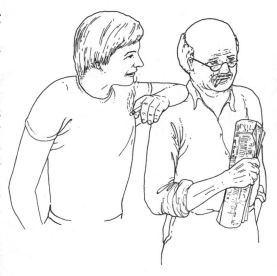

Nurse's problems

When a nurse wishes to change a patient's behaviour, even if it is to improve that patient's health, if the patient is happy with his present state it can be said that it is the nurse rather than the patient who has a problem.

Mrs Maver, in her 70s, considered herself clean. She washed her hands and face every day, had a bath once a month and changed her clothes every week in the summer and every two weeks in the winter. She washed her hair twice a year. On admission to hospital with respiratory disease she was bathed. The nurse identified one of her problems as 'personal hygiene' and planned daily baths in the hope of removing some of the ingrained dirt from Mrs Maver's feet and legs.

The nurse's problem was that she found Mrs Maver offensive because the latter's standards of hygiene did not match her own. Mrs Maver's problem became the daily ordeal of a bath, which she felt 'dried out all the natural oils'. Many old people suffer considerably in hospital from over-cleanliness, and while it is reasonable that for the sake of other patients an individual should be clean, some compromise should be possible between the patient's and the nurse's view of the world.

Stockwell (1972) and Roberts (1984), when doing some research into what makes patients popular or unpopular, found, not surprisingly, that the popular patient is the one who conforms and is cheerful. What is perhaps more worrying is that once a patient is labelled 'difficult' or 'unpopular' this belief tends to generalize to all staff members who care for the patient. Non-conforming behaviour may be seen by a nurse to be a patient's problem. It was seen in earlier chapters that it is possible to expect patients to eat together and socialize when they are in hospital. The shy patient, who prefers to eat alone, may be assessed to have a problem. He may be seen to be withdrawn or antisocial.

It is true that some patients may have such problems, but if the patient says, 'I'm a bit of a loner, I prefer not to mix' then it is not necessarily a nursing duty to change that individual's personality. The problem is the nurse's in that the patient does not fit into the expected mould and may need his meals to be brought to his bedside.

Defining problems

Problems mentioned so far in this chapter have been both global and vague. A newly diagnosed patient with diabetes needs to be stabilized, a patient with respiratory or heart disease needs to be educated, an elderly woman needs to be cleaned up. In taking a nursing history, this is very much the way that problems are offered or observed. What the nurse needs to do is to define each problem in such a way that care can be planned and goals set.

If we return to Mrs Witherington, it can be agreed that her problem was whether to keep a promise to her small child. The nurse, however, while understanding the patient's perspective, will define the problem rather differently in that a patient will be at home for two days with untreated diabetes. Defining the problem in this way allows the nurse to help Mrs Witherington take as few risks as possible before readmission.

In the case of the patient who needs educating, the problem may be defined in terms such as 'patient does not understand link between smoking and present condition'. It can be seen that if the problem is defined in this way, the goals set will be different from those when the problem is defined as 'patient is a smoker', which might lead to a goal of immediate cessation.

With an elderly woman, a problem of 'personal hygiene' may be, as in Mrs Maver's case, a blanket term for a number of problems. If these are defined separately, progress can be monitored more easily.

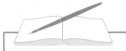

Select a patient who is a smoker. Negotiate some time with him/her and try to gain a picture of his/her beliefs about smoking. Is there motivation to cease? If yes, how can you help? If no, what do you see as **your** responsibility to this patient in terms of his/her behaviour?

Problem anticipation

Although each patient will respond to disease and treatment in an individual way, it is possible to anticipate potential problems in a patient given that the disease process and treatment are understood. Experience of responses to disease may also help a nurse to anticipate problems, though care must be taken not to make assumptions without assessment. The value of problem anticipation is that it can effectively ensure the problem will not arise for many patients and that it will be recognized early if it does arise in others.

Anticipating physical problems

By understanding the symptoms of disease it is possible to anticipate many physical problems. It is to be expected, for instance, that patients with bronchitis may have difficulty in breathing, especially if they are laid flat in the bed. Such knowledge will affect the nursing care of patients with bronchitis. Similarly it is reasonable to anticipate that a patient with arthritis of the hip will have a problem with walking.

Another physical problem which may be anticipated in any illness which affects mobility is that of pressure sores (Figure 6.1). These sores, which start as a redness of the skin at pressure points on the body, and which may break down into open sores, used to be called bedsores. This is a misnomer since pressure can just as easily occur in a chair as in a bed.

In anticipating a problem of pressure it is known from the work of Norton (1975) and others that some patients are more at risk of these sores than others (Table 6.1). The very thin are at risk, for instance, because of the lack of padding between bony prominences and skin, and possibly a poor nutritional state. The very heavy are also at risk because of their weight. Anticipation of the problems of

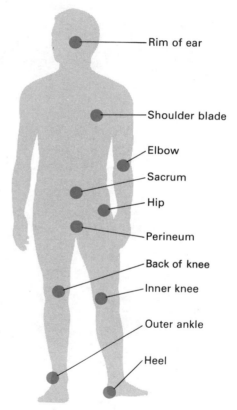

Fig. 6.1 Risk areas for pressure sores.

Table 6.1 The Norton scale.

Physical condition	Mental condition	Activity	Mobility	Incontinent
Good 4	Alert 4	Ambulant 4	Full 4	Not 4
Fair 3	Apathetic 3	Walk/help 3	Slightly limited 3	Occasionally 3
Poor 2	Confused 2	Chairbound 2	Very limited 2	Usually/urine 2
Very bad 1	Stuporous 1	Bedfast 1	Immobile 1	Doubly 1

pressure will lead to pressure area care at regular intervals, so preventing problems rather than waiting for them to arise.

It is possible to anticipate problems in surgical patients in the same way. Post-operative patients, for example, may suffer pain. Foreknowledge of this should ensure that adequate pain control is prescribed before it is needed, so avoiding the problem of waiting for a doctor to prescribe analgesics while the patient is wondering why nothing is done for him. Such knowledge should also alert the nurse to assess post-operative patients for pain since they may be attempting to be 'brave' and uncomplaining.

These and other physical problems may be anticipated on the grounds of knowledge and experience, although each patient will still require an individual assessment to establish the existence of the problem potentially relating to him. In other words, an anticipated problem is one to which the nurse is alerted because it arises in many patients with similar illnesses. This is different from other problems that the nurse will be unaware of until they are elicited from the patient or have been observed and confirmed with the patient.

Anticipating psychological problems

Given what is known about reaction to illness and disease, it is possible to anticipate some of the psychological problems experienced by patients, though again this anticipation does not dispense with the need for careful psychological assessment of each individual.

Stress on admission to hospital has been discussed in Chapter 3. Foreknowledge of this problem allows the nurse to try to alleviate its results, although stress may be compounded both by problems which can be anticipated and by those which cannot. If we remember Mrs Witherington, psychological stress on having to accept her diagnosis could have been anticipated. Without assessment, any signs of stress could be explained in this way. A nurse who identified the problem at this level and aimed to reassure the patient that once she became used to her regimen she could lead a reasonably normal life, would have been wasting her time. Mrs Witherington's mind was concerned with other matters.

Another area where psychological problems may be anticipated is that of mutilating surgery. This is particularly so for women undergoing mastectomy or hysterectomy, both because of the feelings of mutilation and because of associations with femininity. Maguire *et al.*

(1980) and Webb (1982) have given good accounts of how women feel after this surgery and it is known that allowing these patients to explore their feelings may aid psychological recovery.

Any mutilation to the body may engender problems of this sort simply because the patient no longer feels complete as a person. In anticipating problems it is a mistake to think of the problem in proportion to the extent of the mutilation since each patient sees only his own situation. The individual who has lost some toes after an accident with an electric lawnmower is unlikely to feel grateful that he did not lose a leg – and even if he does, his sense of loss and incompleteness may well remain.

Some diagnoses may precipitate problems that can be anticipated, either because they are fear-provoking or because they appear to represent an unacceptable change in life. Diabetes has already been mentioned in this chapter. Many patients faced with such a diagnosis imagine that they will have to be 'controlled by the clock' and will be unable to lead a normal life. Young patients with diabetes, especially, may fight against adhering to a regimen. Anticipating this response to diagnosis and the problems it may cause should alert the nurse to the need for educating the patient to accept a regimen which fits his normal lifestyle as closely as possible.

Perhaps the most fear-provoking diagnosis where problems may be anticipated is that of cancer. Although cancer is not the biggest killer in the United Kingdom, and although many patients survive, this diagnosis is probably the most feared of all. Cancer means death to most members of the lay public and this feeling can only be enhanced if doctors and nurses are not prepared to be as open about this diagnosis as they are about more 'acceptable' diseases. Faulkner (1980) found nurses far more prepared to tell a patient that he had had a 'coronary attack' than they were to tell another patient that he had cancer.

The problems that can be anticipated when a patient does learn he has cancer may be concerned with survival, unacceptable treatment and pain, among others. Fear of the unknown may cause multiple psychological problems. By realizing this, the nurse in her assessment can give the patient an opportunity to voice his individual concerns.

There are many other psychological problems which may be anticipated in a patient once his diagnosis is known. This is yet another area where nursing problems may be generated by a physical disorder as well as by an individual's reaction to admission to hospital.

Anticipating social problems

Although knowledge of a patient's background will help to elicit any social problems, and indeed will put social problems into context, there are some problems which may be anticipated from a knowledge of the disease and its effects on an individual. Many of these problems may not occur until the individual is discharged, but some may affect the patient while he is in hospital.

It was shown in Chapter 2 that society has certain expectations of its members and that these expectations must be met in order for individuals to be acceptable. Disease may affect social behaviour and so problems may be anticipated for the patient.

It is not uncommon for elderly patients to have problems of urinary control, which can, if leakage occurs, lead to odour which is offensive to others. On these grounds alone relatives may not be prepared to take a patient home, since they can foresee a urine-soaked bed, chairs and carpets and a smelly house as a result. Anticipation of this problem may lead not only to better control or suitable waterproof clothing, but to retained dignity for the patient.

Patients who have hip replacements are known to have difficulty in managing to walk up and down stairs. Since there are not normally stairs on a ward, the patient may be unaware of this potential problem. Anticipation should result in physiotherapy, which will not only retrain the patient in his technique on stairs, but will send him home with confidence.

Sometimes the treatment prescribed for patients involves a change in social behaviour. For example, diet may be restricted, or alcohol contraindicated. Although society is more diet-conscious than formerly, and the laws on drinking and driving have raised consciousness about alcohol consumption, hosts are still likely to push 'just one little drink' or 'another helping of Helen's trifle'. By anticipating problems before the patient is discharged to such temptations, he may be helped to understand the seriousness of any restrictions and to develop strategies where he will not be seen to be either a social 'spoil sport' or a 'neurotic' who is always reminding people about his illness.

In anticipating social problems, the patient's return to society may be eased and his chance of reaching full health potential enhanced.

The dangers of anticipation

One of the dangers inherent in the anticipation of problems may be seen to be that, by expecting a problem, it

Choose a patient you are caring for. Given the diagnosis, which problems would you predict? Compare your predictions with the problems listed on the care plan. With hindsight, how would problem anticipation have helped you?

will surely arise. If a patient is asked on every drug round if he has a pain, will he not come to expect and then experience pain? And if a patient after mastectomy is asked her feelings about her body image, will she not begin to feel that she **is** a freak? It is probable, if the questions are asked in this way, that such a risk does exist. What is required is that the nurse is alert to the possible problems but that her questions do not lead a patient to suppose that he should feel a certain way about a particular situation.

Another danger of problem anticipation is that it might trigger inappropriate action on the part of the nurse. It was seen that in the traditional model of nursing every patient would have 'things done', such as temperature, pulse and respiration measurements, whether or not they were necessary. It would be easy to adopt a similar attitude when it is known that a problem is likely. For example, if patients are expected to have a pain postoperatively, should they not be given analgesics as standard routine post-operative care? This sort of thinking would destroy the concept of individualized care. Anticipation of problems should neither lead to the development of problems nor to routinized care. What it should do is alert the nurse to problems that are very possible in a given situation so that she may assess the patient and either count the problem out or make plans for appropriate care.

Formulating aims for care

Table 6.2 shows how problems may be divided into those which are physical, psychological and social and further

Table 6.2 Classes of problems to be identified.

Problems and relationship to disease
Physical
Related to disease (anticipated)
Related to disease (not anticipated)
Not related to disease
Psychological
Related to disease (anticipated)
Related to disease (not anticipated)
Not related to disease
Social
Related to disease (anticipated)
Related to disease (not anticipated)
Not related to disease

subdivided according to their relatedness to a particular disease.

Once identified, problems will need to be ordered in terms of both priority and possibility of action. As in the case of Molly Witherington, priorities will not necessarily be set on problems related to disease, but rather on their importance to the patient's overall needs, given that the greatest priority may be for physical survival or physical or psychosocial well-being.

Some problems which are identified may not require nursing action but may yet affect the patient's interest and co-operation in care. The nurse may give priority to referring these problems in order to relieve the patient's worries, before setting aims for his physical care.

Miss Voyce, an elderly spinster, appeared to have a problem in that she did not wish to stay in hospital for necessary treatment. Further investigation identified the problem as an elderly dependent friend who could not care for himself. Referral to the Social Services resulted in a home-help and meals-on-wheels for him while Miss Voyce was hospitalized.

A number of problems, once identified, will need to be referred to appropriate agencies. Other problems will need to be grouped into those with possible solutions, those which may be alleviated though not necessarily solved, and those where there is no obvious solution.

Problems with possible solutions

Once a problem is identified and a solution foreseen, care may be planned and goals set for steps towards that solution. After a hip replacement a patient may have problems associated with mobility. These may include:

1 Fear of weight-bearing on affected leg (anticipated problem)
2 Difficulty in walking (anticipated problem)
3 Difficulty in managing stairs (anticipated problem)
4 Reluctance to get up (not anticipated)
5 Hostility to hospital personnel (not anticipated)

These problems may all be seen to have a solution and the nurse may, for example, decide that to solve the mobility problems, 4 and 5 must have top priority. Aims for care will take into account goals which can be realistically reached in a given time, and then more ambitious goals can be set. If hostility is a problem, it might be too much to reduce the patient's hostile feelings to all staff at once **and** elicit the underlying cause.

Similarly with walking, the patient will be encouraged if the goals are not too distant. 'We will have you hopping around like a nine-year-old by the time you leave' sounds like a vague promise compared with 'By Thursday let's aim for you to walk as far as Mr Smith's bed and back.' If this is achieved by the stated time, further goals can be set, even though the patient may not actually be skipping by the date of his discharge.

This problem-solving approach to aims for care is possible in many situations. Even if all problems do not have an obvious solution, it is usually possible to formulate some aims for care.

Problems which may be alleviated

Some diseases produce deficits which are permanent. In this respect we talk of chronic disease (of which bronchitis is an example) when identifying problems where it is known that full functioning will not be restored. Here, aims for care cannot be in terms of solutions but in terms of achieving maximum improvement. This calls for a slightly different approach since it is often not known what level of improvement is possible.

Other areas where 'solution' is an inappropriate way to think are where deficits may be rectified but life, as the patient previously experienced it, may be altered. Diabetes is a good example of this in that the deficit, i.e. insulin, can be replaced but the patient may never again take for granted the balance between insulin, food and exercise.

Aims for care here, as in other areas, should have goals that are realistic and reachable, while education for the future may be a large component of the care that is planned. It may be depressing to have to face the fact that one will never be 100% healthy again. A positive attitude on the part of the nurse will encourage the patient to work towards maximizing his potential. Small gains in functioning or learning can act as a spur to greater achievement.

Problems where there is no solution

Patients often present a nurse with problems for which there is no solution. It may be a broken marriage, a chronically ailing child, personal failure, or other problems which may seem unrelated to the present illness but whose stress may well be affecting recovery. In formulating aims for care, time may be set aside to allow the patient to talk through his worries in the hope that he can learn to accept what is inevitable and work positively where possible, though after assessment some of these problems may need to be referred to a social worker or psychiatrist.

The patient who is terminally ill may have physical, social and psychological problems which have no solution other than the patient's death. In formulating aims for care here, death with comfort and dignity may be the goals, to be set alongside goals for dealing with other problems which can be alleviated or indeed solved. Whether aims for care include solutions or not, some goals may always be set for the patient to achieve with the nurse's help. The difficulty which can be experienced by the nurse is of feeling that she has somehow failed if she cannot solve all the problems.

It has to be accepted that most people, well or ill, have a certain number of insoluble problems. Most people can accept this up to a point, though the knowledge may make them sad. In identifying problems of this sort in patients, the nurse should not list problems which the patient has accepted. For example, the patient at the beginning of this chapter who had had trouble with the local council had already succeeded in having her windows replaced and a new hot water cylinder fitted. Her account of the conflict was 'neutral' material, not to be confused with a problem which was affecting her chances of recovery.

Finally, the nurse needs to accept that helping a patient learn to cope with a seemingly insoluble problem can be as worthwhile as solving others, and to accept that knowing when a referral is necessary is also a skill.

Summary

This chapter has considered the identification of problems in terms of whether they are the patient's problems or the nurse's in physical, psychological and social areas.

The anticipation of problems has been discussed, based on knowledge of disease processes and a patient's expected response to his disease. Caution has been expressed in allowing anticipation of problems to lead to routinized care.

In formulating aims for care, the problems need to be identified and given priority before reachable goals are set. Problems have been considered under the headings of those which have solutions, those which may be alleviated and those which have no solutions.

References

Faulkner, A. (1980) *The student nurse's role in giving information to patients.* Unpublished M. Litt. Thesis, Aberdeen University.

Faulkner, A. & Ward, L. (1983) Nurses as health educators in relation to smoking. *Nursing Times*, Occasional papers, *79*(8), 47–48.

Maguire, P., Tait, A., Brooke, M. & Sellwood, R. (1980) Emotional aspects of mastectomy. *Nursing Mirror*, January 17, 35–37.

Norton, D. (1975) *An investigation of geriatric problems in hospital.* Edinburgh: Churchill Livingstone.

Roberts, D. (1984) Non-verbal communication. Popular and unpopular patients. In Faulkner, A. (Ed.) *Recent Advances in Nursing, No. 7: Communication.* Edinburgh: Churchill Livingstone.

Stockwell, F. (1972) *The unpopular patient.* London: Rcn.

Webb, C. (1982) Body image and recovery from hysterectomy. In Wilson-Barnett, J. & Fordham, M. (Eds.) *Recovery from illness.* Chichester: J. Wiley.

Further reading

Barrett, E. (1988) A review of risk assessment methods: care. *Care, Science and Practice*, *6*(2), 49–52.

Carlson, J., Craft, C. & McGuire, D. (1982) *Nursing diagnosis.* Philadelphia: W. B. Saunders.

Carpenito, L. J. (1987) *Nursing diagnosis*, 2nd edn. Philadelphia: Lippincott.

Department of Health (1989) *A strategy for nursing.* London: HMSO.

Gordon, M. (1982) *Nursing diagnosis: process and application.* New York: McGraw-Hill.

Wilson Barnett, J. & Batehup, L. (1988) *Patient problems: a research base for nursing care.* London: Scutari Press.

PART THREE
PLANS FOR CARE

Care Plans

CHAPTER SUMMARY

Components of a care plan, 148
The identified problem, 148
Goals set for care, 149
Care planned to meet goals, 149

When a standard care plan is useful, 151
Limitations of standard care plans, 152

Critical pathways: care mapping 154

Individualized care plans, 158
The format of an individualized care plan, 159

The patient's role in a care plan, 163

The dynamic element of care plans, 169

Summary, 173

References, 173

Further reading, 174

When a patient has been assessed and his problems identified, then care should be planned, if possible, in consultation with the patient so that priorities are set that can be agreed by both parties. The Patient's Charter requests that each local area sets its own standards for care. Care should be planned in accordance with these standards and documented so that a clear record is available of both the patient's progress and the standards of care delivered. This should allow coherent care to be maintained by all members of the health care team involved with each patient.

Care plans may be individual to each patient or may, in certain situations, be standardized. The notion of a standard care plan may at first sight appear contrary to the concept of individualized care. However, it was seen in Chapter 6 that many problems may be foreseen because of their known association with particular diseases. Similarly, problems may, as an example, be anticipated and therefore avoided in patients before and after surgery and other routine procedures. A more recent concept is that of critical path analysis where the care plan has certain standardized elements but there is room for differentiation of problems for each individual.

Although there is a case for a standard care plan in some situations, that risk of routinized care must be avoided, for even with standard procedures no two individuals react in the same way.

Components of a care plan

A care plan should be readily understood by those who are expected to use it. As such it should be succinct and devoid of irrelevant material.

It was seen in Chapter 6 that when a nursing assessment has been made, problems will be identified and given an order of priority. Care is planned on the basis of identified problems which have a solution in nursing care terms. Other problems will be referred to the appropriate member of the health care team and will not necessarily need to be on the main care plan.

This differentiation does not mean that the nurse will lose sight of the problem. For example, Miss Voyce (Chapter 6) will not need the problem of her elderly friend on the care plan, since it has been referred to the Social Services. The nurse, however, will document the problem elsewhere, on a 'communication' or assessment sheet, and check how things are at reassessment.

The components of a care plan include the identified problem, the goals set for care, and the care which is thought most likely to achieve the goals set.

The identified problem

It will be seen that problems are identified at assessment. After this the nurse will require time to decide which problems have a nursing solution, which require referral and which are of immediate importance. For those problems referred, she may also need to know if there are any implications for nursing care.

It is at this stage that the interrelated roles of the nurse and the other health professionals become apparent. For example, a patient with bronchitis may have problems in breathing. This problem will have a medical, a physiotherapy and a nursing solution, and the nurse will be involved in all of these. She will administer drugs and help the patient to follow a regimen prescribed by the doctor and will also participate in the physiotherapist's prescribed care plan, which will include sitting the patient in an upright position. The joint goals of all professionals are that the patient's breathing problem will be eased.

The problem should be stated in an unambiguous way. If the problem is one associated with breathing, for example, the actual problem should be stated. It may be that the problem only arises when the patient is lying flat or that there are difficulties at all times which are exacerbated by lying flat. This precision aids the planning of care. If the problem is stated simply as 'breathing problems' it becomes possible that inappropriate care will be given and that those giving it will not understand the rationale for care.

Goals set for care

Just as problems need to be precisely defined, so do the goals set for care. A goal of 'easier breathing' is ambiguous and impossible to measure. A goal of 'breathing without difficulty' may be evaluated by both patient and nurse – the patient by the way he feels and the nurse from her observations.

It has been pointed out (Chapter 6) that the goals set ideally involve both patient and nurse and should be readily attainable so that further progress may build on past successes. By stating goals precisely, care may be planned for the patient to reach his potential in achievable and measurable steps. Rasmussen and Genglee (1994) describe giving the patient a 'plan of care' form on admission to keep. This is written, and updated, in layperson's language without abbreviation or medical terminology.

It might be argued that if care is properly planned, the patient will reach his potential without goals being set. There is an old saying that if you don't know where you are going, you might end up in the wrong place. Goals not only act as a reminder of what care is about but also act as an incentive to both patient and carer to realize those goals.

Care planned to meet goals

When care is planned for a patient, it generally involves nursing decisions, medical decisions and decisions of other health professionals involved in an individual's care. The most coherent care must involve consultation between all relevant health professionals before decisions are agreed. This multidisciplinary cooperation, particularly between nurses and doctors, need not diminish the status of any health professional. What it should do is to improve interdisciplinary relationships as each member of the team learns to respect the other's view.

It would give a totally false impression if it were implied that different members of the health care team will always see each other's view. A classic situation which may cause problems is that of how much information to give a patient who is wrestling with a frightening diagnosis and perhaps an uncertain future. There have been many studies to show that patients who are properly informed do better than those who are cared for in ignorance of what is happening for them. A classic study, reprinted in 1994, is that of Haywood and Boore. Often it is the nurse who is asked by the patient for information that the doctor has not thought fit to share. These situations require that each health professional is prepared to listen to the other and that the nurse should be assertive for the sake of her patient. This issue of nurse/doctor relationships in particular is important in all aspects of nursing and will be discussed in Chapter 18.

Care planned in isolation from the rest of the health care team may lead to confusion for the patient if he cannot see the relevance of what is happening. McFarlane and Castledine (1982) state: 'Nursing care plans should demonstrate co-ordination with the overall medical and general health care plan for the patient.' This co-ordination and co-operation not only ensures that all health professionals are alive to the patient's problems but should also increase the patient's motivation to co-operate in care.

Faulkner (1981) cites the patient with diabetes who did not co-operate in care prescribed for him because he did not understand the implications of that care. To motivate a patient to co-operate he must be involved. The alternative is to do things to or for the patient in the traditional manner. Planned care must be precise if there is to be a later evaluation. For example, 'attention to pressure areas two hourly' or 'continuity of care' from one shift to another, is imprecise and may lead to a number of interpretations. 'Two hourly turning' is better because the attention to be given is clearly defined as 'turning'.

Knowledge of a patient's diagnosis is important when planning care. For example, two patients, one with bronchitis and one with emphysema, may have difficulty in breathing, yet the concentration of oxygen which may be safely administered to the patient with bronchitis could kill the one with emphysema (Chapter 10). Although oxygen is prescribed by doctors, it is administered by nurses and its use must be understood by them when planning care related to medical prescription.

Knowledge of diagnosis is also necessary when planning care which is not related to medical prescription. For example, if a patient is clinically depressed, emotional care will need to be based on a knowledge of the depression and may require referral. It may be that a nurse thinks a patient should be encouraged to talk through his emotional worries. If the depression is severe, being faced with the cause could tilt the patient's mood towards suicide. In this instance, care should be planned on careful assessment, knowledge of the mental disease, and consultation with the psychiatrist and medical or surgical consultant.

When a standard care plan is useful

The components of a care plan are the same whether the plan is standard or individual. The difference lies in the fact that standard care plans are compiled on knowledge of a particular disease or procedure, while an individualized care plan is compiled on knowledge of an individual gained through assessment.

Many patients are in hospital for a very short stay and for a particular reason – for example, a minor operation. A standard care plan is useful in this situation since it is based on a routine associated with the reason for admission. Further, it leaves the limited time available with the patient for personal assessment.

Mark Jones was admitted for a gastrointestinal endoscopy (Hollanders, 1979). This is a procedure for which a standard care plan is useful. However, individual assessment showed that Mark was unusually frightened.

Plans were made, **in addition** to the standard care plan, to deal with Mark's fears by exploration of the cause. In fact, Mark had known someone who had died after endoscopy and thought that this was a real risk to him too.

The above case illustrates that a standard care plan alone may leave the patient with unidentified problems if it is used without individual assessment. Individual assessment should always be made even if care is commenced using a standard care plan.

A standard care plan is also useful for the unconscious patient where individual assessment is not always possible. In this situation, relatives may be able to furnish relevant details about the individual which may be pertinent to medical prescription.

Limitations of standard care plans

Since it was argued in Chapter 6 that all diseases have related problems, it might also be argued that standard care plans might be possible for all patients. This would bring us full circle – back to treating the disease rather than the person.

In pre-operative care and in nursing care associated with some procedures there are standard tasks to be performed irrespective of the individual. This is not always so when nursing an individual with a disease.

Returning to Mrs Witherington, diabetes is a common disease, causing deficits in the regulation of blood sugar. A standard care plan would cover urinalysis, diet and treatment, including education. The limitations of such a plan are immediately apparent since there would be no chance to explore how Mrs Witherington felt about her diagnosis in relation to her own life and obligations. Further, standard plans for education might not be as effective as individualized plans. An individualized care plan, based on assessment, and incorporating standard elements based on research and best practice, allowed Mrs Witherington to delay treatment in order to deal with more pressing personal problems.

A standard care plan sets priorities in terms of procedures rather than individuals (Figure 7.1). As such it should be used with caution. Another limitation to a standard care plan is that it is generally static – that is, it will list the care to be given and a nurse will sign that it has been given. The plan is not based on assessment and evaluation, and therefore reassessment may not occur. It can be seen that this type of plan may be very suitable for procedures, but on its own is not suitable for pre-planning care for specific diseases.

It will be seen from the example of a standard care plan (Figure 7.1) that problems are not listed as 'patient's problems' but as 'expected problems' – that is, problems which could arise if appropriate care is not given. If care is given according to the plan, the patient will be ready to be escorted to theatre.

It will also be seen that in this example there is some room for assessment in both psychological and physical care. In psychological care there has been no assumption that there is a standard explanation of an operation, rather that the nurse will discover 'where the patient is' in terms of understanding. Similarly with physical care: re-

Name _____ Date of birth _____ Hospital No. _____

Date	Expected problem	Goal	Care to be given	Date	Signature
	Psychological stress due to lack of under-standing of operation	That patient has understanding of operation and post-operation experience	1 Assess patient's level of understanding, give information and check that patient knows what will happen to him		
			2 Answer any questions from patient		
			3 Encourage patient to verbalize fears		
	Physical welfare	That patient's physical state is monitored	4 Record observations of TPR, BP, weight, urine		
			5 Review medical notes and check patient's perceptions of physical problems, e.g. breathing, past operations, allergies		
			6 Report any physical concerns		
	Post-operative complications	That patient undergoes operation with-out complications	7 List any prostheses and remove before operation		
			8 Record and report loose teeth or other potential obstructions		
			9 Starve for minimum of 4 hours before operation		
			10 Ensure that patient is bathed and shaved if necessary		
	Identification of patient for theatre	That the correct patient receives operation	11 Check patient's identification verbally and from band. Review medical notes for completed consent form		
	Unprepared patient	That patient is prepared in time for operation	12 Take custody of jewellery, valuables. Cover wedding ring if appropriate		
			13 Dress patient in theatre gown, pants and socks		
			14 Check and give pre-med		
			15 Check that patient has emptied bladder		

Fig. 7.1 Example of a standard care plan: a standard pre-operative care plan.

cording observations is standard but the nurse is expected to take action if she is concerned about the patient's physiological state.

Another point to note about using the standard care plan is that it may lead to the need for an individualized care plan. For example, if a patient verbalizes fears which are not associated with his operation, plans may have to be made to deal with those fears, either before or after operation. This illustrates the point that, as care is given, assessment should also be occurring even when the care to be given is standard.

Critical pathways: care mapping

A recent move has been to develop care plans which are standard in important respects but which allow room for individual variance of a patient. These are sometimes called care maps and sometimes called critical pathways. The components of a care map are based on local standards for care with measurable outcomes. An important feature is that the care maps are multidisciplinary in that they are filled in by nursing, medical and other staff and that they are particularly useful for standard procedures. Figure 7.2 shows a care map for day case surgery and it will be noted that there are clear pathways that have to be taken by the nursing and medical staff, also that there is a separate page for variance from the map for a particular individual.

Another feature of care mapping or critical pathways for care is that the patient and relatives are involved. Hampton (1993) describes managed care frameworks as a viable approach to improving the quality of patient care. He describes a patient care guide for open heart surgery patients to illustrate the patient and family involvement in care.

A major difference between a standard care plan and a care map is that the standard care plan is based on actions to be taken by a nurse to avoid possible problems, and care maps and critical pathways are based on nursing interventions from the point where the patient enters the ward and is greeted to the time that he is discharged, in a patient-oriented style. Such plans or frameworks may well extend to individualized care in the future. Indeed, Trella (1993) describes the use of critical pathways in the care of frail elderly patients.

CARE MAP FOR DAY CASE SURGERY

B WARD

ADDRESSOGRAPH LABEL

DATE :-

WELCOME

	WELCOME	SG		WELCOME	SG
1.	GREETING–SHOWN TO BED		1.	BLOODS	
2.	INTRODUCTION & CHAT TO WARD STAFF		2.	TEACHING	
3.	DEMOGRAPHIC PATIENT DETAILS		3.	INFORMED CONSENT	
4.	CHECK NOTES–I.D. BAND/PATIENT		4.	CONSENT FORM SIGNED	
5.	FASTED FROM		5.	PRESCRIPTION	
6.	PRE-ADMISSION		6.	EXAMINATION & HISTORY	

ADMISSION

	NURSING INTERVENTION	EVALUATION	SG
1.	TEMPERATURE AND PULSE		
2.	WEIGHT		
3.	EMLA CREAM	TIME POSITION	
4.	LOOSE TEETH	R I L	
5.	ALLERGIES/ASTHMA		
6.	ALLERGY BAND/WRIST		
7.	PREVIOUS ANAESTHETIC		
8.	MEDICAL PROBLEMS		
9.	REGULAR MEDICATION		
10.	ASSESSMENT		
11.	NURSING PROCESS		
12.	ORIENTATE TO WARD		
13.	PRE-OP TALK		
14.	SAFE ENVIROMENT	OBSERVE PLAY/BEDREST	
15.	THEATRE SLIP		
16.	ANXIETY PARENT/CHILD	AM PM	
17.	OPERATION LIST		

PRE-OP CARE

	NURSING INTERVENTION	WARD	SG	THEATRE	SG
1.	IDENTITY BAND				
2.	CONSENT				
3.	FASTED				
4.	ALLERGIES/BAND				
5.	CLOTHING				
6.	JEWELLERY				
7.	HAIR				
8.	LOOSE TEETH/PROSTHESIS				
9.	NAIL VARNISH/EMLA				
10.	X-RAY				
11.	BLOOD RESULTS				
12.	MEDICATION GIVEN				
13.	PRESCRIPTION SHEET				
14.	ESCORT TO THEATRE				
15.	SIGNATURE				

Fig. 7.2 Example of a care map for day case surgery. Reproduced with kind permission from the Practice Development Unit at Seacroft Hospital, Leeds.

CARE MAP FOR DAY CASE SURGERY

B WARD

DATE :-

POST-OPERATIVE CARE

	NURSING INTERVENTION	EVALUATION	SIGN
1.	PREPARE OP-BED		
2.	WARD CHILD SAFETY		
3.	POST-OP CHECK		
4.	WARDED AT :		
5.	CONDITION		
6.	INFORM PARENT/OP		
7.	POST-OP FRESH UP		
8.	POST-OP DRINK		
10.	MEDICATIONS		
11.	POST-OP BREAKFAST		
12.	ELIMINATION NEEDS		
13.	MOBILIZE		

DISCHARGE

	NURSING INTERVENTION	EVALUATION	SIGN
1.	ASSESSMENT		
2.	HOME CARE ADVICE		
3.	GP LETTER		
4.	WRITTEN INSTRUCTION		
5.	MEDICATIONS		
6.	OPD APPOINTMENTS		
7.	GP LETTER IN A WEEK		

THEATRE

TIME	BP	PULSE	O_2

SURGEON :

ANAESTHETIST :

OPERATION :

ANALGESIA :

SWABS NEEDLES INSTRUMENTS :

PACKS :

Fig. 7.2 *Continued*

CARE MAP FOR DAY CASE SURGERY

B WARD

PATIENT'S NAME

DATE	IDENTIFY VARIANCE	REASON FOR VARIANCE	ACTION TAKEN	BY WHOM

Fig. 7.2 *Continued*

Individualized care plans

Both standard care plans and care maps or critical pathways to care come from standard knowledge of elements of care required for patients with particular conditions. Although critical pathways allow for variance from the standard elements of care, they still fall short of being truly individualized to each particular patient. They are, however, based on local standards which offer measurable levels of care. It might be argued that it is more difficult to measure the level of care given on an individualized care plan than on one that is standard. This need not be the case. What is a powerful argument is that any type of standardized care plan, whether or not it allows for variance, can be put into action without assessment of the patient, whereas an individualized care plan requires careful assessment of the patient using effective interactive skills and an assessment form on which the information relevant to an individual patient is recorded.

Where individualized care plans are used either alone or in conjunction with a standard plan, the individualized plan should be based on knowledge both of the patient, gained from assessment, and his disease or treatment, which a nurse will know from experience and research findings.

This will give the possibility of care at two levels – firstly, care which will be related to current problems and deficits, and secondly, care related to potential problems and deficits. Once again it can be seen that knowledge of the patient's disease is an important element in planning care. Therefore, reading the patient's medical history will be a useful adjunct to the nursing assessment that is undertaken.

A major difference between a medical history and a nursing assessment is that the first will give a picture of the patient's physical and mental health over a period of time, as diagnosed by the doctor, while the second should give the patient's perception of, and reactions to, past and current illness as recorded by the nurse. If a nurse uses assessment in the same way as a doctor, i.e. by listing previous illnesses and deficits, she is simply repeating what should have been carried out by medical staff and may well irritate the patient who feels that he has had to repeat everything twice.

Of course there will inevitably be some overlap between medical and nursing assessments. Both professionals are interested in planning the best possible care and each may contribute to the other's knowledge. An example of a nurse contributing considerably to a medical diagnosis was the one who spot-checked Mrs Witherington's urine (Chapter 4) and found glucose present. The nurse, however, could not plan care immediately on the basis of her finding since it is a medical responsbility to confirm diagnosis and prescribe treatment.

The format of an individualized care plan

There is a variety of ways for care plans to be set out. Some wards devise their own to suit the particular needs of a patient group, while some hospitals have a standard format used on all wards.

What is important is that the layout is readily understood and has columns to cover both problems/deficits and the care planned, and has room for evaluation and updating. It is also important that new staff undertaking care of the patient can understand both the assessment and the care plan for each patient. Figure 7.3 gives some headings used in a care plan.

It can be seen from these headings that there is a time factor on goals and a reminder that evaluation is linked to reassessment.

Figure 7.4 shows an alternative format where each problem has its own page with a subsequent page for evaluation. One could argue that this is going to take a lot more paper than a simple page with the date and the current state of a problem on it, but it does mean that each problem stays separate from other problems so that if someone is particularly worried about an aspect of care, they can find the relevant page and fill in the relevant information. This type of care plan is usually kept in a ring binder and often used by all members of the care team.

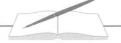

Take a critical look at the documentation for care in your area. What type of format is used? Does it fit with local standards of care?

Borrow your standards of care folder and see how nearly the care plans reflect **two** standards of your choice. Can you suggest improvements to the documentation?

Fig. 7.3 Headings used in an individualized care plan.

Name		Hospital No.		
Date	Problem/Deficit	Care to be given	Goal (with date)	Evaluation/reassess

MULTIDISCIPLINARY CARE PLAN

DATE   PROBLEM No.

PROBLEM/DEFICIT:

GOALS:

ACTIONS:

NAME: WARD: UNIT No.

Fig. 7.4 Example of a multidisciplinary care plan. Reproduced with kind permission from the Practice Development Unit at Seacroft Hospital, Leeds.

EVALUATION

DATE		SIGNATURE

Fig. 7.4 *Continued*

MULTIDISCIPLINARY COMMUNICATION NOTES

DATE		SIGNATURE

Fig. 7.4 *Continued*

Figure 7.5 shows part of the care planned for Mrs Witherington (Chapter 4) and uses the one-page care plan format. This was probably the most useful format for someone who was in fact a day patient and whose subsequent diagnosis of diabetes and her need to go home untreated demanded that a care plan was commenced for her prior to her two days at home. This allowed the nurses to think carefully about problems and deficits and to help the patient avoid a crisis while at home. It will be seen too that the major need was for education over a relatively short space of time.

Although the time spent in hospital by many patients is considerably less than formerly, many do have problems which are not resolved immmediately. In such cases the page-a-problem format is very useful, in that the problem can be readily monitored over a period of time. For example, John Hughes (Chapter 3) had considerable difficulty with meeting the objectives for handling some of his problems. The page-a-problem format suited him extremely well.

That all relevant information is on a care plan is important. For example, when Mrs Witherington was readmitted, although the same nurse was not on duty, another nurse could make immediate sense of the assessment and care plan so that reassessment could occur without being unnecessarily repetitive.

The patient's role in a care plan

It was seen in Chapter 6 that there may be a difference in perception between patient and nurse over what constitutes a problem. If the patient is to have a role in planned care he needs firstly to understand the rationale behind the care, and secondly to agree that the care is necessary. Both aims may best be achieved by involving the patient whenever possible in decisions about care.

The alternative is that an individual becomes a passive recipient of care, and that may indeed be necessary in some cases such as that of the unconscious patient. However, if the patient is **not** unconscious he may become an aggressive recipient of care if he has no idea of what is happening to him or why it is happening.

When John Hughes (Chapter 3) was admitted to hospital with coronary heart disease, he was labelled 'difficult' by the staff and seen as uncooperative. The nurse who had assessed him after admission had decided that some of his

Name	Molly Witherington		Hospital No. 390467	
Date	**Problem/Deficit**	**Care to be given**	**Goal (with date)**	**Evaluation/reassess**
9.8.94	Admitted for liver biopsy	As standard care plan for liver biopsy	–	–
9.8.94 (11am)	Glucose in urine (diagnosed as diabetes)	Discuss problem with Molly	That Molly will accept treatment and remain in hospital	Discussion shows Molly has problem with daughter at home. Feels she must go home today. Willing to come back 12.8.84
	Refused to stay for stabilization			
	Patient going home without treatment	Teach to test urine and report to GP if worried	That Molly will learn to monitor urinalysis and act if ketones appear 9.8.84	Patient can test own urine. No ketones present
		Give advice on low-calorie diet	That high blood sugar will be minimized 9.8.84	Patient has good knowledge of diet. Appears to understand
		Explain symptoms of hyperglycaemia	That Molly will recognize symptoms 9.8.84	Molly unable to recount symptoms
9.8.94		Give telephone number of diabetic nurse	That Molly will have contact if problems arise 9-8-84	Molly and husband both have number and agree to call nurse if necessary
9.8.94 (5pm)	Molly does not appear to understand concept of hyperglycaemic coma	Give written information	That learning will occur at home Reassess 12-8-84	

Fig. 7.5 Care plan for Molly Witherington.

problems were associated with lifestyle. The extract from his care plan in Figure 7.6 gives an example of this.

In fact, John did not want to stop smoking, nor did he see it as a problem. The nurse was correct in identifying smoking as a contributory factor to heart disease and in hoping to stop John from continuing as a smoker. Her error was in making an arbitrary decision without assessing John's knowledge and beliefs, and in failing to gain his co-operation on a planned programme of non-smoking.

A different approach to John's smoking behaviour might have been planned as in Figure 7.7.

The difference between the first plan and the second is that the first prohibits a certain behaviour while the second allows for informed choice.

Some care that is planned does not allow for choice. The patient with retention of urine may need to be catheterized whether or not he approves of the procedure. In this instance catheter care is given as a necessity. However, a nurse will still need to explain what is happen-

MULTIDISCIPLINARY CARE PLAN

DATE 10/4/95   PROBLEM No. 670395

PROBLEM/DEFICIT:

10/4/95 Pt smokes 40 a day.

GOALS:

The pt stops smoking

ACTIONS:

Remove cigarettes

NAME: John Hughes

Fig. 7.6 Care plan for John Hughes.

EVALUATION

DATE		SIGNATURE
12/4/95	Pt uncomfortable. Demanding cigarettes	J. Smith

Fig. 7.6 *Continued*

MULTIDISCIPLINARY CARE PLAN

DATE 10 | 4 | 95

PROBLEM No. 670395

PROBLEM/DEFICIT:

10/4/95 Pt smokes 40 a day.

GOALS:

The patient will decide to give up smoking

ACTIONS:

Discourage from smoking.
Give booklet
Review 17/4/95

NAME: John Hughes

Fig. 7.7 Improved care plan for John Hughes.

DATE		SIGNATURE
12/4/95	Pt has read booklet. Is asking questions	J. Smith

Fig. 7.7   *Continued*

ing and why, in order to help the patient cope with what may be an embarrassing situation.

If decision-making on appropriate care does not include the patient, careful assessment needs to be made. This should ensure that fears and worries will be explored. What is a 'normal' procedure for nursing staff may have fearful connotations for a patient which need to be explored so that all possible reassurance may be given along with clear explanations. Catheterization and aftercare are a part of nursing care 'done to' a patient. Other non-choice care may call for co-operation from the patient. It is essential that the care planned includes motivation and education for the patient, along with reassessment.

Some patients may not wish to be involved in their own care and may indeed refuse care prescribed for them. This may cause ethical problems for the nurse and other members of the health care team. What needs to be remembered is that being in hospital does not take away the rights of an individual to make a logical and rational decision. The responsibility of the health care team is to ensure that the patient has made an informed choice and is mentally able to do so.

It can be seen that involving a patient in decisions about care may be less comfortable for the nurse than making the decisions herself. However, by returning to John Hughes and his smoking, it can be seen that the nurse forbidding the patient to smoke will achieve results which last at most for his hospital stay – and may lead to illicit smoking in the lavatory. Educating John, on the other hand, may possibly lead to a permanent change in his behaviour.

The dynamic element of care plans

The dynamic element of a care plan can be seen in the evaluation/reassess column, as it is here that a nurse will record whether goals have been met by the date given. In this way, care which does not meet the patient's needs will be identified and reassessment will occur. Given that different aspects of care will have different dates for evaluation, it can be seen that the patient's care will be continually under review. In Mr Hughes's case, a week was given for initial education about smoking. That part of his care plan may look like Figure 7.8 after a week.

In fact, in the first week John had reduced his smoking but on discussion with the nurse he felt that he would try a day without cigarettes as long as he had support from the nurse.

Care plans should be designed for easy updating. It can be seen from the examples of John Hughes that the page-a-problem format allows easy updating and does not require that a problem is continually re-written on each assessment date. After review, goals should be reassessed and any new goals clearly stated with the date for review. For example, John Hughes' goal to give up smoking remains, but on 17/4/95 a smaller goal was set that the patient would manage for 24 hours without smoking at all. Until that period of time has passed it is not established if the original goal will need to be redefined or whether the patient will make a conscious decision to continue smoking in some form. Any new plans should be written down clearly by the nurse involved in the patient's care. Different nurses may care for a patient and need to be able to check which care is ongoing and which goals have been reached, updated or changed, as a result of evaluation and reassessment. Occasionally the circumstances which led to care being planned may change and this leads to reassessment before a given date. The nurse who is caring for the patient should change the plan and give her reasons in the evaluation column.

Where care plans are kept may be an issue. Some professionals believe that they should be kept in a central place where all health professionals may have ready access to them. Another belief is that they should be kept by the patient, at the end of the bed, by the locker, or somewhere so that there is no question of muddle about which care plan relates to which patient.

Another issue is that of how often evaluation and reassessment should take place. With the implementation of the Patient's Charter and promises from the Government on what patients may expect in terms of care, there is now more emphasis on the legal issues surrounding patient care. If goals are set and evaluation does not occur for a period of time, it could be argued that this constitutes neglect of a patient. For this reason the proposed date for evaluation should be set clearly with each goal and subsequent action to reach that goal. Where possible, these evaluation dates should be agreed in terms of realism and also in terms of the expected co-operation from a patient. Often the most realistic review dates are set by the patient. John Hughes, for example, decided that he would try 24 hours without smoking and see how it was for him. Similarly, Mrs Witherington agreed that what she needed was two days to sort out her problems at home. She then willingly came back.

MULTIDISCIPLINARY CARE PLAN

DATE 10/4/95   PROBLEM No. 67 0395

PROBLEM/DEFICIT:

10/4/95 Pt smokes 40 a day

17/4/95 Pt continues to smoke 30 a day

GOALS:

The patient will decide to give up smoking

17/4/95 That pt will manage 24 hrs without smoking
7pm – 7pm 17th – 18th

ACTIONS:

Discourage from smoking
Give booklet
Review 17/4/95

Attempt to change situations where smoking is
most likely to occur. 17/4/95

NAME: John Hughes

Fig. 7.8 Care plan for John Hughes after one week.

EVALUATION

DATE		SIGNATURE
12/4/95	Pt has read booklet. Is asking questions	J. Smith
17/4/95	Has reduced smoking by 10 a day. Says he needs help. Has agreed to try 24 hours without smoking	J. Smith

Fig. 7.8 *Continued*

Even if review dates cannot be set by the patient for particular reasons, like regimens of care that have to be prescribed, then they should still be discussed with the patient so that he understands why he is expected to reach a certain goal in a certain time.

The reality of care plans means that assessment, care and evaluation are happening all the time, instead of each stage in the process having to be completed for all the problems of an individual before the next can occur. This dynamic element of the process should lead to high-quality care planned on the basis of ongoing assessment and evaluation.

Summary

In this chapter, care plans have been considered in both standard and individualized forms.

Standard care plans are useful in situations where an individual's problems are known to be common, such as pre- and post-operative care and care of the unconscious patient.

Individualized care plans have the advantage of allowing care to be planned on the basis of a patient's specific problems. It is possible to combine standard and individualized plans for the same patient.

Where possible, care should be planned with the co-operation and understanding of the patient. It should be regularly monitored and updated by the nurse caring for the patient.

References

Faulkner, A. (1981) Aye, there's the rub. *Nursing Times*, *77*(28), 332–336.

Hampton, D. C. (1993) Implementing a managed care framework through care maps. *Journal of Nursing Administration*, *23*(5), 21–27.

Haywood, J. & Boore, J. (1994) *Information: a prescription against pain*. Research Classics from RCN, vol. 1. London: Scutari Press.

Hollanders, D. (1979) *Gastrointestinal endoscopy*. London: Baillière Tindall.

McFarlane, J. & Castledine, G. (1982) *A guide to the practice of nursing using the nursing process*. London: C. V. Mosby.

Rasmussen, N. & Genglee, T. (1994) Critical pathways of care; the route to better communication. *Nursing*, *24*, 47–49.

Trella, R. S. (1993) A multi-disciplinary approach to case management of frail, hospitalised, older adults. *Journal of Nursing Administration, 23*(2), 20–26.

Further reading

Brandrick, J. (1980) Nursing care study: a nursing care plan for convalescence following a cardiovascular accident. *Nursing Times, 76*(29), 1253–1257.

Clark, M. (1978) Planning nursing care. *Nursing Times*, Occasional Papers, *74*(5), 17–20.

Hunt, J. M. & Marks-Moran, D. (1990) *Nursing care plans: the nursing process at work*. London: Scutari Press.

Jaffe, M. (1991) *Medical, surgical, nursing care plans*, 2nd edn. New York: Appleton and Lang.

May, C. (1992) Individual care: power and subjectivity in therapeutic relationships. *Sociology, 26*(4), 589–602.

National Health Service and Community Care Act (1990) London: HMSO.

Richardson, A. (1991) *The Royal Marsden Hospital book of core care plans for cancer nursing*. London: Scutari Press.

8

Maintaining Records

CHAPTER SUMMARY

The documentation required for each patient, 175
Medical records, 175
Drug records, 176
Charts, 179

The nursing record as a legal document, 184
Legal status of nursing records, 187

Co-ordination and the nursing records, 189
Patient transfer, 190

Summary, 190

Reference, 191

Further reading, 191

The documentation required for each patient

From previous chapters it will be seen that there are a number of nursing records required for each patient, i.e. a record of admission and assessment, and a care plan. Some hospitals' documentation incorporates all this information into one document called the nursing record. Others may have a separate assessment form from which the care plan is derived. It is a nursing duty to maintain these and other records and to ensure their safe keeping.

Patients may ask to see their records, and have a right to do so, providing that the Consultant cannot see any contraindication to this. This adds to the responsibility of keeping coherent records that can be readily understood.

Medical records

Each patient will have a medical record in addition to any nursing records. This is primarily the responsibility of the medical staff and will constitute an individual's medical history. It is a statutory requirement that medical records are stored in the hospital for a minimum of eight years after a patient's discharge.

When a patient is admitted to hospital for the first time he is given a hospital number. This number is used on all documents and is a safeguard against individuals with the same name being confused with each other in their diag-

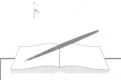

Why do you think it is important to keep patient records? What are the advantages to the patient? What are the advantages for staff responsible for the patient's care?

nosis, treatment and care. Should a patient be readmitted, his medical record will be sent to the ward from the medical records office and he will retain his original hospital number.

The medical record is the property of the hospital. This means that if a patient is moved around the country he could have records in several hospitals. Occasionally, if a consultant requests information about a patient from a colleague in another part of the country, notes will be transferred, but more usually a detailed letter, giving a synopsis of the patient's past medical history, will be sent.

While a patient is in hospital, his medical record is stored in a trolley on the ward, sometimes in Sister's office. Medical records are confidential documents and it is a nursing duty to maintain confidentiality by allowing only authorized personnel to have access to them.

Drug records

Each ward has a drug documentation system which includes a prescription sheet for every patient (Figure 8.1). This sheet contains the patient's name, hospital number and any known allergies. It is used to list current medication, which must be written up and signed by the doctor. Times for drugs are ticked as given, with dates for their administration. There is also space for 'as required' prescriptions and for once only/premedication prescriptions. On the back of the sheet demonstrated here (Figure 8.2) there is a section for non-administration and notes on how to use the sheet.

In the past, drugs have only been prescribed by a qualified medical practitioner and this includes writing the patient's drug prescriptions. However, recent legislation for community nurses has allowed some prescribing authority. In other situations, the UKCC code for administration of medicines does not allow prescribing by nurses. This can occasionally cause difficulties if a medical colleague telephones and asks a nurse to give a drug which is not written up. The doctor may suggest that the nurse writes in the new drug and may also promise to sign the entry later. Such action on the part of the nurse may be against the local policy of the hospital and is certainly against the recommendations of the UKCC code. Under normal circumstances, no drugs except those which can be prescribed by a nurse should be given to any patient unless they are written up and signed by the doctor. This caution helps to ensure that the drug prescribed is the

HOSPITAL/WARD		UNIT NUMBER	AGE
CONSULTANT		SURNAME (Block Letters)	
HOUSE OFFICER		FIRST NAMES	

REGULAR PRESCRIPTIONS	AFFIX CONTINUATION SHEET HERE

MONTH & DATE →

TICK TIMES REQUIRED OR ENTER VARIABLE DOSE ↓

1

Route	Dose	Start	Finish

0900
1400
1800
2200

Special Directions

Signature · Pharm

2

Route	Dose	Start	Finish

0900
1400
1800
2200

Special Directions

Signature · Pharm

3

Route	Dose	Start	Finish

0900
1400
1800
2200

Special Directions

Signature · Pharm

4

Route	Dose	Start	Finish

0900
1400
1800
2200

Special Directions

Signature · Pharm

5

Route	Dose	Start	Finish

0900
1400
1800
2200

Special Directions

Signature · Pharm

6

Route	Dose	Start	Finish

0900
1400
1800
2200

Special Directions

Signature · Pharm

7

Route	Dose	Start	Finish

0900
1400
1800
2200

Special Directions

Signature · Pharm

8

Route	Dose	Start	Finish

0900
1400
1800
2200

Special Directions

Signature · Pharm

Fig. 8.1 A drug prescription sheet. Reproduced with kind permission from the Practice Development Unit at Seacroft Hospital, Leeds.

Fig. 8.2 Reverse of the drug prescription sheet shown in Fig. 8.1. Reproduced with kind permission from the Practice Development Unit at Seacroft Hospital, Leeds.

NON-ADMINISTRATION

MEDICINE	REASON OMITTED	SIGNATURE	DATE

drug given to the patient and it also protects the nurse against possible litigation.

Similarly with cancellation of drugs: these should be cancelled by a doctor, who will sign his name and put in the date. An exception to this may be prescribed courses of treatment. For example, if the prescription states clearly that it is for, say, five days, the nurse will be expected to take responsibility for discontinuation of that drug when the treatment is complete.

The nurse's responsibility for the drug records lies primarily in ensuring that when drugs are given they are accurately recorded on the drug sheet. Both the nurse giving and the nurse checking the drug will sign that the correct amount of the correct drug has been given by the correct route.

Although actual prescribing is a medical responsibility, it is sensible for a nurse to take the responsibility for ensuring that what is prescribed is decipherable. This may sound so obvious as to be unnecessary to mention. In fact, doctors may forget to print the name of the drug unless the nurse requests it, or may use a trade name instead of the generic term. Many drugs have similar names, and mistakes caused by misinterpretation may have serious effects for both the patient and the nurse responsible for the error.

Drug records are now commonly held at the patient's bedside, though formerly stored in the ward manager's office. The ward manager is responsible for keeping these records up to date in terms of patients' names and numbers, and ensuring that the record follows the sequence of the ward plan. There is now extra emphasis on the responsibility of the named nurse, even though the ultimate responsibility lies with the ward manager. There is also a responsibility for ensuring that records are removed from the bed or the container used when the patient is discharged.

Charts

Although drug records may be kept in the ward manager's office, other documentation is now much more likely to be kept by the patient's bedside. Patients have a right to read these documents and it can be argued that this will encourage the individual to be more involved in his care than previously when patients were simply expected to be a relatively passive recipient of care.

Keeping charts by the bedside allows easy access and considerably less likelihood of notes being muddled between one patient and another. Each patient has a number of documents which are normally kept on a clipboard or in a ringbinder which hangs on the bottom rail of the bed. There is considerable variation in documentation from one hospital to another; the charts used in this chapter are for illustrative purposes only, since it would be impossible to include all variations.

Charts for recording temperature, pulse and respiration

Most patients have a temperature, pulse and respiration chart (Figure 5.8) which allows staff to see at a glance if there are abnormal variations in temperature, pulse, respiration and blood pressure. The standard chart was formerly called a BD chart, BD being an abbreviation of the latin *bis in die*, which means twice a day and which is the usual interval for taking temperature, pulse and respiration on general wards. These charts are now more commonly called TPR charts.

On some wards these observations may be taken only

once a day and on wards for elderly patients they may not be taken at all, unless a patient appears to show signs of change.

If a patient has problems or deficits which could affect temperature, pulse or respiration, a second chart may be used to allow four-hourly or more frequent observations to be made. In some instances, e.g. after neurosurgery, a separate chart may be used for recording an individual's temperature, pulse and respiration at frequent intervals (Figure 8.3). Such charts are normally used in addition to the TPR chart.

Charts for recording fluid balance

Another very common chart used for individual patients is the fluid balance chart, on which a record is kept of all fluid intake and output for those patients with actual or potential problems of fluid balance (Figure 8.4).

The nurse is responsible for keeping clear, accurate charts for each patient in her care. There are particular problems with fluid balance charts because patients may be vague in describing how much fluid has been taken, and may occasionally forget to tell the nurse when they have had a drink. In these circumstances it is tempting for the nurse to chart each drink as it is brought to the patient so that it is not forgotten, but if the patient then takes only part of the drink and the cup is taken away by a non-nurse, the chart is no longer an accurate record of fluid balance.

One method of recording fluid balance is to 'top up' the cup or glass with water from the patient's measured jug. This ensures a more accurately recorded intake if any fluid taken from the cup or glass is unfinished. If the fluid balance record is in evidence, all grades of staff will follow this procedure on removing crockery.

The most accurate fluid balance charts are probably those kept by the patient. Any patient who is able to may be encouraged to keep his own record but will need to know the standard measure of the cups and glasses used on the ward. However, allowing the patient to participate in his care does not remove the responsibility for the charts from the nurse.

Charts for recording urinalysis

Some patients may need regular urinalysis. An example of this is the patient with diabetes who needs to know if there are any glucose and ketones in his urine. There are special 'diabetic' charts for patients which will be kept by the patient's bed, and these may also be used to record blood glucose (Figure 8.5).

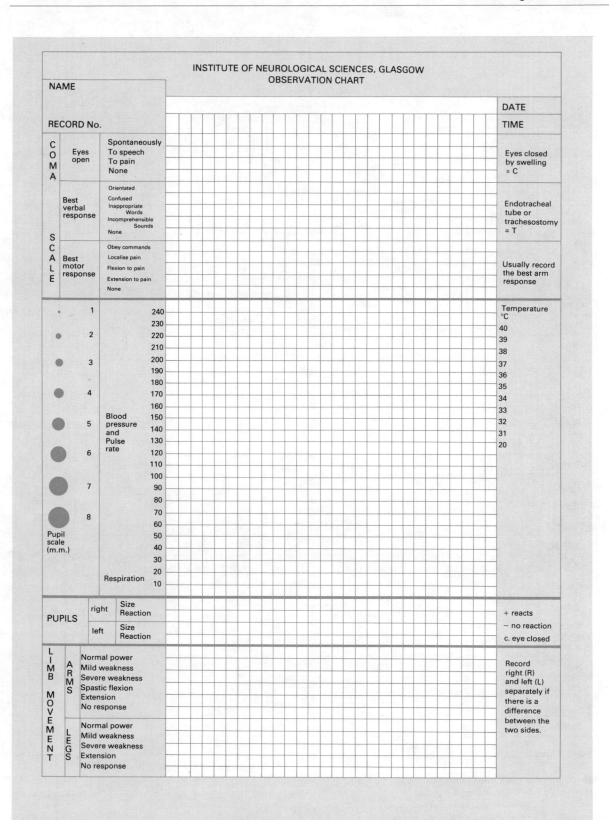

Fig. 8.3 The Glasgow coma scale.

Unit No.	
Surname	
First names	

All measurements in ml.

| Hour | Intake | | | Output | | | |
| | Mouth | Intravenous | | Urine | Vomit | Aspirate | Other |
		Fluid	Volume				
9 am							
10 am							
11 am							
12 M.D.							
1 pm							
2 pm							
3 pm							
4 pm							
5 pm							
6 pm							
7 pm							
8 pm							
9 pm							
10 pm							
11 pm							
12 M.N.							
1 am							
2 am							
3 am							
4 am							
5 am							
6 am							
7 am							
8 am							
Total							

Grand total for intake

Total output

Allowance for insensible loss

Grand total

Record intravenous fluid volume when each bottle has been infused

Date

Balance

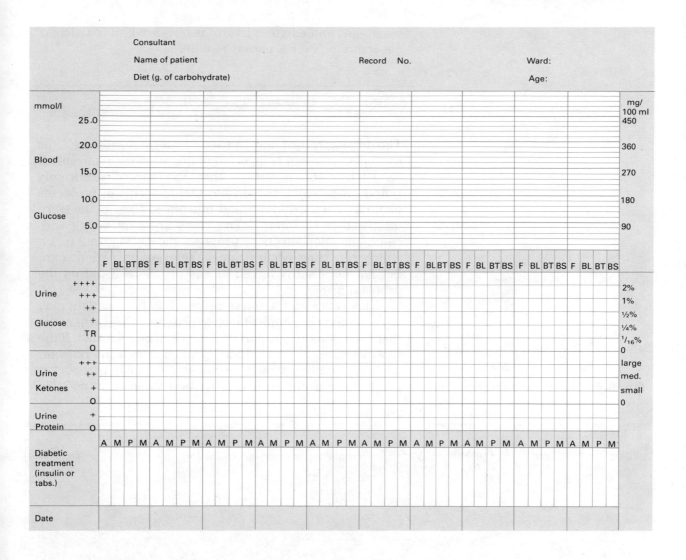

Fig. 8.5 A diabetic chart.

As with fluid balance charts, the best person to fill in a 'diabetic' chart may well be the patient. The patient with diabetes needs to learn how to test his own urine so he can monitor himself at home. If taught how, he will probably keep a more accurate record than one filled in by many nurses. Teaching patients to look after their charts does not remove the responsibility from nurses to ensure that the tests ordered have been carried out.

When a patient is discharged, the charts are usually put into the patient's medical notes along with other nursing records.

The charts discussed here are common to most wards. Other, specialized charts may also be seen on the wards

◀ **Fig. 8.4** A fluid balance chart.

when an immediate picture is required of particular observations over a period of time.

The nursing record as a legal document

The nursing record may be used as a legal document if, for example, a patient is involved in litigation with a hospital. As such it is important that the record accurately reflects a patient's stay in hospital in terms of problems identified, actions taken and outcomes. Care plans were discussed in Chapter 7. The plans are kept, along with communication sheets or progress sheets (Figure 8.6), on which reporting occurs that is relevant to patient care but not necessarily linked to any problems listed on the problem pages.

Theoretically, the nurse responsible for a patient may write on the communications or progress sheet whenever there is anything to report that needs to be recorded. If the report relates to an identified problem, then the relevant problem number should be noted. Obviously a report is much more accurate if it is written as soon as possible

Fig. 8.6 Example of a progress sheet.

Date	Time	Problem No.	Progress, reassessment, evaluation	Signature

Number	Surname	Age	Religion	Diagnosis	Consultant

Date	Time	Problem No.	Progress, reassessment, evaluation	Signature
8-4-95	6 pm	6	Visited husband. Distressed	SB
9-4-95	6 am	/	Slept well after Mogadon II	JE
9-4-95	6 pm		Hair washed. Weepy	SB
10-4-95	6 am		Restless. Incontinent	JE
10-4-95	6 pm		Tired after trip. Very weepy	SB
11-4-95	6 am		Better night	JE

after an event and by the nurse responsible rather than the nurse in charge, but this does not always occur.

Fig. 8.7 Progress sheet for Jessie Mayhew.

Jessie Mayhew, an elderly patient, was admitted to a medical ward when her husband was in a different hospital. This separation was accepted as a problem for Mrs Mayhew, which was to be resolved by arranging for her to visit her husband. A nurse assigned to care for Mrs Mayhew, after several days off duty, read the progress sheet shown in Figure 8.7.

The nurse assumed from the sketchy report that visiting her husband had upset Mrs Mayhew. In fact, Jessie's husband had died on the night after Jessie's visit to him. If this had been reported, the weepiness and upset would have been explained and the nurse would have avoided the further upset of asking 'How was your husband yesterday?' when the patient's visit had actually been to the mortuary.

No matter which form of documentation is used, the aim is that **changes** should be accurately described. In Mrs Mayhew's case her husband's death clearly was of major import and could either have been written on the care plan as a new problem associated with a need to grieve, or subsumed under problem 6, in which the change, i.e. death of husband, should have been clearly recorded.

There is no need to put an entry on a document if there is no change in a patient's condition. The feeling that there should be something written down may lead to the type of entry shown in Figure 8.8, which in fact gives very little indication of a patient's current state.

As with Mrs Mayhew's progress sheet, problem numbers have been ignored in favour of general statements which are meaningless to anyone who does not have personal knowledge of the patient.

Just as in verbal interactions, ambiguous words and vague phrases should be avoided when making written reports on patients. 'Good night' or 'Good day' can mean very different things to different people. For example, a patient who complains of sleepless nights might feel that two or three hours' unbroken sleep constituted a 'good night' while the patient who takes eight hours' sleep a night for granted would consider two or three hours a very poor night. It follows that reports on patients should be relative to each individual's experiences.

Returning to Mrs Mayhew's problem, her progress sheet might have read as in Figure 8.9. This more detailed report of a major problem for Mrs Mayhew means that a new nurse caring for her would quickly gain knowledge of

Fig. 8.8 An uninformative progress sheet.

Date	Time	Problem No.	Progress, reassessment, evaluation	Signature
6.7.95	6 p.m.		No change	A.S.
7.7.95	6 am		Good Night	JB
7.7.95	6 p.m.		Good Day	A.S.

Date	Time	Problem No.	Progress, reassessment, evaluation	Signature
8.4.95	6pm	6	Visited husband. Distressed by his condition. Very tired and dispirited on return to ward.	SB
9.4.95	6am		Difficulty in settling. Mogadon 10mg 10.30pm. Slept until 4am. Appears anxious about husband	JC
9.4.95	11am	6	Received phone call of husband's death. News broken to patient. Appears confused. Unbelieving. Valium given 10mg. 10.50am	SB
9.4.95	4pm		Daughter visited. Patient tearful. Demanding to see husbands body. To visit mortuary 10am 10-4-84	SB
10.4.95	6am		Restless night. Fitful sleep after Mogadon 10mg. 11pm. Withdrawn this am.	JC
10.4.95	12noon	6	Patient visited mortuary. Returned quiet and withdrawn. Daughter who accompanied her, stayed for lunch. Funeral arranged for 12-4-84	SB

the recent important events affecting care. Of course, Mrs Mayhew might have had other problems which would also be documented on the progress sheet if there were changes to report.

Fig. 8.9 Improved progress sheet for Jessie Mayhew.

Legal status of nursing records

Nursing records not only help staff to give co-ordinated care, but may be called for if there are any questions arising about a patient's care. Although most patients appear to be quite satisfied with the care received, complaints are occasionally made to an authority, and sometimes a patient or his relatives will take legal action if they believe that medical or nursing staff have been negligent in their care or treatment. At such times the records that have been kept for a patient are of paramount importance, and if a case actually goes to court, a nurse could well be asked why the story that she gives about what happened to a patient is either not in the nursing record or

Patient transfer check list	
Surname:	Transfer from:
Forname(s):	To:
Date of birth: (use patient label if available)	Consultant:

Next of kin notified?   Yes ☐   No ☐   If yes, name:

Relationship:

Notified by telephone ☐ Letter ☐ Verbal ☐

Reasons for transfer:

Investigations/appointments booked   Yes ☐   No ☐
If yes, specify:

Summary of nursing requirements

Diet   Special ☐   Ordinary ☐
If special, specify:

Pressure areas intact?   Yes ☐   No ☐   If no, specify:

Incontinence	Urinary	Yes ☐	No ☐	Bowel	Yes ☐	No ☐
Ambulent		Yes ☐	No ☐	Specify aids:		
Fire risk		Yes ☐	No ☐			
Property/valuables with patient		Yes ☐	No ☐	If no, location:		
Notes enclosed		Yes ☐	No ☐			
X-rays enclosed		Yes ☐	No ☐			

Special instructions/comments:

(Continue overleaf, if necessary)

Names of medication in use (omit dosage):

Name (in block letters):	Grade:
Signature:	Date:

Fig. 8.10 A patient transfer sheet.

in the nursing record but written in a different, or less clear form. The fact that the nursing record is a legal document and that the person who signs their name against an entry is responsible for that entry means that nurses need to be very careful about accuracy in making any report on a patient in their care.

Mr Abraham was a confused, elderly patient who was admitted to a medical ward for investigations of abdominal cramps. The nursing staff positioned his bed where it could be readily seen from both the ward desk and Sister's office. They also put up cot sides on the bed to guard Mr Abraham from falling out.

One day, Mr Abraham climbed over the cot sides, fell, and fractured his right femur. At the time, Sister was checking drugs with a junior nurse at the far end of the ward and the other two nurses on duty were making beds in a side ward.

Mr Abraham's relatives claimed that the fall was due to neglect on the part of the nurses.

If the nursing record had been vague – that is, if there were statements such as 'confused but slept well' or 'noisy day', it would have been difficult to disprove neglect. A clearly written report, stating that cot sides had been used, that nurses were aware of the confusion and had taken positive action, i.e. moved the bed, could lead to the verdict that what had happened was a regrettable accident which the nursing staff had attempted to avoid.

Questions may still be asked about staff numbers, confused patients on medical wards, and the use of cot sides. The point, however, is to do with producing clear documentation of what has occurred during a patient's stay in hospital.

Co-ordination and the nursing records

Although the progress, reassessment and evaluation chart is used for day-to-day reporting of changes in problems and care, it may also be used to co-ordinate information from other sources.

If a patient is pyrexial, it can be argued that changes will be reflected in the temperature, pulse and respiration chart, but it is also worth noting any major changes on the progress chart using the appropriate problem number; similarly with other observations. This does not make standard observational charts redundant but it does alert a nurse to changes in a patient's state.

Controlled drugs may also be written on the progress chart. In some hospitals, controlled drugs, i.e. those drugs which are defined in the Misuse of Drugs Act 1971

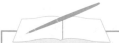

Take the care plan and accompanying documentation for a patient in your care. How precise are the entries? Are all entries signed? How could the records be improved? Would you be comfortable for a coroner to see the entries?

(Connechen *et al.* 1983), are recorded in the ward book for controlled drugs and on the patient's drug sheet. In this case, the drug may be written in another colour, or underlined, on the progress chart together with the dose, route and time given.

If the nursing record is used in this way, it provides a succinct record of day-to-day change and care, which, with a regularly updated care plan, will allow co-ordinated care even with a complete change of nursing staff.

Patient transfer

Occasionally it is necessary to transfer a patient from one ward to another or indeed from one hospital to another. If this occurs it is usual to send information about the patient to the new location. Some hospitals simply send the medical notes, nursing records and a covering letter, while others have a transfer sheet such as that shown in Figure 8.10. If the transfer is from hospital to hospital it may not be possible to send medical notes or nursing records.

Sending adequate documentation when a patient is transferred can ease the transition for the patient, who may be stressed by what is, to him, a further upheaval in his life. Even if the patient is ambulant, it will help to reduce the stress of transfer to a different ward, if a nurse known to him can accompany him and introduce him to his new environment.

Summary

It can be seen from this and previous chapters that there is a considerable amount of documentation required for each patient. Used correctly, this documentation provides an accurate profile of a patient's stay in hospital.

The nursing record contains a care plan along with a communication sheet or progress chart for day-to-day reporting of change in a patient's physical, social and psychological state. This may also be used to note changes which are reported in more detail on a variety of observational charts.

The drug record contains a space for prescribing drugs, which is the responsibility of the medical staff, a sheet for recording drugs given, space to note drugs that were prescribed but were not given, and space for drugs that are given occasionally or perhaps only once, e.g. pre-operative drugs. Any drugs that are given occasionally or on a one-off basis, and any controlled drugs given may be reported on the progress communication sheet to show that change required different measures.

All records for a patient constitute legal documents that may be called upon in case of complaint, sudden death or aberration. For this reason, all documents should be clearly written, dated and signed at all times. The observant nurse will monitor the documentation for each patient and report any change to the nurse in charge of the ward or the doctor responsible for the patient's care.

Reference

Connechen, J., Robson, R. H. & Shanley, E. (1983) *Pharmacology for Nurses*. London: Baillière Tindall.

Further reading

Kolin, P. C. & Kolin, J. L. (1980) *Professional writing for nurses.* St Louis: C. V. Mosby.

Lelean, S. (1973) *Ready for report nurse?* London: Rcn.

NHS Training Directorate (no year given) *Keeping the records straight: a guide to record keeping for nurses, midwives and health visitors*. London: NHS Management Executive.

NHS Management Executive (1991) *Access to Health Records Act (1990). A guide for the NHS*. London: NHSME.

PART FOUR
PROBLEMS AND PLANS FOR CARE

9

Towards Diagnosis

CHAPTER SUMMARY

Diagnostic investigations, 196

Investigations of blood, 196
Glucose tolerance test, 197

**Investigations of bodily excretions/
secretions, 200**
Faeces, 200
Urine, 201
Sputum, 203
Pleural effusion, 204
Ascites, 205
Cerebrospinal fluid, 205

Investigations of body tissue, 206
Endoscopy: general factors, 208
Biopsy: general factors, 211
Investigative endoscopic and biopsy
procedures, 211

X-rays, 219
Routine radiographic views ('straight' films),
219

Specialized radiographic views, 220
Scans, 225

**Investigations recording electro-activity in
the body, 228**
Electrocardiogram, 228
Electroencephalogram, 229

Towards diagnosis: the nurse's role, 230
Blood pressure, 230
Urinalysis, 234
Fluid balance, 236

Co-ordination of information, 238
Reactions to diagnosis, 239
Complementary therapies, 240

Summary, 241

References, 241

Further reading, 242

It was seen in Chapter 5 that deficits in normal physical, social and psychological functioning may lead to an individual being unable to lead the life to which he is accustomed. In many cases the patient's GP may be able to give a rapid explanation for the particular deficit and advise measures which will restore the patient to his previously healthy state.

There may, however, be a number of potential explanations for the presenting symptoms which will cause the GP to suggest investigations, diagnosis and treatment. Similarly he may suggest admission to hospital if the deficits in normal functioning are having a severe effect on the patient. In either case the patient may arrive on the ward with only a provisional diagnosis or no diagnosis at all.

When a doctor makes a medical diagnosis, he is determining the cause of the patient's presenting symptoms. He is helped in his decision making by knowledge of the patient's history, by carrying out a physical examination and by the diagnostic investigations he may make in an out-patient department, or which may be carried out after admission to a ward.

Diagnostic investigations

Diagnostic investigations are requested by the doctor in charge of the patient and may be carried out in specialist departments or on the ward. For all tests a request form is completed and signed by a member of the medical staff and, if the test is not carried out on the ward, the request form should be forwarded to the appropriate department immediately. Even if the nurse is not personally involved in the investigations, she needs to be aware of how and why they are performed so that she can meet the patient's need for explanation and reassurance as he attempts to make sense of what is happening to him.

Investigations may be requested to confirm a diagnosis or to establish a diagnosis. A variety of tests may be required in either event, which will be linked to the deficits described by the patient or his family. No assumptions can be made of the patient's understanding of what is happening to him, so it is essential to make a careful assessment of his knowledge and need for information.

A major problem for nursing staff lies in the fact that most investigations soon become very familiar to them. It then becomes difficult to 'tune in' to a patient's apprehensions or indeed to recognize that such apprehensions are present. This can lead to facetious remarks about investigations when what the patient requires is support and empathy from the nurse.

Investigations of blood

Specimens of an individual's blood can give considerable information about the normal and abnormal functioning of the blood and blood-forming organs and a number of other body systems and processes. Consequently blood tests are often the first investigations to be carried out after admission.

Investigations are usually concerned with the composition of the blood and in some instances, e.g. when liver disease is suspected, its ability to clot. The tests are usually divided into two groups, haematological and biochemical. Haematology is concerned with the measurement of blood cells and clotting, while biochemistry involves the measurement of electrolytes, proteins, enzymes, iron, vitamins, pH, cholesterol, glucose, carbon dioxide, oxygen, hormones, urea and creatinine (Table 9.1). In addition to the above tests, speciments of blood are sent to the microbiology laboratory when infection of the blood is suspected.

The specific blood tests requested by the doctor will depend on the patient's signs and symptoms. A patient who is breathless on exertion and appears pale may be anaemic, and measurement of haemoglobin and the red cell count would be two of the first tests to be carried out. Similarly, a patient who has problems of excessive thirst and polyuria would have tests to measure the glucose levels in the blood to exclude or confirm a diagnosis of diabetes.

Depending on the test(s) required, blood may be collected from an artery, a vein or a capillary. The commonest site is from any readily accessible vein in the arm, usually in the antecubital fossa.

The patient is asked to hold his arm out straight. A cuff, which restricts circulation, is put around the arm above the elbow and the blood is drawn up from a vein into a syringe (Figure 9.1). The cuff is then released, the patient asked to hold a small pressure pad against the puncture site, and the blood is transferred to an appropriate bottle or bottles for the test and taken to the laboratory.

Many people are frightened by the sight of blood and by 'needles' being put into them. The nurse may help by accompanying the doctor and acting in a supportive role towards the patient, by explaining the procedure and by explaining the need for a particular test or tests. If a patient needs to have specimens taken several times during the day or night, or even daily over a period of time, he is more likely to be co-operative if he understands the rationale behind the action.

Glucose tolerance test

This is an example of a combined investigation of blood with another body substance – in this case urine, to give specific diagnostic information about patients with suspected diabetes mellitus.

A glucose tolerance test is performed in order to test

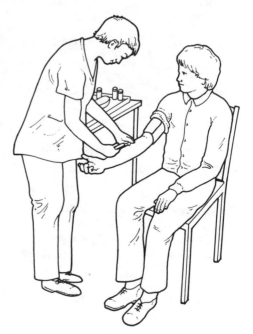

Fig. 9.1 Blood being taken.

Table 9.1 Normal values for common blood tests, with examples of associated diseases.

Blood test	Normal range (SI units)	Raised levels in	Lowered levels in
Haemoglobin – men – women	13.5–18.0 g/dl 11.5–16.5 g/dl	Dehydration Polycythaemia Hypoxia	Anaemias
Red cell count – men – women	4.5–6.5×10^{12}/l 3.8–5.8×10^{12}/l	Dehydration Polycythaemia Hypoxia	Anaemias
White cell count	4–11×10^{9}/l	Leukaemias Bacterial infections	Aplastic anaemia Agranulocytosis Viral infections
Platelets	150–400×10^{9}/l	Generalized infecions Thrombocythaemia After surgery	Idiopathic and secondary thrombocytopenia

Prothrombin time	12–18 s
	(depends on technique)
	  used)
		Liver disease
		Use of anticoagulant
		  drugs	

Clotting time	3–11 min (depends on technique used)	Haemorrhagic disorders	
Erythrocyte sedimentation rate – men – women	3–5 mm in 1 h 4–7 mm in 1 h	Infections Collagen diseases Myelomatosis	Polycythaemia
Sodium	136–148 mmol/l	Cushing's syndrome Dehydration	Addison's disease Vomiting Diarrhoea
Potassium	3.5–5 mmol/l	Advanced renal failure Addison's disease Diabetic coma	Cushing's syndrome Glomerulonephritis Gastrointestinal fluid loss Use of diuretics
Chloride	95–105 mmol/l	Metabolic acidosis Cushing's syndrome Dehydration	Prolonged vomiting Prolonged gastric aspiration Addison's disease
Glucose – fasting	<5.5 mmol/l	Diabetes mellitus Cushing's syndrome Hyperthyroidism	Hypoglycaemia Insulinoma
Urea	2.5–6.6 mmol/l	Kidney disease Dehydration Obstruction of the urinary tract	Liver disease Malnutrition
Creatinine	62–124 μmol/l		
Oxygen (PO_2)	11–13 kPa	Not clinically important	Respiratory diseases, e.g. asthma Congestive cardiac failure
Carbon dioxide (PCO_2)	4.8–6 kPa	Respiratory diseases	Overventilation due to hysteria or during anaesthesia
Total proteins – total albumen	62–82 g/l 50–65% of total protein	Dehydration	Nephrotic syndrome Burns Liver disease
– total globulin	35–50% of total protein	Liver disease Sarcoidosis Collagen diseases	Not clinically useful

the body's ability to clear excess glucose from the blood stream so that the blood sugar is returned to within normal limits (<5.5 mmol/l). In order to do this, specimens of blood and urine are collected as follows:

1 The patient is fasted overnight; then specimens of venous blood and urine are collected to give the fasting glucose levels.
2 The patient is asked to drink 50–100 g of glucose dissolved in water.
3 Blood and urine specimens are collected at a half-hour, one, two and three hours after the glucose has been taken.
4 Laboratory measures are made of the glucose levels in the blood and urine specimens and curves are drawn to show the rise in blood glucose levels and their return to normal, along with the glucose levels in the urine over time.

In patients who do not have diabetes the blood sugar will rise after the concentrated glucose drink but will return to normal within two hours. Urine will remain glucose-free. In the patient who is diabetic, the blood sugar will rise more sharply and take longer to return to normal (up to six hours) (Figure 9.2). Glucose will appear in the urine as a result of the blood sugar rising above the 'glucose renal threshold' in the absence of insulin, which is normally secreted in the pancreas (see Chapter 2, p. 35).

The test is unpleasant for the patient because the

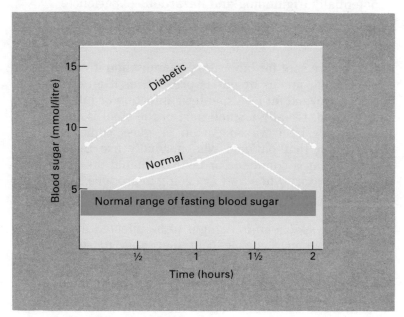

Fig. 9.2 Glucose tolerance curve.

concentrated glucose drink can seem very sickly on an empty stomach and because a number of separate blood specimens are taken. The nurse's role is to make sure that the patient understands the procedure and has any questions answered. It is also important that the patient understands the need to fast until the test is over. The major concern for the patient may be the implication of the results for diagnosis, if this has been discussed. Assessment is necessary to avoid inappropriate information and reassurance being given to an individual.

Investigations of bodily excretions/secretions

Bodily excretions/secretions may be examined in the laboratory for abnormalities: they can give valuable information on the areas from which they come. In general these specimens are collected by nursing staff with the co-operation of the patient. The nurse should check that the patient's particulars, i.e. name, hospital number and ward, are correctly entered on the request form and on the specimen container, and that the patient understands fully what is expected of him. There are some bodily secretions, e.g. those mentioned at the end of this section, which must be removed from the patient by a doctor using specialized equipment and techniques. The nurse's main role is in preparing the patient for what is to occur and in supporting and observing the patient during and after a potentially frightening and hazardous experience.

Faeces

Faeces are sent for laboratory examination if it is thought that blood, mucus or pus is present, or if an absence of bile, abnormal fat levels, enteric infection or infestation is suspected. Usually a small part of the stool is sent to the laboratory in a waxed carton or glass container. It is important that patients who normally use the lavatory rather than a commode or bedpan should take a bedpan to the lavatory when they are going to produce a specimen of faeces, and inform the nurse when they have done so.

If the specimen is thought to be infected it should be despatched in a sterile container and, in some cases, taken to the laboratory immediately (hot stool specimen) so that the micro-organisms can be more easily detected. The nurse should be careful in handling such a specimen to avoid unnecessary contamination of herself and her surroundings: afterwards she should carry out the appropriate disinfection/disposal procedure for the bedpan and its remaining contents.

Occasionally, as in fat absorption tests, the whole stool is requested (a faecal fat collection). The patient is given a diet containing a known amount of fat, and all stools are collected in large plastic or waxed containers for a three- to five-day period; the total fat content is then estimated in the laboratory.

Table 9.2 shows abnormalities of faeces and the implications for diagnosis.

Urine

Many tests of particular aspects of the composition of urine may be carried out on the ward by nursing staff and are considered on pp. 234–236. There are, however, some investigations of urine carried out in the laboratory, e.g. microscopy tests for urinary tract infection, and also tests for excretion of certain products over a time period, which can assist in the diagnosis and monitoring of impaired renal function. As with specimens of faeces, the nurse is responsible for gaining the patient's co-operation and for correctly collecting and documenting the specimen.

Table 9.2 Abnormalities in faeces with possible diagnosis.

Abnormality	Appearance	Possible diagnosis
None	Brown, soft, well-formed stools	
Blood	Bright-red flecks in stools	From colon or rectum Haemorrhoids Carcinoma Ulcerative conditions
	Dark, tarry stools (melaena)	From stomach or small intestine (affected by digestion) Ulcerative conditions Carcinoma
Blood and mucus	Loose stools containing red and creamy flecks	Inflammatory bowel disease, e.g. ulcerative colitis, Crohn's disease
Increased stercobilin and stercobilinogen	Dark-brown stools	Haemolytic jaundice
Absence of bile pigment	Loose, bulky, clay-coloured stools (offensive smell)	Liver disease ⎱ cholestatic Gallbladder ⎰ jaundice obstruction
Increased fat (steatorrhoea)	As above	As above Malabsorption secondary to a number of bowel and systemic disorders

Urine may be collected as a single specimen or as a '24-hour specimen'. In either case the patient needs to understand exactly what is happening so that a test is not spoiled by incorrect technique or an inadvertent visit to the toilet. On the whole, patients are eager to co-operate, and a mistake made through a misunderstanding can lead to feelings of guilt and misery which are often disproportionate.

The 'clean' specimen

A 'clean' specimen is one that is uncontaminated by organisms outside the urinary tract. To facilitate its collection, the external genitalia are cleaned beforehand and the specimen collected half-way through micturition. In female patients, after an explanation has been given, the vulval area is washed thoroughly and may also then be swabbed with a mild antiseptic lotion. Care should be taken to work from front to back to lessen the risk of contaminating the urethral meatus with faecal bacteria. The female patient is asked to sit well back on the bedpan or lavatory with her labia held apart and to commence passing urine: the specimen container is then held beneath the flow and a 'mid-stream' specimen is collected into it, taking care that the inside of the container is not contaminated with the fingers. A sterile jug may be used instead and the urine transferred to the specimen container afterwards. In male patients the glans penis is exposed, urethral meatus cleaned and the specimen collected similarly, except that the male patient will use a urinal. After the specimen is collected, the patient completes micturition into the bedpan, urinal or lavatory. The specimen container is sealed and any excess urine wiped off with tissues before labelling.

The early morning specimen

For the diagnosis of some conditions (e.g. pregnancy, renal tuberculosis), the first specimen of urine passed on waking in the morning is required. For the latter condition the total amount of urine passed is sent to the laboratory.

The 24-hour specimen

A 24-hour specimen comprises all the urine passed during a 24-hour period. The specimen collection is timed from the passing and discarding of an initial specimen of urine (this is usually the first urine passed in the morning). It is complete when urine passed at the same time, 24 hours later, is added to the container. The urine is normally collected in a one-litre plastic container, clearly labelled with the patient's name and the time of commencement and termination of the specimen collection. The nurse should ensure that she knows before the collection begins whether a 'plain' (empty) container or one containing a chemical preservative is required; otherwise the patient may well feel distressed and frustrated at the time wasted obtaining a useless specimen.

If the patient is ambulant he needs to remember that all his urine is to be collected. Sometimes the specimen container is left beside the bed as a reminder, but it can be embarrassing to publicly pour urine into a jar by the bed. It is preferable to keep the container in the sluice and show the patient where it is: he should also be equipped with a clean jug and cover in which he can collect his specimen before transferring it to the container.

At the end of the 24-hour period the laboratory staff will require either the total contents of the container or a well-mixed sample. If the latter, this requirement should be checked before discarding any of the total specimen. Although the ambulant patient will have collected his own specimen, the responsibility for collection lies with the nurse. It is easy to forget to thank patients who co-operate, especially the bedfast individual who says, 'Remember, it's all being collected today'. Nurses can be irritated by such reminders and label the patient as interfering or a busybody, when in fact a reminder can often be extremely useful and should not be discouraged.

With some 24-hour specimens, e.g. for a creatinine clearance test, a sample of blood is taken from the patient during the test: the nurse needs to remember that this must be sent to the laboratory with the urine when the test is completed.

Table 9.3 shows abnormalities in urine and their implications for diagnosis.

Sputum

Sputum is an excess of secretions from the air passages and its production is therefore abnormal. It can be used to assist in the diagnosis of many respiratory and some cardiac disorders and may be required for laboratory analysis. It should be collected directly into a sterile container, preferably on waking, when the overnight accumulation of exudate will make it easier for the patient to cough up a specimen of actual sputum rather than saliva with its accompanying commensal organisms, which could confuse results.

It is worth remembering that 'spitting' is in general socially unacceptable so patients may feel embarrassed

Abnormality	Colour	Smell	Possible diagnosis
Nitrite	Normal	Strong smelling (fishy)	Urinary tract infection Renal calculi
Blood	Red, reddish-brown or smoky	Normal	Acute glomerulonephritis Hepatitis Carcinoma (kidney, bladder) Urinary calculi Trauma Malignant hypertension Haemorrhagic diseases Menstruation
Bilirubin, excess urobilinogen	Dark yellow	Normal	Liver disorders Biliary disorders
Glucose	Normal to pale (increased volume)	Sweet	Diabetes mellitus
Ketones	As above	As above	Uncontrolled diabetes mellitus

Table 9.3 Abnormalities in urine with possible diagnoses.

when asked to sit up in bed and produce a specimen of sputum in front of other patients. Ambulant patients may prefer to take the container to the bathroom while bedfast patients should have screens pulled around the bed.

The nurse may find the collection of sputum unpleasant. It is important that she does not show her distaste as this will only add to a patient's unease. The nurse should observe the amount of sputum expectorated and the effort required to produce it. Table 9.4 shows examples of abnormal sputum and the implications for diagnosis.

Pleural effusion

A pleural effusion is an abnormal collection of fluid between the two layers of pleural membrane: its occurrence is secondary to a malignant or other inflammatory process in the lung. Withdrawal of this fluid can give valuable diagnostic information as well as increasing the patient's comfort on breathing. The latter effect may help the nurse to encourage the patient during what can be an uncomfortable and lengthy procedure.

To remove the pleural effusion the doctor performs a chest aspiration in the ward. This is an aseptic technique performed using local anaesthetic to ease discomfort as the biopsy needle passes through the skin and between the ribs: a two-way Luer Lok tap is attached to the biopsy needle to prevent air entering the thoracic cavity with subsequent lung collapse.

In preparing the patient, the nurse needs to ensure that he knows what to expect and what is expected of him. For example, to cough during the procedure could cause complications, so he should try not to cough or should warn the nurse and doctor if he cannot avoid doing so. The nurse should ensure that the patient can maintain, in comfort, a seated position with the side of his chest exposed: a firm padded table on which to rest his arms and head should be placed in front of him.

During and after the procedure the nurse should be alert to signs of respiratory distress and/or blood-stained sputum. The doctor will label and send the pleural fluid in sterile containers to the laboratory.

Ascites

Ascites is the term used for excess fluid accumulating in the peritoneal cavity: it can occur in conjunction with liver disease, malignancy and severe cardiac or circulatory failure. As with chest aspiration, withdrawal of the fluid can aid diagnosis as well as considerably ease the patient's discomfort. The procedure used for this is called abdominal paracentesis (see Chapter 10).

Cerebrospinal fluid

Cerebrospinal fluid (CSF) is a normal body secretion formed in the ventricles of the brain. The fluid is contained within a sac of meninges which completely surrounds the

Table 9.4 Examples of abnormalities in sputum and implications for diagnosis.

Abnormality	Appearance	Possible diagnosis
None	Clear, thick, copious	Chronic bronchitis Bronchial asthma
Blood and tissue fluid	Watery, pink tinged, frothy	Pulmonary oedema

Blood (haemoptysis)	Ranges from:
	   slight red streaking
	   rust coloured
	   bright red almost pure blood
		
		Bleeding in upper respiratory tract
		Pneumonia
		Bronchial/lung carcinoma
		Bronchiectasis
		Pulmonary embolism
		Pulmonary tuberculosis

Pus (purulent sputum)	Thick, yellow	Bacterial respiratory tract infection (e.g. acute bronchitis, infective exacerbation of chronic bronchitis, bacterial pneumonia)
	As above but copious and fetid	Bronchiectasis Lung abscess

brain and spinal cord, extending about 5 cm beyond the latter. This means that CSF can be aspirated by a lumbar puncture without damage to the delicate nervous tissue. The fluid, when analysed in the laboratory, can give valuable information about disorders of the nervous system.

This is a procedure that patients are often extremely apprehensive about, fearing pain or even paralysis. Procedures performed 'out of sight', as in this case behind the patient, can cause additional anxiety. After the procedure has been explained to the patient, he should be positioned flat on the bed in a lateral position with his knees drawn up to meet his flexed head. This position will flex the spinal column and facilitate entry of the aspiration needle between the lower lumbar vertebrae. The doctor's main task will be to remove the spinal fluid as safely and quickly as possible maintaining strict asepsis throughout.

As the doctor will be working behind the patient it is essential that the nurse is the other side of the bed where the patient can see her, hold her hand and hear her explanations of each step of the procedure. This position enables the nurse to detect any non-verbal indication of discomfort and any signs of drowsiness or respiratory depression which may indicate a rare but life-threatening complication. The nurse is also enabled to help the patient maintain his position when he tires and to prevent sudden movement which could be hazardous with the needle in position.

After lumbar puncture the nurse should continue to observe the patient for any reduction in consciousness level. The patient will almost certainly experience headache and this can be minimized by keeping him flat in bed for 12 to 24 hours until more cerebrospinal fluid is formed and the negative pressure in the system equalized.

Table 9.5 shows examples of abnormal cerebrospinal fluid and the implications for diagnosis.

Investigations of body tissue

It can be seen that body excretions and secretions may be very useful in determining a medical diagnosis as a result of laboratory investigations. Examination of body tissue by direct internal viewing and in certain cases by obtaining samples of the tissue may also give vital

Abnormality	Appearance	Possible diagnosis
None	Clear, colourless	
Large amounts of polymorphonuclear leucocytes	Cloudy	Bacterial meningitis
Increased lymphocytes	Colourless, possibly cloudy	Viral meningitis Encephalitis
High protein level	Yellow, cloudy or clear	Acute polyneuritis (Guillain–Barré syndrome) Multiple sclerosis Spinal tumour
Increased glucose	Clear, colourless	Reflects hyperglycaemia in diabetes mellitus
Decreased glucose	Colourless, cloudy or clear	Bacterial meningitis Carcinomatous meningitis
Blood (fresh)	Uniformly red	Subarachnoid haemorrhage Post-head injury
Blood (after several days in CSF)	Dark yellow (xanthochromic)	As above after several days

evidence to account for the deficits in functioning described by patients.

The relatively recent development of flexible fibre-optic instruments means that internal examination of the body tracts (endoscopy) can be performed more easily for diagnostic purposes. Biopsy specimens, samples of body tissue which can later be examined by microscope for disease type, are often collected in conjunction with these endoscopy procedures with the aid of a device built into the special equipment used.

Some body tissues are not accessible for endoscopic viewing. Biopsy specimens can still be obtained, however, by needle aspiration, e.g. renal and liver biopsies, which may be carried out on the ward while the patient is conscious, or by surgical removal of a small section of the tissue, e.g. biopsy of a breast lump, which is usually carried out in the operating theatre under general anaesthesia.

Endoscopy and biopsy are performed by doctors who are skilled in such specialized techniques, although in some areas routine endoscopic procedures may be performed by specialist trained nurses. However, routinely the nurse's role, as in the techniques for removing body secretions, is in preparing the patient, in observation and, if the patient is conscious, in giving support during the procedure. Her support and observations,

Table 9.5 Abnormalities in cerebro-spinal fluid and implications for diagnosis.

which will vary in detail depending on the procedure performed, will continue afterwards. Post-operative care will be needed for those patients who have been anaesthetized.

Endoscopy: general factors

An endoscope is a fibre-optic instrument which may be rigid or flexible. Its development has made possible the viewing of a large number of body cavities and passages, and more recent developments have allowed not only confirmation of diagnosis, but also non-invasive or minimally invasive surgical procedures. It will be seen in Chapter 11 that the development of endoscopic equipment has revolutionized many surgical procedures in that many investigations and surgery can be completed in a day, without a patient having to stay overnight in hospital.

For investigative purposes, the endoscope is generally flexible and allows the doctor to observe the contents, mucosa and movement of various body tracts which include the nose, mouth, rectum and urethra (Figure 9.3). During endoscopy, photographs, both still and videotaped, can be taken and tissue removed with biopsy forceps. This is important as diagnosis cannot be made with 100% accuracy by observation alone. Many patients will have seen

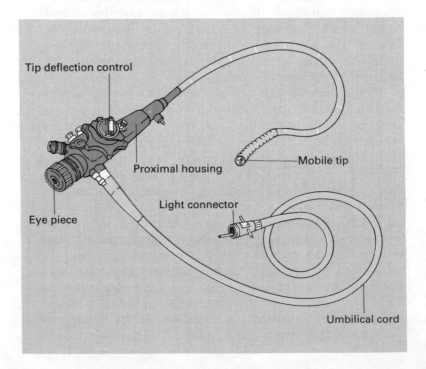

Fig. 9.3 An endoscope.

fibre-optic lamps in homes and restaurants and so may well understand the concept of light travelling down a fine fibre and, therefore, grasp the function of the endoscope more easily.

Endoscopy for diagnostic purposes is performed in a special endoscopy unit or in the operating theatre. It is nearly always performed while the patient is conscious and so it is essential that adequate explanation and preparation are given and a consent form signed before the patient undergoes this procedure.

The idea of lying still while an instrument is passed into a body orifice can be an extremely alarming prospect, particularly in the mouth where retching and a feeling of choking can increase anxiety. As with other areas of patient care, the nurse needs to assess the nature of a patient's fears and give what reassurance she can. For the patient who is worried that he will be unable to co-operate, the knowledge that a tranquillizer (e.g. diazepam) will be given to reduce his agitation before the test, and that a local anaesthetic will be administered at the site where the endoscope will enter, may be of some reassurance. If a nurse who the patient knows can be with him during the procedure, this may act as moral support. It is important to take any fears and worries seriously and let the patient talk them through.

More complex endoscopic equipment includes complete television endoscopy systems (Figure 9.4) (Hill and Summers 1994). These systems have the availability of a number of accessories to include the potential for biopsy, cautery, cutting loops for the treatment of tumours and for the extraction of calculi, other surgical procedures, cytology and biliary drainage.

Rigid endoscopes are generally used for minimal invasive surgery and other therapeutic procedures within the body. The design of the equipment allows simultaneous direct viewing of the procedure with television monitor viewing, so that a particular operation may be combined with a teaching potential. Surgical lasers can also be used during endoscopy. A laser beam is a powerful light which is increasingly used to remove tissue or to seal bleeding points. Because of the intense beam of lasers, safety precautions are required to avoid damage to the eye, particularly of staff who are involved in its use.

There are complications to all endoscopic procedures. Complications are rare but it may be that a particular patient has heard about them and so may need some reassurance on the relative safety of the procedure. In a survey carried out by the British Society for Digestive Endoscopy, it was shown that three people out of a sample

Fig. 9.4 An endoscopic trolley. Reproduced from Hill and Summers (1994) with kind permission of the authors.

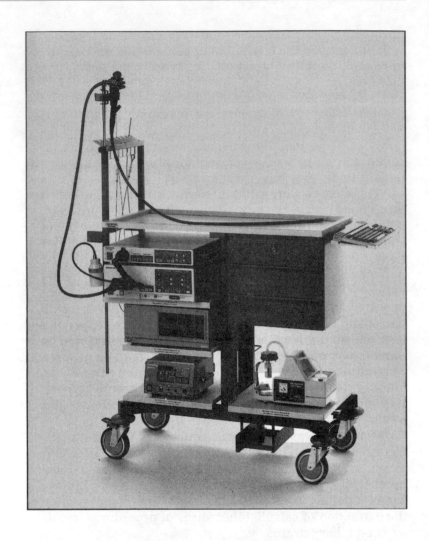

of 24 000 died as a direct result of upper gastrointestinal endoscopy (Hollanders 1979). This means that the investigation is safe providing it is undertaken by an experienced endoscopist. Other complications may include perforation of the oesophageal or stomach wall, aspiration of gastric contents into the lungs, or sensitivity reactions to premedication. Laser treatment may also carry risk to the patient if safety procedures are not observed.

Since a patient is very likely to have been conscious during endoscopic examination, he is likely to be sleepy after the procedure, depending on the extent of reaction to the premedication drug. For some patients, endoscopy will include biopsy and so the factors around potential diagnosis need to be considered.

Biopsy: general factors

In all biopsies an individual is consenting to having a piece of himself removed, often while he is conscious. There are few patients who do not find this alarming at some level. Until the biopsy specimen has been analysed, an answer cannot be given to the patient's questions about the findings. The nurse needs to assess the patient's fears, to point out that nothing can be confirmed or denied until the results of the biopsy come back from the laboratory, and to ensure that when information is available a doctor or nurse will discuss the outcomes and their implications to the individual.

A real difficulty arises if a biopsy and a necessary operation are carried out in sequence on the same day. An example of this is in breast cancer when a frozen section of tissue is taken from the breast, analysed immediately and, if found to be cancerous surgery may be performed. In this instance, the patient will go to theatre unsure of whether she will be having a lumpectomy or partial mastectomy.

In cases such as this, where diagnosis and traumatic surgery may go hand in hand, the nurse needs to allow the patient to talk through the possibilities and, if necessary, exercise her right to consent to the biopsy only at first, so that afterwards, in the light of diagnosis, she may examine the options open to her and be involved in the treatment decisions. Before any biopsy, it is up to the nurse to assess the level of apprehension and take positive action to ensure that the patient suffers the minimum physical and psychological damage.

Investigative endoscopic and biopsy procedures

Upper gastrointestinal tract endoscopy/biopsy

The preparation of patients for upper gastrointestinal endoscopy will be the same whether or not the investigation is of the oesophagus alone, the stomach and duodenum or, as is often the case, all three. The patient is fasted for 12 hours, given an operation gown to wear and asked to remove jewellery and false teeth (any loose teeth or crowns should be described on the consent form). The premedication is given and 15 minutes prior to the examination a local anaesthetic is given in the form of a lozenge or applied using a throat spray.

In the endoscopy unit the patient is made comfortable in the left lateral position and then the endoscope is passed gently over the tongue and down the throat into the oesophagus and stomach. Although the patient will be drowsy he will need continual verbal encouragement and instructions about when to swallow.

Modern endoscope tips can be manoeuvred into all parts of the stomach by the operator and, if necessary, a biopsy specimen of potentially cancerous tissue can be removed using fine forceps via the endoscope.

After the procedure the patient is likely to be sleepy and have a dry mouth. No food or drink should be given until the local anaesthetic has worn off, usually at least four hours, but after that a warm drink may be given provided there are no contrary instructions in the patient's notes. The nurse should be alert to any evidence of complications of endoscopy, which in this patient might present as haematemesis, abdominal pain and distension and/or signs of shock.

Lower gastrointestinal tract endoscopy/biopsy
There are two possible procedures: colonoscopy is the examination of the whole colon using a flexible fibre-optic colonoscope, while sigmoidoscopy is a more common procedure to examine the sigmoid colon only. For the latter a sigmoidoscope is used, which is a rigid, metal, fibre-optic tube approximately 30 cm long. Because the sigmoidoscope is readily portable and the procedure can be performed on the ward or in the out-patients' department its use is less complicated than that of the colonoscope; however, diagnostic information can only be obtained about lower colonic and rectal disease.

From the patient's point of view either experience may be worrying and embarrassing. Adequate explanation should be given and the patient encouraged to verbalize fears and worries. Analgesics may be prescribed for pain, particularly if a patient has haemorrhoids. Further preparation is different for each of the procedures.

Colonoscopy Colonoscopy is carried out so that the colonic mucosa can be examined and biopsy specimens of inflamed mucosa or growths can be taken. It is essential, therefore, that the bowel is cleared. To ensure this, the patient may be given a low-residue diet for four to five days followed by a fluid-only diet on the day before the examination. On the day of endoscopy the patient is given an early morning drink. Enemas used to be given followed by high colonic washout. However, these have been replaced in general by powerful laxatives such as Picolax. These may be taken at home, in which case written infor-

PICOLAX

INFORMATION LEAFLET FOR PATIENTS

Appointment

Please Attend at ....

Date ....

PICOLAX HAS BEEN PRESCRIBED TO CLEAR THE BOWEL PRIOR TO YOUR EXAMINATION
TWO SACHETS ARE TO BE TAKEN THE DAY BEFORE YOUR EXAMINATION
ACCORDING TO THE SCHEDULE OVERLEAF

IT IS IMPORTANT THAT YOU FOLLOW THESE INSTRUCTIONS CAREFULLY

THE SUCCESS OF YOUR EXAMINATION DEPENDS ON THE BOWEL BEING AS CLEAR AS
POSSIBLE OTHERWISE THE EXAMINATION MAY NEED TO BE REPEATED

PLEASE FOLLOW ANY ADDITIONAL INSTRUCTIONS GIVEN BY THE HOSPITAL

Directions for the Preparation of PICOLAX

Dissolve the contents of ONE sachet in a cup of water. Stir for 2-3 minutes and drink the mixture

BE PREPARED FOR FREQUENT BOWEL MOVEMENTS STARTING WITHIN 3 HOURS
OF THE FIRST DOSE

FERRING

Product Licence Holder:
FERRING PHARMACEUTICALS LTD.
11, Mount Rd. Feltham, Middlesex.

Manufactured by:
FERRING AB, Malmö, Sweden.

PICOLAX

SUGGESTED TREATMENT PLAN THE DAY BEFORE YOUR EXAMINATION

DRINK PLENTY OF CLEAR FLUIDS THROUGHOUT THE TREATMENT WITH PICOLAX
TRY TO DRINK AT LEAST A TUMBLERFUL EVERY HOUR DURING THE TREATMENT DAY

WATER, FIZZY DRINKS, CLEAR SOUPS OR MEAT EXTRACT DRINKS MAY BE TAKEN AT ANY TIME.
TEA OR COFFEE SHOULD NOT BE TAKEN LATER THAN MID-AFTERNOON

BE PREPARED FOR FREQUENT BOWEL MOVEMENTS STARTING WITHIN 3 HOURS
OF THE FIRST DOSE

BEFORE BREAKFAST (not later than 8.00 am)
Take the first sachet of PICOLAX dissolved in water as described overleaf

BREAKFAST (8.00 to 9.00 am)
Breakfast, if taken, should be limited to a boiled or poached egg
and/or white bread
a scraping of butter or margarine is allowed, but no jam or marmalade

LUNCH (12.00 to 1.30 pm)
A small portion of steamed, poached or grilled white fish or chicken
may be taken with a very small portion of boiled potato OR white bread
Clear jelly may be taken for dessert

2 HOURS AFTER LUNCH (not later than 4.00 pm)
Take the second sachet of PICOLAX dissolved in water as described overleaf

SUPPER (7.00 to 9.00 pm)
NO SOLID FOOD IS ALLOWED
Clear soup or a meat extract drink may be taken
followed by clear jelly for dessert

NO FURTHER FOOD IS ALLOWED UNTIL AFTER THE EXAMINATION

CONTINUE TO TAKE FLUIDS UNTIL THE BOWEL MOVEMENTS
HAVE CEASED

DRINK AS MUCH AS IS REQUIRED TO SATISFY THIRST

41-41-63

mation will be given to the patient (Figure 9.5) along with the medication. Emphasis needs to be put on adequate fluid intake to avoid dehydration. Consent is obtained. Premedication may be given but it is thought to be less necessary than in upper gastrointestinal endoscopy.

Sigmoidoscopy The preparation for sigmoidoscopy varies. A small phosphate enema or two glycerine suppositories may be given the evening before, but sigmoidoscopy can, if necessary, be performed without special preparation. For both procedures the patient needs to be in the left lateral position with the bed protected by a waterproof pad. The instruments should be lubricated liberally and the patient reassured whilst they are being introduced. The patient should be warned that air will be introduced

Fig. 9.5 Information leaflet on Picolax. Reproduced with kind permission of Ferring Pharmaceuticals Ltd (Copyright acknowledged).

into the bowel to facilitate examination, and that his may lead to a feeling of distension and to expulsion of flatus; such a warning can save a patient much anxiety and embarrassment.

Biopsy specimens taken during either procedure should be sent in clearly labelled specimen pots to the pathology laboratory.

Table 9.6 shows the indications and contraindications for gastrointestinal endoscopy as a diagnostic process (Hollanders 1979).

Respiratory tract endoscopy (bronchoscopy)/biopsy

The broncho-fibrescope (a flexible fibre-optic endoscope used to examine the respiratory tract) can be used to obtain valuable diagnostic information about airway patency and, in conjunction with biopsy, about broncho-pulmonary tumours. It can also be used as a therapeutic instrument to remove an airway obstruction.

Using the flexible endoscope, bronchoscopy can be performed with the patient in a relatively comfortable position. This means that a general anaesthetic is not necessary. However, in some cases, a rigid bronchoscope is the diagnostic instrument of choice, which means that general anaesthesia will be used and the patient prepared accordingly. Preparation when a flexible endoscope is used (in addition to that mentioned on p. 211) includes starving the patient for eight hours prior to the procedure to eradicate the risk of vomiting and aspiration of stomach contents. Dentures should be removed and loose teeth or

Table 9.6 Indications and contraindications for endoscopy.

Indications	Contraindications
Upper gastrointestinal endoscopy	
1 Dyspepsia	1 Uncooperative patient
2 Gastrointestinal haemorrhage	2 Concurrent serious illness
3 Dysphagia	3 Large oesophageal pouch
4 Post-operative symptoms (scarring or distortion)	4 Aortic aneurism
5 Inspection of abnormalities demonstrated radiologically	5 Positive hepatitis B antigen (risk of contamination of endoscope)
Lower intestinal endoscopy	
1 Symptoms where barium enema shows no abnormality	1 Very ill patients
2 Barium enema shows abnormality but nature uncertain	2 Severe inflammation of bowel, e.g. ulcerative colitis
3 ? Carcinoma of bowel for recurrence	3 Pregnancy
	4 Aortic aneurysm

crowns reported. Premedication will be administered, e.g. atropine 0.6–1.0 mg to reduce bronchial secretions and bronchospasm. Diazepam 10 mg may be given to reduce anxiety and sometimes a cough depressant such as codeine may be prescribed.

During the procedure the patient sits semi-recumbent and is asked to keep still whilst the endoscope is passed through one nostril into his trachea. Verbal encouragement will be required from the doctor and nurse assisting him and the patient can be further helped by the local anaesthetic which was previously applied into his nostril and throat. He should breathe through his mouth during the procedure.

After the procedure, any biopsy specimens taken are sent to the appropriate laboratory. The patient is kept in bed, initially in a semi-prone position, as he will still be drowsy from his premedication drugs. He should be given nothing by mouth for four hours or until the effects of the local anaesthetic have passed. The nurse should encourage the patient to cough up any secretions. If a biopsy specimen has been taken the nurse should be alert to the possibility of haemoptysis and should monitor the patient's pulse and blood pressure half-hourly for a few hours.

Urinary tract endoscopy (cystoscopy)/biopsy

This procedure can aid in the diagnosis and monitoring of bladder, ureteric and, in males, prostatic disease. The cystoscope is a rigid instrument and, because of the shape and length of the male urethra, is performed in males under general anaesthesia unless there are strong contraindications. In the female, with a short, straight urethra, the technique can be performed without undue discomfort and risk, providing the principles of local anaesthesia to the urethra and aseptic technique are followed. The position required for this procedure may cause the patient some embarrassment, and the nurse, particularly if known to the patient, can help to encourage her and put her at ease. After the procedure the nurse should be specifically alert to the patient's urinary output and any haematuria.

Renal biopsy

This procedure involves the removal of a small piece of kidney tissue by needle aspiration, in order to acquire diagnostic information about the specific type of renal disease from which the patient is suffering. Renal biopsies are performed on the ward while the patient is conscious. The doctor's role in preparation for the biopsy is to check

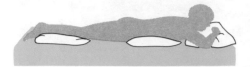

Fig. 9.6 Patient in prone position.

that the patient is not hypertensive, since this is a contraindication to the procedure. He will also need to take blood from the patient for haemoglobin levels and for prothrombin time and bleeding time to be established. He may also take blood for grouping and cross-matching in case a transfusion is necessary, since renal biopsy carries a risk of haemorrhage. An X-ray will be requested to show the size and position of the kidneys.

The nurse's role is to prepare the patient. This is particularly important since his co-operation is vital both in maintaining a prone position for approximately 30 minutes supported by a sandbag under his abdomen (Figure 9.6), which may feel uncomfortable, and by breathing in and holding his breath while the biopsy needle is inserted and the tissue specimen taken.

If a patient seems particularly nervous a mild tranquillizer should be prescribed prior to the procedure. Nervous apprehension may make the patient tremble. This is embarrassing to the patient, irritating to the doctor and potentially dangerous if the procedure has begun. Careful initial assessment of the patient's attitude to the biopsy should establish potential problems in co-operation.

Prior to biopsy the skin is cleaned and a local anaesthetic given. After the biopsy needle has been removed with the specimen of tissue, pressure is applied to the puncture site for at least 30 minutes. Blood pressure and pulse are monitored for 24 hours – every 15 minutes at first, then half-hourly, hourly and four-hourly, if they appear stable.

The patient is kept on bedrest for up to 48 hours and urine observed for the presence of blood. There may be some blood in the urine immediately after biopsy which should clear over 48 hours. Any blood found should be reported, as should bleeding from the puncture site and changes in observations.

Liver biopsy

This is a needle biopsy performed to establish the nature of a patient's liver disease when other tests are inconclusive. From the patient's point of view liver biopsy may be seen to be very similar to renal biopsy in that it is performed on the ward while he is conscious, and his co-operation is required at the actual time the biopsy is performed. Similarly, problems of nervousness on the part of the patient need to be overcome before the biopsy. The following example illustrates the effects of attempting a biopsy without adequate assessment of the patient's ability to co-operate.

Mrs Atkins was suspected of having disease of the liver and a biopsy was requested. This was to be carried out by a Consultant in Tropical Medicine. Mrs Atkins was told that she should not worry because a local anaesthetic would be given. She was, however, very nervous, and when the Consultant attempted to give the local anaesthetic she began to tremble. The Consultant told Mrs Atkins to pull herself together. However, she could not control the trembling and the Consultant left in obvious disgust.

Sister, who had been reproached for inadequate preparation of her patients, told Mrs Atkins that the Consultant would try again the next day and that she really must 'be good'. The patient steeled herself to remain still the following day. On this occasion the Consultant, thinking to get the procedure over quickly, inadvertently punctured the gallbladder. Mrs Atkins was sedated with morphine for 24 hours and refused point blank to submit to further attempts at biopsy.

Some time later in a different hospital a Consultant wished Mrs Atkins to agree to a liver biopsy. He discussed her extreme nervousness with the Sister and she agreed to talk to the patient. She discovered that Mrs Atkins had a real fear of needles and felt guilty for seeming uncooperative. She finally agreed to a biopsy if she had a mild tranquillizer first. Sister went with the Consultant to support the patient and the biopsy was successfully taken with full co-operation from the patient.

Prior to liver biopsy, blood will be taken from the patient for prothrombin time, clotting time, haemoglobin level and platelet count to be assessed in order to ensure that his haemostatic mechanisms are functioning. The blood will also be grouped and cross-matched. These precautions are necessary because the liver is a highly vascular organ and haemorrhage is a significant risk following this procedure. Relative to this the nurse should check blood pressure, pulse and respiration to give baseline data against which post-biopsy observations may be compared, and she should check that a consent form has been signed. She should also assess the patient's need for a tranquillizer and explain the procedure and co-operation required from him.

The patient's position during liver biopsy should be supine, on the right-hand edge of the bed with one pillow beneath his head (Figure 9.7). His right arm should be raised above his head to expose the area to be biopsied (the right hypochondrium). As for renal biopsy, the skin is cleaned, a local anaesthetic given and, when this has taken effect, the biopsy taken with a special needle. The needle is passed through the eighth, ninth or tenth intercostal space. If the liver is enlarged the needle may be introduced below the costal margin. When the biopsy needle is positioned just outside the liver capsule the patient is asked to take two or three deep breaths and then to breathe out and hold his breath until told to breathe again. The biopsy is taken while the breath is held by advancing the needle into the liver tissue and then

Fig. 9.7 Patient in supine position.

withdrawing it quickly: this only takes a few seconds to perform.

After the biopsy the patient is asked to lie on his right side for the first four hours to produce pressure on the biopsy site and then rest in bed for 24 hours. This is essential because of the risk of post-biopsy haemorrhage. During this 24 hours, observations are made of the patient's colour, general condition and puncture site. Blood pressure, pulse and respirations may be recorded at 15-minute intervals for approximately two hours, then every 30 minutes, hourly and then four-hourly if there are no complications. Any pain or rigidity of the patient's abdomen should be reported and investigated medically in case bile or blood has leaked from the liver into the peritoneum.

Tumour biopsy

If a tumour is suspected in an area of body tissue, e.g. if a woman complains of a lump in her breast, a biopsy may be performed to make a differential diagnosis between a benign and a malignant tumour. Although needle biopsies may be performed on the ward or in out-patients it is more usual for a section of the tumour to be taken in theatre under general anaesthesia. The nurse's role is in physical preparation and after-care of the patient (Chapter 11) and in assessment of the patient's perception of what will happen and why so that she can meet expressed needs. This can be a delicate area for the nurse since it is becoming more common for patients to associate lumps, 'growths' or tumours with cancer. This is particularly true for breast lumps (Maguire 1992) where media campaigns have made the public aware that lumps in the breast are possibly due to cancer and should be immediately investigated by a doctor. False reassurance in this situation can reduce the patient's trust in the nursing staff.

Bone marrow biopsy

Occasionally, to investigate blood disorders such as the anaemias and leukaemias, a bone marrow biopsy may be performed so that some bone marrow, which is active in blood cell production and which therefore should reveal any abnormality, may be examined in the laboratory. This is an aseptic technique carried out by a doctor using a specially designed needle with a protective guard to control the extent of its entry into the bone. Even though a local anaesthetic is given to reduce pain and discomfort, the patient may be very apprehensive, as the most usual site for puncture is the sternum. To a lay person, having a large needle inserted into one's chest is very frightening and a nurse should be present to explain the short but real pain on aspiration, and to comfort and reassure as far as possible while the procedure is taking place.

X-rays

X-rays are a valuable diagnostic tool for the medical profession. There are portable machines to X-ray the very ill who cannot be moved, but most X-rays are carried out in a special department within the hospital. It is usual for a porter to collect the patient who requires an X-ray, leave him in the department and take him back to the ward when the X-rays are complete and checked for clarity.

X-rays are photographic negatives taken by the use of electromagnetic waves which are capable of penetrating human skin and showing up internal bones and organs. Since they can produce chemical changes they are used for treatment as well as for diagnosis. Their ability to produce physiological change means that radiographers are at physical risk if they do not take precautions, such as the wearing of lead aprons while the X-ray machines are working.

There are numerous types of X-ray taken for diagnostic purposes; these can be divided into routine radiographic views – sometimes referred to as 'straight' or 'plain' films, e.g. chest and bone X-rays (Figures 9.8 and 12.8(b)) – and specialized radiographic views, which highlight sections of tissue, e.g. tomograms and mammograms, or those which reveal tissue. These latter require the use of a radio-opaque dye, e.g. barium meal or enema, to show structures which do not normally show up on X-ray; these are known as contrast studies. In all cases, however, the patient may simply be told that an X-ray of a particular site has been requested.

Even though a nurse may not accompany a patient to the Radiography Department where X-rays are taken, she has a role both in the preparation of the patient and in meeting his need for information. This latter is important since if the doctor requests the investigation in Sister's office he may fail to inform the patient. This may lead to confusion for the patient when a porter arrives on the ward and calls his name.

Routine radiographic views ('straight' films)

Apart from informing the patient that an X-ray is to be taken and the reason, there is no special preparation of the patient except that he should not be wearing any metal

Fig. 9.8 X-ray of normal chest. Reproduced from Swash and Mason (1984) with kind permission of the authors.

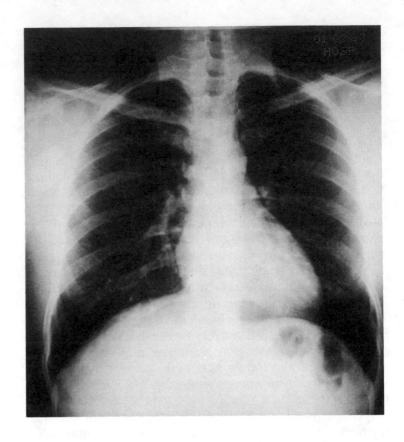

item, such as jewellery or safety pins or zinc oxide plaster, since these will prevent the X-ray waves from penetrating and will obscure the film.

Specialized radiographic views

Tomogram

The word tomography literally means 'drawing a slice'. A tomogram is a multiple X-ray taken at different planes. This allows a section of an organ to be examined in detail where a straight X-ray would be obscured by, for example, the rib cage in the case of a lung tomogram. Tomograms are requested when lesions are suspected, e.g. in tuberculosis (Figure 9.9). Preparation is the same as for routine radiographic views.

Mammogram

This is a useful investigation in the detection of early breast cancer. The same process as for tomography is adopted to show any changes in the breasts. A mammogram may show a lesion too deep to be palpable and will give its size and shape as well as site. The investigation may not yield good results in patients with dense heavy breasts: in such patients a xeromammogram, a newer technique, is more successful. Preparation for both is as for routine radiographic views.

Contrast studies
This term incorporates any X-ray techniques which involve the use of a radio-opaque dye to show up abnormalities in body tissues, tubes and cavities, such as the stomach, bowel, kidney and blood vessels. The following are examples of contrast studies.

Barium meal and 'follow-through' Barium, which is a radio-opaque substance, may be swallowed and its progress monitored through the alimentary tract by a series of X-rays which will show any abnormalities; barium meal is particularly useful in the diagnosis of gastric and duodenal ulcers. Preparation for this procedure commences three days prior to the actual investigation as follows:

  three days prior to examination: all antacids are discontinued
  two days prior to examination: a laxative is given after breakfast and at bedtime

Fig. 9.9 Tomogram of the chest; tuberculosis is shown by the opaque mass at the right apex. Reproduced from Swash and Mason (1984) with kind permission of the authors.

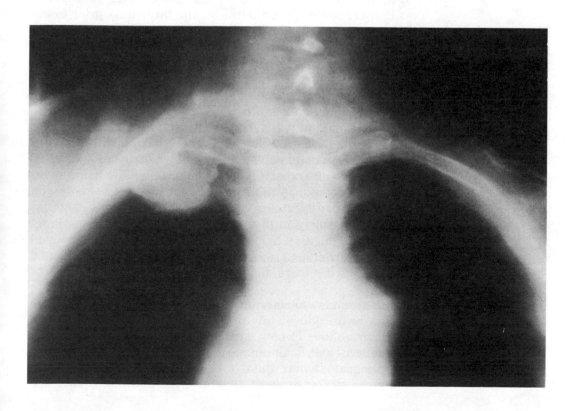

six hours prior to examination: the patient is fasted until the series of X-rays is complete.

Smoking increases gastric motility and so should be discouraged on the day of investigation. The patient will need to understand that a barium meal is more than just an 'X-ray' and will involve some time in the Radiography Department. Barium is unpleasant to swallow, being very 'chalky'. As soon as possible the patient should be allowed a mouthwash and a meal. He should not have to wait until the next 'official' meal time since it will have been some hours since he has eaten.

Monitoring of bowel action is important after a barium meal since the barium can cause severe constipation. It may also reassure the patient if he knows beforehand that stools containing barium are white-coloured and very solid. If only the oesophagus requires investigation, e.g. for dysphagia or in pre-operative assessment for carcinoma of the bronchus, then a barium swallow (just a mouthful of barium) is sufficient and no specific preparation is necessary.

Barium enema   A barium enema is a useful diagnostic tool for showing such diseases as ulceration or carcinoma of the lower part of the intestinal tract (Figure 9.10). Preparation of the patient over the three days prior to the examination may be the same as for a barium meal except that a light breakfast is allowed on the morning of the examination, and an enema is given, though bowel preparation can vary in different units. If the patient's problem is one of diarrhoea the laxatives usually given two days before the enema will be omitted.

The patient will need to understand that when he gets to the Radiography Department the barium will be given as an enema and will be followed by a series of X-rays. As with a barium meal, this will mean some time being spent on the procedure and, subsequently, altered stools and perhaps constipation. The procedure may also be seen as embarrassing and distasteful by the patient. Assessment of his feelings, as before any investigative procedure, will allow the nurse to reassure the patient where possible and to accept his fears and feelings.

Intravenous pyelogram (urogram)   Radio-opaque dye may be introduced into the body through a vein to show up abnormalities in body structure and function with subsequent X-rays. A common example of this is an intravenous pyelogram, where the dye is given intravenously to show up the structure and function of the kidneys. X-rays are

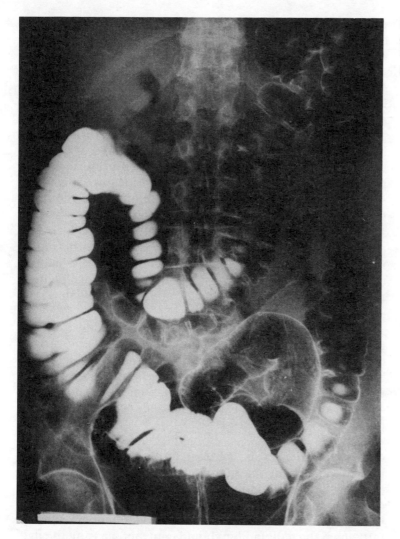

Fig. 9.10 Barium enema of the lower gastrointestinal tract. Reproduced from Swash and Mason (1984) with kind permission of the authors.

taken at intervals to show the concentration of dye in the renal pelvis, ureters and bladder. This investigation may determine the cause of any suspected renal disease.

The preparation of the patient is as for a barium meal although a light breakfast is allowed on the day of the examination and two glycerine suppositories may be given. In addition, the patient should have no fluids for up to eight hours before the pyelogram to allow better concentration of the dye. Since the dye used contains iodine the patient should be screened for allergy before an intravenous pyelogram is performed. He should also be warned that he may feel a hot flush or strange taste in his mouth as the dye is injected and that this sensation will pass quickly. On return to the ward, fluids should be encouraged to counteract their absence prior to the test and the patient given a meal if he is hungry. The nurse should check the injection site for bleeding and be alert to any reaction to the dye, e.g. rash or pyrexia.

Micturating cystogram (urethrogram) This investigation is carried out for patients with abnormalities of micturition. The introduction of radio-opaque dye into the bladder via a catheter, followed by the patient voiding his bladder whilst serial X-rays or video pictures are taken, can reveal abnormalities such as vesico-ureteric reflux and malfunctioning of the urethral sphincters. This is an embarrassing procedure for the patient as he is required to pass urine in a vertical position in the presence of several unknown people. If the nurse does not give adequate warning the embarrassment is likely to be much more acute. The nurse should explain that the people carrying out the investigation will understand his feelings though this will not necessarily diminish his feelings of shame and anxiety.

After the test the nurse should be available to allow the patient to talk through his feelings about the procedure. She should also explain the necessity of a high fluid intake (about a litre over the ensuing ten hours) to assist the passage of dye through the bladder. She should observe urine output and test any passed for the presence of blood.

Cholecystogram This contrast study can give valuable information about the malfunctioning and/or obstruction of the gallbladder and bile ducts. Radio-opaque dye taken orally by the patient is removed from the bloodstream by the liver. This is then stored in the gallbladder. After a fatty meal the gallbladder should contract, passing the dye along the common bile duct to the duodenum. Any obstruction would prevent this process.

The evening before the investigation the patient is given a low-fat meal, after which no food is given, though the patient may drink water or tea and coffee without milk. The following morning the dye is administered orally. If this causes nausea or vomiting, intravenous administration may be required. X-rays are taken throughout the morning, with the final one after a lunch high in fat content. The patient is likely to need much encouragement from the nurse throughout this lengthy and unpleasant investigation.

Angiograms (arteriograms) The injection of radio-opaque dye into arteries can give valuable and unique diagnostic information about aneurysm, stenosis, occlusion or arteriovenous malformation. Such a procedure is invasive, often lengthy and uncomfortable, and not without risk. It follows that the patient needs careful explanation in order to give informed consent. The specific risks and associated nursing observations and care will be associated with invasion, by a foreign substance, of the system being investigated. For example, renal angiography may affect kidney function, carotid angiography alter a patient's consciousness level and coronary angiography precipitate a myocardial infarction. The nurse needs to be knowledgeable and alert to the risks and carry out frequent specific observations after the procedure, as well as assessing the patient's puncture site for bleeding half-hourly for four to six hours.

Scans

Although X-rays are useful aids to diagnosis they do have disadvantages in that:

(**a**) small changes in tissue density do not show
(**b**) repeated or long exposure to X-rays may cause physiological changes in the body, such as alteration of cell constituents and abnormal cell division, necrosis and/ or malignant changes in body tissue.

In recent years computer technology has been developed to assist in medical diagnosis in the form of scanning machines. These machines may use X-rays, as in CT (computerized tomography, formerly called computerized axial tomography) scanning, or gamma radiation, as in radio-isotope scanning. The term 'scanning', however, can be applied to other methods of investigation which, though not radiological, come within the province of the X-ray Department, e.g. ultrasonic and nuclear magnetic resonance scanning. The apparatus required for scanning is very expensive but more and more hospital Radiology Departments are managing to acquire it.

CT (computerized tomography) scans
In this type of scanner (Figure 9.11) X-rays are focused into a fine beam which passes through a small part of the area to be examined. By moving the beam in a pre-arranged pattern over the area, each part of the area is scanned in turn. This process is similar to the human eye moving over the print on the page of a book. After passing through the body the strength of the X-ray beam is measured for each part of the area in turn. This information goes into a computer where it is processed to build up a series of horizontal tomogram pictures of the area under

Fig. 9.11 A CT scanning machine.

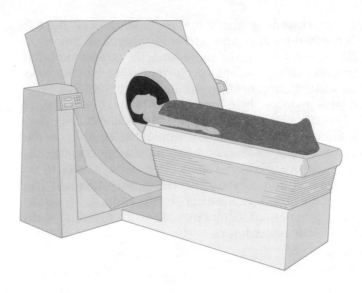

examination. Almost immediate results can be seen on a visual display unit (VDU).

The main advantages of using X-rays in this way lie in the immediacy of a very detailed picture of the body area under investigation without the use of invasive techniques and the accompanying hazards. It was the achievement of a picture not only showing a suspect lesion but giving some indication of its nature that made the CT scanner such a revolutionary new diagnostic tool in the 1970s.

Disadvantages are that, although with modern body scanning machines the patient has only to lie still for a few seconds, with older machines and head scanners the patient has to lie still for at least four minutes while the X-ray tube scans the area under investigation. This may necessitate a general anaesthetic for a child or confused adult. Some patients describe a feeling of claustrophobia during a head scan. Another disadvantage is the immense capital outlay for the scanning machine which has limited the availability of this investigation to all patients, although this is changing as more machines become available.

There is little preparation or after-care for CT scanning other than explanation of the procedure to the patient and warning him that he will be left on his own for a few minutes while the scan is taking place, though the technician will be within easy reach observing him.

Radionuclide imaging

This is a scanning technique which, though less informative than the CT scan, is a relatively inexpensive and safe diagnostic tool. The investigation depends on the use of radioactive substances – isotopes – which, when introduced into the body (usually intravenously), are taken up by particular organs, e.g. brain, lungs, liver. The isotopes used, e.g. technetium (^{99}Tc), have a short half-life to ensure that there is no risk of exceeding a safe radiation dose to the body as a whole; they emit radiation including gamma rays, which can be demonstrated using a gamma camera. Increased uptake of the isotope can reveal a 'hot spot' on the film indicating a tumour or abscess. Conversely, a zone of diminished uptake may be evident suggesting, in the lungs for instance, a pulmonary embolism in cases where the 'straight' X-ray is inconclusive.

The progress of isotopes can also be monitored, e.g. through the kidney tubules, using a Geiger counter, giving information about the function as well as the structure of body organs.

Preparation and after-care of the patient is minimal. An explanation is required and some patients will need reassurance about 'being radioactive'. A drug such as potassium perchlorate may be given to prevent uptake of the isotope by the very active thyroid gland before it reaches the organ being investigated.

Ultrasonic scan (ultrasound)

The term 'ultrasonic' applies to sound waves of frequencies too high to be detected by the human ear. These waves, induced by special transducers, can pass through body tissue at 1500 m/sec but will be partially reflected when a change in tissue density is encountered. Use of a scanning process in combination with measurement of the amplitude and time delay of the reflected waves enables a three-dimensional picture to be composed on a monitor, or on photographic film, of the area under examination.

The procedure has many advantages: it is painless, non-invasive, safer than radiography, relatively inexpensive, easy to perform and has no known side effects. This makes it valuable for mass screening. Valuable information may also be gained about the presence of lesions in organs such as the liver, kidney, pancreas and thyroid. It can be used to study the haemodynamics of the heart and perhaps its most extensive use is in the field of obstetrics, where pregnant women can see their embryonic babies moving about as early as six weeks after conception. Obstetricians can establish the size and therefore the age of the fetus and the position of the placenta, which aids them considerably in the subsequent management of the pregnancy.

Magnetic resonance imaging

Magnetic resonance imaging (MRI) is based on the principle of nuclear magnetic resonance. Since its development in the 1980s, which were evaluated at a few centres in the United Kingdom, it has replaced CT as the investigation of choice in many diagnostic situations.

The advantages of MRI are high intrinsic soft tissue contrast, direct multi-planar imaging, no ionizing radiation, no bone and air artifacts, and no biological hazards (Gillespie and Gholkar 1994). Some patients cannot complete the examination because they become claustrophobic. In addition, patients with prostheses and cardiac pacemakers or any metallic foreign bodies are contraindicated for MRI. Another disadvantage is the limited availability of MRI and the high cost.

Investigations recording electro-activity in the body

Electrocardiogram

The electrocardiograph (ECG) is an instrument which detects very small electrical signals, generated by the cardiac muscle, at the surface of the body. It then amplifies these signals and records them either on an oscilloscope (TV monitor) or a strip of graph paper (Figure 9.12). Electrical impulses from various parts of the heart can be detected by placing electrodes on the skin in different parts of the body, e.g. chest and limbs (Figure 9.13). To allow conduction of the currents from the skin to the electrode a contact jelly is smeared on the skin beneath each electrode.

The ECG can give valuable diagnostic information about cardiac function and is the definitive method of confirming coronary heart disease in most cases. It can also demonstrate cardiac arrhythmias such as ventricular tachycardia and heart block, which themselves may be evidence of underlying cardiac disease. An ECG per-

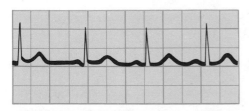

Fig. 9.12 An ECG recording.

formed at rest may show no abnormality and sometimes the patient will be asked to use an exercise bicycle or treadmill to produce extra cardiac effort, after which abnormalities may become evident. An ECG is usually performed by a skilled technician and the tracing of the heart's electrical activity is studied for deviations from normal. Since the machine is portable the investigation is normally performed on the ward.

For the patient the procedure is painless if rather messy. The nurse needs to explain to the patient that the seemingly complex apparatus will do no harm but will give information on the action of the heart. It is not uncommon for patients to believe that electricity flows from the machine rather than to it. The technician should clean the jelly off the electrode sites before leaving the patient, but even then the patient may well appreciate a wash and being made comfortable.

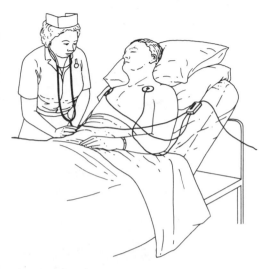

Fig. 9.13 Placing ECG electrodes on a patient.

Electroencephalogram

An electroencephalograph (EEG) records the electrical activity of the brain. As with ECG, the recording is made by placing electrodes on the skin but, whereas with an ECG the electrodes are placed on several parts of the body, for an EEG the electrodes are placed on the scalp and the ear lobes (Figure 9.14). Since the brain in consciousness transmits electrical activity at all times, an EEG can localize tumours and haematoma by recording areas of electrical deviation, either decreased or increased activity. By showing specific deviations from normal activity,

Fig. 9.14 Possible placements of EEG electrodes on a patient. The zone markings shown are of use to the technician.

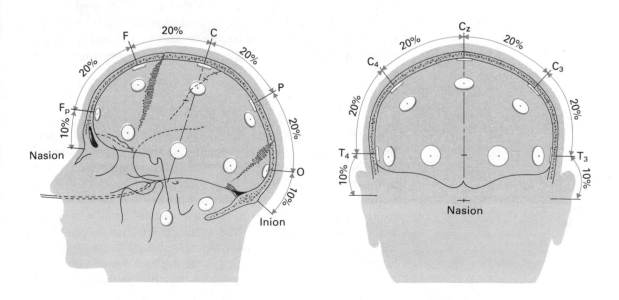

the investigation can also assist in the diagnosis of epilepsy, particularly petit mal.

Although no assumptions may be made on a patient's response to this investigation, concerns may be similar to those for ECG in that it may be a little alarming to feel 'wired up' or there may be fear of electric shock. The nurse should, as in all investigations, be supportive and give explanations and information according to individual needs. EEGs are not performed on the ward but in a room which is screened from outside interference. It is a painless and risk-free procedure and all that the patient may be asked to do is to respond to stimuli so that the effect may be recorded. Otherwise he will sit relaxed until the electrodes are removed.

Towards diagnosis: the nurse's role

The diagnostic investigations described in this chapter do not comprise an exhaustive list but represent the more common tests available to the medical profession as they seek to diagnose a patient's medical condition.

The nurse has a role in this investigative phase of a patient's stay in hospital in preparing him physically and psychologically for the investigations. She also has a responsibility for collecting some of the data which will be used to aid a doctor in making his diagnosis. TPR (temperature, pulse, respiration – Chapter 5) is both an aid to diagnosis and a means of monitoring a patient's progress. Similarly, knowledge of an individual's blood pressure, fluid balance, weight and urinalysis can all contribute to the patient profile, which is built up in order that an accurate diagnosis may be made and treatment planned which will allow each individual to reach his maximum health potential.

Blood pressure

When the heart pumps blood through the vessels in the body, pressure is exerted laterally on the walls of arteries, arterioles, venules and veins: the pressure will vary in the different vessels. Blood pressure is dependent on two main factors. The first is the amount of blood ejected by each ventricle and the heart rate per minute, which together comprise the cardiac output (CO). The second factor is the resistance within the circulatory system as the blood flows through it; this will depend on the calibre and patency of the blood vessels, which may be altered by the action of special centres in the brain to aid the individual to maintain, for example, adequate blood pressure after blood loss from an injury. It may also be altered in conditions such as arterial disease. This resistance within the circulatory system is called peripheral resistance (PR).

Blood pressure (BP) is therefore related to cardiac output and peripheral resistance in the following way:

$$BP = CO \times PR$$

If output drops but peripheral resistance increases, blood pressure will remain constant. If cardiac output remains stable but peripheral resistance increases, e.g. due to arterial disease, blood pressure will increase.

The heart is a muscular organ which pulsates, causing fluctuations in pressure. This pressure is generally measured at the patient's brachial artery in millimetres of mercury (mmHg). The greatest pressure is recorded when the left ventricle of the heart has just contracted and discharged blood into the aorta (the systolic pressure). This wave of pressure is transferred along the artery wall and can be picked up in the brachial artery. Between contractions, when the heart is resting, there is still blood passing through the arteries but it is exerting less pressure. This is the diastolic pressure, which can also be detected in the brachial artery. Measurement of blood pressure can aid in the diagnosis and monitoring of a patient's disease or physiological state.

Measuring blood pressure

A sphygmomanometer and a stethoscope are required to measure blood pressure. The sphygmomanometer is placed level on a firm surface beside the patient. The cuff of the sphygmomanometer is wound around the upper arm above the elbow. It is important to leave a space between the elbow and cuff or it becomes difficult to apply the stethoscope to the brachial artery (Figure 9.15). For accurate results the width of the cuff must be appropriate and this will vary in adults and children. If a patient is very thin, even if a short cuff is used, there can appear to be too much cuff. It should be wound round the arm carefully, covering the previous layer until all the cuff is used, and the end tucked in.

By inflating the cuff the brachial artery is compressed by pressure, which is transferred to the column of mercury in the machine to be read. The cuff is inflated 20 mmHg higher than the point at which the brachial pulse disappears. This occurs when the pressure of the cuff is greater than the systolic blood pressure. It means that circulation is effectively cut off below the cuff. The stethoscope is then placed on the brachial artery and the

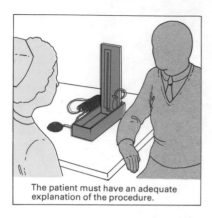

The patient must have an adequate explanation of the procedure.

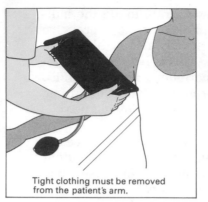

Tight clothing must be removed from the patient's arm.

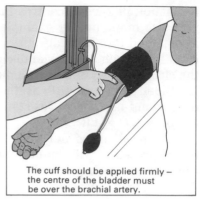

The cuff should be applied firmly – the centre of the bladder must be over the brachial artery.

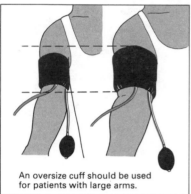

An oversize cuff should be used for patients with large arms.

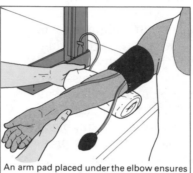

An arm pad placed under the elbow ensures support and relaxation of the arm and accessibility of the brachial artery.

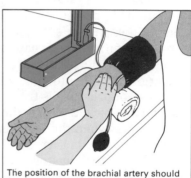

The position of the brachial artery should be established before recording commences.

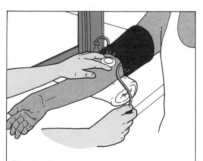

The diaphragm of the stethoscope covers a larger area than the bell and is easier to secure with the fingers of one hand. The stethoscope must not be pressed too hard on the artery – this distorts the artery and may produce false sounds.

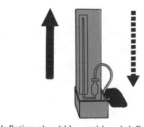

Inflation should be rapid and deflation must be slow (2 mmHg per second). THIS IS VERY IMPORTANT. Too rapid deflation gives grossly inaccurate readings. After noting systolic and diastolic pressures, break the connection for patient comfort and zero pressure. The procedure must be repeated from the BEGINNING if the pressure is missed.

The pressure should be recorded immediately.

It is valuable to take more than one reading. Markedly discrepant readings must be repeated (i.e. if systolic blood pressure equals or exceeds 20 mmHg or diastolic blood pressure equals or exceeds 10 mmHg).

Fig. 9.15 Measuring blood pressure. Redrawn with kind permission of Greta Barnes and the *Nursing Times*.

cuff slowly deflated so that the nurse can hear the beat from the blood pressure through the ear pieces, and observe the column of mercury at the same time. At the first pulse heard (the systolic pressure) the mercury level should be noted. Further slow deflation brings more muffled sounds before the pulse finally fades. There is some debate in medical circles about whether the diastolic pressure should be noted at the point when beats change to a muffled sound or at the point when they disappear. The nurse needs to check which policy is being adhered to in her area.

Most patients will have some knowledge of blood pressure but, as with other procedures, no assumptions should be made on any individual's knowledge of how or why it is taken. Because inflation of the cuff reduces circulation to the arm the procedure should not be prolonged unnecessarily, and the cuff should be fully released as soon as readings have been noted.

Blood pressure is usually recorded on a patient's temperature, pulse and respiration chart, with the systolic pressure noted above the diastolic pressure, i.e. 120/80. Since exercise and emotion may affect blood pressure, measurement is more likely to be accurate if the patient is relaxed and resting. It is possible that small differences in readings will occur between nurses since there will be individual differences in interpretation of sounds and in levels of hearing. Table 9.7 shows normal limits of blood pressure.

Table 9.7 Normal limits of blood pressure.

Age (years)	Systolic range	Diastolic range	Cause of normal variations
70 ↑ 35 ↑ newborn	slight increase ↑ 100–130 mmHg ↑ 55–90 mmHg	slight increase ↑ 60–80 mmHg ↑ 40–55 mmHg	weight emotion exercise age

Table 9.8 Potential reasons for abnormal changes in blood pressure.

Part of circulatory system involved	Change in BP	Possible diagnosis
Decreased intravascular blood volume (hypovolaemia)	BP ↓	Haemorrhage Burns Dehydration Reduced aldosterone secretion
Increased intravascular blood volume (hypervolaemia)	BP ↑	Over-transfusion Increased aldosterone secretion Oral contraceptive therapy
Reduced cardiac output	BP ↓	Impaired cardiac function
Increased peripheral resistance	Systolic pressure ↑ Diastolic pressure ↓	Arteriosclerosis Acute or chronic renal disease → ↓ renal circulation → ↑ renin and angiotensin production

One of the problems in using a patient's blood pressure as an aid to diagnosis lies in the fact that the patient may not have had it measured before he became aware of the deficits which caused him to seek medical help. If an individual's normal blood pressure is 100/60 mmHg, then a hospital reading of 140/90 mmHg would represent a considerable rise, whereas the same reading might be less important in a patient whose normal level is 130/80 mmHg. This is especially so if the blood pressure is taken in the first 24 hours after admission, when Wilson-Barnett and Batehup (1988) have shown that stress levels will be high. Table 9.8 shows some potential reasons for changes in blood pressure.

Urinalysis

A great deal may be learnt about the composition of a sample of urine by simple tests which can be carried out in the ward sluice. When a patient is admitted to hospital it is almost standard practice to test a sample of urine for abnormality. Table 9.9 shows the normal characteristics of urine.

Abnormalities in urine

Urine collected for analysis in the laboratory (p. 201) will be microscopically examined for bacteriological, biochemical and cytological abnormalities. On the ward the nurse will start with a macroscopic examination of the specimen, i.e. colour, odour, specific gravity. This will be followed by biochemical tests for which reagent strips are used (Figure 9.16). A multipurpose reagent strip which tests for a number of abnormalities is used for routine screening of urine on admission.

It is important to read the directions on the bottle and to use a strip from a bottle which has been left with its lid screwed on firmly. If the strip is exposed to the atmosphere for any length of time it may absorb moisture and

Table 9.9 Normal characteristics of urine.

Volume	600–2000 ml in 24 h
Specific gravity	1.001–1.030
Reaction	Acid (pH ± 6)
Colour	Pale amber/like dry sherry
Smell	Aromatic – not unpleasant
Composition	
Water	95%
Urea	2%
Salts	2%
Other deposits	1%

give false readings. Each bottle will have an expiry date on the side. Out-of-date strips should not be used. The bottle should be stored in a cool, dry place but not in a refrigerator.

The most comprehensive reagent strips will give readings on specific gravity, pH, protein, glucose, ketones, bilirubin, blood, nitrate and urobilinogen. The outside of the bottle has a clear guide against which to compare the strip after dipping it into a well-stirred, fresh sample of urine. The time in seconds at which the strip should be read is given against each test and should be strictly adhered to for accurate results. Should abnormalities in urine show up on a reagent multistick, an individual test using a special reagent strip should be performed to confirm the reading. Any abnormalities should be reported.

Individual reagent strips are available to test for protein, glucose, ketones and blood in the urine, while for the urine of a patient with diabetes a combination strip for glucose and ketones is available. Table 9.3 shows abnormalities in urine with possible diagnoses, most of which will be confirmed by laboratory tests.

When collecting a urine specimen for testing on the ward, an explanation should be given to the patient about routine screening on admission and any questions answered if possible. The results of urinalysis on admission are charted on the patient's temperature, pulse and respiration chart and on the nursing report. If

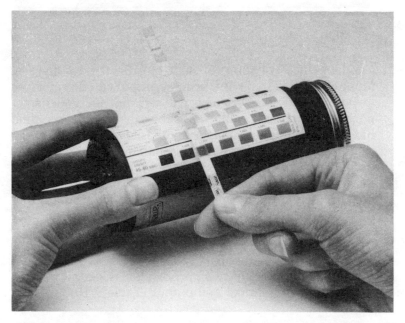

Fig. 9.16 Reagent strips and bottle used in urine analysis. Reproduced with kind permission of Miles Laboratories Ltd.

there are no abnormalities this is noted in the patient's records.

If there are no abnormalities the patient should be told so when the result is charted, for no matter how routine a test is, once it is initiated it is a cause for concern for an individual. If abnormalities are found, a discussion with Sister or the doctor will lead to a consensus on what the patient is told. If, for example, glucose is present in the urine, it would be foolhardy to talk to the patient about diabetes until other diagnostic investigations are carried out.

Of course the patient may not ask about the test. If he does ask, the nurse will need to assess his need for information. A vague answer such as, 'well, things aren't quite right – it may be a minor upset but more tests will be carried out to make sure' may be enough, but an articulate patient may want more information on what it is that is 'not right'. In a situation where a nurse feels unable to divulge more information, she should arrange for a senior nurse or doctor to talk to the patient.

The patient, of course, may have enough insight to jump ahead to a diagnosis.

olly Witherington (Chapter 4) had been told after her youngest child was born that she was pre-diabetic. As soon as she was told that there was 'sugar' in her urine she knew what the diagnosis was likely to be. This did not prevent her from being very upset but it does mean that she would have been unlikely to accept any vague descriptions of the abnormalities found in her urine.

Fluid balance

Fluid balance (Chapter 2) may be affected by disease. Monitoring fluid input and urinary output can therefore be an aid to a diagnosis which will account for deficits reported by a patient. Table 9.10 shows disturbances in fluid balance with implications for diagnosis. It should be noted that oedema will only affect fluid balance if the total body fluid is increased, which is not the case in oedema resulting from increased venous pressure, thrombosis or capillary permeability; in this case it is fluid distribution, not fluid balance, that is affected.

Observations

If fluid balance is disturbed, observation of the patient may be an aid to identifying problems associated with an individual's fluid intake and output (Table 9.10).

Fluid deficit		Fluid excess	
Dehydration	Diagnosis, clinical sign	Oedema	Diagnosis
Loss of fluid	Vomiting/diarrhoea Pyrexia Haemorrhage Uncontrolled diabetes (excess glucose in urine) Acute renal failure (diuretic phase) Chronic renal failure Burns Diabetes insipidus (antidiuretic hormone deficiency)	Reduced glomerular filtration rate	Cardiac failure Acute nephritis Hypovolaemic shock Congestive cardiac failure Cirrhosis of liver
Decreased aldosterone production and sodium loss	Addison's disease	Increased aldosterone production and sodium retention	Cushing's disease
Lowered fluid intake	Coma, cerebral injury (if fluid restriction is required to prevent cerebral oedema)	Increased venous pressure	Cardiac failure Thrombosis

Table 9.10 Causes of dehydration and oedema with possible diagnoses.

Dehydration

Unless dehydration occurs because of coma or cerebral injury where normal thirst regulation is affected, a dehydrated individual will soon show signs of thirst. In diabetes, for example, the polyuria which is caused by the excess of glucose in the urine is accompanied by excessive drinking. The individual will also complain of a dry mouth and sore tongue as the saliva levels are reduced. The patient's skin will be dry and the area around his eyes will look dark and sunken. If the dehydration is not caused by polyuria, urine will be concentrated and the volume reduced (oliguria). Because of this, waste products normally excreted in urine build up so that the patient becomes acidotic, that is, the balance between the alkalinity and acidity of the blood is disturbed. This leads to vomiting, drowsiness and an effect on the breath which is described as smelling of 'new mown hay'. Ketones will appear in the urine and the patient will complain of tiredness and lethargy.

Since evaporation of fluid on the skin helps to maintain body temperature within normal levels, prolonged dehydration will lead to pyrexia. Blood pressure may fall and the pulse become weak. Untreated dehydration may lead to coma and death.

Oedema

Oedema may also cause weakness and apathy but may be characterized by weight gain and swollen tissues, which will pit if pressure is applied. For this reason the term 'pitting oedema' is used.

In some conditions causing oedema there will be decreased urinary output as in dehydration, but where in dehydration this is due to bodily systems conserving fluid, in oedema unnecessary fluid is being retained. If some of this excess fluid is in the lungs (pulmonary oedema) the patient will be dyspnoeic and may have moist sounds in the chest. If an individual is ambulant the first sign of oedema may be in the ankles. For the bed- or chair-fast patient sacral oedema will be evident. Excess fluid in the peritoneal cavity (ascites) may be part of generalized oedema.

Co-ordination of information

A diagnosis is seldom reached as a result of one investigation. Rather the medical staff request a number of relevant specialist investigations and, together with data gathered by the nurse, attempt to reach a decision on the cause of the patient's medical problems. The nurse is not called upon to make a medical diagnosis but is involved both in data gathering and in patient care during the diagnostic period. It is the unique combination of medical and nursing expertise which contributes to patient care during this period while the results of investigations are collated.

Medical diagnosis is not, however, the whole story. The patient may have social and psychological problems which result from or affect his reaction to disease. During the early days in hospital while the doctor is reaching a diagnosis and planning treatment, the nurse will be making a full nursing assessment of the patient and making plans for individualized patient care.

This is not to imply that medical staff are only interested in medical diagnosis. What is true is that the doctor's major responsibility is to reach a diagnosis and prescribe care. He is unlikely to have the opportunity for prolonged personal contact with the patient, who may in any case feel unable to 'waste the doctor's time' with problems other than the immediate medical ones.

The nursing assessment may give insight into patients' problems which will help medical diagnosis **and** plans for nursing care. Similarly nurses need to be aware of and record on the nursing record diagnostic tests which are performed. This is not only so that appropriate nursing care can be given but so that the nurse is alerted to what is happening to the patient, and can identify related problems in terms of fears, anxieties and the need for information.

Reactions to diagnosis

Reactions to diagnosis will vary enormously according to the severity of the problem and also to the expectations of the patients prior to diagnosis. Few patients go to their doctor feeling neutral. Often they have themselves tried to make sense of the signs and symptoms of ill-health that have begun to concern them. This means that the woman who has found a lump in her breast will be aware that it could be breast cancer that is causing the problem. Obviously she will be delighted if what is found is a benign tumour that can be readily excised. Similarly with other diseases, the expectation of patients may be based on their previous life experience, the people that they have known who have suffered from disease and the preparation that they have received from medical and nursing staff.

Many patients, when awaiting diagnosis, realize that what they are facing is potentially bad news (Faulkner 1992). If the diagnosis does constitute bad news for the individual and his family, the reactions may vary from total disbelief and denial through to quiet or angry acceptance. If a patient does not readily accept the doctor's diagnosis, this can cause difficulties both in terms of the reality of the situation and the fact that the patient may wish to go elsewhere and find another opinion or other treatment options. This is most likely to occur if the disease is potentially life-threatening and if the treatment cannot be offered with the certainty of cure. By careful assessment of the patient's problems and in giving the patient an opportunity to talk through his feelings about diagnosis, it may often be possible to move ahead with appropriate treatment and care.

Families too may find it difficult to accept a loved one's diagnosis, particularly if it is life-threatening or carries a stigma, such as AIDS. In such situations, the diagnosis may reveal some element of the loved one's lifestyle that had not been apparent to his family before, and there may be a period when they have to adjust to the reality of the situation. It is not unusual for both the patient and family members to cast around desperately in their minds for something that might help in addition to what is being offered in conventional therapy.

Complementary therapies

Complementary therapies were first known as alternative therapies and were favoured (among others) by patients who had carcinoma where no further treatment options were available to them. In the forefront of the alternative therapy movement was the Bristol Cancer Centre which offered residential care to cancer patients, including special diets and a number of therapies such as acupuncture, relaxation, visualization and others. Some research on the effects of alternative treatment on the patients who attended the Bristol Cancer Centre suggested that those patients did no better than patients on conventional treatment (Bagenal *et al.* 1990). What perhaps was missed was that the type of patient who went to Bristol was someone who was known to have a very small chance of survival and generally where active treatment had been discontinued. The media brought a lot of unwelcome publicity to the role of alternative therapies (Sheard 1990).

From the aftermath of the alternative therapy research, the move has been made to offer such therapies as complementary **to** rather than alternative **from** conventional treatments. This has meant that complementary therapy centres are setting up all over the United Kingdom and often in close proximity to and in collaboration with hospital departments. Woodham (1994) suggests that complementary therapy has made major advances since the first BMA report in 1986. The Osteopathy Bill was enacted through Parliament in 1993 and several Health Authorities have made available complementary therapy services for patients through the NHS.

Nurses are not expected to be complementary therapists, though it is argued that they do have a therapeutic role (Faulkner 1995). What patients may require from nurses is advice on asking for complementary therapy. Given the vast array of complementary medicines on offer (Stanway 1994) it may be difficult for the nurse to give clear advice on (a) what is on offer, and (b) what the claims are for a particular therapy. What is most important is that the patient who is looking for such help understands clearly that, for example, acupuncture or visualization may not actually cure his disease, but may improve his quality of life.

A further difficulty for the nurse is that some complementary therapies are offered by individuals without any clear indication that they will work, and patients do need to be advised to avoid those practitioners who cannot substantiate their claims. For example, a modern complementary therapy offered to cancer patients is shark's cartilage, which is given by injection and is desperately expensive. This is offered with no scientific evidence whatsoever that it will make a difference to a patient who has advanced cancer. Perhaps the biggest difficulty for the nurse in situations like this is in recognizing that every patient has the right to make an informed choice and to spend his money as he wishes. The nurse's role in this respect is to gather the necessary information so that the choice that is made by a patient is truly informed.

Summary

It is argued in this chapter that nurses need to be involved in medical diagnosis in a number of ways. It is necessary to understand the many diagnostic tests available in terms of where, why and how they are performed and then to give adequate care when those investigations are over. The nurse also has a role in observing and investigating patients' problems on the ward, which will aid the medical staff in making a diagnosis in addition to helping the nurse plan individualized care.

A full nursing assessment will take cognizance of the diagnostic investigations in addition to fulfilling the function of identifying an individual's physical, social and psychological problems and their implications for nursing care. In diagnosis, doctor and nurse work as interdependent members in the health care team.

It has been seen that often it is the nurse who picks up the pieces after a patient has learned about his disease and the possibility or not of effective treatment. With a life-threatening disease the patient will often look for alternative options which may include complementary therapies.

References

Bagenal, F., Easton, D., Harris, E., Chilvers, C. & McElwain, T. (1990) Survival of patients with breast cancer attending Bristol Cancer Help Centre. *Lancet*, *336*, 606–610.

Faulkner, A. (1992) *Effective interaction with patients*. Edinburgh: Churchill Livingstone.

Faulkner, A. (1995) The therapeutic role of the nurse in complementary therapy. *The Journal of Complementary Therapy in Nursing*, *1*(2), 37–40.

Gillespie, J. & Gholkar, A. (1994) *Magnetic resonance imaging and computed tomography of the head and neck*. London: Chapman & Hall.

Hill, D. & Summers, R. (1994) *Medical technology: a nursing perspective*. London: Chapman & Hall.

Hollanders, D. (1979) *Gastrointestinal endoscopy. An introduction for assistants*. London: Baillière Tindall.

Maguire, P. (1992) Improving the recognition and treatment of affective disorders in cancer patients. In Granville Grossman, K. (Ed.) *Recent advances in psychiatry 7*, pp. 15–30. Edinburgh: Churchill Livingstone.

Sheard, T. (1990) Letter to Editor. *Lancet*, *336*, 1185–1186.

Stanway, A. (1994) *Complementary medicine: a guide to natural therapies*. London: Penguin Arkana.

Swash, M. & Mason, S. (1984) *Hutchison's Clinical Methods*. London: Baillière Tindall.

Wilson-Barnett, J. & Batehup, L. (1988) *Patient problems: a research base for nursing care*. London: Scutari Press.

Woodham, A. (1994) *HEA guide to complementary medicine and therapies*. London: Health Education Authority.

Further reading

Absten, G. & Joffe, S. (1993) *Lasers in medicine and surgery: an introductory guide*, 3rd edn. London: Chapman & Hall.

Axon, A., Bell, G., Jones, R., Quine, M. & McCloy, R. (1995) Guidelines on appropriate indications for upper gastro-intestinal endoscopy. *British Medical Journal*, 6983(310), 853–856.

Booth, J. A. (Ed.) (1984) *Handbook of investigations. Lippincott Nursing Series*. London: Harper and Row.

Gillespie, J. (1993) *A text atlas of diagnostic imaging of the head and neck*. London: Chapman & Hall.

Krasner, N. (Ed.) (1991) *Lasers in gastroenterology*. London: Chapman & Hall.

Rankin-Box, D. (Ed.) (1995) *The nurse's handbook of complementary therapies*. Edinburgh: Churchill Livingstone.

Reece, L. (1993) *Diagnostic tests in endocrinology and diabetes*. London: Chapman & Hall.

Thompson, D. & Bowman, G. (1985) *Medical investigations. Nurses' aids series*. London: Baillière Tindall.

10

Planning Care: Medical Interventions

CHAPTER SUMMARY

Introduction: the medical ward, 243
Types of medical ward, 244
Medical conditions, 245

Medical conditions associated with deficits in oxygen uptake, 246
Bronchitis, 246
Emphysema, 251
Carcinoma of the lung, 256
Pneumonia, 264
Cardiac failure, 269
Ischaemic heart disease, 274

Medical conditions associated with deficits in nutrition, 281
Peptic ulcer, 282
Ulcerative colitis, 287
Cirrhosis of the liver, 291
Diabetes mellitus, 298

Hyperthyroidism, 310
Hypothyroidism, 313

Diseases associated with fluid balance, 315
Acute renal failure, 316
Chronic renal failure, 319

Deficits associated with rest and exercise, 322
Anaemia, 323
Multiple sclerosis, 330
Rheumatoid arthritis, 334
The unconscious patient, 341

Lifestyle and disease, 346
AIDS, 347

Summary, 350

References, 351

Further reading, 351

Introduction: the medical ward

Patients are admitted to a medical ward for the diagnosis of a disease which has led to expressed deficits in functioning or for the treatment of a known medical disorder. Some of these patients will be admitted via their GP, some from the out-patients' department and some as emergencies (Chapter 3). For many patients the admission will be the first experience of hospital, while for others the ward will be all too familiar. What will be common to all patients is that each will have his personal concerns associated with admission to hospital which may or may not affect the course of the disease and the potential for recovery.

The majority of medical patients face considerable uncertainty – about their diagnosis, the length of stay, the prognosis, and the effects these will have on normal life. There is nothing cut and dried about a medical condition and it is not unusual for a consultant to suggest hospitalization for 'a few days', only for it to be found subsequently that the patient needs to stay for several weeks. Of course, once the diagnosis is known, the time in hospital can be gauged more accurately.

Types of medical ward

Some medical wards are described as 'general', which means that patients may be admitted there with any medical condition. Other wards may specialize in a discrete group of conditions. For example, one ward may take only patients with respiratory diseases; another may deal with metabolic disorders, and another with renal diseases. This division of patients is largely due to the specialization of the medical profession and the grouping of specialist resources. Such specialization may be seen to enhance expertise since, if a consultant treats only patients with diabetes, for example, he is able to keep abreast of current developments in one field in a way which is not possible for every field.

There are advantages and disadvantages for the patient who finds himself on a specialist medical ward. The advantage is that he may expect to receive high-level care from an expert staff. He may also meet other patients who have been treated successfully. A disadvantage is that he might meet patients with complications or whose disease is resistant to treatment. A patient may find this worrying and upsetting. To see someone with the same disease who is very ill may be perceived as a portent of one's own future, and to the patient who is worried about his future this negative view may not be balanced by seeing other patients who are recovering.

A further disadvantage is that the patient may find himself on a mixed-sex ward. Mixed-sex wards are unpopular with many patients because they conflict with what is normally socially acceptable. It is not usual to meet strangers of the opposite sex in night wear. Many patients find it difficult enough to meet their friends and family while wearing night wear in a hospital bed, so to share a room and toilet facilities and to eat meals with unknown patients of the opposite sex can be extremely embarrassing and distressing.

New health service guidelines (DH 1995) for patients state: 'Except in emergencies, you have the right to be told before you go into hospital, whether it is planned to care for you in a ward for men and women. In all cases you can expect single sex washing and toilet facilities. If you would prefer to be in single sex accommodation (either single sex or a 'bay' within a larger ward which offers equal privacy) your wishes will be respected wherever possible.' What is important here is that patients are made aware of their rights rather than that they suffer emotional discomfort.

A nurse may not be able to change the ward system but when she is nursing a patient she should be sensitive to his problems and alleviate any embarrassment. She should understand that he may take measures to avoid the unacceptable; he may, for instance, avoid interaction with very ill patients, and may ask to eat meals by his bed. This should not be labelled as 'unsociable behaviour' without assessing and understanding the individual's underlying problems and beliefs.

Medical conditions

Many medical conditions are labelled 'chronic'. Once present, such conditions are long term and the individual may never return to full physical health. Examples of this are chronic bronchitis, cirrhosis of the liver and chronic renal disease. Other conditions such as diabetes and hypothyroidism are also labelled chronic, though this may appear to be a misnomer since with well-controlled replacement therapy the individual may lead a perfectly healthy life. Such patients have a chronic condition but may object to being labelled 'chronically ill'. On a medical ward, the majority of patients may be suffering from chronic disease. Many of them will have had prolonged periods of hospitalization previously and they may have several weeks of treatment ahead of them.

The other patients on the ward will be suffering from acute conditions such as pneumonia, gastritis or acute pyelitis. Acute conditions usually respond rapidly to treatment so that the hospital stay is shorter for these individuals than for those with chronic conditions.

Because chronic conditions tend to exacerbate with increasing age, and because many patients on a medical ward have chronic conditions, there may be relatively few young patients on the ward. This has implications for the types of social and psychological problem which present in the nursing assessment, both in the patient's reaction to his disease and in his reactions to the ward environment.

Some specific medical conditions will be considered in this chapter together with their possible effects on the individual and the resultant implications for care. Al-

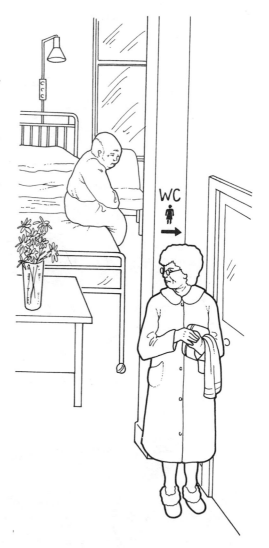

WC

though these conditions will be grouped according to their effects on breathing, nutrition, fluid balance, and rest and exercise, the interrelated functions of the body systems should not be overlooked. For example, diabetes may be considered as a disease which affects an individual's ability to maintain adequate nutrition since it is a metabolic disorder, yet, untreated, it also affects fluid and acid–base balance and, eventually, breathing, rest and exercise.

Medical conditions associated with deficits in oxygen uptake

The major organs associated with the uptake and transport of oxygen are the lungs and heart (Chapter 2). Disturbances in their function can be a threat to life since oxygen is necessary for the functioning of all the cells in the body. In this section some of the diseases affecting oxygen uptake will be examined, and the individual's physical, psychological and social reactions to the effects of the disease process will be illustrated.

A knowledge of the possible effects of a known disease should help the nurse to plan care. The nurse must remember, however, to account for individual differences and to assess each patient not only for known and potential problems, but for problems which may not be related to the disease process but which may affect goals and outcomes.

Bronchitis

THE DISEASE PROCESS

Acute bronchitis is generally a short illness characterized by inflammation of the bronchioles following an upper respiratory tract infection. Untreated, it may progress to pneumonia (p. 264) but in most cases it is treated in the patient's own home with antibiotics and a full recovery is achieved. However, frequent infections and inflammations of this type may lead to the more serious condition of chronic bronchitis, which may also be described as chronic airway obstruction.

In chronic bronchitis the bronchial mucosa is affected by the preceding infections, leading to an increase in the activity of the mucus-secreting glands (Figure 10.1). The extra mucus secreted forms a warm moist base for infective organisms to grow in. Over time, the epithelial lining

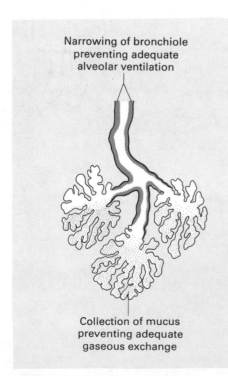

Narrowing of bronchiole preventing adequate alveolar ventilation

Collection of mucus preventing adequate gaseous exchange

Fig. 10.1 Chronic bronchitis.

and cilia in the bronchial pathways are destroyed so that particles normally swept out of the airways remain in the lungs. The mucosa becomes damaged, thickened and oedematous with the result that the airways are narrowed and become blocked by mucus.

In such a situation, inspiration does not take enough oxygen to the lungs while expiration of the carbon dioxide-rich air is also partially blocked. As a result, over time the alveoli become permanently distended and may rupture under the pressure of trapped air.

Because there is an inadequate supply of oxygen to the pulmonary circulation there may be vasoconstriction in the vessels serving the lungs. This localized vaso-constriction may lead to pulmonary hypertension and eventually, because of continued resistance to the efforts of the right ventricle to pump blood through the lungs, right-sided cardiac failure may develop. The inability to exchange gases adequately leads to hypoxia and hypercapnia (too low a concentration of oxygen and too high a concentration of carbon dioxide, respectively).

The disease process in chronic bronchitis is progressive if early treatment does not reverse the situation. Although infection appears to be a key factor, social habits and conditions are also seen to be contributory. Among these are smoking, pollution in the air and living in a cold, damp environment. There appears to be a familial (hereditary) tendency to chronic bronchitis, but it could be argued that families tend to live in similar conditions and that perhaps environmental influences are stronger than hereditary traits.

Physical reactions

As a result of the irritation caused by infection and the increased mucus production, the individual will have a productive cough which may be painful. Early morning coughing is usually the worst because mucus builds up during the night.

Breathing becomes difficult and the respirations are described as 'wheezy'. The patient begins to experience dyspnoea of effort and may reduce his physical activity as a result. In severe cases the patient is unable to walk upstairs without extreme breathlessness, and cyanosis may be present. If breathing is difficult when lying down (orthopnoea), the patient may have to sleep sitting up in bed. Coughing requires effort, and prolonged 'hard' coughing to bring up the copious sticky sputum will leave the patient exhausted. He will feel physically ill and drained. Many individuals will allow the situation to become quite serious before seeking medical help, while others will become concerned enough to seek advice much earlier. Because the disease has an insidious onset, an individual may not realize how much worse his cough and breathlessness have become. It may be that a visitor will make a remark that causes the individual to reassess his own physical state and take action.

Psychological reactions

A patient with bronchitis may become very frightened by his breathlessness and experience feelings of panic. He may be worried about sleeping in case he chokes and stops breathing in the night. This is a very real fear for the individual who slips down the bed as he sleeps and wakes up fighting for breath. Coughing and expectoration may be distressing and lead to fears of being socially unacceptable and repulsive to others. This, along with the physical restrictions caused by breathlessness, may produce feelings of extreme misery for the individual who previously enjoyed life and who now has to face the fact that he is chronically sick. Other reactions may include anger or aggression – towards fate for sending the affliction or towards family and partner because they are well. Such seemingly illogical behaviour may lead to tension in the family and exacerbate psychological problems.

Chronic disease, with no likelihood of a return to normal life, may cause an individual to question his religious beliefs, so that his faith deserts him at a time when it might have helped in accepting the inevitable. In others, faith is unaffected or strengthened, as may be other relationships in such time of affliction.

No assumptions can be made about an individual's psychological reactions to chronic bronchitis (or any disease) without adequate assessment.

Social reactions

Although it is commonly known that smoking exacerbates chronic bronchitis, and is a factor in its cause, smokers often choose to ignore this information. As a result, the patient with bronchitis may not react to the disease by giving up smoking but instead may rationalize its continuation. Many individuals with chronic bronchitis maintain that smoking, particularly first thing in the morning, 'helps to bring up the phlegm'.

Physical and psychological reactions to bronchitis may affect social interactions and relationships, including partnerships, since breathlessness may lead an individual to be diffident about his ability to make love, while his partner may be put off close contact by the patient's physical condition and his cough.

Working relationships may also be affected. Depending on the nature of employment, the individual with bronchitis may often be too sick to work or may go to work but not be able to pull his weight. Employment problems may lead to further psychological concerns.

When the individual is admitted to hospital the inter-related physical, psychological and social problems will be of varying importance. For some patients, admission to hospital may be a relief while for others it will add to the burden of stress they are trying to cope with.

PLANNING NURSING CARE

Physical care

Nursing care will be planned on the basis of the individual's problems and the medical care which has been prescribed for him. Physical problems which may be anticipated in all cases are breathlessness and a productive cough. In advanced cases the bronchial airways can be in a state of chronic spasm (bronchospasm) which is characterized by wheezy breathing. Medical treatment may incorporate antibiotics for the infection and a bronchodilator such as salbutamol in aerosol form. Oxygen therapy may also be prescribed.

The nursing care plan should state the treatment which has been prescribed to deal with the physical problem of breathlessness, since this treatment is carried out by a nurse. The plan should also state the nursing measures taken to relieve breathlessness, such as the positioning of the patient upright in bed, and other plans to aid breathing such as education on how to expectorate sputum more effectively and how to improve breathing techniques. Such tuition may be given initially by a physiotherapist but it is the nurse's role to encourage the patient to practise these skills.

With chronic bronchitis, especially as the disease advances, it is unrealistic to set goals for a return to normal breathing since the bronchial airways are permanently damaged. The patient may have been admitted in an acute phase of the disease with severe dyspnoea. An immediate goal would be to reduce the feelings of panic and alarm which can increase the severity of the dyspnoea. This may be achieved by oxygen therapy and reassurance on the part of the nurse that immediate treatment will almost certainly bring relief. Longer term goals would be that the patient's breathing becomes effective (if not normal) without the aid of oxygen therapy.

Education is important in a number of areas which the patient may not realize are related to his problem of

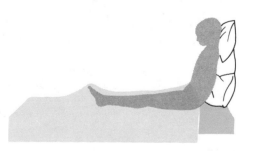

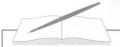

Identify a patient with chronic bronchitis, and define those areas where education could improve his management of his disease.

1 Plan priorities for education.
2 Choose the most important priority and negotiate a way forward with the patient.
3 How could you measure the success of your intervention?

breathing. Poor nutrition, for example, predisposes to infection; obesity puts strain on the heart and lungs; irritants such as tobacco smoke can exacerbate bronchitis by both active and passive intake (Ward 1984) and breathing at night is affected by the change from a warm living room to a cold bedroom.

Plans for educating a patient (Chapter 15) will not only help his condition in hospital but may well allow him to avoid future acute attacks or indeed slow down the advancement of the disease. Assessment is required prior to educating the bronchitic patient to ensure that it is pertinent. For example, a patient who is under-nourished does not need to be taught the dangers of obesity – rather he may need advice on nutrition and on how to achieve his ideal weight, as well as an understanding of the links between diet and infection.

Physical care of the patient with bronchitis will include observation of the amount and type of sputum expectorated, of the temperature and pulse if infection is present, and of respiration and skin colour since cyanosis may be present. It is also important to ensure that fluid intake is adequate and that fluid balance is maintained.

A patient's mouth may need care. Expectorated sputum and oxygen therapy may well produce a dirty, unpleasant taste which the individual is unable to cope with alone. Physical care may also include monitoring the patient's reactions if right ventricular failure is present (p. 269).

Psychological care

The problems which may be predicted are those associated with the breathlessness, the cough, and the inevitability of living with a chronic condition. As medical treatment and nursing care bring an improvement in the individual's health, such problems may recede. It is important that each patient is allowed to talk through his feelings and fears. Learning of the positive measures he can take to reduce the risks of acute episodes may also help the patient, since he should no longer feel a helpless victim of the disease.

The extent to which an individual's self-image is damaged by the bronchitis should be assessed, and steps taken to help him build a more positive picture of his worth. Relatives are important here for they may not realize the nature of the problems and may have been unwittingly cruel about the symptoms such as coughing and spitting or the effects of the disease such as unemployment. Often it is enough if the nurse gets the family to talk over their feelings, for disease affects more people than those who carry it.

There may be a number of psychological problems which cannot be predicted. When identified, they may not have solutions. The nurse needs to identify these problems and to learn to refer where appropriate, help the patient find his own solution where possible and, if the problem is insoluble, talk it through with the aim of helping the patient to adapt to the effects of the problem so that coping mechanisms can be brought into play. This will allow the patient to concentrate on those problems where solutions are possible.

Social care

Social problems may be linked to the physical and psychological problems in bronchitis. As the patient's condition improves, he may feel more able to socialize with other patients, and will consider the social habits and conditions of his life at home in the light of his present condition. For example, breathlessness may make it difficult for an individual to talk, so reducing his ability to socialize with family and friends.

Social interaction cannot be forced on to an individual, but problems with relationships will need to be examined if the patient wishes to discuss them. It is a pity if an individual becomes reclusive because of the physical or psychological effects of his disease.

Problems that are concerned with social conditions, once identified, may need to be referred to an outside agency such as social services. Patients may require information on benefits and services available to the disabled and, if relevant, the unemployed.

THE CARE PLAN

Once identified, problems which have a nursing solution or intervention should be listed in order of priority of action, and realistic goals should be set incorporating the co-operation of the patient and his family, as relevant. Cognizance should be taken of problems associated with the condition and those not associated with it but which could have a bearing on the individual's ability or motivation for recovery. Constant reassessment is required and new goals should be set, remembering that if a condition is worsening the patient's potential may be reduced.

Emphysema

THE DISEASE PROCESS

Emphysema is linked with bronchitis in that there is often a long history of chronic bronchitis prior to the insidious onset of emphysema, and the two diseases are often present in the same patient. The damage caused to the lungs by emphysema is permanent and more destructive than that from chronic bronchitis. Because of its link with a long history of chronic bronchitis, emphysema is more common from middle-age onwards.

The blocking of the bronchioles with mucus and the consequent trapping of air in the alveoli seen in bronchitis lead to loss of elasticity in the lungs and decreased ventilatory capacity. Tissue is destroyed between alveoli with the result that groups of alveoli join together, producing larger spaces in the lungs and increasing lung size (Figure 10.2). The exchange of gases is hampered by pressure on the capillaries in the lungs and by the destruction of alveoli, which reduces the area of lung available for gaseous exchange. This can lead to respiratory acidosis. To balance the low alkalinity in the blood which results from raised carbon dioxide levels, serum electrolyte levels are disturbed – bicarbonate and sodium are raised, while chloride is reduced. The decreased lung capacity leads to the muscles of respiration becoming inadequate, with the

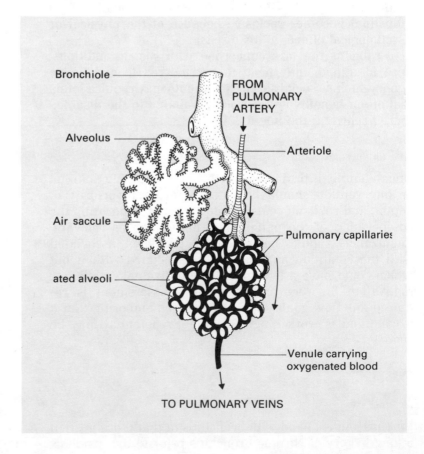

Fig. 10.2 Alveoli in emphysema.

less effective accessory respiratory muscles coming into use.

Physical reactions

For the patient with a history of bronchitis, the onset of emphysema leads to severe dyspnoea, with more and more effort being required for breathing, especially if the individual attempts physical exertion. A cough may be present, although, after years of coughing with bronchitis, the coughing mechanism may be ineffective.

The increased lung size causes the chest to become barrel-shaped and enlarged, while hypoxia, for reasons which are unknown, leads to clubbing of the fingers. With the major muscles of respiration becoming ineffective, respiration is difficult. Breathing may be described as wheezy with prolonged expiration. The patient may have a flushed complexion; this is not due to exertion but to arterial dilatation which results from hypercapnia. As the disease progresses, signs of right-sided cardiac failure may appear for the same physiological reasons as in advanced chronic bronchitis (p. 246).

Although the physical reactions to emphysema are linked with those of chronic bronchitis, it does rarely occur as a primary condition, in which case a long history of ill-health may be absent.

Psychological reactions

The psychological reactions may be similar to, but are more marked than, those in chronic bronchitis. As the severity of dyspnoea increases, feelings of panic about breathlessness may arise. Breathing can no longer be taken for granted but requires continuous, exhausting effort.

The permanence of the disability and its certain advancement may lead to depression because the individual feels powerless to fight his situation and worthless as a member of society. If breathing is an exhausting effort, all other exertion may be abandoned in misery and frustration.

Social reactions

As with bronchitis, the physical and psychological reactions to emphysema may lead to difficulties with social interactions. As the disease progresses, the chances of unemployment will rise, cutting the patient off from friends and colleagues. Dependence on partner or family may disrupt the balance of relationships. The individual living alone may not be able to care for himself adequately and may have to consider giving up his home. This may have repercussions on the family, especially if an alternative home cannot be offered by a family member.

Physical care

Although there is no cure for emphysema, the patient can be educated to lead a less disabling life. Many of the educative measures for a patient with chronic bronchitis are equally pertinent to the patient with emphysema, e.g. learning to breathe and cough effectively may ease the problems of breathlessness. Pulmonary irritants, such as cigarette smoke and polluted air, should be avoided and the patient educated, according to his problems, about nutrition, exposure to infection, and the need to sleep in a warm bedroom.

Although medical treatment may be prescribed, such as oxygen therapy, the use of bronchodilators and antibiotics, the major nursing role will be in giving support to the patient and helping him to gain insight into his physical problems so that he is motivated to learn how to alleviate his breathlessness.

Priorities in planning care will probably lie in relieving breathlessness. In a healthy individual, breathing is regulated by the rise in carbon dioxide in the blood. In the advanced chronic bronchitic and emphysemic patient, the carbon dioxide level is permanently raised and breathing then becomes regulated by the low oxygen level in the blood. This needs to be considered when administering oxygen therapy since a normal concentration of oxygen will raise blood oxygen levels and the patient will cease to breathe (Figure 10.3). Oxygen therapy should always be prescribed by a doctor, but the nurse needs to understand the reason for its administration at different concentrations according to the physical condition of the patient.

The patient will probably be exhausted on admission to hospital. Assessment of what he can do for himself in terms of hygiene will set priorities for physical care while maintaining as much independence for the patient as possible. Physical care and observations will be similar to those for the patient with chronic bronchitis (p. 249).

As with chronic bronchitis, the goals will need to be realistic since there is no possibility of the condition reversing. As the disease advances, admission to hospital, hospice or nursing home may be for terminal care (Chapter 13). In this case it must be remembered that patient potential may be expected to move in a negative direction and that plans for care may include preparation of rela-

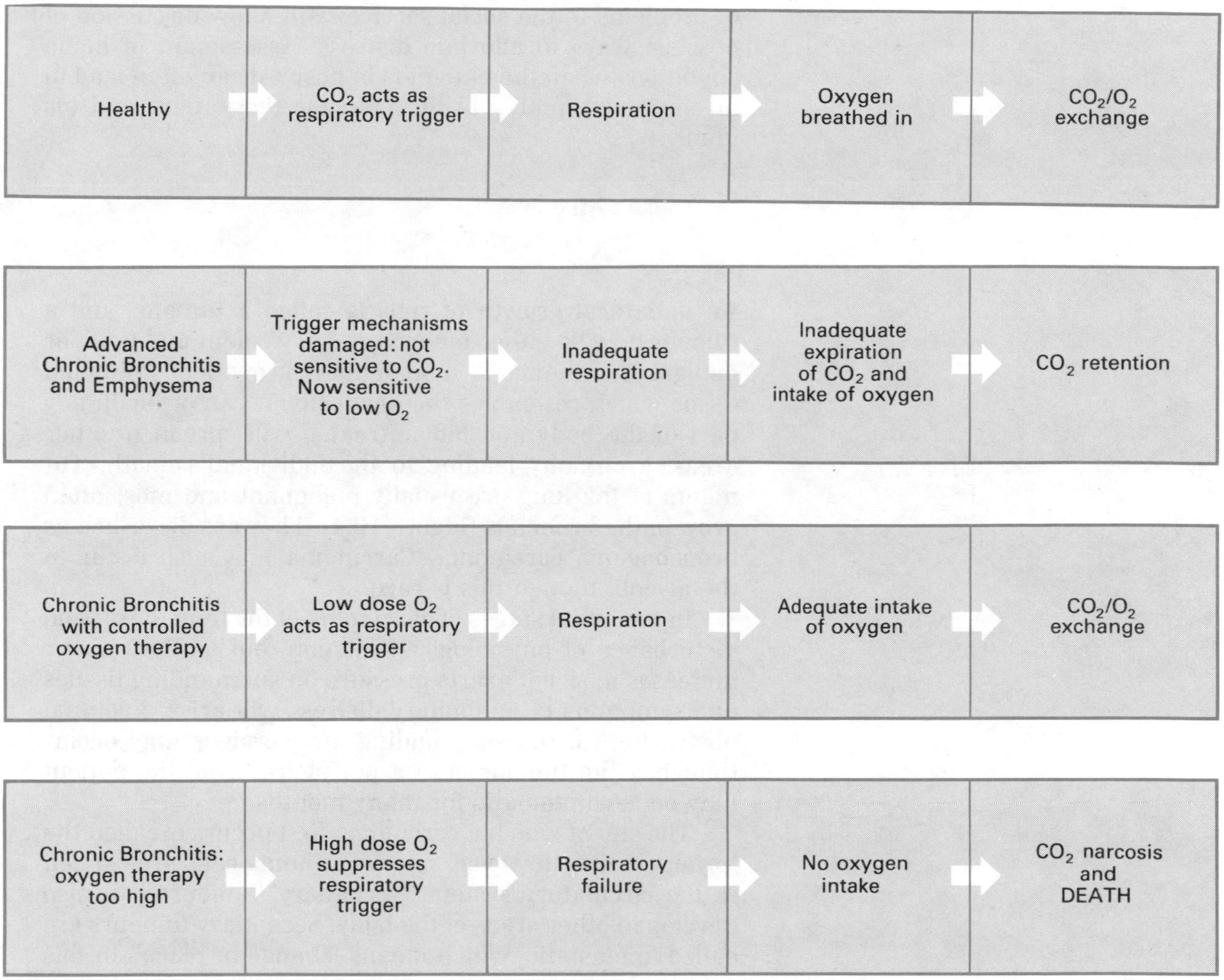

Healthy	CO_2 acts as respiratory trigger	Respiration	Oxygen breathed in	CO_2/O_2 exchange

Advanced Chronic Bronchitis and Emphysema	Trigger mechanisms damaged: not sensitive to CO_2. Now sensitive to low O_2	Inadequate respiration	Inadequate expiration of CO_2 and intake of oxygen	CO_2 retention

Chronic Bronchitis with controlled oxygen therapy	Low dose O_2 acts as respiratory trigger	Respiration	Adequate intake of oxygen	CO_2/O_2 exchange

Chronic Bronchitis: oxygen therapy too high	High dose O_2 suppresses respiratory trigger	Respiratory failure	No oxygen intake	CO_2 narcosis and DEATH

tives for the patient's death. In the earlier stages of the disease, involving relatives in the patient's education to alleviate breathlessness may be considered in planning care.

Fig. 10.3 Mechanisms of CO_2/O_2 balance in health and in chronic bronchitis and emphysema.

Psychological care

Psychological care will be similar to that for chronic bronchitis, though it has to be remembered that problems may become more severe as the disease progresses. Individual problems should be assessed and their relevance to the patient's present condition explored.

Social care

As the disease progresses, social problems may arise in self-care or for relatives who care for the patient. Referral of problems to the social services will allow discussion of possible ways to alleviate distress. Assessment of home conditions when the patient is in hospital can often lead to an improved quality of life both for the patient and his family.

Carcinoma of the lung

THE DISEASE PROCESS

An unnatural growth of cells is called a tumour, and a tumour may be either malignant, i.e. virulent and fatal, or benign. Carcinoma is a malignant growth of epithelial tissue which resembles the host cells. It can occur in any part of the body and left untreated will spread to other areas, eventually leading to the individual's death. Tumours of the lung are usually malignant and most often grow in the bronchus (Figure 10.4). They are described as bronchogenic carcinoma. Carcinoma may also occur in the alveoli, though this is rare.

In the initial stages of carcinoma of the lung there is no disturbance of physiological function, but as the tumour increases in size it exerts pressure on surrounding tissues and symptoms of pulmonary distress will arise. Eventual obstruction of the surrounding air passages may occur, though if the tumour is in a peripheral area the patient may be asymptomatic for many months.

The site at which a carcinoma first occurs is called the 'primary' site. However, since carcinoma cells are carried in the circulatory system, 'secondary' tumours can also develop in other areas of the body. Secondary tumours are called 'metastatic' which means 'change of place', in this

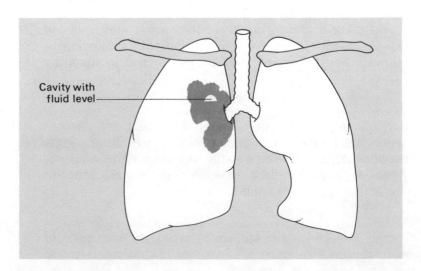

Fig. 10.4 Carcinomas of the bronchus.

Cavity with fluid level

case of cancerous cells. Cigarette smoking is seen to be a key factor in primary carcinoma of the lung (Ward 1984) and a leading cause of death in the UK. Other irritants such as polluted air and chemical gases are also factors associated with the disease.

Those patients who do not smoke but who develop carcinoma of the lung may feel that it is somehow another's fault that they have contracted the disease. 'Passive smoking' is the term used for those who are forced to inhale the smoke exhaled by others, but who do not smoke themselves. This has been taken up as an issue in many places so that it is now possible to travel on an aeroplane and on public transport, and to eat in restaurants in areas that are designated 'Non-Smoking'.

Physical reactions

The physical reactions to an obstructive tumour tend to mimic those of other pulmonary disorders. Indeed recurring attacks of bronchitis or pneumonia may occur due to the build up of secretions and the resultant infections. Coughing and wheezing are also common, along with increasing problems with breathing. Pain in the chest may be present due to pressure of the tumour, the area depending on the site of the tumour. Haemoptysis may occur if blood vessels are eroded.

Much will depend on the site, but it is possible for carcinoma of the lung to be relatively advanced before there are any pulmonary reactions. If this is the case, other reactions to the carcinoma, such as anaemia, loss of weight and tiredness, may be the symptoms which cause an individual to seek help. These latter reactions occur in any untreated carcinoma since the malignant growth acts as a parasite on normal cells. Specific reactions to carcinoma of the lung may include difficulty in speaking if the vocal chords are affected, and oedema of the face and neck if there is obstruction to the superior vena cava.

Psychological reactions

Before diagnosis, the psychological reactions will be those of an individual who faces the fact that he is not well without knowing the reason for his malaise. These reactions will range from attempting to ignore the facts to seeking help, depending on the individual and the severity of his symptoms (Chapter 2).

The diagnosis of cancer may be described as fear provoking in that little is known about its cause. Despite advances in treatment, in many people's minds it is synonymous with a death sentence. Those patients who contract lung cancer as a result of smoking may have fewer psychological problems than those who contract the disease as a result of passive smoking or other undetermined reasons. There may be much heart-searching for a reason for the disease in the absence of any cause and effect. This often leads to feelings of anger that the disease has occurred, guilt if the disease is seen as a punishment, and blame for known or unknown others who may have contributed to the disease.

If the patient is not given a diagnosis he may react with anxiety, especially if he feels that his condition is not improving. Such anxiety will be enhanced if the patient suspects that information is being withheld. It is also true that when the patient is told of his diagnosis, he may have psychological problems in coping with a fear-provoking diagnosis and an uncertain future.

Other psychological problems may arise as a result of a relative's reactions to the diagnosis. It is not uncommon for a consultant to tell the relative the diagnosis while withholding it from the patient, particularly if the prognosis is poor. This may lead to problems of collusion (Chapter 13).

Other psychological reactions will include those arising from admission to hospital and its implications for the personal life of the individual.

Social reactions

Social reactions will be those associated with any illness which involves inability to lead a normal life. Repeated sick leave for chest infections might result in employment problems while tiredness might be interpreted as lack of interest in normal social interactions. The individual may find he lacks the energy to go out with his partner, meet his friends, or indulge in his hobbies.

PLANNING NURSING CARE

Physical care

Care will be influenced by the individual's physical condition and his treatment. In any patient with cancer there is a choice of treatment, from surgery for those cases where early detection and lack of metastases suggest a favourable outcome (Chapter 11) to radiotherapy or chemotherapy as an adjunct to surgery or for inoperable cases. Radiotherapy, where X-rays are used in an attempt to control the growth of the tumour, and chemotherapy, where cytotoxic drugs are used to destroy the malignant cells, may have considerable effects on the patient (see below). These effects have implications for planning nursing care.

Careful assessment of the individual's reactions to his treatment will need to be made, taking into account the course of the disease. Some patients, for example, may have had surgical resection of the lung and then be admitted for treatment of complications caused by metastases in the spine, brain or liver.

Radiation is aimed at destruction of malignant cells. It may also have an effect on normal cells, and may produce local reactions which vary from a redness of skin and temporary loss of hair through to a more severe reaction where blistering and ulceration of the skin occurs with permanent loss of hair and sweat glands. General reactions may include tiredness, nausea and anorexia.

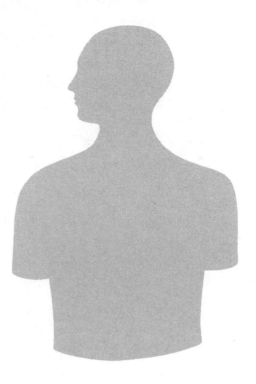

Plans for care will involve preparing the patient for treatment, both in meeting his needs for information and in his acceptance of the treatment. The area to be treated is usually marked out and the patient is told not to wash it or to use creams or ointments on it. A light splash with tepid water may be all that is allowed for some weeks and may mean that the patient is unable to bathe or shower. This may lead to the patient feeling unclean.

Since the treatment causes breakdown of cells, fluid intake is normally increased to help elimination of the resultant waste products. Diet is also important both to promote healing and to resist infection. Both fluid and diet intake may present a nursing problem if the patient is nauseated and anorexic. Small tempting meals and preferred drinks should be offered. Compliance is more likely if the patient understands the importance of nutrition in the treatment of his disease. Hospital food is often refused but it may be that relatives will bring in favourite foods in small portions which will be tolerated.

Mobility may be a problem since the patient may feel too tired after treatment to be very active. Plans for care will need to include encouragement to take gentle exercise. Prolonged periods in bed could lead to problems of pressure sores. Relatives may be anxious about the apparently adverse effects of the treatment and may need help in understanding care. They may interpret nursing actions as heartless as their sick, tired relative is persuaded to eat and drink when he does not want to, and get out of bed when he is obviously (to them) not 'up to it'.

Chemotherapy There are a number of cytotoxic drugs used in the treatment of carcinoma (Neale 1987). They may be administered orally, intravenously, intramuscularly and occasionally intra-arterially, though the latter is a more complex procedure which is carried out in theatre.

A large number of chemotherapy drugs have some effect on lung cancer and usually these are given in combinations of two or more, rather than as single dose regimes. Chemotherapy alone has not been shown to cure cancer but it may help with palliation and in reducing the pressure symptoms associated with lung cancer.

Reactions to cytotoxic preparations are unpleasant and distressing for the patient and preparation of what to expect is an essential part of nursing care. In order to destroy the malignant cells, the drugs are extremely toxic, which leads to physiological effects such as anaemia, nausea and vomiting, disturbance of bowel function, oedema, temporary loss of hair and loss of libido, according to the particular drug used.

In planning care, a balance needs to be achieved between giving a realistic picture of the possible effects of the drug to be used without upsetting the patient who may already be anxious and disturbed about his illness. This requires a positive approach on the part of the nurse. For example, it can be explained that the nausea will be counteracted by the use of an anti-emetic. If hair loss is expected, the patient who can afford to will have a wig made in preparation so that she will not have to be seen bald. It can also be explained that the hair will usually grow again, although it will be the soft vellus hair normally seen in infancy. Some centres offer scalp cooling which may reduce hair loss.

Extreme sensitivity is required when offering reassurance. The nurse who says cheerfully, 'Look on the bright side – you will save pounds at the hairdressers' can be very upsetting to a patient. Exploring feelings and showing understanding of an individual's reactions to aggressive therapy should be an essential component in planning care.

Plans for care during the course of treatment will take into account the side effects and the resultant problems for the patient. For example, nausea, anorexia and bowel function will have an effect upon the patient's co-operation in taking adequate fluids and diet, listlessness will affect mobility, and loss of hair, even with an attractive and well-fitting wig, may affect the patient's desire to get out of bed and interact with other people.

Plans for care will also include nursing action for the deficits produced by airway obstruction, physical disability, according to the level of advancement of the disease, and pain caused by pressure of the tumour on surrounding tissues. Frequent reassessment will be necessary so that realistic goals may be set as the patient's potential changes.

Many patients with carcinoma respond well to treatment, gaining lengthy remissions. The patients seen on a medical ward, however, are generally those who are not responding well or who have metastatic complications. This may lead nurses to take a more negative view of both the disease and the prognosis than is warranted (Elkind 1982) and may affect their attitude to patients with inoperable carcinoma. The problem in carcinoma of the lung is that the majority of patients die within a year of diagnosis because of late presentation of symptoms and lack of suitable treatment.

Psychological care

In planning psychological care for the patient with carcinoma of the lung his reactions to treatment will need to be considered as will his reactions to the diagnosis (if he has been told) or his uncertainty if the diagnosis has been withheld. Added to this are the problems associated with feeling physically ill and others which may or may not be associated with the disease.

Priority may need to be given to the psychological aspects of treatment. Although most patients cannot face the 'no hope' option of refusing further treatment, others may well question the sense of continuing when they have been ill for some time, are aware of their diagnosis and may know that their physical condition is not improving. Treatment in such cases may achieve a little more time for the individual but no more than that.

The patient may feel that the cost of the treatment in terms of reduced quality of life simply outweighs the potential but uncertain time to be gained. This can be a difficult problem for the nurse who will have her own values. Nevertheless, the nurse should be prepared to talk the situation through or refer the problem to someone in whom the patient feels able to confide. Every individual has the right to refuse treatment. The nurse's role is to ensure that patients' decisions are made as the result of informed choice.

The patient may have psychological problems arising from his understanding of the diagnosis. Plans for care should aim to meet the patient's expressed need for information. This may cause difficulties for the nurse if the consultant has a blanket policy of withholding information from all patients (Chapter 13), but the major point to remember is that some patients will not wish to discuss their diagnosis while others will have many questions to ask. An assessment of each individual's readiness to face his diagnosis and prognosis will lead to realistic plans. These plans may have implications for the nurse–doctor

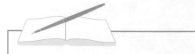

Identify a patient with a diagnosis of cancer and who is having medical treatment.

1 Assess the patient's understanding of the disease.
2 What are the major problems?
3 What help do you think this patient requires to adapt to his disease and its treatment?

relationship (Chapter 18) but essentially they should aim to meet the patient's needs.

Individual problems will be affected by the patient's age, relationships and responsibilities. Some will be insoluble especially if the outlook is poor, but with help, and the chance to talk, the patient may learn to cope with the uncertainties associated with his life. Plans should aim to deal with the patient's spiritual needs as he grapples with what may be the most serious crisis of his life.

Assessment should identify those most able to help with the crisis. It may be the nurse, a minister of religion or a partner. If the illness is prolonged and the outlook obviously poor, depression may occur and the patient may need to be referred to a psychiatrist. In planning emotional help of this sort, the patient must be involved, and agree (a) that he wishes to talk and (b) choose who he wishes to talk to. Psychiatrists, for example, may be seen to carry a stigma and some patients do not appreciate an unsolicited visit from a minister of religion.

Plans for care should also include the concerns of the relatives, who may have psychological problems associated with the diagnosis and prognosis. These may affect their relationships with the patient. Although the nurse's major responsibility is to the patient, his relatives are part of his life. If they are not supported they may withdraw emotionally from him and add to his existing feelings of anger and frustration.

Pain   may lead to fear and apprehension, especially if the patient is dependent on others for its relief. These fears may be relieved by promises that at all times the pain will be controlled. There are wide individual differences in responses to pain. Some people must take an aspirin if they stub their toe while others appear able to bear considerable pain with fortitude.

Assessment of a patient's pain must depend to a large extent on the individual's own reports (Figure 10.5), but bodily position and facial expression may also give clues for the nurse to follow up. In a prolonged illness such as carcinoma, the patient will build up a tolerance to drugs so that larger doses or stronger drugs will need to be prescribed.

The essence of pain control is that the patient feels secure that his needs for analgesia will be met. Fear of pain returning can cause tension which may increase the pain and make it more difficult to control. A prescription for drugs to be given at regular intervals will both reassure the patient and prevent pain from recurring. The individual also needs to know that his own pain threshold

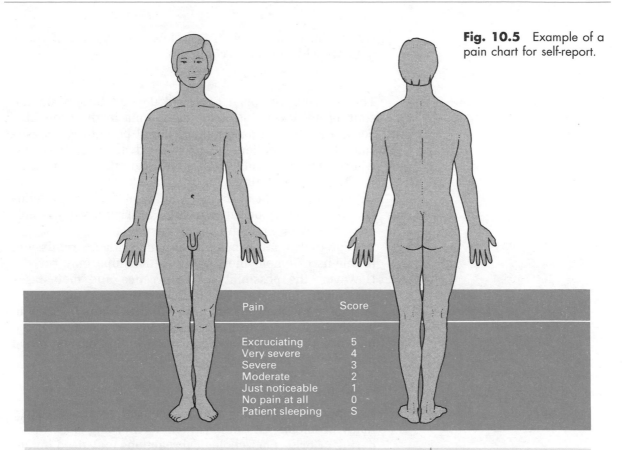

Fig. 10.5 Example of a pain chart for self-report.

Pain	Score
Excruciating	5
Very severe	4
Severe	3
Moderate	2
Just noticeable	1
No pain at all	0
Patient sleeping	S

PAIN OBSERVATION CHART

DATE

SHEET NUMBER

PATIENT IDENTIFICATION LABEL

TIME	PAIN RATING									MEASURES TO RELIEVE PAIN Specify where starred									Initials
	BY SITES								OVER-ALL	ANALGESIC GIVEN (Name, dose, route, time)	Lifting	Turning	Massage	Distracting activities*	Position change*	Additional aids*	Other*	COMMENTS FROM PATIENTS AND/OR STAFF	
	A	B	C	D	E	F	G	H											

will be accepted, even if it is lower than that of other patients with the same condition.

Social care

The planning of social care will depend largely on the state of advancement of the carcinoma in the bronchus. Social habits such as smoking should be viewed realistically, for if the patient's disease is advanced to the point where survival is unlikely, it is futile to attempt to change the habits of a lifetime.

For the patient in the early stage of the disease, education is worthwhile on the effects of irritants to the pulmonary system and smoking in particular.

For individuals whose treatment brings a remission, problems of employment and relationships may recede. However, the possibility of recurrence and metastases does mean follow-up visits to GP or clinic and the acceptance of possible problems in the future. Plans for care in hospital may need to include suitable preparation of the patient and his family and education so that early referral of future problems is assured.

THE CARE PLAN

Carcinoma of the lung and its medical treatment carry many problems with implications for nursing care. In ordering priorities, psychological reactions may need immediate attention in order that the patient understands the treatment options and feels he has made an informed choice. Preparation for treatment and reassurance that side effects will be promptly treated will also need priority.

It is impossible to make assumptions about the range of problems the patient will encounter. Constant reassessment should ensure that care is planned to meet the changing needs of the patient, given the stage of his disease and its manifestations.

Pneumonia

THE DISEASE PROCESS

Pneumonia may be taken as a blanket term for acute infection and inflammation of the lungs which result in the alveoli filling with fluid, which may or may not contain blood cells, irrespective of whether the cause is bacterial or viral.

Pneumonia may be predisposed by social habits such as smoking and alcoholism or social conditions such as overcrowding, lack of ventilation or air pollution. It may also be secondary to another disease such as chronic bronchitis (bronchopneumonia) or influenza (viral pneumonia). It can also result when an individual is debilitated through malnutrition or disease (hypostatic pneumonia).

Pneumonia may affect one lobe of the lung and is then described as lobar pneumonia, or it may spread through the whole of one or both lungs and is then described as bronchial pneumonia. The alveoli fill with fluid so that the affected area becomes consolidated (Figure 10.6). This disturbs the exchange of gases so that the level of oxygen in the blood is reduced. The level of carbon dioxide is

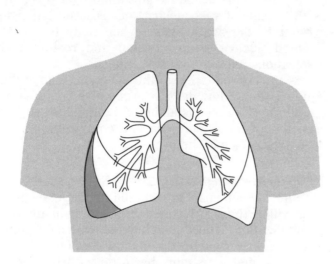

CONSOLIDATION OF ONE LOBE

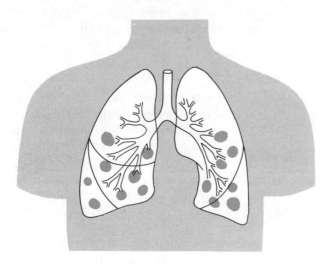

PATCHY CONSOLIDATION

Fig. 10.6 Diagram to show sites of pneumonia.

initially increased but returns to normal if there is enough unaffected lung tissue to excrete it.

Physical reactions

The physical reactions to most infective pneumonias are sudden with a chill, a rise in temperature, pulse rate and respiration, and a dry painful cough; respirations may be shallow and noisy. Viral pneumonia or hypostatic pneumonia have a more gradual onset but in all pneumonias the individual will complain of feeling unwell, with headache and generalized aching pains. In cases where disturbance of gaseous exchange is present, cyanosis of central or peripheral areas such as lips and finger tips may occur as the result of vasoconstriction. Disorientation may be present in the acute phase when body temperature is elevated. Pleurisy may develop and result in shallow respirations and pain on breathing.

As the consolidation in the affected areas of the lungs liquifies after a few days, a productive cough is present. Sputum may be bloodstained and difficult to expectorate, especially if the pneumonia is a complication of chronic bronchitis. Pus may be present.

Psychological reactions

In acute, sudden onset pneumonia, the psychological reactions will be those associated with feeling ill and requiring hospitalization. They may include worries about being sick at an inconvenient time, about responsibilities which cannot be met, or simply be to do with the individual's own feelings of malaise. Some individuals may feel so ill that they fear for their own survival.

If pneumonia is secondary to an existing condition, it becomes one more stress to add to the current burden of worries.

Social reactions

Social reactions will be those associated with needing to take time off from work and being unable to fulfil social functions. The acute nature of pneumonia means that sudden arrangements may have to be made to care for children, animals or other dependants. This may put a burden on other members of the family unit. For example, if a young mother is hospitalized at short notice, her husband may have no choice but to stay at home until he has made alternative arrangements. This in turn will affect the finances of the family and may cause problems for the husband with his employer.

PLANNING NURSING CARE

Physical care

Medical treatment involves treating the infection and dealing with the problems of breathing. Acute infective pneumonias usually respond quickly to the appropriate antibiotic. The nurse's role includes the delivery of care based on assessment and the monitoring of the patient's progress. She will report any deterioration in condition. To this end, a priority in the care plan is observation for any change which has implications for treatment – temperature, pulse and respiration rate, blood pressure, fluid balance, colour and degree of restlessness.

Modern treatment has reduced the risk of complications in pneumonia but the possibility does still exist, particularly in the patient who is already debilitated by other disease or who is very young or very old. If oxygen intake and fluid balance are severely affected, the patient may suffer shock (p. 364). Pulse and respiration will be rapid while temperature will fall. The patient will be pale and cyanosed. Such symptoms need to be reported immediately so that action, such as oxygen therapy, drug administration and possibly an intravenous infusion, may be taken.

Fluid balance is an important element in planning care since pyrexia will result in excess fluid loss from the body, as will rapid respirations and increased pulmonary secretions. The patient may feel too ill to drink or eat, but will need to be gently persuaded. The aim of planned care should be to give fluids and a liquid diet which will appeal to the individual, maintain adequate fluid intake and nutrition, and replace lost salts and water. As the patient responds to treatment, normal diet and fluid intake may be resumed.

Plans for care should include care of the mouth, which may be dry and sore due to the patient's pyrexia and his infection, and the treatment of problems of elimination which may arise through inactivity and loss of fluid. When pyrexia is present, increased perspiration will require that the patient is washed frequently, and has his clothes and sheets changed often.

The individual will need to rest, particularly in the acute stage of the disease. This will help to reduce his need for oxygen at a time when the lungs are unable to function normally. Hospitals are not very restful places but care should be planned so that there is not a constant stream of disturbances to the patient. For example, meeting his need for hygiene, making his bed, giving him a

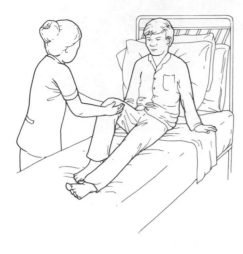

drink and his drugs could be planned to occur together, leaving a long period of rest until the next round of attention.

Pain may interfere with rest, as may psychological concerns. Drugs will be prescribed for pain and should be given promptly to reduce the patient's anxiety. Local application of heat may also relieve pleural pain. Coughing, which is encouraged to aid expectoration of sputum, may be painful, as may moving to change position. The nurse needs to be supportive in these activities and explain the necessity of clearing the lungs of the secretions which are affecting oxygen intake.

As the patient recovers from the acute phase of his illness, planned care should include gradual mobilization. No patient is kept on bedrest longer than required because of the risk of venous thrombosis in the legs. This risk is reduced by active exercise of the legs at four-hourly intervals when other care is being given. As with all patients who have problems of breathlessness, the period of bed rest is spent in an upright, sitting position to aid breathing.

The individual's infection will probably be communicable, that is, it may pass from one patient to others. This has implications for planning physical care. Gowns and masks used to be used as a means of reducing the risk of cross infection but it is recognized that good hygiene, plastic aprons and observance of a high level of nursing are a better option than making the patient feel 'untouchable'. Care is particularly needed when handling and disposing of infected sputum.

Psychological care

The individual with pneumonia will need the opportunity to discuss his fears and worries. If these are ignored, it will be difficult for the patient to rest and relax. The dramatic effect of antibiotics should dispel fears of the seriousness of the disease but the patient may be concerned by residual debilitation. This may lead to feelings of tiredness which are worrying to the patient if he thinks he should be fully recovered.

If the pneumonia is a complication of an underlying disease, psychological concerns may be very much in the area of uncertainty for the future. The nurse should explore any such concerns along with more general psychological problems and, if necessary, refer the patient on to the ward manager or to the doctor.

Social care

While the patient is in hospital, he may need education about the social habits or conditions which predispose to pulmonary disease. This will depend on individual problems such as smoking or alcoholism, and on general living conditions.

Preparation will also be required for convalescence and a return to work. Social interaction may have been restricted in hospital due to the patient's infective condition. Caution must be advised against resuming normal life too quickly to counteract these feelings of deprivation, since resistance to infection is reduced after an acute, albeit short illness.

THE CARE PLAN

In ordering priorities on the care plan, the acute nature of the disease will give priority to physical care and careful observation for signs of change in the patient's condition. Psychological problems will also need to be assessed so that the patient's essential rest is not disturbed by fears and anxieties. Since the patient is likely to be very ill on admission, contributory social habits such as smoking may not be a problem. They may, however, be a potential problem as the patient recovers, and carry a need for education.

Cardiac failure

THE DISEASE PROCESS

Any chronic obstructive airway disease can eventually put so much strain on the heart that it is unable to perform its function of pumping blood round the body. It will be remembered that in chronic bronchitis, for example, there is strain on the right ventricle because of localized vasoconstriction in the lungs, which in turn is due to an inadequate supply of oxygen to the pulmonary circulation. The term 'congestion' is used to describe the build up of blood with which the overstrained heart is unable to cope, and 'congestive cardiac failure' is the result.

Other disorders can cause congestive cardiac failure, by imposing strain on the heart, including ischaemic heart disease (p. 274), anaemia and thyrotoxicosis. In all cases, the initial cause of the congestion is the predisposing disease. Blood usually builds up on one side of the heart only; which side is affected depends on the cause.

Prolonged congestion injures the heart and hence reduces its function further. If left untreated, both sides of the heart will eventually be affected. Oedema results from the increased venous pressure caused by the congestion. If the failure is left-sided, pulmonary oedema will result, which, if untreated, can severely affect respiration, causing hypoxia (Figure 10.7).

Physical reactions

The individual will be dyspnoeic, especially on exertion, and may have a cough due to fluid in the alveoli and bronchioles. These reactions may or may not be associated with the underlying cause of the congestion. If they are, as in chronic bronchitis, the cardiac condition may be temporarily masked.

Other reactions include those relating to inadequate circulation. Body temperature may be lowered and the patient may be pale or cyanosed. Blood pressure may be lowered in left ventricular failure. There may be disorders in fluid balance since venous engorgement will decrease the kidneys' ability to produce urine.

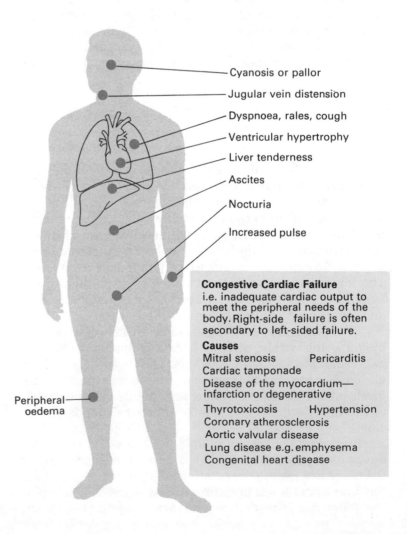

Cyanosis or pallor
Jugular vein distension
Dyspnoea, rales, cough
Ventricular hypertrophy
Liver tenderness
Ascites
Nocturia
Increased pulse

Congestive Cardiac Failure
i.e. inadequate cardiac output to meet the peripheral needs of the body. Right-side failure is often secondary to left-sided failure.
Causes
Mitral stenosis   Pericarditis
Cardiac tamponade
Disease of the myocardium—
infarction or degenerative
Thyrotoxicosis   Hypertension
Coronary atherosclerosis
Aortic valvular disease
Lung disease e.g. emphysema
Congenital heart disease

Peripheral oedema

Fig. 10.7 Congestive cardiac failure: summary of causes and effects.

In right-sided congestive heart failure oedema of the ankles and other parts of the body may occur as the disease progresses. This is accompanied by a gain in weight which is due to the accumulated fluid in the tissues. Anorexia may develop since the individual will feel tired and ill.

Psychological reactions

Individual reactions will include a response to breathlessness, to the underlying condition and to a diagnosis of heart disease. Anxiety may be present, not only in terms of present incapacity but in future prospects for health and normal pursuits, especially if the patient has felt debilitated for some time. There may also be problems associated with weight gain if there is fluid retention.

If the cardiac output is severely reduced and the oxygen supply to the brain is affected, the individual may be disoriented. This can be distressing if the patient is aware of his impaired concentration and ability to function mentally.

Social reactions

Social reactions will be those associated with breathlessness and with the underlying disease, along with the problems of long-term ill-health which affect an individual's ability to lead a normal life and, if appropriate, earn a living.

Since many patients with congestive cardiac failure are elderly, there may be social implications in the family as the individual may need more care. A partner might become quite worn out caring for a relative and individuals who live alone may make moves to ask grown-up children to care for them. This can cause problems as the son or daughter may feel 'pig in the middle' between meeting the needs of the elderly parent and those of a growing family.

PLANNING NURSING CARE

Physical care

Care will be aimed towards reducing the workload of the heart, reducing the effect of pulmonary oedema and consequent breathlessness, and improving cardiac output. Rest is important in nursing care, which will link with medical treatment.

Oxygen therapy may be prescribed to increase the supply of oxygen to the tissues and reduce dyspnoea. Mouth care will be important to alleviate dryness. Bedrest to reduce the body's requirements for oxygen and a com-

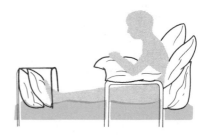

fortable upright ('orthopnoeic') position in bed should also help to reduce dyspnoea. A cardiac bed is particularly useful if right ventricular failure is present since it allows the patient to sit upright with the legs downwards so that oedema is drained away from the abdomen where it might hinder breathing. It should also be remembered that a comfortable, restful position may be obtained in a chair if a cardiac bed is not available.

The potential problems of prolonged rest in the same position need to be considered, such as pressure sores, which are exacerbated in the presence of oedema, and venous thrombosis. Another potential problem is increased patient dependency as he becomes used to a nurse meeting his needs for hygiene and comfort.

The drug digitalis is usually prescribed to strengthen and steady the heart beat if atrial fibrillation is present. Regular observations of temperature, pulse and respiration, blood pressure, colour and cough will show any change in condition, which should be reported. As the rest and treatment bring improvement, reassessment of the patient's ability to be involved in his care will need to be made. Plans may be made to reduce dependency without panic on the part of the patient. This may require that initially the nurse will be present while the patient washes himself so that he knows she will take over if the exertion increases dyspnoea.

Goals should be set that are realistic and which the patient feels are possible. After the acute phase of the disease the return to self-care and ambulation will need to be carefully monitored. By planning mobility within the patient's capabilities, there is less risk of discouragement or feelings of helplessness as yet another attack of breathlessness occurs on exertion.

Oedema is generally treated with diuretics. As these can deplete potassium in the body, oral potassium is often prescribed to retain balance. Paracentesis or venepuncture to drain excess fluid are unpopular because of the risks of infection, but may occasionally be performed. The patient may be weighed daily to monitor the effects of diuretics and other treatments of oedema. Salt in the diet may be restricted since sodium holds fluid in the tissues. There may be problems in persuading an individual to eat a salt-free or salt-reduced diet especially if he is anorexic. Small light meals are encouraged, as the patient may feel unable to attempt a full meal.

If the patient is obese, plans will need to include realistic goals for weight reduction. If the individual understands that excess body weight places undue strain on the heart he may be prepared to co-operate in reducing his intake of fats and calories.

There may be problems with elimination since bedrest and inactivity along with a light diet, may cause constipation, with a resultant strain on the heart as the patient attempts to have his bowels open. A mild aperient may be prescribed or, if necessary, suppositories. A frequent need to pass urine as the result of diuresis may also be exhausting, and plans need to be made to reduce effort where possible. This may require that two nurses help the patient on and off the bedpan or commode.

A further potential problem which is pertinent to the planning of care is that the patient will become a 'cardiac cripple' unnecessarily. Plans may include assessment of the patient's normal lifestyle, assessment of his potential following recovery from the current attack, and the need to educate both the individual and his family so that the quality of life, although partly restricted, is maximized. The relatives play an important part in this educational aspect of care since they can foster dependence if they do not fully understand the situation.

Psychological care

Few people are unaware that the heart is vital to life. A diagnosis of heart disease is thus seen as serious in the extreme and can lead to problems of anxiety and panic as the individual attempts to come to grips with the possibility of his dying. This is particularly true in acute heart failure, where the urgency of treatment may mean that drugs are given intravenously, so underlining the 'life or death' aspect of the individual's illness. Even in those cases where treatment is not necessary, a cure is unlikely because of the underlying causes of cardiac disease. The thought of permanent disability may lead to prolonged anxiety and depression. Added to these concerns are the problems associated with the symptoms of disease such as dyspnoea, which can cause panic, and tiredness, which can cause anxiety as it affects normal functioning.

It is particularly important in heart disease to deal with psychological problems since emotional distress releases adrenaline, which prepares the body for fight or flight (p. 35), placing an additional burden on the heart. Emotional problems should be carefully assessed along with the individual's need for information. Relatives may also need to be involved since their concerns about the future and their resultant anxiety may transfer to the patient.

Allowing a patient and his relatives to talk through problems may help to reduce their anxiety and set realistic goals for the future. Reassurance may be given on the possibility of recovering to the extent that a useful, if restricted, life may be restored to those patients whose disease has not progressed to a chronic inhibiting condition.

When the heart is permanently damaged through congestion due to chronic disease such as bronchitis, the patient may become angry as he realizes the consequent restrictions on his life. Others may ignore advice and shorten their lives as a result. The nurse's role in planning emotional care is to aim to meet needs where possible and to refer problems such as depression to an appropriate agent. In terms of patient decisions, the aim should be that decisions are informed even if they do not conform to the philosophy of the health care team.

Social care

Congestive cardiac failure may require plans to be made for changing an individual's social habits and environment. Smoking should be discouraged while in hospital with a view to permanent discontinuation. If the individual's breathlessness continues to be a problem, social restrictions may remain and need to be planned for during the patient's hospital stay. It may mean that employment needs to be changed or living conditions modified to conserve energy and ensure the safety of the patient.

These changes should occur to help the individual reach his own potential without wasting energy, rather than as a prelude to an invalid's life. A positive attitude on the part of the nurse is essential in planning care to prepare the patient for a restricted return to social activity. Relatives may also need support at this time as they face the implications of a chronic diagnosis, and its potential effect on their own lifestyle.

THE CARE PLAN

Priorities in the care plan may need to be concerned with providing bedrest for the patient and dealing with the problems of dyspnoea and oedema. However, psychological problems may exacerbate cardiac distress and may also need to be given priority. Educating the patient to maximize his potential and avoid the adoption of the role of invalid should be considered, as should solutions to problems which may reduce co-operation in care.

Ischaemic heart disease

THE DISEASE PROCESS

Ischaemia is a term used to describe a deficiency in the blood supply to any part of the body. In ischaemic heart disease, the deficiency is to the heart muscle. It is caused by either obstruction to or narrowing of the coronary arteries, which reduces the oxygen supply to the heart muscle. Nutrients are also reduced but the main concern is the oxygen deficit since the heart muscle cannot function efficiently with less than an optimum oxygen supply.

Narrowing and hardening of the arteries ('arteriosclerosis') is caused by degenerative changes and the build up of cholesterol and other fatty deposits ('plaques') in the vessel wall. 'Atherosclerosis' (Figure 10.8) is the term used to describe the process by which plaques develop and subsequently become fibrotic or calcified. The linings of the arteries become roughened because of the presence of plaques, so reducing the lumen and eventually blocking it. The possibility of thrombus formation arises as the circulation slows down. Should a coronary artery become totally blocked, oxygen to the area of muscle concerned will be cut off. The damage to this tissue is called an infarction and the individual is said to have suffered a myocardial infarction or coronary thrombosis.

When the blood cannot flow freely through the arteries, it may divert through smaller vessels and form what is knows as a collateral or alternative route. Such alternative circulations are unlikely to provide the myocardium, for example, with an adequate oxygen supply.

Ischaemic heart disease is thought to be associated with cigarette smoking, diets high in fats and cholesterol, stress and tension, and diabetes. Heredity factors are also important.

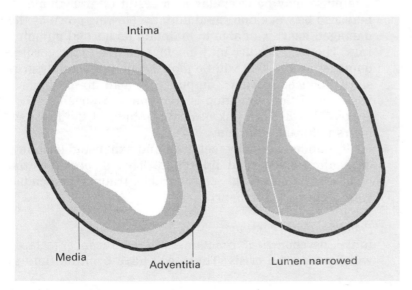

Fig. 10.8 Damage to the arteries in atherosclerosis.

Physical reactions

Angina pectoris is a pain associated with physical exertion or emotional distress in patients with heart disease who have an insufficient oxygen supply to the myocardium. The pain actually comes from the part of the heart muscle which is deficient in oxygen and may be described as tight, strangling or suffocating in nature. It is felt in the chest or it may be felt in the arms or shoulders. Alternatively it may start in the chest and radiate to the arms or shoulders. The pain is usually acute.

Angina is an indication that atherosclerosis is present, and may become more frequent as the condition progresses, depending on the adequacy of alternative circulations.

Myocardial infarction Some myocardial infarctions are small and may go unnoticed. In others the reaction is rapid and serious and may result in death almost immediately. The individual collapses and will be brought to hospital as an emergency, probably being taken initially to an intensive therapy unit (ITU). When and if the patient recovers from the acute stage, he will be transferred to a medical ward. He will have problems of chest pain and dyspnoea; the latter may be related to his pain or due to pulmonary congestion. The pain is more severe than in angina but occurs in the same sites. It may last for longer in the patient with an infarction.

The blood pressure may rise at the time of infarction due to the secretion of adrenaline, but will then drop because of the damaged myocardium's reduced efficiency. The pulse may be irregular as a result of arrhythmia. It may also be weak and rapid initially, slowing down as the damaged heart is unable to maintain its normal pumping rate. The temperature may be elevated due to the cardiac damage but the skin will be moist, cool and possibly grey since reduced cardiac output will lead to peripheral vasoconstriction. Vomiting is common. Cardiogenic shock is possible, and the risk of death is high in the first few hours following infarction.

The individual may feel tired and exhausted for a few days after myocardial infarction. This is probably the body's reaction to the considerable trauma associated with damage to the heart.

Psychological reactions
Initial psychological reactions will be those associated with unexpected crisis. There will have been no time to

prepare for either ill-health or hospitalization, yet both will need to be accepted.

Anxiety may be a major reaction and this may be associated with anger and feelings of doubt about the future. Myocardial infarction often occurs in males at a difficult time of life in that the individuals are in their mid-40s and at the time of realizing their ambitions before they become too old.

The myocardial infarction may have happened at an embarrassing moment. Many men in their 40s see youth 'passing them by' and in order to prove they are still attractive will indulge in extramarital affairs. If, as is not uncommon, the infarction occurs while the patient is with his mistress, there may be psychological reactions with implications for the patient's marriage.

Psychological reactions to the diagnosis of heart disease may be similar to those described for congestive heart failure (p. 271).

Social reactions

No assumptions can be made about the social reactions to a crisis except that the individual may need to consider changes in social habits and conditions in line with the limitations set by the seriousness of the infarction.

PLANNING NURSING CARE

Physical care

In planning physical care following myocardial infarction, priorities will be aimed at resting the damaged heart and relieving pain and dyspnoea. Constant reassessment of the patient's physical state (temperature, pulse, respiration, blood pressure, colour and level of pain) will lead to modifications of goals. Glycerol trinitrate in tablet form is the usual drug prescribed for angina but other drugs such as morphine may be prescribed for the particularly severe pain of infarction. An anti-emetic may be given with morphine. In addition to reducing pain, the management of myocardial infarction aims to reduce the damage to the heart and reduce the possibility of complications. In this, thrombolytic agents such as streptokinase and urokinase are used (Brunner and Suddarth 1989).

Relief of pain may reduce dyspnoea but oxygen therapy may also be prescribed. Total bedrest is essential both to reduce strain on the heart and to reduce attacks of angina of effort. Nursing care will include attention to hygiene since the patient should be relieved of any effort.

Goals for the patient will be aimed towards a gradual recovery, with physical activity to be resumed within the limits dictated by his cardiac condition, and the control of angina. Patient co-operation is important because, after he begins to recover, an individual may resent the physical restrictions placed upon him. Understanding the risks associated with over-exertion in the recovery phase may help compliance.

In patients who deny their condition, or refuse to accept restrictions, a potential problem is that a further infarction may occur. If this happens the patient's heart may stop beating. This is called 'cardiac arrest' and constitutes an emergency on the ward.

Cardiac arrest Although cardiac arrest is considered here for convenience it can happen in disorders other than myocardial infarction. Speed is essential since, if the blood supply is not restored to the brain cells within three or four minutes, irreversible brain damage will occur.

Every ward should have access to an emergency trolley laid up for cardiac resuscitation or a box containing drugs and equipment for resuscitation. When an arrest occurs, one nurse runs to the telephone, dials a special number and, when it is answered, says, 'Cardiac arrest, Cardiac arrest' and then repeats the ward name or number twice. This will prompt the arrival of a team of doctors. On the way back to the patient from the telephone, the nurse collects the resuscitation box or trolley.

Meanwhile a second nurse commences artificial respiration and external cardiac massage (Figure 10.9). This must be done on a hard surface. If the bed base is hard, the patient is left on the bed. If not, he is transferred to the floor or a board is put under the mattress. Difficulties can arise if only one nurse is on duty. In this instance, priority must be given to telephoning for the team since to start resuscitation with no hope of relief is unrealistic.

Thought must be given to the other patients on the ward after the emergency has been dealt with. It can be very frightening to see screens drawn and hear the noises of resuscitation, especially if the patient dies or is taken away to the coronary care unit. An explanation afterwards should help to allay fears about the incident.

The policy on cardiac arrest will vary according to the locality, but in planning patient care it is a nurse's responsibility to know the method of summoning the team, the whereabouts of the box or trolley and the rudiments of resuscitation. The decision on when to discontinue the effort to resuscitate is a medical one.

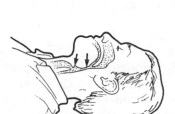

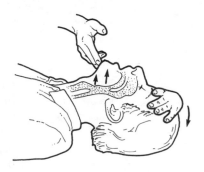

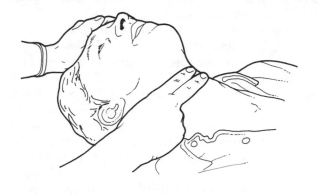

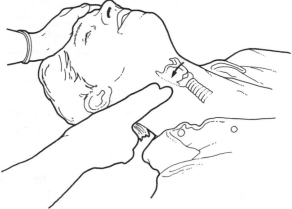

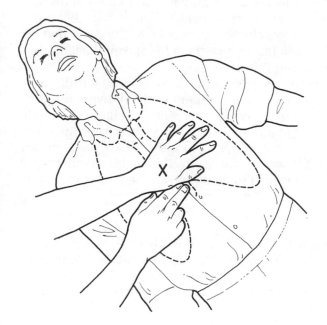

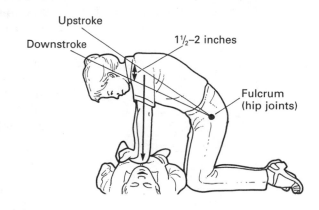

Upstroke

Downstroke

1½–2 inches

Fulcrum
(hip joints)

Fig. 10.9 Diagrams to illustrate
practical procedures in basic life support.

If a patient survives a cardiac arrest he will normally be transferred to an intensive care or coronary care unit.

Psychological care

In planning care the reduction of anxiety must be an aim, given the extra strain placed on the heart by stress. As long ago as 1976, Degree Coustry gave three types of psychological reaction to myocardial infarction during rehabilitation. These are (a) impulsive reactions where the individual denies the seriousness of his disease, acts aggressively and refuses to change his lifestyle, (b) adaptive reactions where the disease is accepted realistically and adaptations made to maximize potential, and (c) regression reactions where the patient exaggerates his limitations and is overwhelmed by fear which prevents a return to any degree of normal living.

In the assessment of each individual prior to care being planned, it is important to establish the patient's reaction to his disease and involve him in the goals to reduce his anxiety and reach acceptance of the necessary restrictions. Those individuals crippled by fear will need to examine the fear, and by education become motivated towards maximizing their potential. Such fear can be encouraged by well-meaning relatives who attempt to place the patient in the role of cardiac cripple. It is suggested that over one-third of patients who have suffered a myocardial infarction do not return to work for psychological rather than physical reasons. Specific psychological problems which may or may not be related to disease but may affect recovery should be identified, discussed and, if necessary, referred. It may be at this time that an individual is also facing a crisis in his spiritual beliefs and may need help in this area.

The severity of myocardial infarction may bring psychological problems for partners and relatives. In planning care, aims should be set to increase their understanding and reduce their fears. Inappropriate reassurance should not be given to either the patient or his family but a positive approach should be taken to the possibility of a return to health given the necessary modifications to avoid a recurrence.

Social care

Assessment will elicit information about the social habits and conditions of the patient. Care should be planned to educate the patient about the dangers of smoking, the importance of diet and the effects of stress. Learning to take life at a more leisurely pace can start in hospital. As with other areas, the patient's decision on how to live his life is a personal one which should be based on informed choice.

Relatives can be supportive to a patient and should be involved while he is in hospital. If, for example, the patient has been advised not to smoke, then relatives can be encouraged to refrain from bringing cigarettes as a present. Similarly they should not worry the patient about events at home or work when he is powerless to take action.

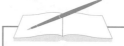

What advice would you give to an individual who wished to reduce the possibility of heart disease? What information would you need from the individual? What factors would influence your advice?

THE CARE PLAN

The priorities on the care plan should be those associated with medical treatment to reduce the physical symptoms caused by myocardial infarction, and the promotion of rest from physiological, social and psychological problems.

As the patient improves, goals should be aimed towards a gradual return to mobility and self-care and the promotion of a healthy and less stressful lifestyle. Relatives should be involved and goals set to reduce anxiety and promote co-operation in helping the patient to return to a relatively normal life.

The Health Education Authority and local Health Promotion Units have booklets that give a simple account of ischaemic heart disease which may help patients to understand how to reduce strain on their heart without becoming an invalid. Such booklets are also useful for relatives to read.

Medical conditions associated with deficits in nutrition

Deficits in nutrition may occur as a result of insufficient intake of nutrients but may also arise as a result of damage to or disease of the alimentary tract or the organs and glands associated with digestion such as the liver, gallbladder and pancreas. Metabolic disturbances such as insulin deficiencies and under- or overactive thyroid glands will affect the rate at which nutrients are turned into energy to meet the body's requirements.

Some of the diseases most commonly seen on a medical ward will be considered, with emphasis on patient reactions and implications for nursing care. It is the responsibility of each nurse to assess not only the individual reactions to the disease process but also those reactions relating to the patient's personal circumstances and life-style before ordering priorities for patient care.

Peptic ulcer

Ulceration, i.e. erosion of an area of tissue, may occur in any part of the alimentary tract. If it occurs in the oesophagus, stomach or duodenum it is referred to as a peptic ulcer. Such ulceration occurs when the hydrochloric acid and pepsin, which are present for digestion, attack the protective mucosal lining of the upper gastrointestinal tract. Since such digestive fluids are present in all people and do not normally cause ulceration, it is thought that the condition occurs when there is an imbalance between the acidity of the hydrochloric acid and the protective alkalinity of the mucosa which is eroded.

The cause of most peptic ulcers has been uncertain until now but predisposing factors may be smoking, alcohol and drugs such as aspirin which, if taken in excess, may harm the mucosa; inflammation such as gastritis, which may damage the mucosa; stress, which may increase gastric secretion, and be due to anxiety, tension or physical trauma; and irregular eating habits, which leaves gastric secretions in the stomach for long periods in the absence of food. Ulcers are now known to be caused by the bacterium *Helicobacter pylorus*, and this may be treated successfully with a course of antibiotics.

Peptic ulceration is more common in men than in women and usually occurs in the age range of 40 upwards; the mid-life crisis. The most common site of ulceration is the duodenum, and the least common the oesophagus. In women, the most common site is the stomach.

Physical reactions

The most common reaction to ulceration is epigasric pain, the timing of which gives an indication of the site of the ulcer. Some individuals do not have severe pain, while in others the presenting reaction to ulceration is haematemesis. In duodenal ulcer the pain characteristically wakes the patient at night. It may also occur from two to four hours after ingestion of food and is relieved very often by taking a glass of milk or a small snack. Oesophageal ulcer causes pain almost immediately after taking food, and a gastric ulcer half an hour to one hour after a meal. The pain of these latter two is normally relieved by antacids. The pain is episodic, often clearing after days or weeks of misery. However, remissions become less frequent over time, and pain more prolonged. Vomiting may relieve the pain but persistent vomiting will tend towards weight loss.

Nutritional deficits are not necessarily present since individuals tend to deal with their pain and continue their normal dietary habits. Vomiting does result occasionally if the ulcer is near the pyloris, but this is an uncommon reaction which is due to narrowing of the tract with a resultant delay in the passage of food into the small intestine.

Psychological reactions

Pain invariably causes psychological reactions, to some extent dependent on the pain threshold of the individual. Other reactions will be dependent on the level of disturbance caused to normal life by the effects of the disease. This disturbance of normal life may be a factor in the individual's decision to seek medical help for his problem.

Social reactions

Since the patient's pain is associated with food this may have an effect on his social life. Eating out or a social evening in the pub may be of little interest if they are followed by pain. This may have an effect on social relationships, as may the pain itself if it affects mood.

PLANNING NURSING CARE

Physical care

The aim of both medical treatment and nursing care is to rest the individual and reduce his gastric secretions so that the ulcer may heal. In planning such care it must be remembered that the individual may not feel ill and may resent the restrictions placed upon him. Involving him in planning care and helping him to understand the rationale behind the prescribed rest and medication should increase co-operation.

Alkalis will be prescribed to neutralize the acid in the stomach while drugs such as cimetidine and ranitidine may be given to reduce gastric secretions. Rest, both physical and mental, will also reduce gastric secretions. Antibiotics will also be prescribed if *H. pylorus* is present.

Diet should be planned to avoid those foods and drinks known to bring on the individual's pain and those known to stimulate gastric secretion, such as alcohol, spicy foods, acid foods and coffee unless it is caffeine-free. If symptoms are severe, fluids only may be given, initially at hourly intervals. After that, meals should be small and frequent, but, as the patient's condition improves, normal meal times can be observed as long as they are regular.

Bedrest may be prescribed for some patients but, given the risks of inactivity such as pressure sores and venous thrombosis, it is likely that the patient will have limited activity, which will increase as the ulcer heals. Goals for rest that the patient is prepared to adhere to should be set. As with all care, the responsibility for ensuring that adequate rest is taken lies with the nurse, who will need to monitor the patient's activity levels.

Plans should be made to educate the individual about the predisposing factors in peptic ulceration in order to dissuade him from smoking, irregular and unsuitable meals, and alcohol.

Psychological care
Because stress is known to be a factor in peptic ulceration, the individual may have psychological problems in addition to those associated with his disease. In planning care, an attempt should be made to identify and work towards solutions to these problems since, if a patient returns to a personal or a work environment fraught with tension, his ulcer may recur or degenerate to a point where complications require readmission to hospital.

If the individual is tense, he may have a mild tranquillizer prescribed to help him relax. This will not reduce the need for the patient to have opportunities to talk through his concerns, with the aim of reducing tension. Problems may vary from those which the patient can deal with to those where professional help may be necessary. Certainly the changes of lifestyle which may be necessary for a return to health can engender tension if they are unpalatable.

Ulceration does occur in individuals who appear to lead tranquil lives. In giving the opportunity to identify and consider stressful situations, a nurse needs to accept that some patients will not actually have problems in their normal life that they cannot cope with. Others will not wish to discuss their problems with a health professional.

Social care
The period in hospital creates an opportunity to set new patterns of social behaviour to replace those which were associated with the peptic ulceration. The motivation for this should arise from the improvement in the individual's

condition as he follows the restful regimen prescribed for him.

Regular meal times, discontinuation of smoking and lack of tension should be the aim after the patient has returned home. This needs sensitivity on the part of the nurse to relate cause and effect without appearing to nag or blame the patient for his condition. An awareness of the constraints imposed by each individual's lifestyle will aid the focus of education for health.

THE CARE PLAN

The priorities for planning care will depend very much on the individual's problems in that either the physical or the psychological reactions may be most important. The individual in severe pain will not feel like discussing plans for relaxation until he is pain-free, yet relaxation is of prime importance in nursing care. Similarly, the patient who is very tense will be unable to meet goals for relaxation and may feel unable to discuss the cause of his tensions until he has relaxed. A first priority for such a patient may be a medical prescription for a mild tranquillizer.

In setting educational aims for care, thought will need to be given to the patient's reactions to hospitalization and his diagnosis. Plans to help the patient decide to give up smoking, for example, may have to be delayed while emphasis is put on diet and rest. This is equally true whether or not the consultant has forbidden the patient to smoke.

Complications of peptic ulceration

It is important when setting priorities for care for the patient with peptic ulceration to plan careful observation for the potential complications. Haematemesis or melaena in an individual is a sign that the ulcer is bleeding, while vomiting related to anorexia and complaints of 'feeling full' indicates an obstruction, usually in the narrow pyloric area which becomes inflamed and oedematous. Sudden severe epigastric pain which spreads to the abdominal area and is accompanied by pallor, rapid pulse and shallow respiration indicates that the ulcer has perforated.

The complications of peptic ulceration require immediate medical attention since they have severe implications for the patient.

Haemorrhage The loss of blood caused by a bleeding ulcer may have mild effects, such as feelings of weakness or restlessness, through to a loss of consciousness, de-

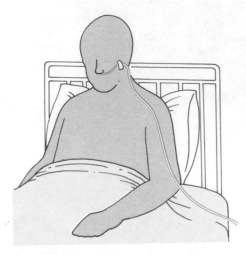

Fig. 10.10 The nasogastric tube.

pending on the severity of the bleed. Nursing care may include total bedrest, oxygen therapy and transfusions of blood and/or parenteral fluids. Sedatives may be required for the restless patient. The priority of care will be to treat the emergency and give psychological support to the patient in what can be a terrifying situation at worst and at best the cause of considerable anxiety. If haemorrhage occurs, an important aspect of care will be the monitoring of blood pressure, pulse, colour and urine output. In older patients, emergency surgery may be required.

Obstruction is usually of gradual onset, wih increasing vomiting. Over time this will cause the patient to become thin and dehydrated. Electrolyte balance may be disturbed and vitamin deficiency arise.

In obstruction the priority in care is to empty the stomach and rest it so that the swelling and inflammation can subside and the obstruction can clear. This will be achieved by passing a nasogastric tube into the stomach and aspirating the contents by continuous or intermittent suction (Figure 10.10). Although the patient will not be allowed to eat during this period, gastric secretions need to be withdrawn to avoid further erosion of the ulcer.

Fluids will be given intravenously during this period. Mouth care will be important, since the mouth may be dry and the nasogastric tube may cause feelings of dryness in the throat. Frequent mouth-washes are essential. When small fluid feeds are introduced, gastric aspiration will precede each feed. These aspirations will give an indication of gastric flow and the reduction of the obstruction. From the volume of the aspirate, decisions will be made on introducing a gradual return to light meals which are free of irritants.

The individual will need psychological support during this period since he may be anxious not only about the manifestations of the complication but also of the aspirations and intravenous fluids. Since surgery is a real possibility for obstruction, fears associated with an operation may also be present.

Perforation is an emergency since the patient may go into shock (p. 364). In the majority of cases surgical intervention will be necessary. If so, the shock will be treated immediately, as will the pain, after which transfer will be arranged so that the patient returns from theatre to a surgical ward. Pre-operative preparation (p. 359) will be given on the medical ward since the aim is to operate as soon as possible.

Medical treatment for perforation is similar to that for obstruction in that the aim of care is to empty and rest the stomach so that healing can occur. A blood transfusion may be given in addition to intravenous fluids. Drugs that may be prescribed are morphine for pain and antibiotics as a cover against possible infection which could be caused by leakage of stomach contents into the abdominal cavity.

Ulcerative colitis

THE DISEASE PROCESS

Ulcerative colitis is ulceration of the rectum and distal colon which may spread upwards to involve the whole colon. The mucosal lining which protects the colon is destroyed. The cause is not certain, although one theory is that it is an 'autoimmune' disease.

Autoimmune process   The body has an immune system (Fuerst 1983) which protects the individual from foreign organisms, such as bacteria and viruses, by producing antibodies specific to the invading agent. This immunity may be 'natural', i.e. the body is resistant to certain organisms from birth, or 'acquired', i.e. the body raises antibodies in response to invasion by an organism so that the individual will be resistant to that organism in future, e.g. the way we become resistant to the childhood infectious diseases of mumps and measles. Acquired immunity may also be gained by vaccination, where inactivated organisms are introduced in a controlled way.

In an autoimmune response, certain types of normal cell in the body are treated as foreign bodies and antibodies are produced against them. The mechanism by which this occurs is not fully understood but the consequences for the individual may be severe. It is this autoimmune response which is thought to be responsible for ulcerative colitis. Antibodies are thought to be formed which destroy the mucosal lining of the rectum and colon, leading to ulceration and sloughing from the damaged tissue.

Physical reactions
Physical reactions are slow since the onset of the disease is usually insidious. Diarrhoea occurs and the faeces contain blood, mucus and pus. Colic accompanies diarrhoea as the involuntary muscles of the colon contract spasmodically, and abdominal pain may also be present.

As the disease progresses, there will be physical reacions to the abnormal loss of fluid from the bowels, from electrolyte imbalance and from malabsorption of nutrients, leaving the individual dehydrated, tired, anaemic and suffering from loss of weight.

Psychological reactions

Ulcerative colitis is a chronic disease. The individual may recover from an episode only to have a relapse at a later date. There is no particular pattern to the disease but episodes are often preceded by psychological upsets.

A stereotype of the psychological manifestations of an individual with colitis shows an immature, dependent, moody person liable to displays of temper and fits of depression. Each of these reactions may be present as the result of long-standing, painful illness, and of the family's indulgence, which may be to compensate for the misery of the disease. The individual, because of his acquired dependence, may fail to cope with the stresses of life so that major distress such as bereavement or the breakdown of a close relationship will precipitate an attack.

There is, however, a danger in stereotyping and it is worth remembering that attacks may also be preceded by infection or inappropriate diet.

Social reactions

Ulcerative colitis most often occurs in young people. Their adoption of a 'sick role' can lead to social isolation since people who are constantly feeling unwell are not seen as fun to be with by their peers.

The reality of diarrhoea and pain will also restrict social interaction, perhaps to a level where the individual fears to leave home. Social reactions may be dependent on the severity of the physical reactions to the disease.

PLANNING NURSING CARE

Physical care

The individual is likely to be admitted to hospital either for diagnosis or during an acute attack of ulcerative colitis. Both nursing and medical care will be aimed at resting the colon and treating deficits such as anaemia, dehydration and loss of weight.

Nursing observation will include fluid balance, weight changes and the pattern and content of diarrhoea. Dietary intake is also monitored and an assessment made of eating habits and of the effects of particular foods on the bowel movements. As in ulceration of the upper gastrointestinal tract (p. 282), the potential problems of haemorrhage and perforation exist along with their attendant risks.

For the patient who is debilitated, life can be exhausting. Physical care will include bedrest, which will have the effect of reducing activity in the bowel. This can be difficult to achieve in a patient with diarrhoea. Medication may include drugs such as propantheline to reduce peristalsis and drugs to reduce inflammation such as steroids or immunosuppressants. The problem with the latter, e.g. azathiaprine, is that normal antibody production is also suppressed so that the patient is very susceptible to infections. Antibiotics may be prescribed for secondary infections.

Bedrest, particularly if the patient is debilitated, carries the risk of pressure sores. Pressure area care is necessary with particular attention to skin around the anal area, which can be reddened and sore from diarrhoea. Position is important to relieve pressure and prevent contractures of the lower limbs. These may occur if the patient, because of abdominal pain, lies curled up and very still for long periods of time.

The colon is also rested if the patient is taken off normal food and drink during the acute phase. Parenteral fluids, nutrition and, if necessary, blood transfusion are given. Electrolyte imbalance may need to be corrected, through the parenteral fluids. If these measures are necessary, mouth care becomes important as the mouth becomes dry and unpleasant for the patient. Frequent mouthwashes should be available. When a normal diet is resumed, an attempt will be made to compensate for the weight loss and to correct the anaemia.

Since the individual may feel too ill to be interested in food, or scared to eat because of the expected resultant diarrhoea, the high-protein, low-roughage diet required may present nursing problems in planning care. Fortified drinks may help to supplement the calorie needs of the small eater, and care should be taken to meet patient's preference for certain foods as far as the constraints of hospital catering allow. Fluids should be encouraged when parenteral therapy is discontinued.

Psychological care

Psychological care needs to be planned to help the individual, who may be tense and anxious, to relax. Tranquillizers may have been prescribed to reduce tension on admission and to facilitate rest. The nurse needs to encourage the patient to express his feelings and concerns so that she can identify problems which may be related to the current episode of colitis, and then refer or plan care as appropriate.

The individual may be dependent, demanding and weepy. A busy nurse may become irritated by such behaviour if she does not understand the problems of chronic debilitating disease. Planning to give time to build trust with the patient may lead to the patient becoming prepared to discuss his problems and perhaps gain insight, so that measures may be taken to reduce the tensions in life and develop more effective coping mechanisms. Referral for psychotherapy may be required for some patients.

Bowel disorders may bring their own embarrassment. Bedpans may be required at mealtimes when other patients are eating. This can cause distress to the patient as he worries about what may be interpreted as antisocial behaviour in terms of smell and irritation to others. This distress will be increased if a bedpan is not brought immediately and soiling of the bed results.

Care can be planned to reduce these concerns. Ideally, the patient may be nursed in a side room with *en suite* facilities. If this is not possible, a clean, covered bedpan can be left at the bedside to reassure the patient between bowel movements, and the patient's bed positioned in a corner so that the minimum number of patients are affected if bedpans are needed at unsocial times. An aerosol air freshener may be left on the locker or an airwick left nearby.

The nurse's attitude is also important because the patient may be sensitive to distaste or impatience and react by feeling that he is personally disliked. He may require considerable reassurance that nurses adapt to giving bedpans and do realize that the patient is not being deliberately difficult. It may not always be easy for the nurse to remain calm, since a patient who needs constant attention can be draining, particularly at the end of a shift, but showing impatience is very damaging to the relationship between patient and nurse.

Social care

Social problems may be longstanding in the patient with ulcerative colitis. A period in hospital is a useful time, not only for the patient but also for his family, to examine relationships with a view to improving problem areas.

Relatives may not realize that they foster immaturity or dependence, and care planned may need to include some education for them to improve the balance in social interactions. Stress or tension in such a family may be creating a vicious circle which open discussion with an objective counsellor may help.

As the physical condition improves, the patient may be prepared to indulge in social interaction. Gaining the assurance to do this can start in hospital as nurses help the individual to improve his self-concept.

The priorities in the care plan should be directed towards resting the colon. This requires medical treatment and nursing care that aims to help the patient to rest physically and mentally. Psychological problems should be given priority on the care plan if they are likely to interfere with the patient's rest.

Problems which may be factors in the disease should be identified and care planned with goals set to help the patient gain insight and improve his ability to cope. The involvement of relatives is important since they may need help in learning to interact more successfully with the patient.

Cirrhosis of the liver

THE DISEASE PROCESS

Cirrhosis of the liver is a chronic degenerative disease which is popularly believed to be associated with alcoholism. In fact one of the causes **is** chronic alcoholism and the damage occurs because of a lack of adequate nutrition to buffer the toxic effect of the alcohol. Chronic drinkers often fail to eat regular meals because they do not feel hungry or, as is often the case in the chronic alcoholic, all available money is spent on alcohol.

Other causes of degeneration of the liver are a prior episode of acute hepatitis where damage from the inflammation has left scarring which leads to cirrhosis, and obstruction of the flow of bile over time due to infection, inflammation or obstruction in the bile ducts. Auto-immune reactions may also lead to cirrhosis, as may drugs and metabolic disorders.

Whatever the cause, there is destruction of the parenchymal cells and the liver becomes scarred so that the pathways of the bile, blood and lymph are blocked. This results in congestion within the liver. Congestion and damage to the circulation in the liver lead to a collateral circulation developing and to portal hypertension. Liver function is reduced because of the reduced number of active cells.

The liver is able to regenerate tissue but not in the previous pattern of distribution, so regenerative tissue forms in nodules on the surface of the liver as the original tissue mass is reduced in size by the contraction of scarred areas (Figure 10.11). The end result is an enlarged liver that feels hard and 'knobbly' on palpation.

Physical reactions

There may be no physical reactions to cirrhosis for many years after the onset of the disease since the liver is considerably larger than the body's requirements. This is a disadvantage in real terms since it generally precludes early diagnosis and treatment.

When reactions do occur they are often vague. The individual may feel tired, have slight digestive upsets or lose weight. There may be feelings of nausea and slight anorexia but no alarming symptoms. As the disease progresses, jaundice may appear as the damaged liver releases bile pigment in the blood, and ascites may be seen as the result of congestion of the portal circulation. Generalized oedema may occur as reduced liver function affects the osmolarity of the blood.

The patient may become anaemic as a reaction to deficits in nutrition, and may feel tired and listless. Anaemia may also result from bleeding from oesophageal varices which form as the result of portal hypertension. The individual's abdomen may enlarge as a reaction to splenomegaly, which is also caused by portal hypertension. Peripheral blood vessels may dilate to cause spider angiomas on the skin.

The severity of the reactions is dependent upon the level of liver involvement. The most serious reactions, which are characteristic of advanced cirrhosis, are haemorrhage from oesophageal varices and hepatic coma as a

Fig. 10.11 Normal liver (*left*) and cirrhosis of the liver (*right*).

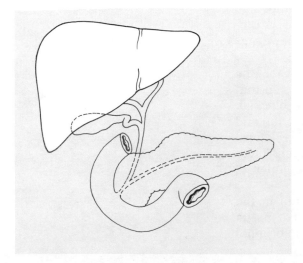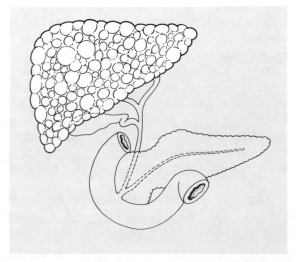

reaction to the impaired liver's inability to convert ammonia into urea. Haemorrhage may also result from the underproduction of clotting factors in the blood, which are normally produced in the liver.

Psychological reactions

Psychological reactions will depend on the cause and severity of the disease. Alcoholism, for example, is thought to develop from its use as a means of dealing with stress. Individuals who use alcohol in this way could be seen to have pre-disposing psychological problems and perhaps be less able than others to cope with deficits in functioning.

The early vague feelings of being unwell may cause psychological problems because the individual cannot make sense of his feelings. Odd, unexplained 'aches and pains' may be interpreted as neurotic, rather than physical, and the individual will feel frustrated that he cannot 'pull himself together'. In patients such as this a diagnosis which makes sense of his symptoms can come as a relief initially, since many people are very threatened by any suggestion of mental illness.

More advanced disease which brings with it jaundice and oedema can cause psychological reactions to the possibilities of serious disruption to normal life and the concurrent threat to survival. There may also be reactions to the diagnosis, given its association with alcoholism and the implied stigma of being unable to cope with the stresses of life.

Social reactions

Social reactions will also vary according to the severity of the disease and its effect upon social functioning. The individual suffering from alcoholism may have so many social problems that ill-health makes little practical difference to his life. However, the idea of hospitalization will cause anxiety because of the restrictions which will be placed on alcohol consumption.

For the individual who feels vaguely unwell, social interactions and partnerships may suffer during the worrying period prior to diagnosis. Relationships at work may also suffer if the symptoms cause days to be taken off for undiagnosed sickness on a fairly regular basis.

The more seriously ill individual may have social problems associated with prolonged sickness, hospitalization and the threat to employment and finance in the family.

PLANNING NURSING CARE

Physical care

Since cirrhosis is a chronic degenerative disease, medical and nursing care will be aimed towards alleviating reactions to the degeneration, and slowing its progress by educating the patient. Much will depend on the stage of the disease and its cause.

If the cause is associated with deficits in nutrition, whether or not they are linked with alcoholism, attention will be given to a change in dietary habits. Fats are not tolerated well in cirrhosis, since the liver normally plays a major role in their metabolism, and should be avoided if the patient is jaundiced. A high-protein, high-carbohydrate but low-fat diet should be encouraged though fat may be eaten if no cholestasis is present. Additional vitamins may be prescribed including B_{12} if anaemia is present. There should be no salt added to the diet if oedema is present.

If the patient is anorexic, there may be difficulty in persuading him to attempt to eat. Food drinks made with skimmed milk may supplement small meals, attention being paid to patient preference where possible. Co-operation is more likely if there is understanding of the role of nutrition in both the cause and treatment of cirrhosis.

If alcoholism is a predisposing factor, the individual may need specialist help in dealing with the problem, for alcohol should not be taken at all by a patient with cirrhosis. Sudden cessation can cause 'withdrawal' reactions such as hallucinations and should not be attempted on a medical ward. The patient may need to be transferred to a detoxification unit, which is usually sited in the psychiatric wing of a hospital. The patient's admission to such a unit must be voluntary.

Medical treatment may include drugs to deal with infection, and vitamins. If the cause is thought to be autoimmunity then an immunosuppressant such as azathiaprine may be given. Diuretics may be prescribed for oedema with a potassium supplement to maintain electrolyte balance. Drugs which need to be detoxified by the liver should be avoided. These include tranquillizers such as diazepam, opiates and the drugs used in general anaesthesia. Should the patient require surgery it is essential that the anaesthetist is aware of the liver condition.

In planning care the nurse needs to monitor the patient's reactions to medical treatment carefully.

Azathiaprine, for example, lowers the resistance to infection while diuretics may affect electrolyte balance, leaving the patient complaining of headaches and tiredness. Other observations included in the care planned are recordings of fluid balance and weight to monitor oedema and response to nutrition, and of temperature, pulse and respiration for early signs of infection. The faeces should be inspected for signs of internal bleeding. The patient's level of fatigue should also be monitored and opportunities found for adequate rest.

Advanced disease If the disease is advanced, care planning should include bedrest and the patient should be monitored for haemorrhage due to ruptured varices and for neurological reactions to the liver deficiency. If these latter are present, e.g. confusion, memory deficits, reduced awareness or hand tremor, protein should be withdrawn from the diet.

Abdominal paracentesis Oedema may be generalized with ascites and the care planned may include abdominal paracentesis to drain fluid from the abdomen, although this is avoided if possible. Paracentesis is an aseptic technique performed by a doctor. The nurse's role is in preparing the patient for the procedure and in giving support, since the patient may be frightened. Assurance can be given that a local anaesthetic will be used and that the procedure ought not to be painful. Other concerns should be identified and dealt with or referred to a senior nurse or doctor.

The nurse needs to observe the patient's blood pressure, pulse and colour for signs of shock in reaction to the fluid removal, which reduces intra-abdominal pressure. One to two litres of fluid may be withdrawn which will contain plasma proteins. These proteins may later be replaced by an intravenous blood transfusion. When the procedure is complete, a sterile dressing is applied to the puncture site. Frequent observations of the dressing, blood pressure, pulse and colour are made for four to six hours after the procedure or until the patient's physical condition is satisfactory.

Hepatic coma may follow neurological reactions to cirrhosis, eventually rendering the patient unconscious. If this occurs the condition is probably terminal and care is planned as for an unconscious or dying patient.

Psychological care

Psychological care will be planned with the aim of facilitating rest and gaining co-operation in physical care. Particular problems may be identified according to the level of advancement of the disease. For the individual who is newly diagnosed, the relief that there is a cogent reason for the ill-health may be followed by depression as a lifetime of chronic illness is envisaged.

Care should include education towards maximum health. This will include helping the patient in planning regular nutritious meals, giving up alcohol (if necessary) and avoiding stress. Practical help of this sort can reduce psychological distress by offering tangible measures to improve health.

Every effort should be made to avoid the individual labelling himself 'chronically sick', particularly in a disease where long periods of healthy living are possible after diagnosis. Individual differences should be observed, but the intelligent patient who follows a sensible regimen but refuses to attend clinic is in effect not allowing the disease to interfere with his life. This choice should be respected, as should that of the patient at the other end of the continuum who gains comfort from medical check-ups on a regular basis.

As the disease advances, care may need to be planned to deal with the psychological distress associated with the increasingly obvious physical reactions to the disease. Oesophageal haemorrhage, in particular, can be very frightening and may require a patient to be admitted to hospital as an emergency. The bleeding may be controlled by vasopressin, which constricts arterioles; this reduces portal pressure and blood flow. If the use of vasopressin is unsuccessful, or contraindicated as in patients with cardiac disease, an inflatable Sengstaken–Blakemore tube may be inserted into the oesophagus (Figure 10.12) – again a very frightening experience. Psychological reactions should be clearly identified so that the patient's needs are met for information, comfort, reassurance (where possible) and the need to verbalize fears and worries.

Social care

In order to maximize his health potential, the individual with cirrhosis will need to consider changes in his social life, particularly in a society where drinking alcohol is an integral part of many social interactions, and where many people eat scrappy irregular meals as part of their daily work pattern. Plans while in hospital will be aimed towards helping the individual to make informed choices about lifestyle. Involvement of relatives may make even-

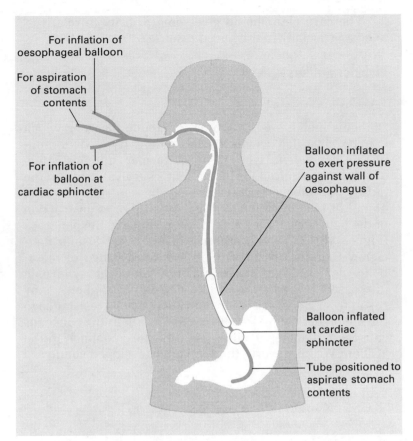

For inflation of
oesophageal balloon

For aspiration
of stomach
contents

For inflation of
balloon at
cardiac sphincter

Balloon inflated
to exert pressure
against wall of
oesophagus

Balloon inflated
at cardiac
sphincter

Tube positioned to
aspirate stomach
contents

Fig. 10.12   The Sengstaken–Blakemore tube.

tual discharge a more positive experience by giving support to the resolutions made in hospital.

For the patient who had problems with alcohol prior to diagnosis, hospitalization may well offer the opportunity to deal with both the problem and its underlying causes. Such individuals may need considerable help on discharge to rebuild their place in society as a person of worth. The social and welfare services may need to be involved.

THE CARE PLAN

Priorities on the care plan will be affected by the physical condition of the patient, unless there is an overruling psychological problem which could influence co-operation in care. Dependence on alcohol is such a problem. Other priorities should have goals towards educating the patient towards a lifestyle to maximize health.

In advanced disease priorities may need to be set to reduce psychological reactions to the obvious worsening of health, including complications such as haemorrhage, jaundice, ascites and neurological reactions.

The care plan should give some priority to relatives' needs, especially in advanced disease.

Diabetes mellitus

THE DISEASE PROCESS

Diabetes mellitus is a chronic metabolic disorder which can be classified as insulin-dependent (type I) or non-insulin-dependent (type II); in the former, administration of insulin is required for the patient's survival, while in the latter, the effects of diabetes may be controlled by diet alone. In insulin-dependent diabetes there is destruction of the beta cells of the islets of Langerhans in the pancreas (Figure 10.13), which produce insulin, and insulin deficiency therefore results; there follows a range of metabolic defects that make up the diabetes syndrome (discussed below). Non-insulin-dependent diabetes may result from a decrease in insulin excretion or resistance to the action of insulin. Debate continues about the cause (or causes) of diabetes mellitus but it is more common in the affluent Western world than in underdeveloped countries.

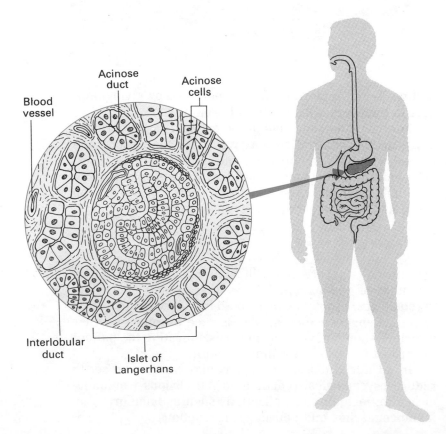

Fig. 10.13 Microscopic struc of the pancreas.

There is thought to be a hereditary factor in diabetes but this has not been proven. If there is, it may merely give a predisposition to the disease and environmental factors may also be involved. In insulin-dependent diabetes there is thought to be an autoimmune destruction of the beta cells which may be triggered by viral infection. In non-insulin-dependent disease there is thought to be a hereditary element which may be associated with obesity.

In the absence of insulin, glucose taken in the diet is not metabolized by the tissues and builds up in the blood as a result. This is termed hyperglycaemia. When blood is filtered in the glomeruli of the kidneys some of the excess glucose is removed from the blood into the filtrate. Water filtered out with the glucose is not reabsorbed into the blood because of the increased osmolarity of the filtrate. This loss of water during filtration will lead to an electrolyte imbalance and dehydration.

Insufficient insulin activity leads to the breakdown of fat in adipose tissue into glycerol and fatty acids, which are then metabolized to produce energy, water and waste products. Ketones build up from the metabolism of fatty acids, causing acidosis. In the absence of fat, the protein in muscle may be broken down as a compensatory mechanism for the production of energy.

Physical reactions

Young people Although the insulin deficit is chronic, the onset of diabetes mellitus in the young is usually acute. The high osmolarity of the glomerular filtrate leads to an increased urinary output, which may contain glucose and ketones. This is paired with excessive thirst (polydipsia), a reaction to the dehydration, which leads to increased fluid intake. In females, the glucose in the urine may adhere to the vulval area, causing inflammation and irritation and providing a medium for infection (vaginitis). Males may suffer inflammation of the glans penis (balanitis).

There is loss of energy as a result of the decreased ability to utilize glucose, and loss of weight as a reaction to the breakdown of adipose tissue. Muscle wasting occurs as protein is broken down.

If the acute reactions to disease are ignored, hyperglycaemic ketotic coma may result.

Mature people Diabetes in later life may have an insidious onset, and reactions to the disease process may be so mild as to go unnoticed. In such instances an individual may remain undiagnosed until a complication of the disease process causes him to seek medical advice, or until glycosuria is discovered in a routine medical examination.

When the diagnosis is made by chance in an older person, an assessment often shows that polyuria and polydipsia, although not severe, have been present for some time.

Although insulin-dependent diabetes is seen most commonly in young people, and non-insulin-dependent diabetes in older, obese patients, the distinction is not clear-cut. For this reason, use of the term 'maturity onset' diabetes has been discarded.

Psychological reactions

Psychological reactions will be in response to the malaise preceding the diagnosis and to the diagnosis itself. The latter can cause severe stress as the individual grapples not only with a long-term health problem but with what he may initially interpret as the need for a rigidly controlled, regimented life.

Much will depend on the individual's level of knowledge of the disease, for reactions can be coloured by fear of the complications of diabetes, such as blindness and circulatory problems, or of treatment, which may be expected to include frequent injections. Alternatively, interactions with stable diabetic patients, such as an aunt or grandfather, may remove some of the fears of the diagnosis.

The individual's family will also react to the diagnosis, perhaps with concern over their role in management of an individual's specialized diabetic needs, or perhaps with guilt if they feel responsible for passing on a genetic disability.

Fear may be present in both the patient and his family that the disease is too complicated for them to manage, or may rule their lives, or both. Young diabetics may fear that the disease carries a stigma which makes them unacceptable to the opposite sex and unfit to become a parent.

Social reactions

Social relationships may suffer as a result of the individual's reaction to the disease process, in that tiredness and lethargy may cause the curtailment of normal pursuits.

In acute-onset disease, the reactions will be those in response to a sudden unexpected disruption to life, with implications relative to the patient's responsibilities and the timing of the disease. This can have an effect not only on the individual but on family and friends.

PLANNING NURSING CARE

Physical care

Nursing care will be aimed towards returning an individual to physiological stability, and teaching him how to maintain that control within his own normal environment with a minimal risk of complications arising.

Since reactions to disease in diabetes mellitus are caused by a lack of effective insulin action in response to the ingestion of carbohydrate, medical treatment includes the prescription of drugs to improve the body's capability to produce sufficient insulin, or the prescription of insulin itself. Diet and exercise need to be controlled so that there is physiological balance between insulin, diet and energy output.

Treatment without insulin   Diabetes mellitus which is not acute may often be controlled by diet alone so that nutrition does not exceed the individual's capacity to produce sufficient insulin. In other cases of mild onset, drugs may be given orally which either augment the secretion of insulin, e.g. glibenclamide, or enhance the effectiveness of the insulin which is secreted, e.g. metformin. These drugs are used in conjunction with dietary control, metformin being used primarily with overweight patients whose beta

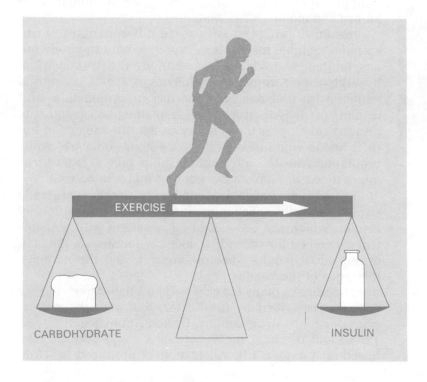

EXERCISE

CARBOHYDRATE   INSULIN

cells are producing some insulin. In some cases, both types of drug may be used together.

Treatment with insulin   Insulin cannot be given as an oral drug, since it is a protein and as such would be digested, but has to be given parenterally. In normal health, insulin is secreted as an automatic reaction to the ingestion of sugar. Once insulin has been prescribed, a careful balance must be kept between the level of insulin in the body and the level of carbohydrate ingested. Too much carbohydrate in the absence of insulin will lead to hyperglycaemia and the attendant risk of hyperglycaemic coma, while too much insulin in the absence of carbohydrate will lead to hypoglycaemia and the risk of hypoglycaemic coma.

Exercise is a vital part of the balance since unexpected or excessive exertion will increase the rate of carbohydrate metabolism, leading to hypoglycaemia, and a reduced exertion level will mean reduced carbohydrate metabolism, leading to hyperglycaemia.

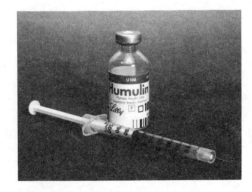

Insulin preparations   There are many different insulin preparations available, primarily produced from pork pancreas, but other animals may also be used in cases where the patient is allergic to pork or beef, or religion forbids their use. If patients are allergic to pork insulins, synthetic alternatives which closely resemble human insulin are commonly prescribed.

Insulin is produced with three different rates of absorption. Soluble insulin acts rapidly within the body but has limited duration. It is useful in the treatment of hyperglycaemic coma, in stabilizing a newly diagnosed patient with diabetes, and for use in conjunction with insulin of longer duration. Isophane and semilente insulins take up to three hours to act after injection but their action continues for up to 24 hours or more, while protamine zinc and ultralente insulins take at least three hours to act but have a duration of up to 36 hours.

Insulins are produced under a number of trade names, and the particular insulin or combination of insulins which are prescribed for a patient with diabetes will depend on the individual doctor's decision, in the light of individual factors affecting control, and the patient's tolerance of the insulin.

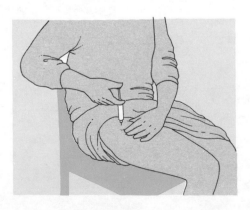

The nurse's plans for care will be related to giving the drug as prescribed by the doctor, following the correct procedure for drug administration (Connechen *et al.* 1983), and teaching the individual how to give his own injection (Chapter 15). All insulin is produced in 10 ml bottles of a strength of 100 units to each 1 ml, and should only be given with an insulin syringe. These are produced in 0.5 ml and 1 ml sizes marked up to 50 units and 100 units, respectively.

A patient with established diabetes, who is in hospital for another reason, or for restabilization, may well prefer to draw up and give his own insulin injections unless he is very ill. This aspect of self-care should be encouraged but does not diminish the nurse's responsibility to ensure that the drug is being given correctly.

For individuals on a combination of soluble and medium-acting insulin, injections are usually given half an hour prior to breakfast and half an hour prior to the evening meal. The pre-breakfast dose will be a combination of both insulins, while the evening dose will normally be of medium-action insulin only. In combination injections, the soluble insulin should be drawn up first, followed by the medium-action insulin, and the injection given immediately. Failure to do this may lead to a change in the molecular structure of the insulin and affect its action after injection.

Insulins with a long duration of action may only be prescribed once daily for the pre-breakfast injection; cover for the breakfast carbohydrate is provided by the previous day's insulin. Although it is usual for all patients on insulin to have breakfast half an hour after the injection, this is less crucial with a once-a-day long-acting insulin than when soluble insulin is given, which commences action in half an hour and will cause hypoglycaemia in the absence of carbohydrate.

Diet Plans for care will include dietary control. Each individual will be prescribed a diet which is related to his energy requirements and the oral drugs or units of insulin taken daily. There is no such thing as a standard 'diabetic diet', rather the individual's calorie intake, particularly carbohydrate, is controlled, with the aim of achieving and maintaining an appropriate weight and maintaining a balance between insulin, diet and exercise.

Carbohydrate comes in many forms. Sweets and sugar for instance are rapidly metabolized and provide energy fast, while bread and potatoes take longer to convert into energy. Individuals with diabetes mellitus are advised to take their carbohydrate from high-fibre, less concentrated sources such as wholemeal bread than from concentrated sources such as sweets and sugars.

In planning care related to the individual's nutrition, education should aim towards his learning the value of the carbohydrate in different types of food so that he can learn

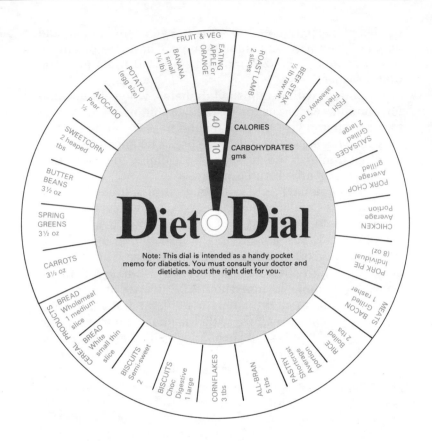

to 'exchange' items in order to vary his diet. This concept of exchange will be taught by the dietitian but the nurse has a role in helping the patient to understand the rationale behind dietary control.

An apple can be seen as a portion of carbohydrate, as can a small slice of wholemeal bread or two cream crackers. Each individual's diet will contain a number of carbohydrate exchanges for 24 hours, which will be divided between meals. From a list of foods he will be able to select what he eats and can choose, for example, to avoid potatoes with his dinner so that he can have a pudding.

Learning to understand the system will help prepare the patient to lead a normal life at home. In terms of diet, an individual should be able to function at home and on social occasions without having to divulge his condition unless he wishes.

Assessment of the patient's ability to understand dietary control will help set the aims in planning care. Some individuals may have difficulty in understanding and may need considerable help, while others will quickly adapt to the restrictions. It is really important that the patient eats regularly in accordance with the insulin action so that blood sugar levels remain within normal levels.

This regular approach to life does not mean 'living by the clock' so much as taking a sensible attitude to the balance between insulin and diet. For example, an individual who wants to stay in bed for a while at the weekends, but who usually has breakfast at 7 a.m., can still remain physiologically stable if he has his insulin and breakfast later on. The important point is that the relationship between the time of taking both remains unchanged. Similarly with evening injections. An invitation to dinner need not cause alarm about the timing of the meal as long as the usual relationship between food and injection is maintained.

When planning care for nutrition in hospital, the individual's normal eating patterns should be taken into account and followed as far as possible as should his food preferences, with the constraint that the newly diagnosed individual will need to train his palate away from sweet foods. There are commercial 'diabetic' products such as chocolate and jams but they are expensive, fattening and do not help the individual to adapt to more savoury flavours. Further, they label the individual as 'different' from others with whom he is eating.

Exercise   Controlling physiological balance can be difficult in hospital since less energy is used than in normal day-to-day living. Care planned should take normal energy expenditure into account and aim towards resumption of normal activity, within reason, on discharge from hospital.

Education is required to give an individual the best possible chance of leading a normal life. Most patients learn to increase carbohydrate intake before extra exertion. As with diet, regularity of exercise is the aim for balanced living but occasional over- or under-exertion can be tolerated as long as the relationship between carbohydrate intake, insulin and energy expended is maintained.

Observations   The care plan for the patient with diabetes mellitus will include monitoring for physiological stability in order to evaluate the success or failure of a prescribed regimen. Monitoring may be achieved by urinalysis and by regular blood glucose analysis. The latter may be carried out on the ward using a glucose meter (e.g. Glucometer) and a reagent strip (Figure 10.14).

A glucose meter is a battery-operated device with a digital readout. Peripheral blood is taken from finger or

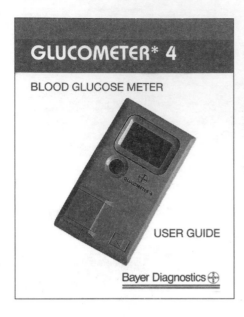

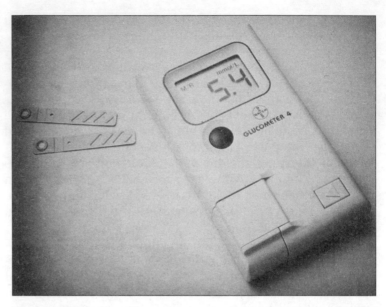

Fig. 10.14 The Glucometer.
Reproduced with kind permission of Bayer
Diagnostics.

earlobe, and, by following clear instructions which come with the machine, an immediate reading of glucose (in millimoles) in the blood can be gained. This allows a profile to be charted so that adjustments may be made if the glucose levels fall outside normal limits.

It is becoming very common for patients to learn to use a glucose meter and to buy their own for use at home in conjunction with urinalysis. By encouraging the patient to make these specific observations of physiological stability, they are encouraged to take more personal care of their own health. Patients also need to learn how to recognize a hypo- and a hyperglycaemic attack so that coma may be avoided.

Table 10.1 shows the different physical reactions to hypo- and hyperglycaemia with possible historical factors. In hypoglycaemia the individual should take rapidly absorbed glucose such as sweets or glucose tablets to correct physiological imbalance, and should always carry one or other so that prompt action may be taken. Hyperglycaemia requires extra insulin (soluble) to restore the physiological balance.

Psychological care
Planning psychological care is extremely important since stress reactions result in energy being expended as the body prepares for 'fight or flight'. In the patient with diabetes this reaction can affect physiological stability.

Initially the stress may be related to the diagnosis. If the reaction is one of anger and bitterness, co-operation in care may be absent while the individual rails against fate, or struggles with changes in his spiritual beliefs. Stress may also be caused by a concern over responsibilities and about the future, which may lead to feelings of hopelessness. Care needs to be planned to deal where possible with the underlying causes of the psychological reactions, with the goal of restoring emotional balance.

Education towards understanding the disease, its treatment and future prospects may do much to restore a sense of perspective about life. This education should be sensitively planned, and empathy shown towards the effects of restrictions and of oral drugs or injections. To assure an individual that taking tablets or giving an injection every day becomes no worse than brushing one's teeth is a sweeping generalization. Many people particularly dislike injecting themselves. They accept the necessity but do not need to have the personal cost diminished.

Young people may find particular difficulty in adjusting to the diagnosis. This can cause problems for peers

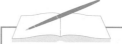

A patient, newly diagnosed with type I (insulin-dependent) diabetes feels overwhelmed with his diagnosis, the necessary life changes and the new skills that have to be learned. How would you plan to work with this patient? How would you order the priorities?

Table 10.1 Differences between hyper- and hypoglycaemia in patients with diabetes mellitus.

	Hyperglycaemia	Hypoglycaemia
Onset	Slow (2–3 days)	Rapid
History	Has not taken insulin/ acute infection	Taken insulin $\frac{1}{2}$–4 h previously, but has not eaten/has eaten but had unusual burst of energy
Patient reactions	Thirst Nausea Abdominal pain Constipation Vomiting	Irrational Bad tempered Disorientated (may be mistaken for drunk)
Leads to	Ketoacidosis Drowsiness BP ↓ Pulse weak and rapid Skin dry Tongue dry	Respirations normal No drowsiness BP normal Pulse normal Skin moist Tongue moist
Leads to	Coma	Coma
Needs	Insulin Restoration of fluid balance	Glucose
Avoided by	Recognition of early symptoms and taking appropriate action	

and family if the rebelliousness is turned outwards. Plans for care may need to include education and support for the family.

In dealing with psychological reactions to the diagnosis, there is an infinite variety of ways in which the situation can be handled. To achieve psychological acceptance is crucial if the individual is to have a full and rewarding life. What needs to be remembered in planning psychological care for the newly diagnosed patient with diabetes mellitus is that a change in self-image will have to be made, from being normally healthy and like one's peers to being **permanently** 'different'. To a certain extent, any illness causes such a change but the reaction is more intense when a label such as 'diabetic' is applied.

The time an individual takes to internalize these changes will vary according to his ability to cope with stressful situations, his knowledge, his personal beliefs and the feedback received about himself as a person. The youngster who rebels seems almost to be saying, 'OK, so I am different. I will show you how different I can be.' The older, more secure person may have greater faith in himself so that he can internalize the change in a relatively short time.

Signs of adjustment may be seen in changing attitudes towards the disease. Individuals who tell everyone their diagnosis and make much of diet and 'differentness' have probably not adapted any more than the person who will not discuss it at all. The well-adjusted individual will discuss diabetes, as any other facet of life, when and as appropriate, without embarrassment.

Social care

Social care will be planned with the aim of an eventual return to normal life. Many individuals fear that their total lifestyle will have to change, including their employment. In fact, people with diabetes mellitus can be found in most employments except those where the physical nature of the work would make control difficult, or where there is a risk to others if hypoglycaemia occurred.

The individual will need to talk through concerns about home, work and responsibilities. Changes required may be little more than those associated with physical health, which involve adjustments to eating habits and exercise.

It should be reassuring to most individuals to find that on discharge they will be able to continue most of their normal pursuits. Relatives need to be involved in learning about lifestyle and diabetes, since ignorance may lead to unnecessary worry and prejudice about the effects of the diagnosis.

Prejudice does exist in some areas. For example some employers are hesitant about offering work to a 'diabetic', and some insurance firms charge extra for vehicle insurance. While the individual is in hospital, he can learn about the British Diabetic Association, which fights for normal treatment of the individual with diabetes mellitus.

THE CARE PLAN

In setting priorities for the care plan, much will depend on the physical condition of the patient. If the patient is comatose, priorities will be set for treating the cause of the coma and for giving physical care as for any unconscious patient.

If hyperglycaemia and acidosis are the cause of the coma, soluble insulin will be given and other necessary measures taken to restore physiological balance. These will include administration of intravenous fluids to correct dehydration and electrolyte imbalance. If the cause of the coma is hypoglycaemia, glucose will be given by intravenous infusion in order to restore physiological balance. If the cause of coma is poor management of diabetes, education will need to be given a priority in order to reduce the risk of further crises.

If the individual is admitted for stabilizing, priorities will include dealing with physical, psychological and social problems which may be affecting control. Observations will be important so that the treatment regimen can be monitored and evaluated, both in hospital and on discharge.

In setting priorities for education, other factors such as physical pain or psychological stress need to be acknowledged. Learning is unlikely to occur unless the individual is motivated and relaxed. Reassessment will determine readiness to learn.

Although priorities for the care plan will be ordered in the light of current needs, potential problems from complications of diabetes will need to be remembered. Major complications are diabetic retinopathy, myocardial infarction due to atherosclerosis, gangrene in the lower limbs due to poor circulation, and nephropathy due to changes in the structure of the kidneys. Education for long-term care to diminish the risk of these complications will be a priority before discharge from hospital.

As long as the patient is able, priorities will be directed towards fostering self-care. Many individuals are better informed about an effective regimen than the nurse who cares for them, but others may need considerable help if they have to adjust to a change in treatment. As in any care plan, priorities will only be set after a careful assessment of each individual.

Hyperthyroidism

THE DISEASE PROCESS

The hormones thyroxine and tri-iodothyronine are produced in the thyroid and in health act to increase the body's level of metabolism. In childhood, the hormones are crucial for normal growth, mental development and maturation. In hyperthyroidism there is over-secretion of these hormones. This is more commonly seen in women than men, and is rarely found in childhood.

Over-secretion of the hormones means that oxygen intake and heat production will be increased in the body. Cellular activity will also increase and may lead to hyperplasia of the thyroid gland, that is the organ will increase in size through the development of extra, normal cells. Alternatively, adenomas (non-malignant tumours derived from epithelial tissue) may develop in the gland.

The exact cause of hyperthyroidism is not known but the condition may be preceded by emotional or physical trauma.

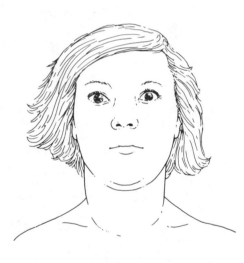

Physical reactions

Appetite is increased as a reaction to increased metabolism, with an accompanying loss of weight if the increased consumption of food is less than required. This metabolic acceleration produces excess heat in the body which leads to vasodilatation, with the result that the individual complains of being too warm; her skin is moist and warm and her diastolic blood pressure is lowered.

Breathlessness, palpitations and a rapid pulse are all reactions to increased metabolism and lead the individual to feel tired and weak. These feelings may be excerbated by diarrhoea, which is a reaction to increased activity of the gastrointestinal tract.

Physical changes may be seen in terms of an enlarged thyroid gland and bulging eyes (exophthalmia); the latter may be due to increased tissue growth which pushes the eye forward (Edwards and Boucher 1991).

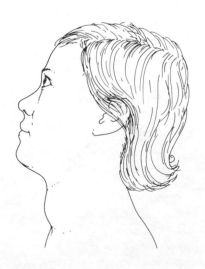

Psychological reactions

The individual is restless, and often very excitable. She may appear nervous and apprehensive. These emotional feelings may be a reaction to the increased metabolism for, with the exception of vasodilatation, they are similar to the reactions of 'fight or flight' (p. 35), i.e. increased heart rate and metabolic rate.

If the condition has been preceded by emotional crisis, reactions to the crisis may also be present.

Social reactions

Physical reactions may have caused emotional instability, affecting the individual's relationships. Tiredness may have affected the individual's personal and working life. She may have felt restless and suffered continual hunger.

As the individual accepts the reality of her ill-health, social problems may arise from the need for hospitalization, in terms of its timing and the patient's responsibilities. The family may be very concerned since they may have worried about the changes in the patient. Weight loss is associated with malignancy in many people's minds, and emotional instability with mental disorders or 'brain tumours'.

PLANNING NURSING CARE

Physical care

One of the choices for treatment is surgical removal of the thyroid gland (thyroidectomy). If this is advised, the individual will be transferred to a surgical ward. Medical treatment includes drugs to reduce the activity of the hormones, or radioactive iodine treatment. In planning care, nursing responsibilities include monitoring the effect of treatment.

The most usual treatment is an anti-thyroid drug which inhibits thyroxine synthesis. Carbimazole may be the drug of choice, which is given once daily until normal functioning is restored. After this a maintenance dose is given for at least a year. Symptoms of hyperthyroidism are generally treated with Propranolol, which reduces tachycardia, breathlessness, sweating and tremor. Nursing observations aim towards effective treatment without side effects from these drugs, which are very toxic. Side effects include rashes, pyrexia or less commonly hepatitis with accompanying jaundice. Other observations planned will be those associated with reactions to the disease such as temperature, pulse and respiration, blood pressure, weight and fluid balance.

Planning will include the meeting of the patient's needs for food and fluid to replace those lost by the accelerated metabolism. Frequent high-calorie meals are required until physical stability is restored. They should be high in carbohydrate to provide ready calories and high in protein since the individual may well be emaciated.

Fluid needs to be given in large quantities, not only to replace that lost through increased perspiration, but to ensure that the increased waste products of metabolism are adequately diluted. In planning to give extra fluids, the individual's co-operation needs to be sought through adequate explanation, for, although she will feel very hungry most of the time, she may not feel so thirsty.

Understanding is also required of the need to avoid stimulating drinks at a time when the body is already over-stimulated. Contraindications to large fluid intakes are cardiac or renal problems which may or may not be associated with the hyperthyroidism.

Although care planned will not normally include bedrest, activity should be restricted in an attempt to slow the metabolic rate. This may be difficult to plan for a restless individual, for even if she understands the rationale and agrees to rest, she may find herself pacing the ward in agitation. Reading and other quiet diversions may aid relaxation.

Frequent cool showers, and a bed space near an open window will help when planning care for an individual who constantly feels too hot, as will cotton nightwear and light bedclothes.

Education for physical health should be planned since, once the individual feels better, she may not understand the need to continue a maintenance dose of her drug for the usual period of one or two years. Further, education is required for the patient and her family to recognize the side effects of treatment and the possibility of hypothyroidism.

Psychological care

Restlessness and emotional instability may be medically treated with a mild sedative or tranquillizer during the day, and sedatives at night. Nursing care should aim towards providing as tranquil an environment as possible with the minimum of stress and frustration.

Underlying psychological problems may need to be talked through, along with current worries and fears, for although medication may relax the individual it does not diminish the problems, which may be a bar to relaxation. It may, however, be easier to talk through the causes of stress once the individual is more relaxed.

Because some of the reactions to disease are emotional, the patient may not understand her feelings, especially if they include mood swings. It may be reassuring to her if she can uncerstand that there are physiological causes for her nervous tension.

There may be fears for the future from both the patient and her relatives. Reassurance can generally be given that the treatment will eventually lead to recovery, although regular screening may be necessary to ensure that normal physiological functioning is maintained.

Social care

As the disease process is reversed, it is possible that the social problems that were associated with the hyperthyroidism will also be resolved. In planning care, other social problems may require attention or referral which could have an effect on the individual's ability to recover.

THE CARE PLAN

Priorities for care will include the delivery and monitoring of medical care, and the provision of a tranquil environment to help the individual to relax. Priorities will also be ordered towards restoration of physical deficits and the alleviation of discomfort caused by excess body heat.

There may or may not be psychological and social stresses which affect the individual's response to treatment. Priorities will be established in the light of the patient's total needs.

Hypothyroidism

THE DISEASE PROCESS

In adults, hypothyroidism, a state caused by a deficiency in thyroid hormones, results in a slowed metabolic rate. It is associated with myxoedema, a thickening of the subcutaneous tissues which is due to the deposition of mucin, which has a propensity to hold water.

There are a number of causes of hypothyroidism, which include autoimmune disease (p. 287), destruction of the thyroid gland, iodine deficiency and total thyroidectomy. There may, in addition, be disease processes that inhibit the pituitary gland from producing the stimulatory hormones necessary to trigger the thyroid gland to secrete its hormones.

Myxoedema is most commonly seen in women of middle-age and older. A congenital form of hypothyroidism may occur in infants and young children and is known as cretinism.

Physical reactions

A general physical slowing down occurs as a reaction to the reduced metabolic rate. This may be observed in a lowered temperature, pulse, respiration and blood pressure, poor appetite, weakness, paleness and sensitivity to cold. There may be a weight gain since the metabolic processes which normally turn food into energy are affected.

The individual looks oedematous though there is no 'pitting' on pressure. The skin becomes dry and rough since the reduced metabolism leads to vasoconstriction and an absence of perspiration. The face is puffy, especially the eyelids, due to the mucin deposits, and the individual sounds hoarse.

Psychological reactions

A general slowing down of mental processes occurs as a reaction to reduced metabolism. These include poor memory, reduced mental reactions, apathy, drowsiness and slow monotonous speech.

The individual is unlikely to have psychological problems associated with her reactions to disease because of the mental apathy. Since the onset of the disease is slow, it is also possible that relatives and friends who see the individual day-to-day may not notice changes for some time, though they may start grumbling about forgetfulness or slow reactions to stimulus.

Often, diagnosis is made after a visitor or friend comments on the apparent change in the personality and looks of the individual.

Social reactions

Slowed physical and mental functions may produce changes in social behaviour. Apathy may lead to neglect of family, friends and work responsibilities. There may be little attempt to feed or keep warm. As the disease progresses, more time may be spent sleeping.

PLANNING NURSING CARE

Physical care

Medical treatment is concerned with replacement therapy. The hormone thyroxine is given (e.g. as Eltroxin), in small doses to start, which are increased over time until the individual returns to normal functioning. She is then kept on a maintenance dose for life. The individual may not require hospital treatment.

Undiagnosed disease may lead to cardiac failure, hypothermia and coma. If any of these occur the individual will be admitted to hospital and care will be planned to deal with both the individual's reactions to disease and the complications which have caused the admission.

Psychological care
As the individual is restored to physiological balance, psychological balance should also be restored. The care planned may need to include the relatives, who may be feeling guilty for having failed to recognize that there were problems. If they can understand the insidious onset of the disease they may be less inclined to blame themselves for neglect.

Both relatives and patient must understand the need for compliance in treatment, for there is a risk that when the patient feels physically and mentally well, she will fail to grasp the need for continued treatment unless she understands the concept of replacement therapy.

Social care
A recovery in general health should lead to a resumption of social activity.

THE CARE PLAN

If the individual is admitted to hospital the care plan will give priorities to monitoring medical treatment and planning care to deal with problems attributed to the disease process. This will include skin care, mouth care, provision of warmth and attention to diet given the weight gain and a sluggish digestive system. A low-calorie, high-fibre, high-protein diet may be prescribed.

Diseases associated with fluid balance

Some of the diseases described in earlier sections, such as cardiovascular disease and diabetes mellitus, are associated with a disturbance of fluid balance. Similarly, the diseases described in this section may have effects on other physiological functioning, in addition to fluid balance, though the disturbances mentioned here are in the organs most closely associated with the regulation of fluid in the body.

The problems considered are normally those associated with the disease process. This does not mean that other problems may not be present in each individual according to his personal background.

Acute renal failure

In acute renal failure, there is almost always an underlying disease which causes the complication of tubular necrosis. Disease processes which lead to vasoconstriction, such as cardiac failure, dehydration or haemorrhage, are common causes of the renal ischaemia which precedes necrosis.

Other reasons for tubular necrosis are toxins which destroy epithelial cells and cause swelling and oedema of the kidneys. Examples of these are sulphonamides and salicylates, drugs taken with suicide intent, i.e. in large doses, and incompatible blood transfusions where haemoglobin acts as an endogenous toxin. Myoglobin is another example of an endogenous toxin when released from muscle cells after 'crushing injuries'.

Physical reactions

Although acute renal failure affects both kidneys, there may not be any immediate reactions to the disease process for a few days. The first physical reaction is a decrease in urinary output (oliguria) which may be followed by absence of urinary output (anuria). These deficits are caused because the damaged kidneys are unable to filter the blood and maintain fluid balance. Further physical reactions result from fluid retention and electrolyte imbalance. These include oedema and respiratory problems caused by cardiac involvement.

Because the waste products of metabolism remain in the body in the absence of renal filtration, uraemia may occur. In effect, the waste products have a toxic effect physiologically and cause reactions of anorexia, nausea, vomiting, headaches and weakness. Untreated, fits, muscular twitching and drowsiness may lead to coma.

Psychological reactions

If the condition is a complication of another disease process, reactions will be those in response to the underlying condition with the added reaction to impeded recovery and to being acutely ill. The failed suicide may leave an individual reacting angrily to the failure or with gratitude for another chance to solve his problems.

Social reactions

These too will be those associated with the underlying cause. The complication of acute renal failure will undoubtedly extend the period in hospital and may affect the chances of a return to normal life.

Physical care

The patient may not recover from acute renal failure but may progress to coma and die. In this instance care is planned as for an unconscious (Chapter 13) and dying patient. However, unless it is confirmed that recovery is unlikely, care is planned towards dealing with the problems of both the underlying cause and the renal failure.

The underlying disease process may be so serious as to preclude recovery and will certainly be a factor in the state of the patient, who will need bedrest both to slow his metabolism to reduce the production of waste products and to conserve his energy.

Plans for care will include meeting the individual's needs for hygiene and giving attention to pressure areas because of the potential problem of pressure sores. Depending on the severity of the reactions to the renal failure, self-care will not be encouraged even if the patient is independent. It may be necessary to explain the need for rest, and energy conservation to some individuals, while others may feel too ill even to contemplate self-care.

Observations will be part of the care planned. These will include fluid balance, urinalysis, temperature, pulse, respiration and blood pressure. Observations for oedema and signs of uraemia such as nausea, vomiting, persistent headache and increasing weakness will also be made. These observations are important since they monitor the course of the condition. The disturbed electrolyte balance may lead to an increase in potassium levels (hyperkalaemia) which can affect cardiac functioning and lead to arrest. Pulmonary oedema is also a risk with fluid retention and a resulting failing heart. Observations of any urine passed is also important for signs of recovery, which is accompanied by a diuresis. Temperature is important since the individual will be prone to infection, especially to pneumonia, while fluid is retained in the body.

Medical care may include frequent blood analysis to monitor electrolyte balance and urea levels. Anaemia may be present as a result of overproduction of leucocytes, and this may be treated with a transfusion of packed cells. Fluids will be restricted to those lost by the body. If no urine is passed, 500 ml only will be given to replace perspiration and respiration losses. The fluid may be given intravenously and constituted to adjust for deficits in physiological balance and nutrition.

Care will be planned to monitor treatment and give explanations to the patient. If he is vomiting, no food will be given orally. Any diet prescribed will be low in protein to reduce nitrogenous waste but will include carbohydrate to avoid the breakdown of body tissue for energy. Lack of oral nutrition and fluid intake will mean that mouth care is important. The individual's mouth is likely to be dry and a nasty taste may accompany uraemia. The lips may be cracked and provide a site for infection. Care planned should include mouth cleansing and frequent mouthwashes.

In planning care in the recovery phase, it must be remembered that when the tubules recover they will not be fully efficient immediately. Filtration will be impaired, resulting in a loss of potassium, salt and water, which could lead to electrolyte imbalance and dehydration. This means that the diuresis phase must be monitored carefully so that losses can be replaced and physiological balance restored. As recovery progresses, plans include a gradual return to normal diet and exercise.

For those individuals where conservative measures do not lead to recovery, renal dialysis may be necessary. The patient will then be moved to a dialysis unit if this is thought to give him a chance of recovery to a healthy life.

Psychological care
Psychological care will be planned with the aim of reducing anxieties and problems which inhibit the individual from relaxing. The seriousness of the patient's disease may be very apparent both to himself and to his relatives. Explanations of the measures taken and the reasons for restrictions on activity, diet and fluid intake may reassure the patient who is alert enough to resent the regimen.

Associated problems should be identified. The individual who has attempted suicide may welcome the chance to explore his problems, perhaps with a psychiatrist, while the individual recovering from a 'crushing' injury may be anxious about his future and any permanent damage from the trauma.

Plans may need to include attention to relatives' reactions to the condition or the underlying cause. Suicide, for example, may leave relatives with feelings of guilt over actions which exacerbated the problems or for not noticing that problems existed. Serious illness, complicated by renal failure, may cause extreme anxiety.

The care planned cannot always lead to a resolution of problems, but a chance to explore problems and increase knowledge can improve the chances of patient and relatives learning to cope with their anxiety and with the possibility that the patient may not survive.

Social care

The patient who is seriously ill may need rest to the extent that he is put into a room by himself. He then depends for social interaction on those who come to him. Nursing care should include time to interact in order to diminish feelings of isolation.

Relatives will need to understand that too much interaction is tiring and should prepare for the time when the patient is discharged in terms of a gradual return to normal activity.

Underlying social problems may need to be considered and action taken so that, on discharge, the individual's recovery is not hampered by a poor environment, risk of infection, or financial problems. Referral to a social worker may be necessary.

THE CARE PLAN

In acute renal failure, priorities for care will be the individual's survival or his peaceful death. Care will be centred on reactions and problems which could inhibit recovery and will include observations to monitor progress.

If recovery occurs, plans will give priority to a gradual restoration of physical, psychological and social functioning for both patient and family.

Chronic renal failure

THE DISEASE PROCESS

While the disease process is reversible in acute renal failure, chronic failure results from permanent damage to nephrons, which, over time, leads to physiological imbalance as metabolic waste products build up in the blood. The cause of chronic renal failure may be prolonged chronic infection or inflammation of the kidneys such as pyelonephritis or glomerulonephritis. It may also occur as a complication of disease elsewhere, such as diabetes mellitus, where the risk of renal disease is high, or where hypertension or atherosclerosis are present.

Prolonged renal failure appears to be linked with problems in the uptake of vitamin D. This can lead to a metabolic disease of bone (osteodystrophy) where decalcification of bone tissue occurs, and hypercalcaemia results.

Physical reactions

Initially there may be no physical reactions to suggest a renal disorder. This is because the kidneys' ability to function is far in excess of the body's needs. As chronic disease progresses, compensation is possible until a considerable area of kidney tissue is involved. Diagnosis may be by chance urinalysis, which may reveal proteinuria and lead to further investigations.

Early reactions will vary according to the underlying cause of the disease and may include headache, nausea and vomiting, diarrhoea and polyuria. In chronic renal disease, polyuria occurs initially because electrolyte imbalance and raised blood urea (uraemia) cause an osmotic diuresis; also, the tubular reabsorption is affected. Other reactions may include those associated with anaemia, i.e. tiredness and lassitude, or hypercalcaemia, where headache, nausea, vomiting, tiredness, and bone pain may occur.

As the destruction of the nephrons increases, there will be reactions related to the renal failure. The individual will become uraemic as a result of the build up of metabolic waste products, which will present as muscle weakness, neurological disturbances and a progression to drowsiness, convulsions and coma. Generalized oedema will be present, as may a tendency to bleed, which is a reaction to an abnormal prothrombin time. Other reactions include pruritus (itching) due to retained phosphates in the skin, amenorrhoea, loss of libido and impotence.

Complications associated with increasing hypertension and fluid retention are cardiac failure and cerebrovascular accident.

Psychological reactions

Chronic renal disease is progressive over months or years. Reactions will include those associated with the underlying cause, plus the response to increasing signs of failing health.

Reactions may also be expected to a diagnosis of chronic disease, and these may include anger, despair, loss of faith and guilt before acceptance is reached. There may also be a fear that dialysis or transplant surgery may not be offered, or may come too late to be of value to the individual.

Social reactions

Social reactions may include curtailment of normal activity, depending on the stage of the disease, with a resultant effect on relationships and employment.

PLANNING NURSING CARE

Physical care

Education is required for the newly diagnosed individual with chronic renal failure so that he may lead as normal a life as possible for as long as possible. Normally, the individual will not be admitted to hospital until the disease process has advanced to the uraemic stage, unless it is for treatment of the underlying condition. The responsibility for maintaining health and for early recognition of complications rests with the individual and his family, who must understand the need for the regimen; the patient is regularly monitored by the general practitioner or consultant. Some individuals may be considered for dialysis or kidney transplant.

In planning care in the advanced stage of the disease, the individual's physical need for care and observation will be similar to that of an individual with acute renal failure.

Psychological care

Psychological care will need to be based on the individual's reaction to his diagnosis and the reality of his failing health. There may be particular reactions to the neurological disturbances if memory or concentration are involved.

Allowing the individual to talk and ask questions is an essential element in nursing care. As with any life crisis, some individuals will cope with the problem and adjust quite rapidly while others may react with varying degrees of upset. A particular problem arises in the patient who denies his condition since this lowers the chance of compliance in care.

Denial and non-compliance on the part of the patient should not be confused with informed choice. Much will depend on the individual and the way in which he perceives the restrictions on his life.

Plans for care should include the relatives, who may themselves need support and information and who may be supportive to the patient.

Social care

If a return to home is possible, care in hospital must be aimed towards preparing the individual and his family for

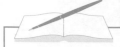

Adaptation to a chronic or life-threatening disease may be very difficult, both for the patient and his family. List the strategies that have worked for you in communicating with two patients of your choice.

1 Which of these strategies was most helpful?
2 How did each patient affect your approach to the problem?

a return to social interaction and pursuits. Problems identified which could affect maintenance of the best possible health should be referred as soon as possible.

As with any chronic disease, plans should be made to prevent the individual adopting a 'sick' role. This may involve education of the relatives, who might undermine the patient's independence with the best of intentions. A balance needs to be achieved by the relatives between smothering the individual with attention and ignoring his problem to the extent that important deficits and reactions are missed.

The individual may react to his current situation with anger or other extreme emotions, or indeed he may go into denial. The care planned to prepare the patient for a return to as normal 'a life as possible may need to be delayed while these emotions are talked through and anger diffused, or denial tested. Until the individual has worked through his emotions, it is unlikely that he will be prepared to learn to handle his disease.

Similarly with relatives: the relative who is encouraging the patient to take on the sick role will need to be assessed so that the best chance of a change of attitude will be possible. At times of stress brought on by disease, the individual's faith may be shaken and he may need to be referred to a minister who will work with him to sort out his problems of faith.

THE CARE PLAN

Priorities for care will depend on the stage of advancement of the disease. In advanced disease, priorities may be similar to those adopted for the patient with acute renal failure. If the disease is diagnosed by chance, and the individual feels reasonably healthy, priorities will be aimed towards educating the patient and his family so that maximum health may be maintained, and a normal life pursued, given the constraints of the necessary regimen.

Deficits associated with rest and exercise

Any condition which results in deficits in oxygen, nutrition or fluid balance can also cause deficits in rest and exercise. Rest may be disturbed by pain, anxiety or physical reactions such as nocturia, coughing or nausea. Exercise may be curtailed by breathlessness, lethargy or the adoption of the 'sick' role.

In this section, some conditions will be considered which have a major effect on rest and exercise, but may also have effects on other individual needs. The unconscious patient will be considered here although it is accepted that loss of consciousness may lead to deficits in all areas of basic human needs.

Anaemia

THE DISEASE PROCESS

Anaemia may be described as a condition in which there is a decrease in the oxygen-carrying capacity of blood as a result of a reduction in the number or size of erythrocytes (red blood cells). It may be due to a deficit of one of the components required to manufacture erythrocytes, or to depressed bone marrow activity which, because this is the site of erythrocyte production ('erythropoiesis'), also has the effect of reducing the quantity of erythrocytes in circulation. Anaemia may also be caused by an accelerated breakdown of erythrocytes due to physiological defects, drugs, infection or autoimmune disease. Anaemia may, in addition, result from haemorrhage, where blood loss exceeds replacement capacity.

Table 10.2 shows the types of anaemia and their causes. Anaemia is a generic term and in all instances the specific type and cause are important in prescribing care. If the anaemia is secondary to another disease, e.g. renal failure, then the disease process becomes part of a larger physiological disturbance than that caused by the anaemia alone.

Lack of adequate erythrocytes results in reduced metabolism because of the resultant hypoxia. This is common to all anaemias. The disease process is influenced by the type and cause of anaemia, but the general physical reactions to all anaemias will be similar.

Table 10.2 Major types of anaemia.

Manufacturing deficits (decreased erythropoiesis)	Excessive destruction (haemolysis)
i Iron deficiency	A Hereditary
ii Vitamin B_{12} deficiency (pernicious anaemia)	i Sickle cell anaemia
	ii Thalassaemia
iii Folic acid and vitamin C deficiency	B Acquired
iv Depressed bone marrow activity (aplastic anaemia)	i Autoimmune disease
	ii Infection
	iii Toxins

Decreased erythropoiesis

Iron-deficiency anaemia The causes of iron-deficiency anaemia may be increased demand for iron (as in pregnancy), nutritional deficits, bleeding (as in ulceration) or malabsorption. The erythrocytes are smaller than usual and contain less haemoglobin. There may also be a reduction in the number manufactured.

Pernicious anaemia Pernicious anaemia results from vitamin B_{12} deficiency, the cause of which is almost always malabsorption resulting from a deficiency of the 'intrinsic factor' in the gastric mucosa. Intrinsic factor may be deficient because of an autoimmune response (p. 287) or there may be a hereditary predisposition to gastric secretory deficits which affects the intrinsic factor. Pernicious anaemia may also follow gastric surgery or nutritional deficits of vitamin B_{12} intake.

When there is a vitamin B_{12} deficiency, there is a reduction in erythrocyte production and wide variations in erythrocyte size. Very large cells are formed called megaloblasts, which contain excess haemoglobin, but the high oxygen-carrying capacity of the megaloblasts does not balance the reduction in erythrocyte production.

Folic acid and vitamin C deficiency may be caused by increased demand (as in pregnancy), nutritional deficits or malabsorption. Production of erythrocytes is reduced since these vitamins are interdependent in that vitamin C improves the catalytic action of folic acid.

Depressed bone marrow (aplastic anaemia) Anaemia caused by depressed bone marrow is rare, and is due to deficits in the function of the marrow or an insufficient quantity of marrow to produce enough erythrocytes. Deficient production of leucocytes and thrombocytes may accompany this condition. Causes may be carcinoma, drugs, chemicals or radiation, although it is possible for the disease to occur for no known cause.

Excessive haemolysis

Hereditary defects In **sickle cell anaemia** the haemoglobin is abnormal due to a recessive hereditary factor. The disease is named after the shape of the erythrocytes, which are distorted due to the formation of crystals from the abnormal haemoglobin (Figure 10.15). These cells are more readily destroyed than normal erythrocytes, and are formed in times of crisis especially when hypoxia is present. Sickle cells can lead to ischaemia since they are more sluggish in the circulation than normal erythrocytes. It is most common in Afro-Caribbeans.

Thalassaemia is caused by a genetic defect in erythrocyte production. The cells are small, easily destroyed and irregular in shape and contain low levels of haemoglobin. It is sometimes called Mediterranean or Cooley's disease and is found primarily in Mediterranean or Asian people.

Acquired anaemia In acquired anaemia, haemolysis occurs as a result of an abnormal action on the erythrocytes which speeds up the destruction of the cells in excess of the manufacture of new ones. The causes are autoimmune disease, infection and toxins.

Blood loss
In small blood loss such as a cut finger or small nose bleed, production of new erythrocytes to compensate for the loss will soon occur. However, in prolonged slow bleeding, trauma or haemorrhage, blood loss may exceed cell production, so causing anaemia.

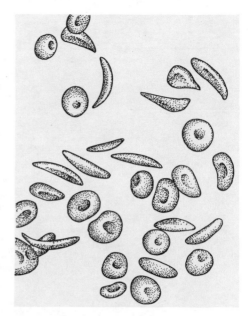

Fig. 10.15 Shape of erythrocytes in sickle cell anaemia.

Physical reactions
General Extreme tiredness, loss of energy and breathlessness on exertion are reactions to the reduced metabolic rate in all anaemias, as are feelings of being cold in relatively warm surroundings. Vasoconstriction, which occurs in the extremities to conserve the oxygen supply to the vital organs, is shown as paleness in the skin and mucous membranes.

Insufficient blood supply may cause reactions such as headache and faintness. The cardiac rate will increase due to the hypoxia, resulting in an increased pulse rate and palpitations. In untreated anaemia, the deficient blood supply may lead to deficits in renal function, so that the individual will become oedematous.

Specific reactions Reactions to iron deficiency may include soreness and inflammation of the mouth (stomatitis) and tongue (glossitis), difficulty in swallowing, and anorexia. Since iron is necessary for healthy nails, they become brittle, thin and eventually concave in its absence (koilonychia).

Reactions to vitamin B_{12} deficiency will be linked with gastrointestinal changes and may include anorexia and a sore tongue. Vitamin B_{12} is required for the health of the nervous system and its lack may cause degeneration of myelin and spinal and peripheral nerves, leading to reac-

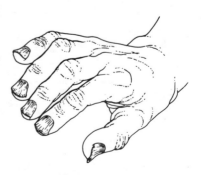

tions of coldness or tingling in the extremities, muscular weakness, loss of co-ordination, and paralysis. If the deficiency remains untreated, damage to the optic nerve may result in blindness.

There are no specific reactions to folic acid and vitamin C deficiency in addition to the general reactions to anaemia.

Although aplastic anaemia may present gradually with the general reactions to anaemia, it may also have a sudden onset with fever, bleeding from throat and mouth, lesions and infection, causing the individual to feel seriously ill.

In addition to the general reactions to anaemia, acute episodes of sickle cell anaemia (sickle cell crisis) occur, which are usually linked with stress and hypoxia. Since there is less oxygen at high altitudes, an episode could occur in an individual on a mountain top or in an aeroplane. The reaction is local to the area where the sickle cells form and causes circulatory stagnation but may include pain and swelling. Localized reactions may mimic other disease reactions, according to their site. The general reaction to the crisis includes weakness, pyrexia and mood change. Since sickle cells have a short lifespan, jaundice may result as a reaction to the increased haemolysis.

There are no specific reactions to thalassaemia in addition to the general reactions in the adult form of the disease.

Psychological reactions

Psychological reactions will include those of any debilitating disease where living itself becomes such an effort that it is difficult to be interested in normal pursuits. This may lead to depression if the disease is untreated.

The disease may be chronic, as in vitamin B_{12} deficiency or the hereditary disorders. This may lead to reactions of anger or denial in response to a change in self-image or to the resultant restrictions which may be imposed, such as curtailment of activities in sickle cell anaemia or a lifetime of replacement therapy in vitamin B anaemia.

There may be personal psychological problems which are attributable to the debilitating disease. For example, there may be marital friction or problems with children if the anaemic parent is too tired to give love and attention or maintain discipline.

Social reactions

Tiredness and breathlessness on exertion may affect normal activity and employment. Time may be lost from work or performance decreased to an extent that an employer will comment. This can add to psychological problems and speed the decision to 'go sick'.

Since activity is an effort, the individual may cut off social contacts and make less effort over personal appearance and responsibilities.

Physical care

Many individuals who are anaemic do not require hospitalization. Once the cause of the condition is found, steps are taken to replace deficits or avoid the causal agents. For example, iron may be replaced by oral administration and by improved nutrition. Similary with folic acid and vitamin C. Vitamin B_{12} can be replaced by maintenance doses, which must be given parenterally since the digestive system cannot absorb it. The individual with sickle cell anaemia may be educated to avoid those situations which provoke a crisis.

If an individual is admitted to hospital either because of the severity of the anaemia or for treatment of a condition in which anaemia is present, care will be planned with the aim of increasing the oxygen-carrying capacity of the blood and helping the patient to improve his physical health. Medical treatment will be prescribed according to the cause of the anaemia.

Rest may be important if the anaemia is severe, to conserve available energy and reduce breathlessness. If breathlessness is present at rest, oxygen therapy may be required. Care planned will need to include attention to pressure areas, particularly in the undernourished patient. Extra bedclothes may be necessary if the individual feels the cold, but these should not be heavy or produce pressure on the patient.

Diet is important in helping the individual build up strength and providing the necessary vitamins and protein for the production of erythrocytes. If the individual is anorexic it is particularly important that the diet ordered should be appealing. Large helpings can be very off-putting. It is better to serve several small nutritious meals than one large helping and say, 'Eat what you can'.

Fluids are important, especially where the mouth and tongue are sore. Soreness of the mouth and tongue will be alleviated by attention to the mouth. Frequent mouthwashes should be given, particularly after meals, to reduce the risk of infections due to stale food lodging in sore areas of the mouth and throat. If eating is difficult because of soreness, fluids may include food supplements. Fluids are also important in sickle cell anaemia, where the circulation is sluggish.

Careful observation of the individual is required for early identification of the attendant problems of anaemia. In addition to monitoring nutrition, fluid balance and the condition of the mouth, observations should be made of the skin so that if jaundice, pruritus or the painful swellings of sickle cell anaemia are present, for example, care can be planned to relieve the problem.

Regular monitoring of temperature, pulse and respiration is also necessary to show changes in either direction. Temperature may rise in infection, to which the anaemic patient is prone, while pulse and respirations are expected to steady and return to normal as a result of rest.

In pernicious anaemia, observations are made for neurological involvement. The individual's self-report is important here, as it is if the general reactions to anaemia include headache and pain. Analgesia may be prescribed but care planned should also aim to reduce the tension and discomfort associated with the pain.

In severe anaemia, blood transfusion and/or intravenous administration of fluids may be prescribed. Observations will then be needed to note the individual's reactions, observe the site, and take frequent note of the pulse and respiration. Any change should be reported.

Education may be required on a number of issues. As soon as the patient responds to treatment, a gradual return to self-care should be commenced. Each individual will need to understand the rationale of his particular regimen. This may include the importance of adequate nutrition, the need for stress reduction and the need for any long-term treatment. Increased knowledge may help the patient to accept any temporary or permanent limitations imposed by his state.

Psychological care

Generally, as the individual's physical health improves, those psychological reactions which accompanied the feelings of tiredness, lassitude and breathlessness will recede. Depression should lift as an explanation is found for the physical deficits and the cause is treated.

However, any psychological problems that arose during the depressed and tired period prior to treatment may not disappear. If there were marital tensions, for example, the relationship may have been damaged to an extent that considerable effort is required on both sides to restore harmony. Care planned may need to include relatives, because if they understand the cause of the problems they may be more prepared to make a fresh start. In assessing psychological problems, the nurse should be aware of the effect of prolonged periods of ill-health on relationships and, if necessary, offer referral to a counsellor or psychiatrist.

For the individual with chronic anaemia, such as pernicious anaemia, psychological care will need to pay attention to the problems associated with a chronic disorder and the need for regular injections. The individual will need an opportunity to talk through his feelings and strategies for coping with a constant reminder that he is no longer a 'whole' person.

Similarly with anaemias where drugs need to be taken for prolonged periods, as in autoimmune disease – the individual has to remember a regimen. If there is a resistance to acceptance of ill-health, then drugs may be 'forgotten'. Care will need to include planning a regimen which minimizes the chances of non-compliance, such as linking drug taking with other daily activities so that one triggers off the reminder of the other.

In haemolytic anaemias, the spleen is sometimes removed (splenectomy) since this will reduce the destruction of erythrocytes. Problems and plans for care of the patient undergoing surgery are discussed in Chapter 11.

Social care

A return to physical and emotional health should be partnered by a reduction of social problems. Care planned, however, should take social background into account to ensure that there were not social reasons for the anaemia. For example, in iron-deficiency anaemia, poor nutrition is often a factor. If this has been due to financial difficulties, the social worker may need to assess the situation. If, on the other hand, the anaemia is due to toxins or infection, it has to be ensured that a return home will not also be a return to the causative agent.

THE CARE PLAN

Priorities for care will depend on the severity of the anaemia, the underlying cause, and the physical reactions to the disease. Priority will also be given to psychological and social problems which accompany the condition.

Although each individual is different, anaemia requiring hospital treatment is almost always accompanied by feelings of exhaustion. Priority must be given to treating the disease and relieving the exhaustion and any pain before other problems that are pertinent are dealt with.

This makes sense since, when the individual is rested and pain-free, he will feel more able to discuss his various problems, whether they are family problems or problems of loneliness, finance, or merely of understanding his reactions to ill-health.

Multiple sclerosis

THE DISEASE PROCESS

There are many conditions of the nervous system which affect an individual's ability to undertake normal exercise and rest. Multiple sclerosis is one example of deficits in the nervous system which are a result of degenerative disease.

In multiple sclerosis, areas of the myelin sheath, which cover the nerve fibres of the spinal cord and brain, are destroyed. After the sheath has been destroyed there is rapid reproduction of neurological cells in the area. The affected area becomes scarred and damaged, so blocking the transmission of nervous impulses to and from the brain.

The damaged areas are disseminated, i.e. scattered, and irregular, the cause being unknown. Possible causes are autoimmune disease or viral infection, though neither has been proven. The disease process is intermittent, but the damage done during the active phases of the disease is cumulative.

Physical reactions
In the early stages of the disease, physical reactions may be vague and will depend on the areas affected. Vague tingling sensations may be experienced in any or all of the limbs, as may numbness and feelings of weakness. There may also be problems of double vision (diplopia) or blurring of vision.

When the disease is not active, the individual may be said to be 'in remission'. There is no pattern of relapse and remission nor any prediction of physical reactions from one relapse to another. However, as the areas of damage accumulate, reactions become permanent and severe, including permanent loss of sensation, paralysis, double incontinence, and problems with speech and swallowing (dysphagia). Eyesight may be permanently damaged and respiratory distress may occur as the result of damage to the nerves associated with the muscles of respiration.

These reactions will emerge according to the areas and extent of the damage and may take many years to reach the stage where the individual is helpless and confined to bed and wheelchair.

Psychological reactions

Psychological reactions attributable to the disease process include mood swings from over-optimism to depression and displays of irritability and temper. As the disease progresses the individual may undergo personality change and loss of intellect.

On learning of his diagnosis, the individual may experience feelings of anger and despair as he contemplates an uncertain life of remission and relapse, which will eventually lead to mental and physical helplessness. The effect on the patient's self-image may be severe, and personal faith may be affected.

Relatives and partners will also react to the diagnosis. These reactions will vary according to the closeness of the relationship and the understanding of the disease process and its implications.

Social reactions

Initially, the reactions may be those associated with irregular bouts of ill-health. These may mean only temporary disruption to normal life patterns, although, as the disease progresses, a poor record of health may have more severe implications.

Once the diagnosis is known there may be effects on social life in terms of realistic plans for the future. Career prospects may be affected as may more personal issues such as marriage and the advisability of pregnancy for female patients. Relationships may become strained, especially when the patient's mood is uncertain. Knowing that someone is ill does not necessarily make them easy to live with if they are moody and difficult and prone to outbreaks of irritability.

As the disease has more serious effects, the individual may become unemployable leading to further depression and possible financial hardship. There may be difficulties with accommodation once a wheelchair is necessary and incontinence becomes a problem. This may have effects on the whole family.

PLANNING NURSING CARE

Physical care

The individual with multiple sclerosis will be admitted to hospital in times of relapse when the disease has progressed to a stage where care at home is difficult. This means that nurses in hospital are unlikely to meet patients

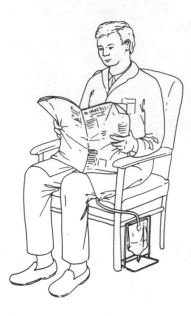

in the early stages of the disease where few symptoms are obvious during remission. Medical treatment is symptomatic since there is no known cure for the disease. Empathetic nursing care and education can help the individual to deal with the problems of his diagnosis and gain maximum benefit from his remissions.

During relapse, rest is important. Nursing care will include attention to pressure areas, and those elements of hygiene, such as bathing and mouth care, which the patient is unable to manage for himself. As the disease progresses, the individual will be able to manage increasingly less self-care. Nursing care should be aimed at meeting needs without loss of dignity for the patient.

Occasional urinary incontinence may occur fairly early in the disease, progressing to total loss of control as the individual becomes helpless. Initially, risk of incontinence may be reduced if the nurse remembers that the patient may have little warning of his needs for elimination. Later, when urinary incontinence is inevitable, the patient may be catheterized. Care plans will need to include catheter care and observations for signs of urinary tract infection.

Faecal incontinence may also present problems, as may constipation. A high-fibre diet and adequate fluids will help to overcome the weakness of the abdominal muscles. Suppositories may be given in an effort to control bowel action.

Physiotherapy may be useful in helping the individual to maintain mobility for the maximum period of time. As mobility decreases the individual will need to learn how to get himself from the bed to a wheelchair with the minimum of help. As sensory deficits increase he will also need to learn how to protect himself from damage which can occur if limbs, for example, are positioned to cause pressure, or if heat that cannot be felt could cause burns to skin.

Plans for nursing care will include monitoring the individual's mobility and sensations, and reinforcing education towards self-care and independence for the maximum period possible. Education may include help for relatives, who may wish to have the patient at home for as long as possible. Knowing how to lift, and when to help the patient without precipitating early dependence, can not only increase harmony in the family but also put off the time when institutional care may be necessary.

Psychological care

Psychological care is crucial for the individual with multiple sclerosis, not only because of the psychological changes attributable to the disease, and those associated with the disease, but because stress may precede a relapse.

The individual has much to be upset about. Often he is young with a family and unfulfilled ambitions. Concern about his future and his responsibilities can exacerbate the depression associated with the condition to a point where suicide is contemplated. Nursing care planned should include monitoring of psychological state. Changes in sleeping, eating and weight patterns should be noted, along with tendencies to weep or withdraw. The opportunity to talk through problems may be helpful but referral to a psychiatrist, with the patient's permission, may be necessary.

Stress should be minimized in that the physical care needed should be given promptly to avoid frustration, which can bring on displays of irrational temper. Later the individual may be ashamed of the outburst, adding to his feelings of depression. Although in a busy ward it is not always possible to pre-empt patients' needs, all efforts should be made to maintain the tranquillity which is an aid to recovery from a relapse.

Religious faith may be affected. Not all nurses feel able to deal with this aspect of care, especially if they themselves do not have a belief. Efforts should be made to allow the individual to raise the subject, after which referral to a minister may be considered. As with so many psychological problems, being allowed to talk matters through with a non-judgemental listener is really important.

Increasing physical disability may lead to emotional stress. It is difficult to accept the changing self-concept, especially when it incorporates loss of control of limbs and bodily excretions. Care planned needs to be sensitive to the patient's feelings. It is easy to treat an incontinent patient like a naughty child, which can be very humiliating to the receiver of care.

Relatives, especially partners, may also need psychological care as they try to deal with the realities of the situation. Knowledge of the disease and the factors which predispose to a relapse can give a positive outlook to relatives and patient, thereby having a beneficial effect on the progress of the disease. Care must be taken, however, not to attach guilt if, for example, relatives cannot always stay calm in the face of an outburst of temper.

The important point in psychological care is to attempt to emphasize positive measures such as freedom from stress, infection and fatigue in prolonging remissions, while accepting the reality of individual problems and concerns. As with any disease, vast individual differences will be seen in the ability to cope with and accept the increasing limitations of a degenerative disease.

Social care

Psychological changes may affect relationships both at a social and a personal level. Care planned should have increased understanding of the features of the disease as its aim, along with encouragement for normal social interaction to continue for as long as possible.

As the disease progresses, help from the Social Services may be necessary to deal with problems of financial hardship, structural implications associated with a wheelchair at home, and the problems of relatives who may find living with a helpless patient a considerable strain.

There is a shortage of institutional accommodation for the young chronically sick individual. If care cannot be maintained at home there may be social problems from being admitted to a place where the other patients are elderly.

Care should be planned to include relatives so that they are aware of the help that is available to them in maintaining social interaction for themselves and the patient while he is at home. The provision of nursing services, holidays and financial help may mean that the individual can remain at home for the maximum period.

THE CARE PLAN

Priorities for care while the individual is in relapse should aim towards physical and emotional rest and the identification of problems that might militate against co-operation in relaxation.

Priorities should also be given to educating the individual and his family with the aim of extending the periods of remission by avoiding factors that precipitate a relapse.

Help in the form of Social Services should be planned early during the patient's hospitalization to enhance his chances of remaining at home as the disease progresses.

Rheumatoid arthritis

THE DISEASE PROCESS

Rheumatoid arthritis is a chronic inflammatory condition affecting peripheral joints in association with systemic disturbances. There is swelling of the synovial membrane

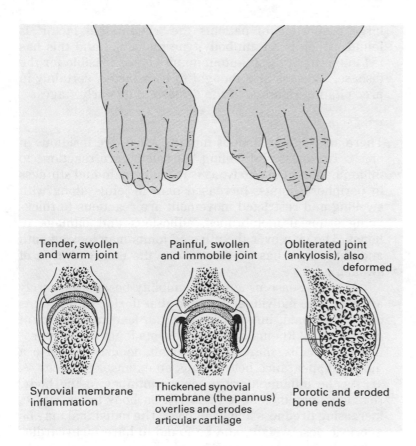

Fig. 10.16 Appearance and progression (*left to right*) of rheumatoid arthritis.

Tender, swollen and warm joint

Painful, swollen and immobile joint

Obliterated joint (ankylosis), also deformed

Synovial membrane inflammation

Thickened synovial membrane (the pannus) overlies and erodes articular cartilage

Porotic and eroded bone ends

and the tissues surrounding joints. Untreated, erosion of cartilage and bone may occur with wasting of muscles. In the early stages of the disease, swelling and congestion of the synovial membrane is present (Figure 10.16). This may progress to a thickening of the membrane (pannus) as the tissues granulate as a result of inflammation. Adhesions may form across the joint space between these thickened layers. As the disease process continues there may be abnormal consolidation of joints (ankylosis) due to the fibrous adhesions and involvement of bones, leading to deposits of bone cells in the fibrous adhesions. Muscle wasting will occur at the affected areas.

Degeneration of connective tissues may occur in other parts of the body including lungs, heart and blood vessels. Anaemia may be present, as may leucocytosis in response to the inflammatory process.

In the early stages, the progress of the disease is erratic with periods of remission and relapse. During the active phases, there is effusion of synovial fluid into the joint spaces.

The cause of rheumatoid arthritis is not known. In a

large proportion of patients the 'rheumatoid factor' is found, which is an antibody-type molecule, and this has led to the theory that autoimmunity is responsible for the disease. Stress is also thought to be a factor, certainly in precipitating relapses of the disease in its early stages.

Physical reactions

There are vague reactions initially which are insidious in onset. Tiredness and feeling 'off colour' are reactions to inflammation in the body, as is morning pain and stiffness in peripheral joints. Increased pain in joints along with swelling and restricted movement are reactions to thickening synovial membranes, adhesions and damage to bones. The skin over the affected joints may look smooth and shiny as it has to stretch over the enlarged area of swollen joint.

As the disease progresses, mobility becomes severely affected. The individual may find that flexion of the joints diminishes pain, but this in turn can lead to permanent contractures. Rheumatoid nodules, made up of degenerative tissue cells, may appear subcutaneously and give a 'lumpy' appearance below joints on extensor surfaces.

As the inflammatory process continues in the body, reactions may include a slight rise in body temperature, increasing tiredness and weakness. The individual may be anorexic, lose weight, and be found to have tachycardia.

Psychological reactions

In the initial stages of the disease process, psychological reactions will be those associated with vague ill-health and occasional pain. Some individuals may react with concern while others may simply take aspirin for the pain and attempt to ignore the fact that all is not well. As the disease progresses, psychological reactions may include anxiety and depression, which will increase as mobility decreases and body image is affected.

When the diagnosis is known, reactions will be those associated with facing a chronic crippling disease. Each individual's ability to cope with a painful permanent disability will vary but there may well be a period of anger and frustration.

Spiritual beliefs may be under strain as the individual tries to make sense of why he should have to accept such suffering. This may also be associated with feelings of guilt.

Social reactions

The age range for rheumatoid arthritis is 30 to 60 years and the disease is most common in women. This means that disability may well occur while the individual has the responsibilities of children, a partner and employment.

Increasing disability will curtail pursuits, not only those associated with exercise but those needing manual dexterity, such as food preparation and many aspects of self-care. Employment may be affected, causing financial hardship. Eventually, walking may be impossible. Life in a wheelchair may cause social deprivation and hardship.

Physical care

In the early stages of the disease process the condition is reversible. However, once joint tissue is destroyed and the bones become involved, the disease may be said to be degenerative. Medical and nursing care is then aimed at reducing inflammation, maintaining effective joint function and reducing the risk of deformity. The possibility of meeting these goals will depend on the co-operation of the patient and the stage of the disease process.

Drugs that may be prescribed are often those which, if taken regularly, have both an anti-inflammatory and analgesic action. The most common of these is aspirin. For patients who do not respond to this type of drug, or whose disease is rapidly progressing, steroids or immunosuppressants may be prescribed.

In planning nursing care, monitoring the patient's re-

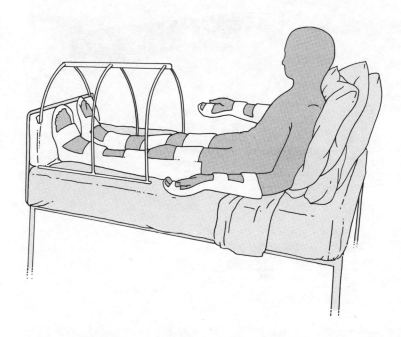

actions to these drugs is an important component. Aspirin, taken over a long period, may lead to gastrointestinal irritation and bleeding, especially if taken without food. Steroids may have side effects such as fluid retention, susceptibility to infection, and the development of a 'moon face'. Immunosuppressants, by their nature, leave the patient susceptible to infection.

Joints may need to be rested in the acute inflammatory phase of the disease process. Splints may be applied and should not only have a resting effect but should help to reduce pain by immobilization and to prevent contractures since flexion is not possible. In planning care to rest joints, it is important that the patient understands the rationale for such restrictions, since stress can exacerbate the condition. He may accept the necessity for splints more readily if he knows that as soon as possible they will be removed during the daytime and only be put on at night.

Bedrest may be necessary in the acute phase of the disease process. A hard mattress or fracture board should be used to give support to the spine and hip joints. Frequent turning will be necessary to prevent the development of pressure sores. The individual is encouraged to become mobile again as soon as possible.

Physiotherapy may be prescribed to aid mobility. Passive exercises will be carried out during the inflammatory acute periods. When inflammation has subsided, active

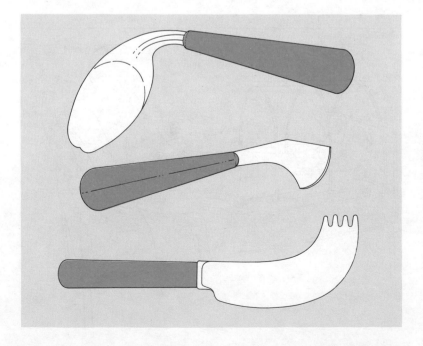

Examples of adapted cutlery

exercise is aimed at maintaining mobility for as long as possible. Nursing care should reinforce the work of the physiotherapist by encouraging regular exercise, and monitoring its effect. Each patient will need to find his own balance between rest and exercise, according to his level of disability.

For individuals with some level of deformity, self-care is very slow, tedious and painful. Nursing care should be aimed at fostering self-care even if it would be easier for a nurse to wash or dress the individual. A number of aids are available which foster self-help such as clothes which fasten with Velcro instead of buttons, implements with fat handles, and tongs which extend to pick things off the floor for people who find bending difficult.

Heat treatment may be prescribed, such as wax baths, to reduce muscular spasm, stiffness, pain and swelling. This may be carried out in the physiotherapy department. Nursing care will be directed towards helping the patient to understand the treatment, and towards monitoring the effect of the treatment. Burns may be a potential problem in heat treatment.

If the individual has anorexia, weight loss and/or anaemia, nursing care will be aimed towards encouraging adequate nutrition. Small, tempting meals should be offered to stimulate appetite, and the patient's weight monitored. Overweight patients should be encouraged to reduce weight and so reduce strain on the joints.

Education for physical health should be part of the nursing care planned so that the individual will co-operate in a regimen which will ensure physical mobility for a maximum period.

Psychological care

Psychological care will be aimed at helping the individual to cope with his present and his future. Rheumatoid arthritis is a common disease so most patients may know of someone crippled in a wheelchair and become very depressed at the prospect.

It is not possible to reassure the patient that his disease is not progressive but it is possible to take a positive attitude. The level of degeneration **can** be slowed down by treatment, rest and exercise so that a near-normal life may be resumed. Much of this is in the patient's hands, thus helping him to feel at least partly in control of the situation. In those instances where the disease progresses rapidly in spite of a regimen, the individual needs to understand that he is not to blame, and that he can still adopt a regimen to maintain some mobility.

Psychological problems may arise in relationships as

the disease progresses. Love making may be difficult and painful, and the patient may avoid physical contact because he feels unattractive as a result of a changed body image. The partner may also need to talk through such problems before they can discuss matters with the patient.

Advice may be necessary, not only on suitable positions for love making which reduces strain on the patient, but on other methods for the couple to give each other love and satisfaction. Nurses may not feel qualified to discuss these matters. However, they should give opportunities for the subject to be raised and then referred.

Similarly with problems of spiritual belief and of depression. Talking to a nurse may help, but the problems may be such that they should be referred, with the patient's permission, to a minister in the case of spiritual problems and to a psychiatrist for depression if the patient appears unable to cope.

Psychological stress may result if the patient cannot meet his responsibilities in relation to employment or child care, feeling that he is useless. Again, talking through the feelings, understanding the frustrations, and offering positive help and advice may restore perspective to the situation.

Relatives may also need help as they too face the prospect of the patient's uncertain future which carries the prospect of increasing disability.

Social care

In the progressive stages of the disease process, the individual may need help from the Social Services to adapt his home and provide aids to rehabilitation. Eventually a wheelchair may be required along with supportive services such as aids with bathing, holidays to give relatives a rest, and home help.

However, in the earlier stages of the illness social life should be maintained for as long as possible, including employment and leisure pursuits. Later, adjustments may need to be made to accommodate increased disability such as a change of job, reduction to part-time employment or indeed giving up work altogether.

Care may need to include education of both the patient and his family so that help may be obtained when necessary, and every effort made to maintain social interaction.

THE CARE PLAN

The priorities on the care plan will be aimed towards early rehabilitation except in very advanced stages of the disease process. This will include giving and monitoring medical treatment, resting the joints during the inflammatory stage, and helping the individual progress towards a regimen of balanced rest and exercise which is, as far as possible, pain-free.

Priority will also be given to reducing physical and psychological stress, both of which can exacerbate the condition. Referral to a counsellor, minister or psychiatrist may be a priority, depending on how well the individual is able to cope with his problems.

As rehabilitation commences, priority will be given to helping the individual towards self-care, with such aids as he may require, and education for him and his family to help maximum mobility to be maintained.

The unconscious patient

LOSS OF CONSCIOUSNESS (COMA)

The state of being conscious is something which most people take for granted. In the conscious state individuals respond to stimuli and form memories which shape thinking and actions. Only in sleep is the individual unaware of his surroundings, and even then a rapid return to consciousness will occur in response to stimuli such as shaking, loud noises or light.

An individual may be described as unconscious when he cannot be aroused by the above stimuli, because the neurones in the cerebral cortex are not responding to incoming signals or because there is an interruption of the signals in the reticular formation of the brain. Unconsciousness will occur if there is a lack of oxygen or glucose supply to the neurones. It can also occur as a result of trauma and anaesthesia. It may be described as intracranial or extracranial, the latter when unconsciousness is secondary to disease affecting other parts of the body.

In this chapter, some conditions have been described which, if left untreated, may lead to unconsciousness. These include hyper- and hypoglycaemia, renal failure, cardiac failure and respiratory failure. Other extracranial causes of unconsciousness include severe infections where toxins affect the neurones and other toxins in large amounts such as alcohol and narcotics.

Intracranial causes of unconsciousness include cerebrovascular disease, which may be due to haemorrhage, thrombosis or embolism, infection of the meninges (meningitis), pressure on the brain cells due to carcinoma or abscess, or trauma.

Patients' reactions to unconsciousness

The unconscious patient shows few reactions, depending on the depth of coma. He will be largely unaware of outside stimuli and as such is at extreme risk. Automatic responses to threat are absent so that in the absence of care by others the individual may die. Breathing may be affected since the patient does not automatically maintain a clear airway. The respiratory centre may be depressed, as may the cough reflex. Further, the tongue may relax and cause obstruction.

Nutrition is affected because nutritional needs are not met and also because metabolism is slowed and circulation impaired. In the absence of fluid intake dehydration may occur, which in turn may lead to electrolyte imbalance.

Sensation is lost so that there is a risk of pressure sores developing, and control of bladder and bowel movement is lost, leading to incontinence and the attendant risks to skin, vulval or penile and anal areas. Eyes are at risk in the absence of normal reflexes and a lack of secretions. If the eyes remain dry for any period of time, ulceration may occur.

In unconsciousness, although there appears to be a total lack of response to stimulus, it is thought that the last sense to fail is that of hearing. This has importance when planning nursing care.

Since the individual is unable to respond, the major focus is on physiological reactions until consciousness is restored. The unconsciousness may, however, have both a psychological and social impact on the patient's relatives, especially if the condition occurred rapidly and unexpectedly.

PLANNING NURSING CARE

Physical care

Unconsciousness may be transitory or prolonged. Medical treatment will depend on a rapid assessment of the cause. If, for example, unconsciousness is the result of hypoglycaemia, glucose will be prescribed and the patient's return to consciousness will be almost immediate. If, on the other hand, the unconsciousness is due to cerebrovascular haemorrhage (stroke) the unconsciousness may last for some hours or days.

In planning nursing care, the aims will be to maintain and protect bodily function until the individual either returns to normal or partial functioning or dies, for if unconsciousness is prolonged there is a real threat to life.

Priority must be given to maintaining a clear airway. This may be established by placing the patient in a lateral position. This allows drainage of mucus and prevents obstruction by the tongue (Figure 10.17). It may also be necessary to use an artificial airway if breathing remains difficult or if the lateral position is contraindicated (Figure 10.18). Suction may be required on admission for clearing mucus collecting in the mouth or for clearing vomit.

Fluid balance and nutrition will be maintained by intravenous infusion and/or by nasogastric feeds. The unconscious patient must not be given anything by mouth since the swallowing reflex will be affected and could lead to food or fluids being aspirated into the respiratory tract. Care of the mouth, and of the nasal area if a tube is used, are essential to prevent soreness and infection.

False teeth may be removed but only if their presence is hindering breathing. Otherwise, they should be cleaned regularly and put back into position. Relatives may be very worried by unconsciousness and, if they have not seen the patient without teeth, they may be even more stressed by his appearance.

Loss of sensation puts the total responsibility for care of the skin onto the nurse. Daily sponging with warm water to maintain hygiene is necessary along with regular attention to pressure areas. Frequent turning to encourage circulation and remove pressure is required, as is particular attention to positioning of the feet and hands which, with diminished reflexes, are at risk of injury, contractures or 'drop', i.e. inability to keep the foot or hand at the correct angle as a result of paralysis.

A special bed may be used, e.g. air or water, to aid protection of the skin. Since incontinence is a risk to skin integrity, an in-dwelling catheter may be used. Catheter care will then be essential to avoid infection. Prompt attention to incontinence of faeces is required. Suppositories, aperients or occasionally an enema may be given in an attempt to regulate bowel movement.

Care of eyes is necessary. Regular irrigation with sterile normal saline will reduce the risk of damage to the cornea. Eye drops may be prescribed to lubricate and guard against infection.

Observations are crucial in the care of an unconscious patient, both to ensure that vital body functioning is maintained, and to monitor the level of consciousness.

Respirations are monitored along with temperature

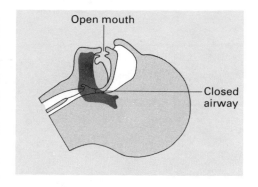
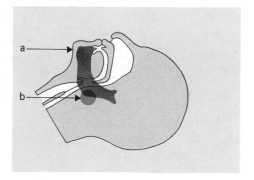

Fig. 10.17 Obstruction of airway by tongue when mouth is open (*top*). Closing the mouth by gently pressing on the chin (a) or at the angle of the jaw (b) will keep the airway open.

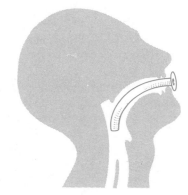

Fig. 10.18 An artificial airway in position.

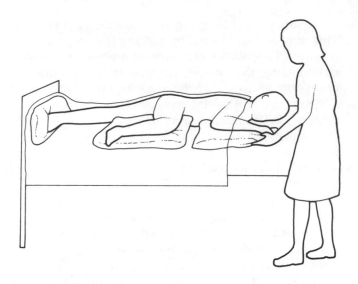

and pulse at regular intervals as prescribed. Changes noted should be reported immediately so that necessary action may be taken.

Fluid balance is recorded and note taken of signs of dehydration such as dry mouth and skin. The general condition of the skin is also observed for signs of pressure or damage. The individual may be nursed naked to aid care and observation.

The level of consciousness is monitored by noting responses to stimuli. These may be spoken, e.g. 'Hello Miss Booth. Can you hear me?', or by testing reflexes, e.g. noting if pupils respond to light or if eyelids close when the cornea is gently touched: squeezing a hand gently or touching the sole of the foot will also bring response as consciousness returns.

In unconsciousness, the patient's state may change in either direction. Any change in any observation should be carefully noted and reported so that a coherent account is built of the individual's progress.

Psychological care

Although unconscious, the individual should at all times be treated with respect, and his dignity should be maintained as far as possible. For example, although it is common to nurse unconscious patients naked, they should be covered with a sheet when their relatives are present. Some elderly married couples, for example, have never seen each other undressed, and may be appalled at the idea. Indeed, in some cultures being seen undressed is not allowed.

Attention to appearance is also important, both for the patient and for his relatives. The image of a toothless, unconscious person with untidy hair may leave lasting memories with a relative and cause unnecessary distress, since the patient has been depersonalized due to thoughtlessness and careless nursing.

Speaking to the patient may seem silly if he is unconscious but in fact hearing is often the first sense to return between consciousness and unconsciousness and many patients can remember what has been said to them when they return to consciousness. Gentle talking may well be therapeutic but it is equally important not to discuss the patient in his hearing, especially in pessimistic or derogatory terms. As the level of consciousness increases the individual may show signs of confusion. Talking in a calm voice, explaining where he is, and that he is being cared for may help in the struggle for complete consciousness.

Most individuals have at some time in their lives had a nightmare of the type in which something awful is happening and yet they know it is a dream. They struggle to wake up but cannot. Patients have described returning to consciousness in very similar terms. In talking to the semi-conscious patient, a nurse or relative may be of considerable help. Psychological care of the unconscious patient must include the relatives. Their problems in coping must be appreciated so that they can talk, ask questions, and gain support from the health care team.

Social care
The social implications of unconsciousness depend on the cause, its duration, and any impairment of function once consciousness has returned.

THE CARE PLAN

Priorities in care must be the maintenance of physiological functioning in the absence of consciousness. Top priority must be given to maintaining a clear airway. The other vital elements of life – fluid and nutrition – should be re-established within 24 hours.

Care planned should also give priority to relatives in terms of assessing their problems and helping them to cope with a difficult situation, and in maintaining an acceptable image of the patient in terms of physical appearance as far as is possible.

As consciousness returns, priority must be given to

helping the individual to re-orientate himself and deal with his 'lost time'.

Lifestyle and disease

Many of the diseases mentioned in this chapter are related to lifestyle. For example, the 40-year-old with ischaemic heart disease may be a workaholic who does not take enough exercise, has an inappropriate diet, smokes and drinks too much alcohol. Similarly, a patient with small cell cancer of the lung may be a smoker. The patient with cirrhosis of the liver may be an alcoholic and the anaemic patient may not have taken proper care over diet.

Health promotion initiatives abound. When watching television, travelling on a bus or underground train, or visiting the cinema an individual may see hoardings or advertisements exhorting him to give up smoking, to eat a healthy diet, to cut down on cholesterol and to moderate drinking. One of the difficulties is that it is possible to get heart disease without living a stressful life, it is possible to get carcinoma of the lung without being a smoker, and similarly with other diseases that are seen to be associated with lifestyle and what are perceived to be unhealthy attitudes to one's body. This may cause difficulties for the patient who feels that he is being punished when he has actually taken good care of himself. These feelings of frustration and distress can affect the way the patient responds to his disease, the diagnosis and the prognosis, particularly if the prognosis is poor.

Some diseases can only be acquired from another person already suffering from that disease. Influenza is a good example of this, although not everyone who comes into contact with someone who is incubating influenza will 'catch' the germ. Again, lifestyle can affect who becomes infected in that those who are in peak health are less likely to succumb to infections than those who are debilitated in any way. This may include poor housing, poor level of nutrition and those suffering from other diseases.

A relatively new infectious disease in the Western world is acquired immunodeficiency syndrome (AIDS). This disease has caused considerable concern particularly in the media, partly as it can be associated with alternative lifestyles. Statistically in the UK, the most vulnerable groups who become infected with HIV (human immunodeficiency virus) and then go on to develop AIDS are male homosexuals and drug abusers.

AIDS

The disease process

The infection which may lead to full-blown acquired immunodeficiency syndrome (AIDS) is called the human immunodeficiency virus (HIV). This is one of a family that carries the genetic material in ribonucleic acid (RNA) rather than deoxyribonucleic acid (DNA). What HIV does in the body is to affect the genetic material of infected lymphocytes. These lymphocytes then reproduce more HIV instead of more lymphocytes. This means that the amount of HIV in the body can increase and so affect more and more body cells through the lymphocytes.

HIV is known to be transmissable from one person to another in three ways. These are through blood-to-blood contact, which includes drug abusers who share needles, through semen and through a pregnant mother to her unborn child. There has been some debate about infection through other bodily secretions, but to date no cases have been identified that were infected in this way.

In the early 1980s when the disease was new in the United Kingdom, some patients were infected by having blood transfusions from individuals who carried the HIV virus. Measures to test all blood given by blood donors have now diminished the probability of this happening to patients requiring blood products.

The disease affects primarily young people and the majority of these **at present** are male homosexuals. This picture may change with an increasing number of heterosexuals being infected and more drug abusers, in spite of Government legislation to provide free syringes to reduce the risk of needle sharing.

There is speculation that it is possible to be HIV positive without developing AIDS. Those people who are seen to be at risk of developing the disease can have an HIV test, and many people who are at risk will ask for that test. Those who are discovered to have an HIV-positive result will be monitored; currently there are people who have carried the virus for over 10 years without developing AIDS. They may feel perfectly well and lead perfectly normal lives but they are able to infect other people.

Physical reactions

When someone who is HIV positive develops AIDS, their symptoms may include deficits in oxygen uptake, deficits

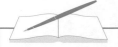

A patient on your ward tells you that he has had a brief affair. He is very concerned that his temporary partner may have been HIV positive.

1 In your assessment of this patient, what aspects of his relationship with his partner would be important to you?
2 What strategies would you use to help this patient to make the decision on whether or not to take a test that will tell him if he is in fact HIV positive?
3 How would you make sure that your own feelings about this situation did not colour the way you interacted with this patient?

in nutrition, neurological involvement, chronic illness and malignancy. The patient is also open to opportunistic infections (Flaskerud 1989).

Psychological reactions

Psychological reactions to both a positive HIV test and to AIDS itself will vary according to the way in which the infection was contracted, many individuals having to deal with a double shock. For example, the woman who finds herself to be HIV positive and at risk of AIDS may have to accept along with this devastating diagnosis the fact that her husband may be bisexual. This can cause tremendous problems, not only for the patient, but for other family members. Any disease that is known to come from another person through infection can cause tremendous emotional responses including anger and blame, with many individuals also feeling extremely guilty for having put themselves in a position where they could develop this disease, and pass it on to other people whom they love.

The patient and other family members will need to be properly assessed to identify exactly what the psychological problems are and whether there are solutions that the individual can work through with their loved ones. One of the difficulties for staff in assessing psychological and other problems in those who are HIV positive and those who develop AIDS is that it is often difficult but essential to be non-judgemental of individuals whose lifestyle and sexual proclivities are very different from one's own.

Social reactions

Social reactions may be very much affected by the way that family members react to the disease. Parents of a young man who is found to have AIDS may again be dealt a double blow. They may, in the past, not have accepted their son's lifestyle and are suddenly faced with the knowledge of the disease together with the truth that their son is homosexual, or a drug abuser.

A male patient may have a strong relationship with another man. Very often at the time that AIDS is diagnosed and the patient is admitted for care, parents may try to exclude the lover from the illness and from visiting the centre where the patient is being cared for. The patient himself may feel caught in the middle of a situation that he does not feel able to deal with in his debilitated state.

Those patients who have developed AIDS as a result of contaminated blood or because they did not know that their husband was sexually unfaithful, possibly with another man, may be shunned by former friends and colleagues because the stigma attached to this disease has been applied to themselves, even though they are neither homosexual nor drug abusers.

Another element which may affect the social life of the patient with AIDS is that there are many misconceptions that lead to the belief that AIDS can be caught by any contact with an infected person.

Physical care
There is currently no cure for HIV or for AIDS itself. Physical care will include treating opportunistic infections and hopefully helping the patient to prevent further ill-health. If malignancy is present, it is very likely to be Kaposi's sarcoma, which is a rare form of cancer but common in AIDS patients. Treatment is currently experimental and cannot ensure success.

Overall, physical care will be concerned with dealing with symptoms as they arise and keeping the patient comfortable in terms of skin care, nutritional deficits and oxygen deficits.

Psychological care
The patient may need to talk through psychological problems following assessment. These are particularly likely to include relationships with partners and family, and perhaps dealing with frictions that have arisen as a result of the illness. Those patients who feel that the disease is a punishment for past misdemeanours may need help and counselling to work their way through the many emotions involved. Family members may also need help in accepting the reality of both the disease and, occasionally, its cause.

Many health professionals find difficulty in working with AIDS patients because of the lifestyle that may precipitate the disease. As with all diseases, professional care must be offered without judgement. There may be conflict between a nurse's belief system and the fact that some sex relationships are new legal in many societies. A judgemental response has not been helped by media coverage, particularly in the early period when AIDS became a reality in the Western world, and was linked with promiscuous homosexuality.

Social care
Social care may well be involved in relationships, helping family members to adapt to the traumatic news and helping the patient to feel that they are being treated the same

as any other patient who requires care. The patient himself may feel that he is socially unacceptable. Many of these patients are cared for in designated wards or hospitals rather than in general wards. This may reinforce the notion that the patient is socially unacceptable to others.

In the early days of the disease, this notion that the patient was socially unacceptable was reinforced with barrier nursing and the patient not being touched by anyone who was not wearing a gown, gloves and a mask. Thinking has changed in recent years as awareness has grown that the risk to any health professional of being contaminated by HIV is minimal if high standards of hygiene are observed.

The care plan

The care plan will reflect the current symptoms of the patient. Emphasis will be placed on maintaining balance in physical function such as nutrition, fluid and electrolyte balance and oxygen intake. Because the patient is likely to be debilitated, particular care should be planned in terms of maintaining skin care, mouth care and general physical care.

The relatives of the patient and the partner, if there is one, need to be apprised of the situation and treated with equal respect. If admission is for terminal care, the plan should reflect the need for meeting patients' wishes for handling unfinished business and for spiritual care.

Summary

In this chapter, nursing on a medical ward has been considered. Some common diseases have been described to illustrate patients' physical, psychological and social reactions to physiological deficits.

Care planning has been considered which accepts every patient as an individual who may have a variety of problems associated with his disease. Other non-disease-related problems have also been identified.

In all cases, nursing care includes the ordering of priorities in care and the referral of problems which cannot be dealt with to specialist help.

Relatives are part of most patients' normal life. Their needs have been considered in accepting diagnosis and prognosis, as has their potential to support the patient.

References

Brunner, L. & Suddarth, H. (1989) *The Lippincot manual of medical surgical nursing*, 2nd edn. London: Harper & Rowe.

Connechen, J., Shanley, E. and Robson, H. (1983) *Pharmacology for nurses*. London: Baillière Tindall.

Degree Coustry, C. (1976) Psychological problems in rehabilitation programmes. In Stocksmeier, U. (Ed.) *Psychological approach to the rehabilitation of coronary patients*. Berlin: Springer-Verlag.

Department of Health (1995) *Health Service Guidelines*. 13, Annex A (March 1995).

Edwards, C. R. & Boucher, I. A. (Eds.) (1991) *Davidson's Principles and Practice of Medicine*, 14th edn. Edinburgh: Churchill Livingstone.

Elkind, A. K. (1982) Nurses' views about cancer. *Journal of Advanced Nursing*, *7*, 43–50.

Flaskerud, J. (1989) *AIDS/HIV infection, a reference guide for nursing professionals*. Eastbourne: W. B. Saunders.

Fuerst, R. (1983) *Microbiology in health and disease*. Philadelphia and London: W. B. Saunders.

Neale, M. (1987) *Medical pharmacology at a glance*. Oxford: Blackwell Scientific Publications.

Ward, L. (1984) *Facts about smoking. A trainer's manual*. Manchester: TACADE.

Further reading

Adler, M. (1993) ABC of AIDS, 3rd edn. London: B.M.J. Publishing.

Anderson, K., Anderson, L. & Glanze, W. (1994) *Mosby's medical, nursing & allied health dictionary*. St Louis: Mosby.

Andrews, C. & Smith, J. (1991) *Nurses' aids series: medical nursing*. London: Baillière Tindall.

British National Formulary (regularly updated). London: British Medical Association and the Pharmaceutical Society of Great Britain.

Cahoon, M. C. (1982) *Cancer nursing. Recent Advances in Nursing, No. 3*. Edinburgh: Churchill Livingstone.

Friedman, E. & Moshy, R. (1986) *Medicine. The bare bones: a comprehensive systematic approach*. Chichester: Wiley & Sons.

Kacmarek, R., Mack, C. & Dimas, S. (1990) *The essentials of respiratory care*. St Louis: Mosby Year Book.

Kasner, K. and Tindall, D. H. (1990) *Baillière's Nurses' Dictionary*, 21st edn. London: Baillière Tindall.

Purchese, G. and Allan, D. (1984) *Neuromedical and neurosurgical nursing*. London: Baillière Tindall.

Resler, M. M. and Bovington, M. M. (1983) *Diabetes mellitus. The Nursing Clinics of North America*. Philadelphia and London: W. B. Saunders.

Royal Marsden Hospital (1984) *Manual of clinical nursing policies and procedures*. London: Harper and Row.

Shillitoe, R. (1988) *Psychology and diabetes: psychosocial factors in management and control*. London: Chapman & Hall.

Trounce, J. (1990) *Clinical pharmacology for nurses*, 13th edn. Edinburgh: Churchill Livingstone.

11

Planning Care: Surgical Interventions

CHAPTER SUMMARY

Introduction: the surgical ward, 353
Types of surgical ward, 354
Surgical conditions, 355

Control of infection, 356
Cross-infection, 356

General care of patients on a surgical ward, 359
Pre-operative care, 356
Post-operative care, 363

Wound care, 371
Asepsis, 371
The Central Sterile Supply Department, 371
Healing, 372
Dressings, 374
Haemorrhage, 376

Surgery affecting body image, 377
Mastectomy, 378

Hysterectomy, 385
Bowel stoma formation, 390

Surgery for a potential threat to life, 397
Appendicectomy, 398
Peritonitis, 398
Repair of hernia, 400
Cholecystectomy, 404
Prostatectomy, 409

Replacement surgery, 414
Physical problems, 414
Ethical problems, 415
Psychological problems, 417

Summary, 419

References, 419

Further reading, 420

Introduction: the surgical ward

The patients on surgical wards, in contrast to those on medical wards, have usually been admitted for a specific purpose and should have a realistic idea of their length of hospital stay. With improvements in medical technology (Hill and Summers 1994) and improvements in surgical techniques, the length of stay may be as little as one day. This is a situation undergoing rapid change with some hospitals reporting 60% of surgical interventions being carried out on a day case unit. Although there are patients who undergo a number of operations, there is less likelihood of there being either long-stay patients or regular readmissions on a surgical ward. The result is a rapid turnover of patients.

This situation has two advantages. Firstly, there is less uncertainty about the duration of stay for the patient, who will have been able to make plans for a specified time away from home. Secondly, he will usually, though not always, know what is likely to happen to him, in terms of the type of operation for which he has been admitted.

This knowledge is not necessarily without stress. For example, the individual who is to have gallstones removed may yet be frightened of the impending surgery, even though he understands the necessity for it. The fear of being 'cut open' may be coupled with other stresses surrounding admission (Seers 1987) including non-comprehension of the information given.

The disadvantage of a rapid turnover of patients is that there is less time for systematic assessment. This is particularly true for those patients admitted for day surgery where they are admitted early in the morning but sent home again the same evening following their operation. Those patients admitted for a longer period of time may come to the ward less than 24 hours prior to surgery. For day-care or longer-stay patients, the notion of their forthcoming surgery may be very stressful and an opportunity should be made to identify problems and clarify any misconceptions before the operation. For some patients, follow-up in the community may be necessary to identify post-operative concerns and explore coping mechanisms.

A busy nurse may well feel it is pointless to identify problems in situations where there is little time to plan care. However, it is important to give each patient an opportunity to discuss both needs and concerns and remember that care can continue in the community for patients who are at risk of physical, psychological and social problems.

Types of surgical ward

As with medical wards, surgical wards may be general or specific. The latter allows a concentration of expertise and resources. As a result a patient who is admitted for a colostomy, for example, will find other patients who have undergone bowel surgery at various stages of recovery in the same ward.

The same problems exist for surgical patients as for those on medical wards in that, although it is encouraging to meet other patients who are recovering well, it may be worrying to see patients whose surgery has been more radical or less successful. This can undermine the patient's confidence that his surgery will be a success.

As surgical procedures improve, more specialization may be seen, not necessarily within particular wards only, but within units in particular hospitals. For example, microsurgery is a particular specialty in Manchester, while heart transplants are a specialty in Cambridge.

Geographical specialization may mean that the patient is a long way from home for the period of hospitalization. Potential difficulties include maintaining links with family and friends, financial hardship and social problems. If a partner or relative stays near the hospital during surgery and recovery, he too may have problems. A patient may be too proud to discuss these problems unless a nurse gives the opportunity for them to be raised.

Surgical conditions

'Surgery' is an operative procedure whereby an individual has diseased tissue removed manually, an injury repaired or bypassed, replacements given, or cosmetic changes made. Surgery may be planned ahead, i.e. 'cold', when the patient is admitted from a waiting list. Such operations are seen as necessary but not urgent. Surgery may also be performed shortly after diagnosis if the operation is seen to be essential to life, and as an emergency to save life.

Surgery may be exploratory in the absence of a clear diagnosis. Before the improvements in medical technology, exploratory surgery, often abdominal, involved a laparotomy, that is an incision of the abdominal wall so that internal organs could be investigated. This was very stressful for the patient because they were facing the unknown as well as surgical intervention. It was seen in Chapter 9 that much diagnosic work may now be undertaken without invading the body or with minimal invasion.

Surgery may be relatively minor, as in the removal of the appendix, or major, as in colostomy. It may also be major and uncertain, as in transplant operations. What has to be remembered is that each individual will view his own operation, no matter how safe or small, in the light of his illness prior to admission and from his own life experiences, rather than by its seriousness in surgical terms. His fears will be central to him and should not be diminished by comparing them to other patients' more serious concerns.

Control of infection

Control of infection is important on any ward but is of particular importance on a surgical ward where there are open wounds with exudate at the perfect temperature for organisms to incubate. These may include the patient's own flora and other, additional organisms, which will have a direct route into the body via the wound. Hospitals contain many organisms to which the new patient will not have acquired immunity. Many of these will be carried by hospital staff or by other patients who have acquired immunity. The transference of organisms by a carrier or the spread of infection from one patient to another is called cross-infection.

Cross-infection

Cross-infection may occur by touch, through the air when dust is raised (airborne), and by moisture (droplets) expelled by coughing and sneezing, or even simply by breathing (Figure 11.1).

Most hospitals have an Infection Control Nurse to teach staff how to minimize the possibilities of infection, to monitor infections, to trace sources and to recommend action once a source of infection is identified. It is also the responsibility of every nurse to reduce, as far as possible, the chances of cross-infection by her own behaviour and by educating the patients, particularly about their wounds.

The nurse

Personal hygiene is important for the nurse since she can carry organisms in her hair, her skin and her clothes from one patient to another, even when she herself feels fit. Hospital uniform is very different today from that in the past. Hats used to cover hair totally and a voluminous apron covered the uniform dress. Nowadays hats, if worn, are no more than a decoration and most nurses' uniforms do not include an apron. The responsibility rests with each nurse to keep her hair tidy, her skin clean, and to wear disposable or plastic aprons when carrying out procedures where her uniform requires protection from organisms.

If the nurse has a cold or other infection she may transfer this to the patients, especially if she coughs. And any hospital patient may have lowered resistance to infection. Nurses who have infections should consider the ad-

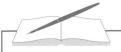

Look up your local standard for wound care. How many elements of the standard refer to (a) personal hygiene and (b) avoiding infection risks?

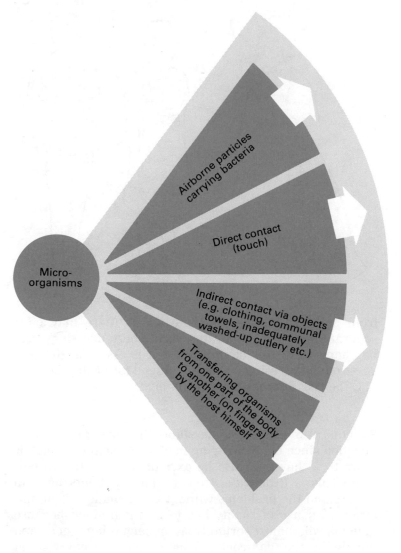

Fig. 11.1 Modes of infection transmission.

Microorganisms

Airborne particles carrying bacteria

Direct contact (touch)

Indirect contact via objects (e.g. clothing, communal towels, inadequately washed-up cutlery etc.)

Transferring organisms from one part of the body to another (on fingers) by the host himself

visability of reporting for duty. It is often felt that taking time off when unwell is frowned upon by senior staff, yet, if a nurse comes on duty when she has an infection, she is not only a risk to patients and other staff, but may also prolong her own illness or fall prey to a more serious condition.

Although nurses do not clean the wards, they can ensure that beds are made without raising too much dust and that one patient's bedclothes are not put onto another bed during bedmaking. Similarly, wounds should not be dressed while the domestic staff are cleaning the wards or while beds are being made. Damp dusting to beds and furniture prevents dry dust and the attendant organisms

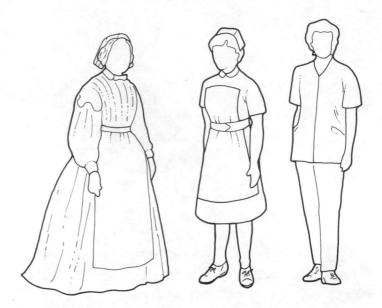

from being circulated. In some wards there may be a separate area away from the ward where dressings may be changed. In this circumstance it is essential that the sheet on the dressing couch is changed for each patient. If not, the risk of cross-infection is high.

The patient

Patients also need to understand the concept of cross-infection since by exchanging books, newspapers, food or cigarettes, they may also be exchanging infective organisms. This is a delicate area, because patients need to understand the problems without being made to feel 'unclean'. A sense of reality has to be maintained because patients will almost certainly sit on each other's beds and mingle in the day-room. This is the normal risk of interaction.

The abnormal risk lies in the variety of organisms at large and the open wounds which need protection. Wounds should be properly covered with a sterile dressing or protective spray and not tampered with by the patient or staff. Teaching the value of not touching the wound, not comparing it with those of other patients, and not showing it to family or friends is important, as is the need for scrupulous personal hygiene especially after micturition or defecation. Genito-urinary tract infections are exceedingly common because of the close proximity of the anus and the urinary tract. If hands are not washed, these infections may be spread rapidly by the hands themselves or via objects handled.

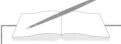

1 Prepare a plan to teach an elderly patient the risks of wound infection. What do you consider the most important aspects to cover? How could you evaluate the impact of your teaching?
2 Implement the plan with a patient of your choice and evaluate the outcomes. For reference, see Pike and Forster (1995).

General care of patients on a surgical ward

Although care is individualized for each patient according to his deficits and needs, there are also general principles of care for every patient undergoing surgery. These principles cover pre- and post-operative care and the care of wounds.

Pre-operative care

There is no standard time for admitting patients prior to surgery. Much will depend on the proposed operation, the beliefs of the surgeon and the general policy of the hospital. As a result, individuals may be admited as day-patients, 24 hours before the operation or several days before the expected surgery.

Pre-operative care should commence on admission. The standard care plan on p. 153 gives the elements of general pre-operative care which should be followed for each patient.

Understanding the operation

No assumptions may be made about a patient's understanding of his operation without assessment. The doctor may have explained what will happen but this does not mean that the patient understands or knows what to expect. He may have been under stress at the time of explanation or may not have understood the language used.

In planning pre-operative care, the nurse should assess the patient's current knowledge and his need for information. The classic work of Hayward (1975) showed that informed patients need less analgesia and recover more rapidly from surgery than patients who lack information. Many other studies show similar results and this is easy to understand, since fear of the unknown can cause stress and tension, which lead to pain. A patient in pain may take longer to return to self-care than a patient who is relatively relaxed.

The level of information given should depend on the individual's needs and ability to absorb information. Some patients may wish to understand the actual mechanics of the operation while others will be more interested in its effect. All patients will need to know when they are going to theatre, the details of the necessary preparation and what to expect on their return to consciousness.

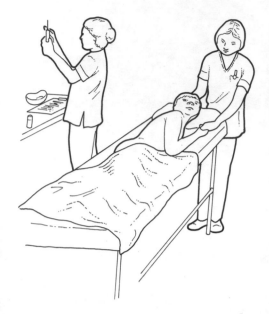

Each surgeon will produce a 'list' for his operation days. This list will give the order in which the patients will go to theatre. There may be variations, but it is common for large operations to be listed early in the day and for minor operations to be put at the end.

The ward sister is usually aware of the time the surgeon takes for specific operations so that each patient should have an approximate idea of when he can expect to be taken to the operating theatre. For the patient who is admitted some days prior to surgery, it will be important to know if the operation is listed for morning or afternoon.

Occasionally, an operation may take longer than expected or an emergency may take priority over list cases. This may mean that patients at the end of the list are delayed or taken off the list altogether for that day. In these instances, good communication is vital between surgeon and ward staff so that patients may be informed of the changed plans as soon as possible. Otherwise the patients may worry that a mistake has been made and their operations forgotten.

Most patients will understand the reasons for delay if they are informed. However, some may become very upset, particularly if they are highly nervous and feel they have to go through the same tension again on another occasion. A chance for the patient to verbalize concerns of this nature may result in his being placed earlier on the next list.

It is often stated that there is no time to assess day-patients and little point, since they will soon go home. In fact a day-patient may be just as tense as an in-patient. It takes very little time to ask, 'How do you feel about your operation?' and 'What are you expecting to happen to you?'. The nurse can then give such information as is necessary. If the patient appears very stressed, a comment such as 'You look worried' might elicit the cause of the tension, which may be something that can be dealt with promptly, or referred if necessary.

Information alone will not necessarily make a patient happy, particularly if his operation will have a severe impact on his life. However, the chance to talk through fears and gain insight into what to expect should reduce the tension associated with the actual process of surgery.

If a patient is to be shaved, have an enema, or other pre-operative procedure, an explanation should be given of the reason for this. The reason for withholding food and drink for some hours prior to operation should also be explained. Understanding will increase compliance and the patient's belief that staff are treating him as a thinking individual.

Premedication, which involves giving a drug by mouth or by injection to make the patient drowsy before he is taken to theatre, should be explained. He should also be told that he will be given drugs to send him rapidly to sleep in the reception area of the theatre, and that he will know nothing of the operation until it is over and he is in the recovery room. It is standard practice in some operations that the patient has intravenous fluids and oxygen therapy post-operatively. If the patient does not know of this he can become very alarmed, believing that 'things have gone wrong' and he is seriously ill. Adequate explanation **before** surgery of what to expect on recovery will prevent distress.

Each patient has to sign a form consenting to a specific operation. The form states that the patient understands the operation and that it has been explained to him. There is often a rider which gives the surgeon the right to perform other necessary operative work. The consent form may be completed in the presence of a nurse. She must be certain that the patient does understand the operation and has thoroughly read the form. He may decide to cross through permission for any measures other than the operation he is expecting. This is evey patient's right.

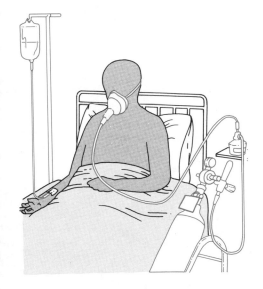

Observations

Pre-operative observations are important because they give baseline data against which post-operative progress may be monitored. They also alert staff to problems which might indicate that surgery would be unwise until they have been treated or referred to an appropriate agency.

The anaesthetist may examine the patient in addition to the ward observations of temperature, pulse, blood pressure, weight and urinalysis. This will allow him to assess the individual's tolerance to anaesthesia and to make any adjustments in response to the patient's general condition.

It is not always possible for a patient to be in perfect health before an operation. Individuals with liver disease, for example, may be in need of a hysterectomy, and patients with diabetes may need an operation. The consultant and the anaesthetist should always be aware of those underlying conditions which might affect the patient's reactions to surgery and anaesthesia.

Avoiding complications

High-quality nursing care pre-operatively can help reduce post-operative complications. It is particularly important

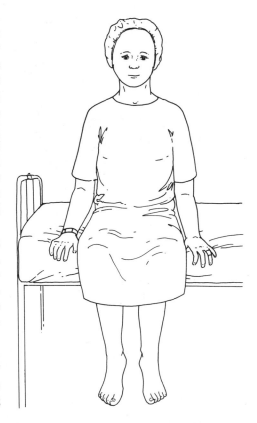

that any prostheses are noted such as false teeth or eyes or a wig. A patient may be distressed to give these up and fearful that relatives will see him 'warts and all', and be affected by it. The nurse should recognize the individual's concern about his appearance and should promise that these items will be restored as soon as he has regained consciousness, and that he will not be seen by friends and relatives while unconscious. It may be easier for a patient to accept the need for removal of prostheses if the rationale, i.e. his safety, is understood.

The cleanliness of the patient is important in reducing the risk of wound infection. Most patients are able to bathe themselves but, if not, a nurse should help them. The bed should have clean sheets and the patient wear a clean gown and sometimes operation socks. All jewellery should be removed and put into safe keeping. The exception to this is the wedding ring, which may be retained if it is covered with surgical tape. Patients are reassured that their valuables will be safe while they are unconscious.

Patients should have their pre-operative bath or shower close to the time of operation and be encouraged to empty their bladder. After this, they should try to relax in bed in preparation for the premedication. Preparing an individual too soon may mean that he goes to the toilet in his theatre gown and risks taking infection to the operating theatre.

Receiving the correct operation

It is not unknown for a patient to receive an incorrect operation. This may occur through mistaken identity or because of incomplete or inaccurate information about the site or nature of the operation.

The nurse should take responsibility for checking the patient's name by comparing the name and hospital number on the wrist band with those on the medical notes, and then asking the patient to state his name. If this procedure is followed there should be no risk of mistaken identity.

If there is the possibility of a mistake in the operation site, i.e. whether the left or right side, the surgeon may mark the patient before the operation. The nurse should check that any such marking is in the correct place and has not been washed off.

The reasons for such a catechism and the importance of double-checking to avoid mistakes should be explained to every patient. If, for example, a patient was to have a diseased right kidney removed and the left was removed by mistake, the consequences would be extremely serious.

What the surgeon does is not the direct responsibility of nursing staff, but nurses do have a role in monitoring the patient, in preparing him for surgery and in reporting any observed anomalies.

A further responsibility of the nurse is to ensure that the patient receives the correct premedication at the correct time, so that he is relaxed when the theatre trolley arrives.

Although porters take patients to the operating theatre, the nurse should accompany and stay with him until the theatre nurse relieves her. The presence of the nurse is usually reassuring to the patient and, ideally, the same nurse should be able to promise the patient that she will be there when he wakes up.

Post-operative care

It is common practice for theatre staff to telephone the ward when the patient is ready to return. Usually the patient regains consciousness in the recovery room, although rarely he may still be unconscious on his return to the ward. The nurse is responsible for the patient's safety both on the journey back from theatre and until he regains consciousness. While he is unconscious, the care given will be that for any unconscious patient (p. 341) with priority given to maintaining a clear airway.

Observations

Temperature, pulse, respiration and blood pressure will be observed for variations from pre-operative recordings. Initially, quarter-hourly observations may be made of the patient's pulse, which, if steady, will gradually be increased to one-hourly, two-hourly, four-hourly and then twice daily. Blood pressure is an important observation because of the risk of bleeding from the operation site and the resultant risk of shock.

If intravenous fluids are given, these should be observed regularly to check the rate of flow and to ensure that prescriptions are accurately followed. The cannula site should also be inspected since a restless patient may dislodge the tube from the vein and so cause the fluids to go into surrounding tissues. If this occurs, a doctor should be notified so that the cannula may be re-sited.

If oxygen therapy is prescribed, it may be discontinued when the patient regains consciousness. A semi-conscious patient may attempt to remove the mask. The nurse should observe that the mask is in place and that the oxygen is being administered as prescribed. The patient's colour should be observed and any signs of cyanosis

Table 11.1 Potential post-operative problems.

Potential deficit	Potential problem
Breathing	Obstruction – embolism – thrombosis – secretions
Circulation	Cardiac failure Thrombosis – coronary artery – deep vein – leg – arm – pelvis Shock Haemorrhage
Nutrition	Vomiting Constipation Obstruction Adhesions
Fluid balance	Dehydration Renal failure Retention of urine
Mobility	Nerve injuries Cerebrovascular accident Pressure sores Pain
Wound healing	Infection – abscess – burst wound – peritonitis Septicaemia Low prothrombin levels Anaemia Poor surgical technique

reported. Suction may be necessary to clear secretions which could cause obstruction to breathing.

Dressings should be checked at regular intervals, according to local policy, for any bleeding from the operation site. Dressings should not be removed because of the risk of infection but extra, sterile dressings should be put on top of the existing ones and the bleeding reported to the doctor. Severe bleeding may cause the patient to go into shock. This is a potential post-operative problem, although it may occur for other reasons.

Shock

Shock occurs when there is a severe drop in the blood pressure which leads to an inadequate supply of oxygen to the tissues. It may result from major trauma (cardiogenic shock), where stimulation of the vagus nerve slows down the heartbeat by acting on the sinoatrial node, or from an insufficient volume of blood in the circulatory system (hypovolaemic shock) following haemorrhage. Hypovolaemic shock may also occur as a result of dehydration, burns, or in response to allergenic antigens, when it is termed anaphylactic shock. In this latter case, enzymes such as histamine are produced in response to the antigen–antibody interaction and these cause vasodilatation. In all cases of shock except anaphylactic, there is decreased cardiac output; in anaphylactic shock, the peripheral resistance is reduced. Both states result in a lowered blood pressure.

The post-operative patient is at risk of some degree of shock as a response to the anaesthesia, because of emotional or physical reactions to the operation, or through loss of blood. Observations should give early warning of the likelihood of shock. The patient's reactions to severe shock may be restlessness, irritability and eventual loss of consciousness due to hypoxia, which is the result of a decrease in circulating blood. The skin may be pale, grey, cold and clammy, with cyanosis. This is caused by vasoconstriction in the extremities, which occurs so that the core blood supply, to the heart and the brain, may be maintained. Such changes should be noted and reported so that immediate action may be taken.

To compensate for the reduced blood volume there is an increase in the heart rate, giving a rapid, irregular and weakening pulse. The temperature will be subnormal due to the peripheral vasoconstriction, and respiration will be rapid and shallow because of hypoxia resulting from vasoconstriction in the lungs. Urinary output will be decreased as a reaction to vasoconstriction in the kidneys. Fluid balance may be disturbed as a result of the lowered blood volume and its effect on the osmolarity of body fluids. This will lead to the patient becoming very thirsty.

If shock is not treated as an emergency, the patient will become acidotic as a result of the hypoxia, the blood pressure will fall further as the heart weakens, coma will develop and the patient may die.

In planning post-operative care, the knowledge that shock is a potential problem should lead to preventive measures being taken. These include reduction of emotional stress pre-operatively, since mental trauma can lead to shock; adequate fluid intake until four hours prior to the time of operation to avoid dehydration; and attention to keeping the patient warm on his return to the ward.

Medical precautions to avoid shock include completing the operation skilfully in the minimum time to reduce physical trauma; prescription of drugs to alleviate pain, which can cause shock; and administration of intravenous fluids to maintain hydration. Oxygen may be prescribed if the patient's breathing is slow.

The patient in shock is likely to be very frightened, especially if it is due to post-operative bleeding which he can see. The nurse should remain calm and attempt to reassure him. Care includes rest, both physical and mental, and warmth, since his metabolic rate will be slowed and he will feel cold. The foot of the bed should be raised to help maintain circulation to the cardiac and cerebral areas, and the patient should lie flat in a comfortable position.

If the patient is cyanosed, oxygen therapy may be prescribed to help counteract the hypoxia. Intravenous fluids may be administered to maintain fluid balance and, if the shock is due to haemorrhage, a blood transfusion may be given. This may be infused at a slow rate to avoid a sudden rise in blood pressure, which could trigger off further haemorrhage at the wound site. It is standard procedure for patients to have their blood grouped and matched prior to operation.

The patient may be in pain. Care must be taken in administering drugs since the peripheral blood vessels will be constricted. Subcutaneous injections will not be absorbed and may build up to have an effect when vasodilatation occurs. Morphine may be given intravenously by the doctor, or intramuscularly by the nurse. Observations of the patient's general condition and of pulse and blood pressure will give an indication of the patient's physical state. As the patient's condition improves, the pulse becomes stronger and the blood pressure rises. Respirations should deepen, colour improve and restlessness decrease.

Observation of the patient's colour is important. Although he needs warmth, caution should be exercised, for if he is made too warm his peripheral blood vessels will dilate and 'steal' blood from the heart and brain. He may also perspire, so losing more fluid and adding to the risks of dehydration and electrolyte imbalance.

The patient should be kept informed of the improvement in his condition. This should reassure him and so reduce his tension. If he asks questions, the nurse should answer them as well as she is able or refer them to a senior person. It must be remembered that shock can be a threat to life. Self-interest on the part of the patient is a perfectly natural reaction to a fear-provoking situation.

Fluid balance

Fluid balance needs monitoring post-operatively. Major surgery leads to excess production of the anti-diuretic hormone by the pituitary gland (Colmer 1987). Because of this, urine production is decreased for up to two days after operation, and this must be remembered when considering fluid intake for the patient.

Adequate fluid intake should be ensured up to four hours prior to operation for all patients unless contra-indicated by the predisposing condition. After operation, fluid intake should not exceed three litres during the first 24 hours, being gradually increased as normal renal function returns.

The low urinary output in the first day or two post-operatively will be accompanied by reduced excretion of electrolytes. This is relevant for the prescription of intravenous fluids, since if normal saline is given the excess salt in the body will lead to oedema. Intravenous fluids given post-operatively are usually 5% glucose solutions. Although the nurse does not prescribe such fluids, an understanding of electrolyte balance and the post-operative effects will alert her to the risks involved, so that she practises intelligently and questions when a prescription seems in doubt.

Anaesthesia may affect the muscle tone in the bladder, leading to retention of urine, so the patient should be encouraged to pass urine. He may be frightened that straining to urinate will damage his wound or cause him pain. He should be helped to sit up and reassured that he will not harm his wound and that, if he has pain, analgesics will be given.

Observation of distension of the abdomen or pain should be reported, as should an inability to pass urine. If there really is difficulty and the patient cannot pass urine at all, catheterization may be considered, though this is usually resisted because of the risk of infection. Hearing running water may help a patient to urinate but this may be difficult to arrange in the middle of a large ward. It is more important for the nurse to be relaxed for, if the patient feels pressured, he will become tense and less able to micturate.

Pain

Post-operative pain may be due to surgical intervention, fear, anxiety or tension (Smiddy 1991). Pain must always be taken seriously in a patient and dealt with promptly since, if it is severe, it may precipitate shock. Further, and just as important, the patient will lose faith in the health care team.

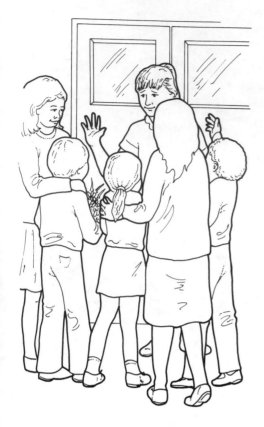

Analgesia will be prescribed for each patient before his operation, so that immediate action can be taken if he has post-operative pain. The aim of any pain control is to avoid severe pain all the time (Aronoff 1985). If this is not fully achieved, the patient may become very tense as his analgesia starts to wear off in anticipation of the return of pain.

Pain may be avoided by careful observation and by being prepared to listen to the patient's self-reporting. Asking 'Would you like some painkillers?' is not useful because the patient may accept them as an insurance, even if he is not in pain at the moment. Careful observation will give clues to the patient's level of pain. The facial expression may be tense, and the body held very still. Necessary movements may be accompanied by grimacing or catching of the breath. The patient may be tearful if the pain is severe.

Each post-operative patient should be assured that he does not have to suffer pain, and that he may, without censure, call the nurse if he is uncomfortable. Open questions from the nurse such as 'How are you feeling now, Mr Jones?' or 'How is the pain now?' will give the patient a chance to express his feelings honestly.

Analgesia will be prescribed initially by the anaesthetist in line with the drugs used in theatre. Those which depress the respiratory centre or lower blood pressure are usually avoided. This includes most of the narcotic drugs, although pethidine has less effect on breathing and blood pressure than stronger drugs such as morphine.

If a drug is prescribed for four-hourly administration it should be given as prescribed even if the patient is not uncomfortable at the time of administration. If he has pain before the four hours are up, the doctor should be consulted for a possible change of prescription.

Pain may be avoided or relieved by tranquil nursing care and attention to the patient's physical, psychological and social comfort. Small things like a rucked-up undersheet can cause a patient to be restless and can bring on pain, as can fears and worries and too many visitors. It is easier for a nurse to screen a patient from an overload of visitors than it is for the patient himself to ask people that he loves to leave.

Constipation may be a problem after operation due to inactivity, dehydration and the effects of anaesthesia on muscle tone. This may cause a different sort of pain, which may be exacerbated by a build up of gases in the bowel. Observations should be made of the individual's abdomen and of any bowel movement. Ideally the patient should have his bowels open within three days of the operation.

Flatulence may be relieved by the use of a flatus tube (Figure 11.2). Constipation should not be allowed to continue for more than a few days ater operation. An aperient may be prescribed by the doctor or suppositories may be given. The aim of care is that the bowels can be opened without strain. Analgesia should not be necessary for the pain caused by flatulence or constipation.

Mobility

It is general policy to get a patient up and walking as soon as possible after operation because of the risks of deep vein thrombosis and pressure sores which result from inactivity. The time at which the patient is mobilized depends on the type of operation, its site and severity, and on the beliefs of the surgeon.

For the individual who has to stay in bed, foot and leg exercises should be encouraged along with regular movement to prevent continuous pressure on one area. All movement should be gentle and unhurried to avoid pain and anxiety.

When a patient is allowed up from bed, care should be taken to ensure he is stable on his feet. Even a few days in bed can leave a person feeling very weak after an operation. Care should also be taken over patients who are allowed up soon after regaining consciousness.

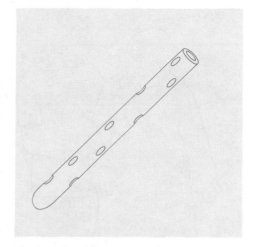

Fig. 11.2 A flatus tube.

Sally Arnold had been admitted for a minor operation and had been starved from midnight, although she did not have her operation until after 4 p.m. the following afternoon. At 6 p.m., Sally asked the nurse if she could go to the lavatory. The nurse said 'Yes' and helped Sally put on her dressing gown and slippers.

Walking to the toilet caused feelings of dizziness but there was no one around, so Sally held onto the wall. On the way back she blacked out and was found on the floor by another patient. A combination of low blood sugar due to starvation, hypotension caused by a day in bed, and the effort of walking caused the problem.

All patients, when first walking after an operation, need supervision.

Some patients may resist efforts to mobilize them after their operation. If this occurs the nurse needs to explore the reasons, rather than insisting on the patient's compliance. It may be that the patient is frightened of pain or some imagined disaster. Once this is identified, reassurance can be given that it is safe for the patient to get up.

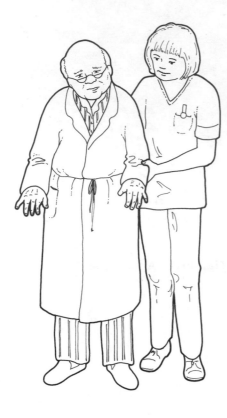

The patient may genuinely feel too ill to get up. For example, the patient with undiagnosed liver disease may react badly to anaesthesia. In this case, assessment will identify the patient's feelings and may lead to medical examination and subsequent investigations.

Some patients may wish to take advantage of the opportunity to lie in bed. The busy mother, for example, may see her operation as a chance for the first real rest she has had in years. Such feelings should be acknowledged, and education given on the need to move about to prevent complications and improve muscle tone.

In mobilizing individuals, it must be remembered that surgery constitutes trauma and will result in reactions of tiredness of some degree in most patients. When a patient is up for the first time, he should be observed for signs of fatigue and not left to become exhausted. A gradual programme should be planned for a return to full mobility within any physical constraints present.

Knowledge

The individual's pre-operative concerns are usually associated with the operation itself. 'How long will I be unconscious?' 'What exactly will they do?' 'Will it hurt?' and 'Will I feel anything?' are common questions, though no assumptions should be made of the patient's concerns in the absence of a preliminary assessment.

After the operation, the patient has time to think of the implications of his surgery and may have concerns for his future that he would like to discuss. The patient with a hip replacement may worry about his future – how long before he can drive his car or dig his garden? The patient after hysterectomy may have similar concerns plus those associated with her sexual relationship. A chance to talk a few days after operation will allow the nurse to assess each patient's concerns and meet his needs for knowledge or refer his problems to another agency. No matter how trivial the problem may seem, it should be taken seriously.

Sometimes there may be no solution to a patient's concerns. If, for example, a patient with a stoma asks, 'Will my wife want me to love her with this?', it would be quite wrong to say, 'Of course she will – it's you she loves, not what you look like.' It is better to let the patient talk through his concerns and suggest that he talks to his wife to explore how she feels. He may need help from a skilled counsellor if he and his wife are not used to discussing personal matters.

Patients may also need information on the help that is available to them on discharge in terms of Social Services

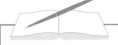

Choose a patient who is recovering from major surgery.

1 Assess the individual's level of knowledge of the operation.
2 Identify any problems/concerns expressed by the patient.
3 How would you plan to work with this patient to improve understanding and reduce anxiety?

and nursing services. Health education may be necessary if aspects of lifestyle militate against a return to health.

Wound care

Asepsis

Wounds are dressed using an aseptic technique. This means that the wound and anything that touches it should be free from any micro-organisms. Some methods of preventing organisms from contaminating wounds have been discussed in the section on control of infection. However, for dressings which are to be applied to open wounds, more vigorous steps are taken to ensure that **all** micro-organisms are absent, not only from dressing materials but from instruments, containers and solutions too.

For micro-organisms to be destroyed, sterilization is necessary. A crude method of sterilization is boiling for five minutes, but the temperature of boiling water (100°C) will kill only bacteria; viruses and bacterial spores survive up to 115°C. For this reason materials for dressings are either autoclaved by steam or treated with gamma radiation.

Such methods are expensive and quite unsuitable for individual wards. As a result most hospitals or groups of hospitals have their own sterilization units, which may be called the Central Sterile Supply Department, shortened to 'CSSD'.

The Central Sterile Supply Department

The CSSD does not simply sterilize materials required on the ward, but puts them into a variety of packs for specialist use. For example, there will be small, medium and large dressing packs, and packs for catheterization, intravenous infusion, biopsies and other procedures (Figure 11.3). There will also be subsidiary packs of cotton wool balls, swabs, etc. to supplement other packs.

To save cost and inventory problems, most items are disposable (Figure 11.4). Dressing towels are made of paper, containers of foil, and instruments of plastic. It is still possible to get sterilized scissors but disposable blades have replaced scissors for removing sutures.

Each CSSD pack is double-wrapped, the outer wrapping being sealed with tape which shows a striped pattern after autoclaving. Packs should not be used unless there

Fig. 11.3 A CSSD pack.

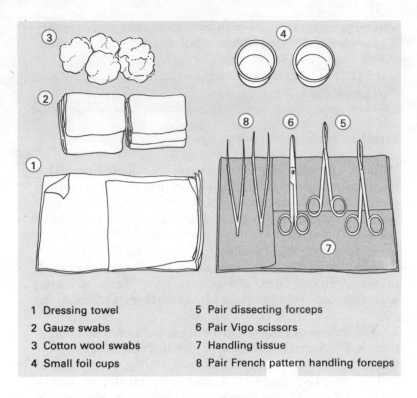

1 Dressing towel
2 Gauze swabs
3 Cotton wool swabs
4 Small foil cups
5 Pair dissecting forceps
6 Pair Vigo scissors
7 Handling tissue
8 Pair French pattern handling forceps

are such stripes on the seals. Each ward keeps a supply of a variety of CSSD packs according to its spcific needs. It is usual for a 'top-up' service to be offered by the CSSD department for standard packs. More specialized packs need to be ordered as required.

It is not possible to sterilize dressing trolleys or a nurse's hands, but both should be clinically clean before and after each dressing. Dressing techniques vary but basically a non-touch technique is developed where the hands do not touch the wound or the contents of the inner CSSD pack except to lift the forceps, and the instruments used to discard dirty dressings are not used to touch clean dressings. Sterile gloves may be worn if the wound is difficult to dress.

Healing

In a healthy individual, wounds caused by penetration of the skin or infection heal quite rapidly. First, blood clots in the wound and leads to the formation of granulation tissue in which new capillaries and fibroblasts grow (Figure 11.5). A good blood supply is necessary for growth of the new tissue. As healing occurs the blood supply is reduced and a scar is formed. As the healing completes the scar contracts, the scar tissue falls off and new skin is seen beneath it. This is called healing by 'secondary intention'.

Most surgical wounds heal by 'first intention' since the skin is incised under aseptic conditions. This means that the edges of the wound unite without visible granulation.

Depending on the size of the incision or wound, a permanent mark may be left on the skin after healing. Surgeons are often proud of the neatness of their incisions

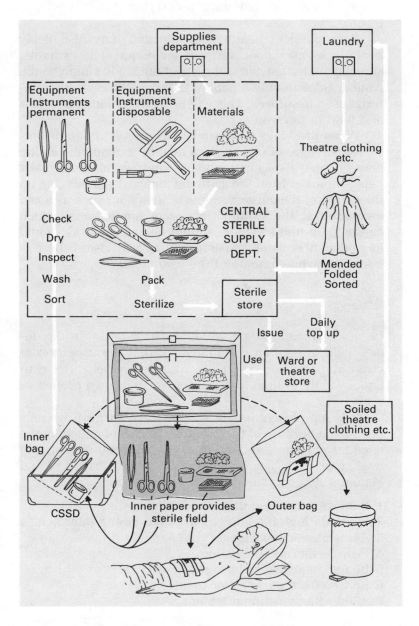

Fig. 11.4 Recycling/disposal of equipment and clothing.

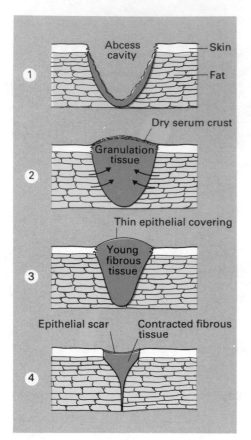

Fig. 11.5 Stages of wound healing by 'secondary intention'.

and stitching which leaves the minimum disfigurement to the skin. An ugly scar may affect an individual's self-image, particularly if it is on the face or a part of the body which is usually uncovered.

Healing may be affected by the patient's age and health. As a general rule, the young heal more quickly than the elderly because of the more rapid growth of new cells. Some physical conditions may also affect healing. A delayed prothrombin time such as occurs in some liver diseases will delay healing, as will anaemia, where reduced oxygenation of the damaged area will occur because of the reduced oxygen-carrying capacity of the blood.

Poor physical health and infection may also delay healing, as may poor surgical technique. For example, suturing under tension will restrict the blood supply to the wound. Occasionally a patient may be allergic to the material used in sutures. This will bring irritation, antibodies and fluid to the wound.

When dressings are performed wounds should be observed for signs of change. In a healthy individual, healing may be seen to occur within a week, stitches normally being removed from the sixth day onwards, depending on the extent of the surgery. Signs of infection, such as a red sore area at the wound site, or of haematoma, which causes pain and swelling, should be reported, as should any other abnormality. Temperature may rise if there is infection or haematoma at the wound site.

Dressings

In small abrasions and wounds which occur in day-to-day living it is often recommended that the area is kept clean and uncovered. This is because air helps the exudate from the wound to dry and to form its own protective scab.

It is not always practicable to leave surgical wounds uncovered because of their depth, the risk of infection, the need for pressure, and the need for protection during the healing process. The function of dressings (Pritchard and Mallett 1992) should be to:

1 Remove excess exudate and toxins.
2 Maintain high humidity at wound/dressing interface.
3 Allow gaseous exchange.
4 Provide thermal insulation.
5 Be impenetrable to bacteria.
6 Be free from particles or toxins.
7 Allow change without trauma.

Modern dressings protect from infection by covering the wound while maintaining moistness underneath, so allowing healing to take place.

Dressings are secured in a number of ways. A number of adhesive plasters is available, and the range includes elastic adhesive, zinc oxide strapping and Micropore. Observations need to be made for allergic reactions to adhesive tape. Bandages are still used though less frequently since the advent of cotton tubular bandages of various widths, which are put on via a special applicator. This type of bandage is very useful for limbs and head wounds because it conforms to shape without difficulty, and is light and porous.

Current practice in the care of dressings favours leaving the dressing intact for several days providing that there is no excessive bleeding or a rise in the patient's temperature to suggest infection or haematoma. The argument is that the less the wound is disturbed, the less the chance of infection occurring. If there is oozing from the wound it should either be covered with a sterile pad or, if it is very damp, redressed, since organisms may get into the damp dressing and travel to the wound site.

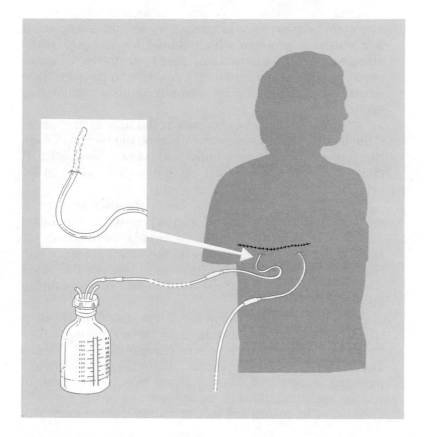

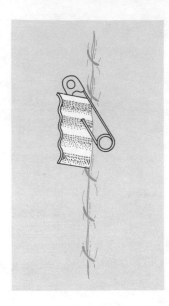

Some wounds have drainage tubes inserted if they are deep and there is a risk of blood or other fluid building up. Drainage tubes may be of the Redivac type, which drain into a disposable bottle. Drainage may also be achieved by a strip of corrugated rubber inserted into the wound, which drains fluid into a thick dressing.

Drainage tubes are inserted in theatre. They may be kept *in situ* by a stitch or by a sterile safety pin passed through the tube to form a stay. There is a risk of granulation attaching itself to a drain, and, in order to avoid this, drains are rotated, or shortened every two days or as requested by the surgeon. To shorten a tube, any stitch should be removed and the tube gently drawn back a short distance. A new sterile safety pin should be inserted each time near the skin to prevent the drain moving back into the wound and carrying organisms with it.

Dressings are normally discontinued as soon as possible. A spray may be used which protects the wound, and the patient will then be encouraged to bathe or shower. Observations of the area should be made to note any breakdown or reactions at the scar site.

Haemorrhage

Although haemorrhage after surgery should not occur, it is a potential problem which should be accepted when planning care of any patient post-operatively. A nurse needs to understand a patient's reaction to haemorrhage so that the problem may be promptly identified and action taken.

Primary haemorrhage occurs at the time of operation. If the loss is small, as in minor surgery, the body will soon compensate providing the individual is in normal health. If there is considerable blood loss, a transfusion will be prescribed to compensate and avoid shock.

Bleeding may also occur some hours after surgery. It may be that the trauma of surgery reduced the blood pressure so that the peripheral circulation became restricted. As the patient recovers, the blood pressure will rise and this increased pressure may remove the blood clots which have formed in the incision space, causing bleeding.

Secondary haemorrhage is the term used for bleeding which occurs some days (usually seven to ten) after trauma or surgery and is due to erosion of blood vessels. The cause is usually infection, though carcinoma may have the same effect. Haemorrhage may be *external*, in which case it can be seen by observation of the patient's dressing or by oozing and lack of wound healing at the site of operation. It may also be internal, in which case more general observations will alert the nurse to the fact that all is not well.

The reactions to haemorrhage are those of shock, the severity depending on the volume of blood lost from the circulation. If the bleeding is abdominal, the irritation and pressure of the blood in the peritoneal cavity will cause pain. Localized bleeding into the tissues will result in bruising or haematoma, which may be painful in the wound area.

Nursing care

For severe haemorrhage, nursing care will be that planned for the patient in shock. If bleeding does not stop spontaneously, the patient may need to be returned to theatre. If bleeding is external, local pressure may be applied with effect. In all cases of post-operative haemorrhage, a doctor should be informed, who may prescribe drugs to aid clotting of the blood, or may make the decision to return the patient to theatre for investigation and treatment.

A number of common operations are described below to illustrate the effects of surgery and the possible needs of the individual in addition to standard pre- and post-operative care. The separation of topics under specific headings is for ease of description but it should be remembered that any operation may, for example, pose a threat to life or affect body image. The examples chosen are those where the effects on the patient, such as problems with body image, are well documented.

Similarly, many of the operations for which preparation is described may, in certain circumstances, be performed as an emergency. If this occurs the patient may go straight from the out-patients' department to theatre and only arrive on the ward post-operatively.

Surgery affecting body image

It can be argued that any surgery may affect body image since even the most minor operation leaves a scar. There are, however, some operations which are known to have a potentially serious effect on an individual's body image. They may be performed because of a threat to life, as in carcinoma of the breast, or because they are having a serious effect on a patient's general health, as in heavy uterine bleeding.

Some common operations will be described to illustrate the effects of mutilating surgery and the implications for nursing care. It must be remembered, however, that every individual's self-image will be affected by surgery to some extent, whether or not it is seen by professionals as 'mutilating'.

Mastectomy

THE OPERATION

Removal of the breast is usually performed because of the presence of a carcinoma. The breast is the most common site for cancer in women in the United Kingdom, most women being well aware that any abnormality of the breast such as lumps or hard areas to the touch may be due to malignancy. It could be assumed that this knowledge would persuade women to examine their own breasts regularly and seek help if lumps are found, but this is not necessarily so.

The first symptoms of a possible cancer in the breast are usually detected by the individual herself. She may find a small painless lump or a change in her skin, or even nipple retraction. If the woman does not go to her doctor on finding these first signs of a problem, there may be nipple discharge or enlarged axillary glands. In recent years there has been a growth of screening clinics for breast cancer and women between 50–61 years of age are invited through their general practitioner to attend a clinic.

Many women, on finding a lump or any other abnormality in the breast, will delay going to their general practitioner and there are a considerable number of women who do not respond to an invitation to go to a screening clinic. This reluctance to seek help is linked with the fear of cancer and the fact that, while one might be worried about what is happening, until someone confirms it the hope remains that it may be 'just something small that will go away'. As with any other cancer, there is no pain or discomfort at the early stages which might accelerate the process of seeking advice.

When a lump is referred to the doctor by an individual, attention is prompt because of the potential diagnosis and the life-threatening nature of carcinoma. The diagnosis is usually made by an excisional biopsy of the entire mass under local anaesthetic. A cutting needle biopsy may be done but the value of needle aspiration (for cytology) is debatable (Abernathy and Young 1991). The biopsy of the lump may be performed as part of a two-stage operation where the affected breast is also removed.

If surgery is the treatment of choice, the type of mastectomy will depend on the assessment of the tumour and its potential spread. Radical mastectomy is the most extensive operation with removal of breast, pectoral muscle and axillary glands. This used to be the operation of choice for carcinoma of the breast, but is rarely performed in modern surgery, although the axillary glands may be removed with the breast to reduce the risk of spread through the lymphatic system. The most commonly performed procedure with the most solid data regarding benefit (Abernathy and Young 1991) is **modified radical mastectomy**. In this operation the breast is completely removed with the underlying pectoralis minor and some of the adjacent lymph nodes. The pectoralis major is not excised. The operation is performed for treating early and well localized malignant neoplasms of the breast.

There is a move to less mutilating surgery for breast cancer in that lumpectomies rather than mastectomies are being offered to patients. The benefit of a lumpectomy is that it is considerably less mutilating than removing the breast but it may leave an indent in the breast, which many women find in itself disfiguring. Lumpectomy is most suitable for those patients who have clinically negative axillary nodes.

Radiotherapy or chemotherapy may follow mastectomy, especially if there is intercostal or glandular spread of the disease. In some cases, radiotherapy may precede surgery to contain the tumour, but this is not common since radiotherapy may affect wound healing.

Surgery for breast carcinoma does not promise a cure, particularly if an early diagnosis has not been made. The proximity of the breast to the axilliary glands increases the risk of spread, with involvement of bone being common. Metastases may occur in the ribs and the spine and, as bone tissue breaks down, hypercalcaemia occurs.

The chances of survival for more than five years following mastectomy are 50%, much depending on the stage of the disease at operation and the age of the patient. The disease is more aggressive in younger patients due to the higher rate of cell formation, which decreases with age.

Physical reactions
There should be few physical reactions to the operation of mastectomy except those associated with wound healing. There may be oedema of the arm (lymphoedema) on the side of the operation site due to surgery and some limita-

tion of movement of the shoulder due to pain. There may also be difficulty in breathing because of anxiety and pain.

Psychological reactions

Psychological reactions to mastectomy may be severe because of the effect of the mutilation on body image and the association of the breasts with sexuality. There are also psychological problems associated with diagnosis and prognosis.

Many women describe themselves as 'lopsided freaks' and some use the term 'castrated' to describe their feelings. Others seem to accept the operation as a preferable alternative to death. There is no particular reaction according to age. Reactions which are linked to sexuality include doubts that the patient will still be desirable to her partner or indeed be able to attract a partner. Many women feel that their partners will cease to love them because of the mutilation.

Women often agree to the operation in the belief that the cancer will be removed totally with the breast. If they later find that chemotherapy or radiotherapy has been prescribed, they can feel cheated and upset at the thought that cancer cells are still present.

It is well documented that clinical anxiety and depression may occur in over 25% of post-mastectomy patients (Tarrier and Maguire 1984). A similar percentage may have body image problems and many couples have sexual problems.

Social reactions

Social reactions will be those associated with hospitalization, often at short notice, and, after the operation, with the perceived effect on body image. Many women dislike leaving the house after mastectomy for fear that others will notice their change of shape. Loose, baggy clothes may be worn. Even when a breast prosthesis (false breast, see Figure 11.6) is fitted, the individual may curtail her social life.

There may be a reluctance to return to work following recovery unless confidence is restored. Metastases may cause tiredness and necessitate readmission to hospital, so disrupting normal social life and responsibilities. If the patient has young children, considerable social problems may arise during the period in hospital and subsequently. The partner, or relative, may need help and support while he struggles with the stress of the patient's illness and the practicalities of working, looking after the children, and visiting the hospital.

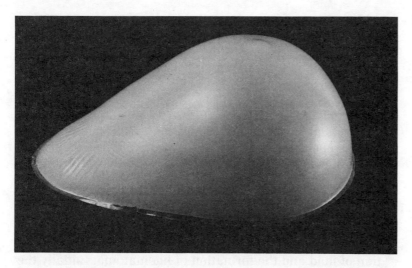

Fig. 11.6 A breast prosthesis.

PLANNING NURSING CARE

Pre-operative physical care
General pre-operative care should be given (pp. 359–363), remembering that admission may be no more than 24 hours prior to operation. If a two-stage operation is planned, it should be pointed out to the patient before she signs the consent form so there is no risk of horrified surprise when the patient who expected a biopsy awakes without a breast.

The axilla is shaved on the affected side, and an X-ray or mammograph is requested, which should be taken, with the patient and her notes, to theatre.

Pre-operative psychological care
The individual should have the opportunity to verbalize her fears and concerns. There are particular problems with such patients since they do not know if they will still have a breast after surgery. Patients should go to theatre with realistic expectations. The nurse can point out that the breast will only be removed if necessary and that the operation will provide a good chance of a return to normal health.

The concept of the prosthesis can be explained so that the patient realizes she can look 'normal' soon after operation. Some surgeons offer reconstructive surgery by implantation of a prosthesis some months after mastectomy. However, this is not suitable in all cases so false hopes should not be raised.

The emphasis of psychological care pre-operatively is to deal with immediate concerns. These are different for each patient. If an individual really cannot face the uncertainty of a two-stage operation she may insist on biopsy alone followed by mastectomy at a later date when she has had a chance to consider all the options. This is every patient's right, even though it is less convenient for hospital organization.

Pre-operative social care
If a patient is concerned about her social commitments before operation, she should have a chance to discuss them. It is more usual for such issues to arise after operation, when the uncertainty has been resolved.

Post-operative physical care
General physical care will be given. The individual may have a corrugated drain *in situ* to prevent the accumulation of fluid and the formation of haematoma. Initially the arm on the affected side should be kept still so as not to put strain on the operation site, or cause unnecessary pain.

Potential problems in breathing and in mobility of the arm should be accepted and plans made to encourage

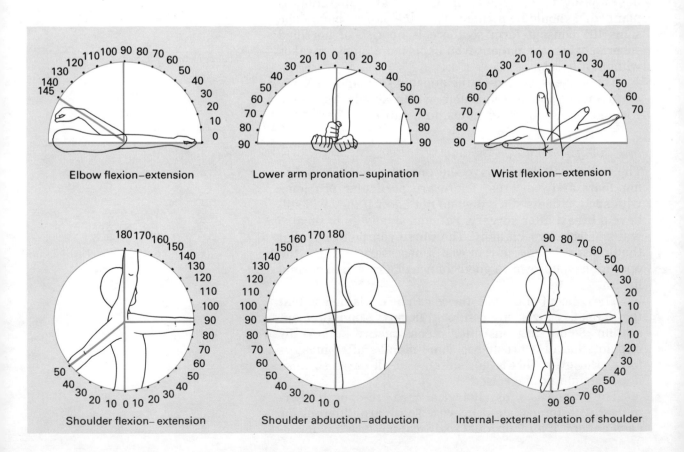

Elbow flexion–extension

Lower arm pronation–supination

Wrist flexion–extension

Shoulder flexion–extension

Shoulder abduction–adduction

Internal–external rotation of shoulder

breathing and teach the patient arm exercises. The patient should be kept pain-free.

A specialist nurse or technician will explain the choice of prosthesis to the patient and give her an idea of when a fitting will be made. Initially a pad, often called a 'softie', will be worn in the bra. Information on suitable bras for use with a prosthesis will be given.

The patient, while in hospital, should understand the need for any follow-up treatment. It can be very upsetting to think one is cured, only to receive a postcard calling for attendance at a radiotherapy department. Explanation should also be given on the need for the patient to attend follow-up appointments after the operation. It is important that an early diagnosis is made in the case of metastases, and that the individual is thoroughly satisfied with a well-fitting prosthesis.

Post-operative psychological care

No assumptions should be made about an individual's concerns. Rather, each patient should be encouraged to verbalize her own anxieties. The feeling that there is no one to listen or understand can lead to depression, whereas the chance to air problems in a non-judgemental atmosphere can help a patient to see her problems in a new light and learn to cope with them.

False or premature reassurance should not be given. If her problems are to do with partnerships then the patient should be encouraged to talk to her partner as soon as possible. Many problems are due to poor communication between a couple – the patient rejecting her partner because she feels unattractive, and the partner holding back out of consideration. Plans for care may need to include aiding a partner to understand his role in helping the patient to regain self-confidence.

Expert counselling may be required for an individual following mastectomy. Plans for care should include monitoring eating and sleeping patterns for signs of change, and observation of mood. Patients who complain of not sleeping, are very weepy and refuse to look at their scar may be at risk of clinical depression. Some people eat less when they are unhappy while others 'grief eat', i.e. eat to comfort themselves.

A problem in psychological care of the post-mastectomy patient is in making a decision between unhappiness, which should pass, and depression, which may become severe and lead to thoughts of suicide. If there is any doubt about the level of an individual's misery, a referral should be made, with the patient's permission, to a psychiatrist.

The patient after mastectomy has, in addition to the problem of body image, a fear-provoking prognosis. Initially after the operation the individual may be so relieved that her cancer has been removed that she is euphoric. Later, anxieties may arise about the lost breast and the chance of recurrence.

In recent years there has been an increase in specialist mastectomy nurses to follow patients into the community. Such nurses need to be skilled in effective interaction so that they may identify the patients' problems and concerns when they get back into family life (Faulkner and Maguire 1994). Many areas also have groups of mastectomy volunteers. There are women who have had a mastectomy themselves and wish to help other people who are recovering from the operation. Such groups need clear guidelines on how best they can help the individual recovering from a mastectomy and adapting to life with a changed body image. Other health professionals who follow up the patient on discharge, such as community nurses, could also have a role in monitoring these patients during the often difficult weeks following discharge from hospital (Faulkner 1984).

Post-operative social care
Plans for care will need to include helping the patient to regain confidence in herself as a person so that she will wish to resume her normal social life. This can be aided by education about prostheses, clothing and a gradual return to normal pursuits. Breast Cancer Care exists to help individuals return to a normal life and volunteers are often recruited by the BCC to work at both a psychological and social level. It is important that such volunteers are helped to develop skills that will encourage the patient to look for ways to return to normal, rather than being prescriptive and sometimes giving negative messages. It is all too easy for both volunteers and staff to work from their own experience rather than encouraging the patient to identify her own problems and seek solutions that will work for her.

Relatives need to be involved in plans for care. Initially the patient will need help with chores, encouragement to go out and loving understanding about resuming sexual relationships. However, a balance needs to be maintained between neglect and smothering, which will hinder a return to a full social life.

Each patient's particular problems should be assessed. Some will require nursing intervention while others may need to be referred to specialist agencies.

THE CARE PLAN

The care plan will give priority to pre- and post-operative care to ensure that the patient is not harmed during her hospital stay. Priority must also be given to allowing each individual to voice her fears and worries. Patients seen to be at risk of anxiety or depression should be referred for specialist help.

Relatives need to be included in the care plan so that they may understand real and potential problems, and be able to ease the transition from hospital to home. They may also have problems associated with the patient's hospitalization and illness, with which they need help. These should be of concern to the nurse. It may be that solutions to the problems cannot be given but support and referral may help a relative to cope with a difficult situation.

Hysterectomy

THE OPERATION

Hysterectomy is performed because of large fibroids forming within the uterus and causing heavy bleeding, dysmenorrhoea, abdominal distension, and possibly sterility. It is also performed when carcinoma is present in the uterus or cervix. Carcinoma of the uterus is more usual in older women and is characterized by post-menopausal bleeding, whereas carcinoma of the cervix is more common in women over 35 years of age. The incidence of carcinoma of the cervix has decreased dramatically since the introduction of the cervical smear test which is available regularly to all women over 30 years old. If pre-cancerous cells are present, a cone biopsy may be performed to remove part of the cervix and arrest the spread of the disease.

If a hysterectomy is performed because of the presence of cancer, the whole of the uterus, cervix, ovaries and fallopian tubes are removed (total hysterectomy with bilateral salpingo-oophorectomy). However, removal of the ovaries is avoided where possible since their secretion of oestrogen is responsible for female sexual characteristics. Total hysterectomy is the removal of uterus and cervix, while subtotal hysterectomy is the removal of the uterus without the cervix.

Hysterectomy may be performed abdominally or vaginally. If the operation is performed vaginally, the wound is normally stitched with catgut, which will be absorbed into the body. This is because of the difficulty

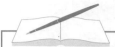

Identify a patient at risk of body image problems following surgery, and assess his/her current concerns. What potential solutions were generated by the patient? How did you help to set goals for working towards solutions? What practical support can you offer this patient?

associated with attempting to remove sutures from the vagina. As a general rule, hysterectomy is performed abdominally for carcinoma, either abdominally or vaginally for fibroids, and vaginally when the uterus has prolapsed.

Physical reactions

A hysterectomy constitutes major abdominal surgery. Physical reactions may include post-operative pain and the risk of shock and haemorrhage. There is also a risk of paralytic ileus, i.e. an absence of peristalsis in a section of the intestine which leads to obstruction of the ileum. This is due to the disturbance of abdominal organs during surgery.

Psychological reactions

Psychological reactions to hysterectomy may be similar to those of the patient after mastectomy in that the operation has affected the individual's sexual image. It might be thought that hysterectomy would not affect body image since the person does not look any different, but Webb (1982) points to many studies which suggest that body image may be affected.

In some ways the loss may seem more severe than that of a breast, since the operation concludes the function of childbearing which is central to many women's feelings of femininity. Fears may be expressed that a partner will feel that the patient is 'no longer a woman'.

If a diagnosis of carcinoma is known there are possible reactions to the threat of recurrence. The dual concerns of body image and prognosis carry the risk of anxiety and depression.

There is a reaction to major surgery which can be described as 'post-operative blues'. The individual feels unhappy and weepy for no apparent reason. These feelings usually wear off after a few days and should not be confused with anxiety and depression related to specific problems.

Social reactions

Social reactions to hysterectomy may be related to partnerships since, in younger women, plans to start or complete a family cannot be realized. This may cause tension and marital difficulties.

The individual who is anxious and depressed may be loath to resume normal social activities. Sick leave from employment, depending on the nature of the work, may be required for up to three months.

Tiredness and lethargy, for whatever reason, may mean that normal activities are neglected. Many women believe that they may not drive their car, do their normal chores or have sexual intercourse for some months, rather than six weeks or so, after operation. They may be irritable with their partner and children and feel unable to cope with day-to-day responsibilities.

PLANNING NURSING CARE

Pre-operative physical care
Pre-operative physical care will be that given to any patient. Admission may be two or three days prior to surgery, the patient being encouraged to rest and relax. Adequate explanation should be given about precisely what is to be removed. It is not uncommon for a woman to consent to hysterectomy without understanding that she will not be able to become pregnant in the future.

Pre-operative psychological care
Fears and worries should be explored prior to operation. Many women admitted for hysterectomy have left dependants at home and may be concerned about their time in hospital and any disability on their return home. There may also be problems associated with the operation itself.

It is always worth asking a patient if she has known other people who have had the operation, since knowledge will affect her reactions. The individual who had a friend who died two months after the operation may need reassurance on the comparative safety of the surgery. Further questioning may show that the reasons for operation were different or that there were other complications which affected recovery.

The nurse's willingness to listen to pre-operative concerns will assure the patient that she is cared for and taken seriously. Questions should be answered where possible and referred if they are beyond the ability of the nurse to answer.

Pre-operative social care
It may help a patient to talk to others who are recovering well from a similar operation if she is at all concerned about her own. Any problems should be aired, particularly to do with home circumstances. If necessary, the Social Services may be contacted. It is important that patients facing major surgery should be as tranquil as possible.

Post-operative physical care

General post-operative care will be given. The patient may have drainage tubes in but this is not always the case. Similarly the patient may have been catheterized prior to surgery, and require catheter care.

Because of the risk of thrombosis, early mobility is encouraged, though the time out of bed should be carefully monitored so that the patient does not become overtired. The patient should be encouraged to exercise her legs regularly and to carry out exercises to help her breathe deeply to avoid pleural complications and aid circulation.

Post-operative psychological care

When the operation is safely over and the patient begins to feel stronger, she may start to worry about her future, particularly in relation to sexual functioning. If extensive surgery has been necessary because of carcinoma, sexual problems may be expected, and the patient needs to understand and discuss the reality in positive terms. If both the ovaries have been removed in a young woman, premature menopause will occur in the absence of oestrogen. If oestrogen therapy is contraindicated, the patient will need to be prepared for the manifestations of the menopause.

Occasionally, surgical intervention includes removing part of the vagina if the cancer has spread. This means that normal sexual relations will not be possible. Advice is needed to help the individual and her partner to find satisfactory ways to demonstrate their affection for each other. Sexual counselling of this nature may need to be from an expert since it is important not to offend a couple's sense of decency. Assessment of the couple's attitude to sexuality and love play is essential in order to help them re-think their relationship.

For the individual who has had a total hysterectomy, normal sexual functioning may be resumed. It is standard practice to advise couples to wait for six weeks after operation before attempting to make love. However, each person is different and a better rule is that sexual relations should be resumed when the patient feels like it: if it feels right, it should be safe.

Care planned may need to include the partner who should understand that if union is painful for the patient it should be left for a little longer. A partner may also need to explore his or her feelings about the operation itself. There is a myth that hysterectomy makes a woman frigid when in fact it may have the reverse effect. A woman who has been tense previously due to fear of unwanted pregnancies may well relax and enjoy lovemaking when the risk is removed.

While in hospital, the patient should be monitored for signs of anxiety and depression, and given a chance to talk through her problems. If the operation is performed on a childless woman, then some difficulty may be found in facing a barren future since, on the whole, women are socialized to believe that their most important function is to bear children.

Fears concerned with femininity and with the diagnosis and prognosis of the disease should be explored and reassurance given where possible. The patient should be encouraged to talk to her partner, the nurse offering to act as an intermediary if this seems necessary.

Post-operative social care

Education for a return home should commence soon after the operation. Although the patient may need some time to convalesce at home, she should not feel an invalid. Relatives may need help in appreciating this. Initially they should take over heavy chores but they should also encourage a gradual return to normal social functioning.

Time limits should be guidelines only. Advice such as 'don't lift bags of potatoes for six weeks' and 'don't drive the car' deny individual rates of recovery and strength. The principle of a return to social functioning is that the patient should not strain herself until healing is complete. If she feels able to drive after three weeks at home, and feels no ill effects, there is no harm in driving. A different individual may still feel too weak to drive four to five weeks after discharge.

Rest is important in convalescence and the patient needs to understand that a certain level of tiredness after major surgery is inevitable, but that a gradual return to strength should occur.

THE CARE PLAN

Priorities in care will include pre- and post-operative care to ensure the patient's safety. Priority will also be given to specific problems of each individual in terms of her femininity and sexual and social functioning.

The individual will be monitored for post-operative complications such as paralytic ileus, which should recover spontaneously within 24 hours, and for anxiety and depression, which may need to be referred to a specialist.

Bowel stoma formation

A stoma is an artificial opening created from the intestine to the abdominal wall. The opening may be from the colon (colostomy), the ileum (ileostomy) or the caecum (caecostomy). A stoma may be necessary in the small bowel because of adhesions from prior abdominal procedures, incarcerated or strangulated hernias or cancer (Cohen and McIntyre 1991). The major reason for large bowel obstruction is carcinoma although a small percentage may be caused by diverticular disease.

The first sign of bowel cancer may be that blood is passed in the stool. This can be very frightening for an individual and would usually mean his visiting the general practitioner to share his concerns. If the bowel becomes obstructed for any reason, the patient will complain of abdominal pain, constipation and also nausea and vomiting.

The Operation

The aim of the operation is that intestinal contents should be discharged through the new opening rather than the anus.

Stomas may be temporary or permanent. Temporary stomas may be needed if an individual has acute intestinal obstruction, inflammation, fistula or trauma affecting the intestines. Often the aim in temporary colostomy is to remove an affected loop of bowel and eventually close the stoma. In fistula or trauma, intestinal contents are diverted to reduce the risk of infection and to allow subsequent surgery.

Permanent stomas will be formed if there is cancer in the anal, rectal or rectal–sigmoidal area, or damage to the rectum such as prolapse or trauma which is beyond surgery. In these instances, a colostomy will be performed. Permanent ileostomy may be performed when there is chronic inflammatory disease present such as ulcerative colitis or Crohn's disease. It may also be performed in cases of carcinoma of the colon. A caecostomy is usually performed for acute intestinal obstruction and involves the insertion of a large tube to release the intestinal contents. It is not permanent.

Stomas are sited on the abdominal wall, their position depending on the type of stoma which is formed (Figure 11.7). Care is taken that the stoma is not placed where clothes will restrict it, a preferred site being the left lower quadrant of the abdominal wall. The nearer the surgery is to the rectum, the more the stoma excretion will resemble a normal bowel action. It follows that a colostomy will

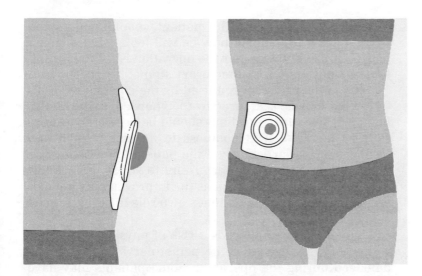

Fig. 11.7 An example of a stoma.

produce a formed stool, whereas caecostomy and ileostomy will produce liquid excretion.

Bowel preparation will include a low-residue diet for several days prior to surgery and a strong laxative such as Picolax on the day prior to surgery, which may be on the day of admission. Antibiotics may be given to sterilize the intestinal tract.

Other preparations will include an ECG, the taking of blood for cross-matching and visits from personnel such as the anaesthetist, surgeon, specialist nurse and physiotherapist.

Patients with chronic bowel disease may be anaemic and underweight. An attempt will be made to improve their nutritional status before operation. A high-calorie, low-residue diet will be prescribed with vitamin supplements. Parenteral fluids may be prescribed to correct dehydration and, if the patient's haemoglobin is very low, blood transfusions may be prescribed.

PLANNING NURSING CARE

Pre-operative physical care

In addition to general and specific pre-operative care, the individual will need education about his impending operation. Most districts have specialist nurses in stoma care who visit the patient, but the general nurse should also be prepared to answer questions and give information.

It is usual to mark the abdomen before surgery, taking into account waistline, previous scars and folds of skin plus other factors which could affect the comfort and function of the stoma. The patient should understand what is going to happen, how he will look, what a stoma bag looks like and whether the operation is for the formation of a permanent or temporary stoma.

The patient may be confused by the complexity of his future but may be reassured by the knowledge that he will be taught self-care. Questions should be answered as honestly as possible. It is pointless to lie about smell and inconvenience, particularly if the patient knows someone with a stoma. It is, however, useful to stress the positive aspects of the situation such as the improvements in modern stoma bags and the patient's own role in his care, such as dietary control.

In male patients there is a risk of physical impotence if the nerve pathways to the penis (nervi erigentes) are damaged during the operation. Some patients may have heard of this and become concerned. The nurse can assure the patient that this does not always occur and that, when it does, it is usually temporary. It is in fact less likely in ileostomy than colostomy (Kolodny *et al.* 1980) where there is a small risk of permanent impotence.

Pre-operative psychological care

In general, defecation is a private and personal affair. It is undertaken in isolation and is certainly a taboo subject in normal conversation. Further, it is normally under total control in adulthood.

For these reasons, the idea of a stoma is particularly hard for an individual to accept, for not only is the site of excretion brought to view on the abdomen, but the previous control will be lost. There is likely to be a severe affect on body image. The patient may wish to talk through his feelings pre-operatively, both to explore his concerns and to increase his understanding of the operation to which he is consenting.

Problems of acceptability to loved ones may arise. It may seem impossible to visualize lovemaking with a plastic bag of faeces in the way (even if one of the available cotton covers is worn), or taking the children swimming, or wearing normal clothes. Sometimes it helps for the patient to meet someone with a stoma who is coping. The major stoma organizations provide visitors who have a stoma themselves and are trained to provide help to others who are adjusting to a difficult diagnosis and a change of body image. Such visitors may also be identified and utilized by the stoma care nurse. At other times it may just be helpful to let the patient talk through

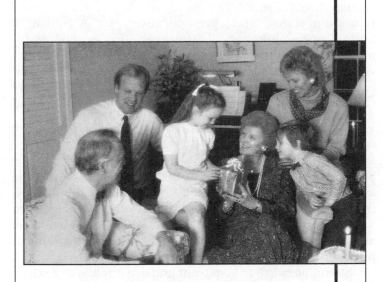

UNDERSTANDING

colostomy

A guide for new patients

his particular areas of concern and gently correct misconceptions.

Pre-operatively, there may also be concern about the operation itself, the length of hospital stay and the chances of a return to a normal life. The nurse should be encouraging since many stoma patients are able to lead a normal life.

If the operation is due to carcinoma, the individual may need to discuss diagnosis and prognosis. Some patients may feel that a stoma is a small price to pay for the chance to survive, where others may feel that life is hardly worth living with a stoma. Each individual should be given an opportunity to discuss his feelings in a non-judgemental atmosphere.

Pre-operative social care

Education should start pre-operatively for a return to normal social functioning. However, this is a stressful operation and much that is explained before the operation will need to be reiterated post-operatively. If the operation is being performed for a chronic condition, the stoma may represent a chance to lead a fuller social life than had been possible previously.

Post-operative physical care

Specific post-operative care of the patient with a stoma is aimed at care of the stoma and education of the patient. Initially the stoma will look red and swollen with oedema, and there will be little drainage. The patient should be assured that the stoma size will decrease, having a moist pink appearance.

Stoma bags are transparent and are applied to a sticky pad which surrounds the stoma and remains in place for some time (Figure 11.8). This avoids damaging the skin by constant removal. Bags may be emptied *in situ* several times before applying a new one and should be emptied when they are no more than half full. The skin may become excoriated, particularly if the patient has diarrhoea. A silicone- or lanolin-based barrier cream should be used, which will heal the area without damaging the stoma appliance.

Most patients soon learn to change a bag and to care for the skin around the stoma, but many need considerable help initially, particularly if they are loath to look at the stoma itself. Help is also required when learning to empty drainable bags and reseal them. After discharge, patients should learn to carry soft swabs and tissues since many public lavatories supply only hard paper which is not suitable for tidying up after emptying a bag.

Disposal of the bags themselves should also be discussed while in hospital, since they should not be flushed down the toilet but wrapped and sealed and deposited in a dustbin. Female patients away from home may empty the bag and seal in one of the paper bags provided for soiled sanitary towels. Men will need to wrap the package up well and find a rubbish bin.

Modern bags are deodorized so there should be little fear of offensive smells. The risks of odour may be further reduced by dietary control. There is no special 'stoma diet', although it is known that some foods such as onions

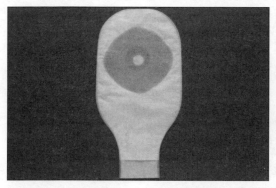 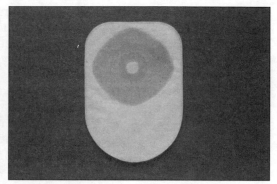

Fig. 11.8 Examples of stoma bags. Reproduced with kind permission of Convatec.

and peas should be treated with caution because of the likelihood of causing 'wind' and odour.

Generally, the individual should be advised to eat a normal diet, avoiding only those foods which seem to upset stoma functioning in terms of composition, odour and flatulence. Foods with a high cellular content may not be digested in the patient with an ileostomy and may need to be avoided because of the risk of obstruction.

Every effort should be made to help the patient view himself as normal in every respect apart from his bag, which can be as private to him as his bowels had previously been, except where his partner is concerned – and even here much will depend on whether the couple are used to seeing each other in the nude.

Post-operative psychological care

Care planned post-operatively should include the aim that the patient will accept the stoma. It is not uncommon for patients to refuse to look at the stoma or become involved in self-care. To make a patient look when he is not ready will only increase his apprehension. A sensitive approach is required with the individual having the opportunity to express his concern and any feelings of horror engendered by his new body image.

Anxiety and depression are possible following the operation so the patient should be monitored for signs of these. Relatives may need to be included in care plans so that they can be helped to understand what is happening and find ways to help the patient return to normal life. Partners, in particular, may need help in accepting the changed body image.

Many couples worry about the effect of the stoma on their sexual activity. Impotence may be physical or psychological in cause. If it occurs, talking through feelings may help, as may skilled counselling, taking into account the couple's normal practices. A major concern may be the effect of the bag on lovemaking. If the couple uses only the missionary position, advice may be required on other acceptable positions which will allow lovemaking but will not squash the bag. If a nurse feels unable to offer such advice, the patient's questions should be referred to a senior member of staff, a counsellor, or a specialist stoma nurse. It might be suggested that the couple read *The Joy of Sex* (Comfort 1975) which is a classic and sensitively written book with illustrations of different positions for lovemaking.

After the patient has adapted to his stoma, he will find that there are definite times of day when it acts and definite times of day when it is dormant. This may mean that for many patients there are periods of the day when they choose not to wear the bag. This would allow them to go swimming, to take a bath and perhaps to make love without wearing the bag. This knowledge can be very reassuring to a patient who, in his imagination, sees the bag constantly being dripped into from the stoma.

Other potential problems include those associated with the response to illness in general, such as feelings of guilt and questions associated with religious beliefs, especially if the stoma is associated with another prolonged illness or a diagnosis of cancer. Each patient will be different and careful assessment will be necessary in order to plan care directed to each person's specific problems.

Post-operative social care

After convalescence from his major surgery, the stoma patient should be able to return to full social functioning. He should be able to bathe, with or without his bag according to preference, wear normal clothes and undertake normal functioning. Employment would need to be changed only if the work is heavy and the surgery extensive.

Partners can be a great help in aiding an individual to return to normal and should be involved in the nursing plans for care so that they may learn the realities of living with a stoma. They may then feel confident in encouraging the patient to swim, eat out, go on holiday and resume normal pursuits.

Relationships need not suffer. There is no need for separate beds or curtailment of normal loving interaction. If there is long-term or permanent impotence, a counsellor may be needed to help the couple discover ways to express their feelings without intercourse. Sexuality has both psychological and social implications since impotence leads a man to feel a failure. He may believe that he will lose his partner's love and respect. This, coupled with frustration on the part of the partner, may lead to tension which will affect the whole family.

Women with stomas are less likely to have physical sexual difficulties but their problems with body image may affect their social behaviour. Plans for care should include reassurance that a person with a stoma is acceptable socially and can function without fear of stigma. Specialist associations exist which offer help and advice to individuals with stomas, but these may not appeal to all patients.

THE CARE PLAN

Priorities for care will include adequate preparation of the individual, both physically and psychologically, for major surgery and the acceptance of a stoma on a temporary or permanent basis. Education of the patient should be a priority, covering self-care, the potential for a return to normal social functioning, and the absence of stigma.

Psychological problems should be identified and action taken to reduce the risk of anxiety and depression. Partners and relatives may need to be included in the care plan so that their concerns may be dealt with and so that they may help the patient readjust to normality. Problems with changed body image and sexuality should be discussed and referred if necessary.

Surgery for a potential threat to life

Carcinoma in, for example, the breast or intestines, constitutes an actual threat to life and as such warrants early treatment which may include surgery. Some other conditions do not threaten life in themselves but may be a potential threat in that, if they are not treated, complications may occur which are dangerous. In these situations the patient, once diagnosed, is put on a waiting list for surgery but stands the chance of emergency admission. Some common operations of this type, e.g. appendicectomy, hernia repair and cholecystectomy, will be described below.

Appendicectomy

Appendicectomy is the most common of all abdominal operations. The appendix is not required for any bodily function but it is prone to infection and obstruction. The operation is normally performed after an attack of acute appendicitis, which is characterized by colic and varying degrees of digestive upsets. There may be a history of mild attacks which may have resulted in the patient being put on a waiting list for surgery. These reactions may mimic those of other abdominal disorders and a correct diagnosis may not be made before surgery.

If acute appendicitis is due to infection, the individual will be pyrexial. Conservation treatment is instituted to reduce the infection and will include antibiotics and rest. The operation will be performed some time in the future when the individual's condition is stable. The risk of leaving a patient with a diseased appendix is that it may rupture and lead to peritonitis.

If abdominal surgery is performed for other reasons, the appendix may be removed at the same time, even if healthy, because of the potential of obstruction or infection. However, if the patient goes to theatre specifically for an appendicectomy, a small transverse incision will be made to avoid weakening the abdominal wall. This means a shorter convalescent period will be needed.

In recent years a new procedure has begun to replace the traditional open appendicectomy. This is called laparoscopic appendectomy. In this operation, a laparoscope is used to remove the appendix electively and in the acute setting. To date, it is thought that the appendix with minimal inflammation is more amenable to laparoscopic removal but there have been reports of laparoscopic removal of severely inflamed appendices. This operation is still seen to be in the early stages and is not yet universally recommended (Abernathy and Gallagher 1991).

Peritonitis

Acute peritonitis, i.e. inflammation of the peritoneum, is a serious, life-threatening situation. It may be generalized due to a perforation or localized if adhesions seal off an area of the peritoneum.

An individual's reactions to acute peritonitis include acute abdominal pain in response to both the inflammation and the fluid which accumulates in the cavity. The individual may complain of nausea, vomiting and distension as a reaction to inflamed immobile intestines which fill with fluid and gas. Respirations will be rapid and shallow to avoid pain produced by movement and by the abdominal distension. The abdomen will be rigid and board-like, and the patient pale and clammy. The pulse is rapid as a reaction to a lowered blood volume in the presence of electrolyte and fluid imbalance. This may lead to shock.

Surgery to deal with the cause and to drain the peritoneal cavity is essential to save the patient's life. If the condition is treated early, no wound drain will be inserted, but patients with severe cases of peritonitis may return from theatre with a drain in position. A Ryle's tube is usually passed into the stomach for aspiration of gastric and intestinal contents and is not removed until peristalsis recommences. An intravenous infusion may be prescribed to help restore fluid and electrolyte balance.

PLANNING NURSING CARE

Pre-operative physical care
For appendicectomy without peritonitis, general pre-operative care is given. If peritonitis is present with vomiting, a Ryle's tube may be inserted pre-operatively to allow suction of the gastric contents, and an intravenous infusion may also be commenced. Observations will include the maintenance of a fluid balance chart.

Pre-operative psychological care
Problems will be those associated with hospitalization and the thought of operation. Although appendicectomy is usually a relatively simple operation, it may be viewed quite differently by the individual concerned. He is as much in need of an opportunity to discuss his concerns and ask questions as those patients undergoing more serious surgery.

Pre-operative social care
Social care should include giving information on the effect of the operation on normal lifestyle. If the operation is an emergency, the major concerns will be to do with the operation itself, though there may also be problems concerned with unfulfilled responsibilities as a result of the rush to hospital. The patient should be assured that key people will be informed and steps taken to deal with immediate problems which might include children returning to an empty house, an unfed cat, or the organization of the local youth club.

Post-operative physical care

General post-operative care will be given. In uncomplicated cases, the patient may return home within a few
days with his stitches in. There needs to be someone at
home to care for the patient, however, because although
he will be encouraged to return to full mobility, he may
need to rest for a few days. Stitches will be removed by the
district nurse.

For the patient who has had peritonitis, a longer stay
in hospital may be necessary since there may be a need to
treat infection and debility. The rate of recovery will be
affected by the individual's general health and the severity
of the peritonitis.

Post-operative psychological care

The patient who has had peritonitis may have been badly
frightened by the experience and needs reassurance
about his health. In uncomplicated appendicectomy there
are no specific psychological problems expected, but no
assumptions should be made. Assessment should be made
as carefully for a patient undergoing simple surgery as for
those with more serious conditions.

Post-operative social care

The individual may expect to return to normal social functioning, including a return to work, four to six weeks after
operation. This time period may be extended a little if
peritonitis was present. In the weeks following operation,
a gradual return to normal pursuits should occur, though
the patient should rest if he feels tired.

THE CARE PLAN

The priorities will be to give general pre- and post-operative care and to identify problems pertinent to each individual. If the operation is an emergency, priority should be
given to identifying concerns associated with the sudden
admission to hospital and reassuring the patient, if possible, that action will be taken.

Early mobilization will be planned with the aim of
early discharge if home conditions are suitable.

Repair of hernia

THE OPERATION

A hernia is a protrusion of an organ or part of an organ
through the tissues which normally contain them. The
most common hernias are abdominal, with part of the
intestine protruding through a weakness in the abdominal

wall. Hernias may be noticed as a lump under the skin. They are named according to their site and may form in the inguinal, umbilical, femoral and diaphragmatic area (Figure 11.9). They may also occur where there has been an incision for previous surgery. A hiatus hernia occurs when there is a weakness in the diaphragm and part of the stomach pushes up through the oesophageal space.

Some hernias can be pushed back into position and are described as 'reducible'. They may be controlled by the wearing of a truss, or disappear when the individual lies down. Other hernias may be described as 'irreducible' since they are held in place by adhesions. In both cases the hernia is not seen as a threat to life although the patient may experience some discomfort.

Operation for repair is usually planned and the patient may have to wait for some time before he is admitted to hospital. The potential risk of such a wait is that the hernia may strangulate.

In strangulation, the neck of the sac which holds the hernia tightens and causes obstruction to the loop of bowel. This obstruction causes the blood supply to the hernia to be reduced, which can lead to gangrene, infection and peritonitis. Hernia then constitutes a risk to life and immediate operation is necessary.

In planned hernia repair operations, the hernia is removed from the sac caused by the weakness in the diaphragm or abdominal wall, and the weakness repaired with strong suturing. Some surgeons use strips of fascia removed from the thigh, though suitable man-made materials are also available. This is an operation seen to be suitable for day surgery.

PLANNING NURSING CARE

Pre-operative physical care

Pre-operative physical care will include specific attention to breathing and bowel movement to prevent the postoperative strain involved in coughing and constipation. It is desirable for any patient to reduce smoking prior to any operation but it is particularly important when a hernia is to be repaired. Some surgeons refuse to operate on patients who do not give up smoking completely. Other patients may need help and encouragement from the nurse to reduce smoking in a period of pre-operative stress.

Chest infections should be treated and cleared prior to operation and the physiotherapist should teach breathing exercises. The nurse should encourage all patients to

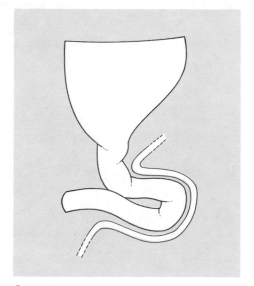

Strangulated hernia

Fig. 11.9 Hernia sites.

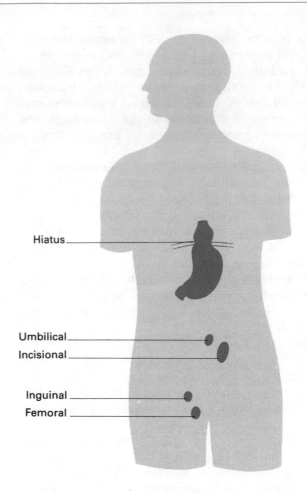

Hiatus

Umbilical

Incisional

Inguinal

Femoral

practise breathing exercises and help them understand the rationale so that they will be motivated to co-operate. A mild aperient may be prescribed for a patient who is constipated, both before and after operation.

Pre-operative psychological care
Problems anticipated will be those associated with major abdominal surgery, but each patient should be assessed and encouraged to discuss specific problems.

Pre-operative social care
In preparation for surgery, the smoker is asked to change his habits at a time of stress. The nurse and the relatives need to understand the strain this may impose, although the situation may be used to encourage a cessation of smoking on a permanent basis.

Problems associated with normal social interaction and responsibilities should be explored, especially if the patient has a strangulated hernia and has been admitted as an emergency. Time may be short pre-operatively in this situation, but adequate time should be spent with the patient to elicit problems since anxiety may affect post-operative recovery.

Post-operative physical care

General post-operative care will be given with particular emphasis on breathing exercises and leg movement. It is usual to get the patient out of bed on the day after operation and gradually increase the exercise. Antibiotics may be prescribed if the hernia was strangulated. The patient should be encouraged to support his wound when laughing or coughing.

Post-operative psychological care

The patient may be anxious about his wound and fearful of moving. He should be encouraged to move but his concerns should not be belittled. The presence of a nurse when he gets out of bed or walks to the toilet should encourage and reassure him that he is 'safe'.

Displays of temper or tension due to nicotine withdrawal should be treated with understanding, and relatives should be helped to understand and to deal with these outbursts. In the final analysis, it must be remembered that the patient has the right to make an informed decision on smoking.

Other psychological problems may arise and if so should also be included in the care plan.

Post-operative social care

In preparing the patient for a return to social activity, it needs to be understood that any strain on the wound by excessive coughing, constipation or heavy lifting should be avoided for at least six weeks after operation. Really heavy strain, as in manual work, needs to be avoided for three months. This should not preclude the individual from returning to employment within a few weeks, though manual labourers may need light duties for a while.

Other social pursuits should be resumed as the individual feels able. Early return to lovemaking should be gentle since this too can put strain on the abdominal muscles.

THE CARE PLAN

The care plan will include specific plans to educate the patient to avoid post-operative strain during the recovery period. This may include education to help the individual give up or reduce smoking, and the development of regular bowel movement without strain.

Although few psychological and social problems may be anticipated, those identified will be included in the care plan or referred to other agencies.

Relatives may need help in understanding both the operation and the individual's reactions to nicotine withdrawal if he is a smoker.

Cholecystectomy

THE OPERATION

Cholecystectomy means the removal of the gallbladder. It is usually undertaken in patients who have a history of inflammation of the gallbladder (cholecystitis), which is generally associated with gallstones although it may also occur in the absence of gallstones. Gallstones are formed from calcium cholesterol and bile pigments and, although their formation (cholelithiasis) is little understood, they are associated with infection. A gallbladder may contain one large stone or a number of stones of various sizes. They are more likely to occur in women of middle-age but do also occur in males.

Gallstones may cause no reaction until one moves and obstructs part of the common bile duct (Figure 11.10). If this occurs the individual may become jaundiced as bile is diverted into the bloodstream instead of into the duodenum. Severe colic may occur in the right hypochondriac region as a reaction to the stone blocking the duct. The pain disappears when the stone returns to the gallbladder. This pain is called 'biliary colic'. It may be felt as a referred pain between the shoulder blades.

The lack of bile in the duodenum will disturb digestion, especially if a meal contains fatty foods. The individual will react with nausea, vomiting and flatulence. Lack of bile also affects the absorption of vitamin K, which is essential for blood clotting. The prothrombin level will be reduced as a result.

In response to inflammation, there may be some pyrexia and a rise in antibody formation. The reactions to obstructive cholecystitis are often so severe that the individual is admitted to hospital. As with other inflammatory conditions, the usual treatment is conservative until the symptoms settle. Antibiotics may be given, along with rest and a fat-reduced diet. Penicillin is contraindicated since it is not excreted in bile.

After an acute episode has subsided, the individual will go on a waiting list for a planned cholecystectomy, where the gallbladder, which acts solely as a reservoir for bile, will be removed. The patient sometimes likes to keep the stones as a memento of the operation.

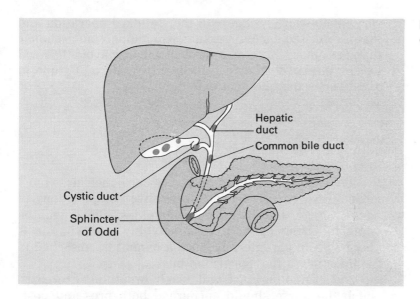

Fig. 11.10 Sites of gallstone obstruction of the bile ducts.

Attacks of cholecystitis do not always subside. The infection may suppurate (empyema of the gallbladder) leading to toxaemia. Individual reactions include rigor and the signs of shock if peritonitis results. Immediate surgery is necessary if either empyema or peritonitis is present.

It may be possible to deal with gallstones without recourse to surgery. One method which is called extra-corporeal shockwave lithotripsy (ESWL) can be used to fragment the gallstones and permit their passage out of the gallbladder into the duodenum. To be suitable for this treatment, the patient must have a stone of less than 3 cm in length and fewer than three stones. It may take several weeks for the fragments of stones to be passed out of the gallbladder and the patient may need to take an oral agent for gallstone dissolution for a period of time after the first treatment.

A newer operation than the standard removal of the gallbladder with the stones is the laparoscopic cholecystectomy. This has been made possible by the con-siderable improvement in laparoscopic techniques and in the improved technology of the cameras. The operation is performed by having a fibre-optic camera introduced into a small incision in the abdominal wall and the dissection of the gallbladder is performed under guidance from the camera either with a laser or by electro-cautery. It was assumed that by 1995 more than 95% of cholecystectomies would be performed through the laparoscope (McNoble and Abernathy 1991). These newer techniques will mean that the patient's stay in hospital is very much shorter than with the standard operation and that a return to normal pursuits will happen much sooner than previously. Such an approach will also avoid the need for the patient to return from theatre with a 'T' tube *in situ* to keep the bile duct patent.

PLANNING NURSING CARE

Pre-operative physical care

In addition to general pre-operative care, measures must be taken to reduce the post-operative complications of haemorrhage and breathing difficulties. Blood will be taken for grouping and cross-matching, and vitamin K may be given parenterally since it cannot be absorbed in the intestine in the absence of bile.

The physiotherapist will teach breathing exercises, which the nurse should encourage both pre- and post-operatively. The patient should be told of the risk of breathing problems which are due to the site of operation and the almost involuntary shallow breathing which reduces pain. Assurance should be given that the pain will be controlled.

A low-fat or fat-free diet will be continued or prescribed. Many individuals find for themselves that fat is nauseating, especially in obstructive episodes, so are willing to co-operate in dietary control.

Pre-operative psychological care

Problems will be those associated with major surgery and a history of ill-health and pain. Individuals will react differently and their particular concerns will be coloured by experience. Jaundice may be very frightening because in many people's minds it is associated with terminal cancer. For many patients, the operation itself may not pose problems since it offers the chance of a return to a pain-free and healthy life.

There may be problems with relationships if there is a history of ill-health. Early signs of cholecystitis are often vague and may lead to tension in the home if a partner is unsympathetic. Hospitalization may exacerbate these problems, particularly if relatives feel guilty that they had not taken previous complaints seriously.

Plans for care need to include the relatives, who may be confused and frightened by the thought of surgery, especially if it is at a time when relationships are strained. Few people realize how hard it is to live with an ailing partner. A nurse, in listening to a relative, may help simply by showing interest and appearing non-judgemental.

Pre-operative social care

The patient's social interaction and work may have suffered during the period between attacks and operation. The operation should promise a return to normality, but it is still necessary to identify social problems which may or may not be associated with the patient's clinical state.

Post-operative physical care

If the standard cholecystectomy operation has been performed, the individual may return from theatre with a 'T' tube *in situ* to keep the bile duct patent. This usually drains into a disposable bag. However, with the increase in laparoscopic operations, this is seen very rarely.

General post-operative care should be given to the patient with particular emphasis on the potential problem of post-operative haemorrhage. A nasogastric tube may have been passed to avoid vomiting and this is aspirated two-hourly before small oral feeds are given.

For patients who have the traditional operation, wound care is vitally important. A corrugated drain my be in position which will necessitate daily dressings. The drain is gradually shortened and then removed on the instructions of the surgeon. The drain is situated in the gallbladder site to channel any leakage of bile. Observations should be made and excessive leakage reported.

If a 'T' tube has been inserted at the wound site into the bile duct, it will remain in position for up to ten days. Bile drained into the bag is measured daily, though its loss from the digestive tract may affect appetite. Faeces are observed for colour. If they are normal a few days after operation, it is assumed that bile is reaching the duodenum. A cholangiogram is performed to confirm the patency of the bile duct a week after operation. The 'T' tube is then clamped off for periods of time and if the patient does not complain of pain, it is assumed that the bile duct can deal with all bile being produced. The 'T' tube is removed on the tenth day after operation.

A potential problem for all operations on the gallbladder is peritonitis due to leakage of bile into the peritoneum. Since biliary peritonitis constitutes a risk to life, observations are particularly important so that reactions may be identified early and action taken.

Post-operative psychological care

If a traditional operation has been performed, the individual may be fearful of moving after the operation and may need considerable psychological support from the nurse in both breathing and moving. In helping the patient to take deep breaths the nurse may observe the effect of this and identify pain if it occurs. The patient should be encouraged to report pain and discomfort.

The removal of the T-tube may also cause apprehension for, although the pain is only momentary, the thought may be terrifying. When explaining to the patient that the tube will be removed, an analgesic may be offered an hour prior to the procedure, which should have a calming effect. The patient will be reassured if he knows that the nurse is experienced and that the procedure is over quickly.

Problems which have been identified, in terms of relationships or in response to a history of feeling unwell, should be included in the care plan or referred to someone more senior.

If a laparoscopic operation has been performed, the patient will be discharged much sooner than previously. The patient who has had the traditional operation may be discharged after the 'T' tube is removed but with sutures still in; these will be removed by the district nurse.

No matter which way the operation was performed, convalescence will include a gradual return to activity and to normal diet, the individual being expected to monitor his own tolerance to fat.

Post-operative social care
Since the operation should bring an improvement in general health there may be no more than residual social problems which may improve as convalescence progresses. The individual should understand that he has had major surgery and will need a gradual return to normal activity. Relatives should be advised how they may help the individual return to normality without making him dependent.

The patient may be concerned about resuming normal pursuits. As with any abdominal surgery, time needs to be taken for healing to occur so heavy work or strain should be avoided. In the main, if the individual does not become overtired, activity should be continued. Each individual will learn his own comfortable pace for a return to chores, leisure activities and sexual activity and should be guided by general principles rather than set rules.

THE CARE PLAN

Pre-operatively, priorities will include education and preparation of the patient to avoid post-operative complications. Individual concerns will be explored and action taken where possible.

Post-operatively, the emphasis will be on observations so that complications may be identified early, and in supporting the patient emotionally to aid early recovery and mobility. Education may be required to aid a comfortable and successful convalescence.

Relatives should be included in the care plan so that they may understand the nature of the operation and their own role in ensuring a return to normal activities.

Prostatectomy

THE OPERATION

Prostatectomy, i.e. removal of the prostate gland, is usually performed because of benign or malignant enlargement of the gland which may lead to genito-urinary problems and risk to life.

Benign enlargement is common in later life, but the cause remains obscure. New tissue thickens the thin encapsulating membrane of the prostate gland until pressure is exerted on the urethra and bladder. It is at this point that the individual reacts to the disease process. Difficulty in passing urine will be experienced; it may be hard to start micturating and impossible to empty the bladder as much as before. Because there is always a larger than usual amount of residual urine in the bladder, the resultant reduced bladder capacity will lead to frequency. This can not only disturb daily functioning but may also affect sleep patterns, the individual needing to micturate several times in the night.

The residual urine makes an excellent culture medium for organisms and may lead to cystitis. Urinary tract infections will increase and cause pain and a 'burning' sensation on micturition.

There is a risk to life if the condition becomes severe and remains untreated. The bladder may become distended and weakened and urine may build up in the ureters (hydro-ureter) and in the pelvis of the kidneys (hydronephrosis). Kidney involvement may lead to uraemia.

The patient may be admitted to a medical ward in the first instance with acute retention of urine. This condition is treated by catheterization. The urine is released slowly to avoid shock, which could happen if blood rapidly filled the vessels which had previously been constricted by pressure. A decision may be made to remove the prostate gland while the patient is in hospital, or he may be treated conservatively and readmitted at a later date for surgery. If the cause of enlargement is carcinoma, chemotherapy may be prescribed as an alternative to surgery.

Suprapubic prostatectomy (Figure 11.11) is performed through the bladder, an incision being made over the bladder. This operation poses no threat of subsequent impotence but it has two disadvantages: the patient requires continuous urine drainage after operation, and has a suprapubic fistula to heal. The operation may also be performed **retropubically** (Figure 11.12), which does not necessitate opening the bladder. Instead the capsule of the prostate is incised. After removal of the gland, the capsule is repaired and a corrugated drain left *in situ*. A urethral (Foley type) catheter is inserted before the patient leaves theatre. There is again no risk of impotence after this operation.

A less popular operation is that of **perineal** prostatectomy. Here, the perineal body is incised and the prostate removed through the prostate capsule. The advantage of this technique is that the abdominal wall remains intact, but the disadvantages are potential impotence and a risk of urinary incontinence. In some cases of carcinoma of the prostate with obstruction, **transurethral** resection (Figure 11.13) is the operation of choice. Here the prostate is resected by diathermy through an endoscope inserted per urethra. This operation does not remove the whole of the prostate gland and may need to be repeated at intervals.

PLANNING NURSING CARE

Pre-operative physical care
General pre-operative care is given. In addition, antibiotics may be prescribed if infection is present. The patient should be given an explanation that the antibiotic needs time to take effect, especially if he has to wait a few days before having his operation. Blood urea levels should be established by the medical staff and the anaesthetist be informed of the results, since a high urea level may have implications for the type of anaesthesia used. Renal function is also assessed and electrolyte abnormalities corrected.

Pre-operative psychological care
Specific attention should be given to any misconceptions the patient may have about the operation, particularly those associated with sexuality. The vasa deferentia are often tied during operation leaving the patient sterile. If this decision has been made the patient may need assur-

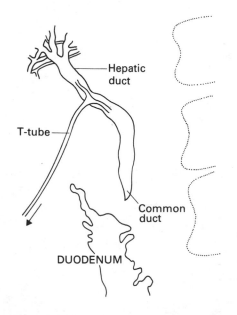

Fig. 11.11 Suprapubic prostatectomy.

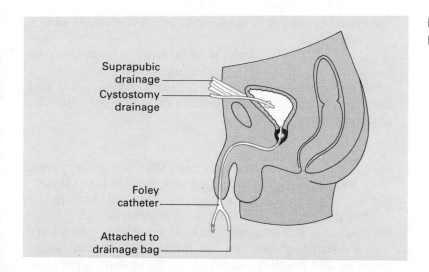

Fig. 11.12 Retropubic prostatectomy.

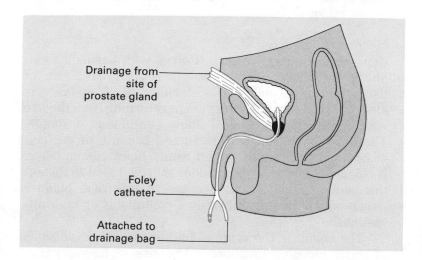

Fig. 11.13 Transurethral prostatectomy.

ance that sterility does not mean impotence. Similarly, there may be fears derived from the belief that prostatectomy itself causes impotence. An explanation that current methods of operation do not carry this risk should put the patient's mind at rest. No assumptions should be made about the age at which patients cease to be concerned with their sexuality. Many couples continue a satisfactory sex life well into old age.

Other psychological care may need to be given in response to concerns about the operation itself and whether it will 'cure' the problems which the patient has experienced. Much will depend on the state of the patient's kidneys but in most cases it should not be too optimistic to offer a considerable improvement in health after operation.

If the patient is elderly, both he and his family may be concerned about the dangers of anaesthesia, especially if other physical disabilities are present. Explanation can help to reassure, as can attention to individual concerns and questions.

Pre-operative social care

Operations involving sexual organs may be embarrassing to an individual since discussion or exposure is not generally socially acceptable. A sensitive approach is required so that the patient can discuss his concerns without embarrassment. It is possible that frequency and cystitis have had a disruptive effect on the individual's normal social pursuits and possibly employment, so that the operation will come as a relief. Social problems associated with hospitalization should be identified and the appropriate action taken.

Post-operative physical care

General post-operative care is given with particular emphasis on observations, since there is a real risk of haemorrhage following prostatectomy. Fluid balance is also observed carefully, the patient returning from theatre with a catheter *in situ* to allow continuous drainage. The flow should not be interrupted because of the risk of blood clots forming, which would block the catheter. If blood clots form in the bladder they will lead to distention and possibly shock. Because of this risk, bladder irrigation will be prescribed on a continuous or intermittent basis.

The colour of the urine should be observed and signs of frank bleeding monitored. The risk of haemorrhage remains for several days after operation, so the patient needs educating that he must not strain to open his bowels as this would in turn put a strain on the wound. An explanation to the patient that his urine will be blood-stained after the operation should allay any panic that something has gone wrong. It is also important that the patient tells the nurse if he experiences feelings of 'fullness' or pain in the bladder since this may indicate clot formation or haemorrhage. If antibiotics have been given prior to operation, the risk of post-operative infection is reduced. Meticulous attention to catheter care will further reduce the risk.

When the catheter is removed, the patient may have problems in regaining full control of continence although this will be affected by the method of operation and the

patient's history. Retropubic prostatectomy gives good results for a return to normal control providing that prolonged obstruction has not caused damage to the bladder.
If the patient has problems of frequency or incontinence
he may need educating for better control. The nurse
should offer a bottle hourly, and gradually increase the
interval until a satisfactory measure of control has been
regained. At night the patient will be reassured if he is
able to have a urinal by his bed.

Post-operative psychological care

If the patient understands the reason for post-operative
blood-stained urine, and is kept free from pain, he should
feel that his recovery is satisfactory. Problems may arise
when the catheter is removed for, if he finds he does not
have adequate control over his bladder, he may feel that
the operation has been a failure. In this instance the nurse
will need to be sensitive to any anger on the part of the
patient, and positive in her explanations of the need to re-
learn control. If an individual shows excessive anxiety,
having a bottle available at the bedside all the time may
help in the first few days until some level of control has
been achieved.

The patient may need considerable help and reassurance while he is recovering from the operation. He should
be encouraged to express his concerns. In learning to
control bladder activity he should not be left tense and
nervous. This will be most likely to occur if the intervals
between offering urinals are extended too rapidly.

Relatives may need reassurance that post-operative
recovery is proceeding satisfactorily. If other conditions
are present which predispose to complications such as
uraemia or cardiac failure, explanations will be given of
any setbacks and their implications for the patient and his
family. The relatives need to be assured that the patient is
receiving the best possible attention.

Post-operative social care

As the patient recovers and gains control over micturition,
many problems of social functioning may disappear altogether or at least diminish in intensity. For example, if
sleep patterns had been disrupted prior to operation,
tiredness may have led to strain and tension in the family
and reduced efficiency at work. Similarly, bouts of cystitis
and frequency may have led to a reduction in social activity, and had an effect on sexual functioning.

There may be some social problems associated with a
period of time off work. If there are complications such as
uraemia, this period may be prolonged. Relatives may

need advice if there is financial hardship as a result. Referral to the Social Services may be necessary in these circumstances.

Personal relationships may be affected for, although modern surgical techniques do not physically impair sexual potency, there may be psychological problems. This is especially likely if the patient has been sterilized. If this occurs, the help of a skilled counsellor may be required for both the patient and his partner.

THE CARE PLAN

Specific priorities will be in pre-operative care, which will prepare the patient for the reality of his operation, including sterilization if this is likely to be necessary. Post-operative care will aim to return him to the best possible functioning. This will include care to diminish the risks of residual clotting or post-operative haemorrhage, and education towards improved bladder control.

Relatives may need information and reassurance about the nature of the operation and its implications for both the patient and his family. In many cases an improvement in quality of life may be expected after convalescence.

Replacement surgery

Many disease processes are irreversible and affect body mechanisms which are essential to normal healthy functioning. Over time, the individual becomes chronically ill or disabled and is faced with a life which may include pain, restriction, medication and a progressive deterioration of health.

In some such circumstances mechanical replacement may be considered. For example, replacement of the head of the femur in cases of osteoarthritis is a long-established and safe surgical procedure which will enhance life for those who receive it and for their families. Also in recent years there has been a steady development in organ replacement surgery using donor organs (homografts). Organ transplantation does, however, pose physical, ethical and psychological problems for the caring professions and for society as a whole.

Physical problems

The major physical problem in organ replacement has been the rejection of the new organ by the patient. Rejection occurs because the body (host) treats the replacement organ (graft) as a foreign body to which it mounts an immune response. This does not happen in corneal transplantation because the replacement cornea is protected from antibodies, which are carried in the blood vessels, by the fluid in the eye. It is not possible to arrange this type of protection for organs such as the kidney and heart since their functions are totally connected with the blood supply of the host.

In early work on kidney transplantation it was thought that a relative's kidney would be more readily acceptable if the blood groups matched. More recently it has been found that the important factor is that tissue types should match. Even so, problems of rejection remain and are largely dealt with by the use of immunosuppressants such as azathiaprine. These drugs may cause problems since they lower the immune response to all antigens and leave the patient susceptible to infection.

Other physical problems include the availability of suitable healthy organs for the patients who need them. Kidney transplants are so common that patients awaiting the operation are listed on computer with all details including tissue type documented. Donor kidneys can then be made available very quickly to the patient for whom they are most suitable.

The improvement in microsurgical techniques means that transplant operations are safe if carried out by a specialist. For example, in 1984 a heart transplant was successfully completed on a baby girl only a few days old. The problem remains one of survival, the baby in question dying at less than one month old. In the USA at a later date, the heart of a baboon was used to replace a man's heart; again it was not successful, although the patient lived for some weeks after surgery. The chances of survival after transplantation continue to improve, but even with a kidney transplant, which is a well-established surgical technique, the survival of the patient cannot be presumed.

Ethical problems

A major ethical issue is that of securing donor organs. In the case of kidneys, it is possible for a relative with matching tissue type to donate a kidney while alive since one kidney is adequate for normal health. The donor may make an informed decision about the risks of halving his chances of survival in the event of subsequent renal disease and of the operation itself.

In the case of other organs such as the heart, liver or

pancreas, it is only possible to obtain them after death. Not only does the donor need to be dead but very recently dead if the organs are to be healthy. There have been many cases in the press of outraged bereaved relatives who have heard of the death of a loved one and have immediately been asked for permission to remove the deceased's organs.

There are two major problems. One problems is how to show acceptable sensitivity to the bereaved at this time, the other is how to decide when an individual is actually dead. Both pose enormous problems for health professionals whose responsibility is both to the living and to the relatives of the dying or dead person. For these reasons, two doctors must independently certify that the patient is brain dead before organs may be removed.

The matter is further complicated by the fact that patients who are critically ill yet may have healthy organs are often kept alive after they would have died by respirators and life-support machines. It used to be thought that death occurred when the heart stopped beating and the patient stopped breathing. In fact, when individuals died at home, it was not unusual to hold a mirror over the patient's mouth. If there were respirations, the mirror would cloud over, and a clear mirror would mean that the patient was dead. The advent of machines which can sustain cardiac rhythm and respiration has led to an enormous debate on the meaning of 'death', since other body tissues may now cease to function before the heart and lungs 'die'. Brain death is currently considered to be a better determinant of death given the above problems. As long ago as 1978, Capron stated, '. . . a human body with irreversible cessation of total brain function, according to usual and customary standards of medical practice, shall be considered dead'.

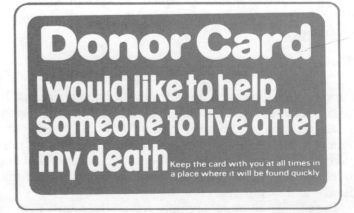

The problem of showing acceptable sensitivity to be-reaved relatives is particularly difficult because many po-tential donors die in accidents. Their relatives will not have had time to adjust to the idea of the donor's death, as is possible in a prolonged or chronic illness. A request for organs may be extremely painful at such a time. One way to overcome the problem is to educate the public about the potential benefits of transplant surgery. Organ donor cards are now more common which may make it easier for relatives to give consent for transplantation. It is also possible to make a will leaving the entire body to a medi-cal institution for research.

From 1995 there has been an Organ Donation Register established to hold information on computer of potential donors and the organs they are prepared to donate (Fig-ure 11.14).

Psychological problems

Even though organ transplantation is increasingly suc-cessful, many people have problems in accepting what may be seen as 'surgical experimentation'. It might be argued that this is both an ethical and a psychological problem. In the case of the baby girl mentioned earlier, her heart was so malformed that survival without opera-tion would have been impossible. A heart was donated, the surgeon was willing to operate and the parents wished to give their child the chance of survival. There was in fact no discord over the operation itself.

It may have been that, if the child had survived, there would have been no public censure. In the event of her death there was considerable comment suggesting that the operation had been an experiment and as such was unacceptable. There are, of course, two sides to this de-bate – the surgeon, the nurses and the parents all believed that the baby had not died in vain, but this begs the question of the quality of her short life.

Similar problems arise in the matter of using animal organs, both from the psychological effects on the recipi-ent of feeling 'part animal' and in the light of the contro-versy on animal rights. At present such controversy is linked with experimentation but, as surgeons become more successful, real decisions will need to be made on the ethics of breeding animals to provide spare parts for humans. To some this may seem no more unethical than breeding animals for food, but to others it may be one more unacceptable sign of human arrogance.

For the individual awaiting a donor organ, there may be many problems, not least the uncertainty of whether an

Fig. 11.14 Organ donor register form.

This form can be used to record your wishes on the NHS Organ Donor Register or to amend your record.

Please complete this form in BLOCK CAPITALS and tick as appropriate.

☐ Please register me on the NHS Organ Donor Register as someone whose organs can be used for transplantation purposes after my death. **(fill in sections A and C)**

☐ Please amend my records on the NHS Organ Donor Register as shown below. **(fill in sections A, B or C as necessary)**

☐ Please remove my entry from the NHS Organ Donor Register as I no longer wish to be a donor. **(fill in section A)**

A

Surname _____

Forename(s) _____

Date of Birth ☐☐ ☐☐ ☐☐
         day month year

Sex ☐ Male ☐ Female

Current Address _____
_____
_____
_____

Postcode _____

Continued overleaf

B

Previous Address _____
(if amending NHS Organ Donor Register) _____
_____
_____

Postcode _____

C

I request that after my death

☐ Any part of my body

OR my ☐ Kidneys ☐ Heart ☐ Liver

☐ Corneas ☐ Lungs ☐ Pancreas

may be used for the treatment of others

Signature _____

Date _____ | **REG** |

The form should be put in an envelope and sent to

NHS Organ Donor Register
FREEPOST (BS 8793)
PO Box 14
Patchway
Bristol
BS12 6BR

There is no need for a stamp

BY ALLOWING YOUR ORGANS TO BE USED FOR TRANSPLANT AFTER YOUR DEATH, YOU WILL BE GIVING SOMEONE ELSE THEIR LIFE BACK.

organ will become available in time and if the operation will be successful. Even in established transplant surgery there is a risk of rejection and each patient has to make an informed decision on whether or not he wants to take the risk or continue with a chronic condition and a limited life expectancy.

Partners and families will also be involved, and concerned. A personal problem for anyone awaiting a donor organ for himself or for a loved one is that, in wishing for one life to be saved, he is also inadvertently wishing for a stranger to die. If an organ does become available, there may be an interest in the donor which will not be satisfied.

It seems reasonable to expect that organ transplant surgery will continue to develop and expand. Any patient undergoing such surgery needs the chance to express his particular concerns and to gain understanding of the nature of his operation and the costs in terms of subsequent chemotherapy and other necessary restrictions.

The ethical debate will continue, particularly in the area of child recipients, since here the decision is made by others. At present, denial of the necessary surgery to a child can result in that child becoming a ward of court. This means that the right to make decisions about what is

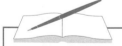

Imagine that two patients are awaiting a life-saving transplant organ. One is female, 28 years old, and the mother of a five-year-old daughter. The other is a 21-year-old male, who is unemployed and lives with his parents.

1 To whom would you give priority for receiving the next available organ?
2 Give reasons for your decision.

best for a child is denied to the parents and invested in the court.

Summary

In this chapter the care of patients on a surgical ward has been considered. It has been seen that many operations are now performed on a day case unit, whilst surgery overall has been revolutionized by the improvement in laparoscopic techniques. This means that many patients' stay in hospital will be considerably shorter than previously and responsibilities for aftercare will be transferred to the community.

Some of the more common operations have been described to illustrate the physical, psychological and social effects of surgery and the nurse's role in planning care. For those patients attending for day surgery, it is particularly important that good relations are established between the hospital and the community.

Although the problems discussed are generally those associated with surgery, other problems should be explored. Relatives' needs have been discussed in general terms to alert staff of the need to support the patient's family when possible and to refer where necessary. It has been seen that some conditions have their own associations which provide volunteer visitors to help support both the patient and their family.

Replacement surgery has been raised as an issue of growing importance to patients and their families, potential donors and the whole health care team.

References

Abernathy, C. & Gallagher, C. (1991) Appendicitis. In Abernathy, C. & Harken, A. (Eds.) *Surgical secrets*. Philadelphia: Handley and Belfus.

Abernathy, C. & Young, M. (1991) Primary therapy for breast cancer. In Abernathy, C. & Harken, A. (Eds.) *Sugical secrets*, pp. 200–203. Philadelphia: Handley and Belfus.

Aronoff, G. (1985) *Evaluation and treatment of chronic pain.* Baltimore: Urban & Scharzenberg.

Capron, A. M. (1978) Death, definition and determination of legal aspects. In Reich, W. T. (Ed.) *Encyclopaedia of bioethics, Vol. 1.* New York: The Free Press.

Cohen, M. & McIntyre, R. (1991) Small bowel obstruction. In Abernathy, C. & Harken, A. (Eds.) *Surgical secrets*, pp. 146–149. Philadelphia: Handly and Belfus.

Colmer, M. (1987) *Moroney's surgery for nurses*, 16th edn. Edinburgh: Churchill Livingstone.

Comfort, A. (1975) *The joy of sex*. London: Quartet Books.

Faulkner, M. A. (1984) Teaching non-specialist nurses assessment skills in the aftercare of mastectomy patients. Steinberg Collection. London: RCN.

Faulkner, A. & Maguire, P. (1994) *Talking to cancer patients and their relatives*. Oxford: Oxford University Press.

Hayward, J. (1975) *Information. A prescription against pain*. London: Rcn.

Hill, D. & Summers, R. (1994) *Medical technology, a nursing perspective*. London: Chapman & Hall.

Kolodny, R. C., Masters, W. H., Johnson, V. E. & Biggs, M. A. (1980) *Textbook of human sexuality for nurses*. Boston: Little, Brown.

McNoble, D. & Abernathy, C. (1991) Gallbladder disease. In Abernathy, C. & Harken, A. (Eds.) Surgical secrets. St Louis: Mosby.

Morris, T., Greer, H. S. & White, P. (1977) Psychological and social adjustment to mastectomy. *Cancer, 40*, 2381–2387.

Pike, S. & Forster, D. (1995). *Health promotion and health education*. Edinburgh: Churchill Livingstone.

Pritchard, P. & Mallett, J. (Eds.) (1992) *Royal Marsden Hospital, manual of clinical nursing practice*, 3rd edn. Oxford: Blackwell.

Seers, C. (1987) Pain, anxiety and recovery in patients undergoing surgery. Unpublished PhD thesis, King's College, University of London.

Smiddy, F. (1991) *Tutorials in clinical surgery in general*. Edinburgh: Churchill Livingstone.

Tarrier, N. & Maguire, P. (1984) Treatment of psychological distress following mastectomy. *Behaviour Research and Therapy, 22*, 81–84.

Webb, C. (1982) Body image and recovery from hysterectomy. In Wilson-Barnett, J. & Fordham, M. (Eds.) *Recovery from illness*. Chichester: J. Wiley.

Further reading

Abernathy, C. & Harken, A. (1991) *Surgical secrets*. Philadelphia: Handley and Belfus.

Anderson, K. & Anderson, L. (1995) *Mosby's pocket dictionary of nursing, medicine and professions allied to medicine*. London: Mosby.

Gray, C. (1989) Patients' perceptions of anxiety. *Surgical Nurse, 2*(3), 12–17.

Harvey Kemble, J. V. & Lamb, B. E. (1984) *Plastic surgical and burns nursing*. London: Baillière Tindall.

Jennet, W. B. (1983) Brain death. *Practitioner*, 227, 1377, 451.

Purchese, G. & Allan, D. (1984) *Neuromedical and neurosurgical nursing*, 2nd edn. London: Ballière Tindall.

12

The Elderly Patient

CHAPTER SUMMARY

The ageing process, 424
Physiological ageing, 424
Psychological ageing, 426
Social effects of ageing, 426

The needs of the elderly patient, 427
Mobility, 428
Incontinence, 429
Safety, 432
Dignity and identity, 434
Sexuality, 435
Loneliness, 436

Confusion, 437
Nutrition and warmth, 440

Specific disease in the elderly, 441
Cerebrovascular accident, 441
Parkinson's disease (paralysis agitans), 447
Osteoarthritis, 454

Summary, 458

References, 458

Further reading, 459

It is not unusual in Western society to separate the elderly from the rest of the population. There is a cut-off point at which an individual no longer works to support himself and he then becomes the potential responsibility of others. There is no hard and fast rule about the age at which a person becomes 'elderly' but in general it appears to be linked with the average age of retirement. The danger here is that ageing will be seen as a disease (Shukla 1994) when in fact it is a normal phenomenon. Many individuals, when they are no longer obliged to work, take on new hobbies and pastimes and generally have a new lease of life. Others resent having to give up work and may in fact go through a very difficult period of adjustment to a life that does not include the work ethic.

In the past, responsibility for the elderly was generally taken by the working members of the family. In cases where there was no family, support was grudgingly given by society with measures such as the Poor Laws of 1795–1834, which put destitute old people into workhouses. A Royal Commission which reported on the Poor Laws in 1834 recommended that poor relief should be organized on harsher lines (Marshall 1968). The problem for the elderly in the past was that they were not considered separately from those who were thought to be able but unwilling to work.

Although efforts were made to differentiate between poverty which was self-inflicted and that which was unavoidable, it was not until 1908 that old age pensions were introduced. There are still people alive whose parents may have threatened them with the horrors of the workhouse as the lot of the poor and lazy. Unfortunately, many of these old workhouses were taken over as hospitals for the aged and chronically sick, and many elderly people saw admission there as 'being put in the workhouse', with the attendant connotations of fear, hardship and personal insult.

It was not until after the introduction of the National Health Service in 1948 that geriatric medicine emerged as a specialty. Previous to this, the elderly had been neglected in terms of diagnosis and treatment, many being kept in bed with no attempt made for rehabilitation. Nursing the elderly emerged as the province of the State Enrolled Nurse and was not included in general nursing training until 1973. At that time it was an optional experience for learners but in 1977 it became part of the General Nursing Council syllabus.

'Geriatric' means 'care of the old' and comes from the Greek for old age (*géras*) and physician (*iatros*). Another word used to define nursing the elderly is 'gerontology' with the wider definition of 'the study of old age and the ageing processes'. In recent years, however, there has been a move away from such labelling of a section of society to the more general term of 'care of the elderly'.

This care is organized at different levels. There are **assessment wards** where investigations and diagnoses occur, and where treatment may be prescribed and decisions made for the future, in consultation with the patient and his family. **Rehabilitation wards** are concerned with helping patients reach their potential with the aid of education, physiotherapy and occupational therapy, while **long-stay wards** are for those patients who need continuing care. There are also **day centres** for those patients who live alone or with relatives, where interaction with peers is organized along with some nursing care, such as bathing and hair washing.

NHS reforms which have brought changes to long-term care of the elderly now demand that a differentiation is made between those elderly people who need acute hospital care and those whose needs are more social than acute. As these reforms are implemented, there are patients who appear to fall between two stools. A classic case was that of a former executive engineer in telecommunications. He had a stroke 20 years prior to his death but before he died he also suffered from Alzheimer's disease, psoriasis, ulcers and chronic renal failure. This patient was deemed one of those whose needs were social in spite of his physical disabilities and so he was discharged from hospital 18 months before his death. The Social Services in his area refused to take responsibility for him, arguing that his needs were considerably more than social. He spent the last six months of his life in a community hospital near his home. Other patients who are in similar situations often spend their last few months in nursing homes at considerable cost to either themselves or their relatives.

Such cases do raise the issue of whether hospital care for elderly patients should be seen to be different in terms of criteria for admission than it is for younger people. MacGuire (1993) found that 50% of nurses' time in caring for the elderly was spent on direct care, that is washing, dressing, taking patients to the toilet and things that many patients are able to do for themselves. It is this balance between the need to be cared for in terms of normal daily activities and the need for acute care that is under discussion as the NHS reforms are implemented.

The ageing process

Physiological ageing

There has been a steady rise in the number of elderly people as a proportion of the total population, since, as standards of living and health care have improved, more people survive to and beyond the 'three score years and ten' described in the Bible. In the UK for instance, in 1901 only 6% of the population were above retirement age. By 1975 this figure had risen to over 19% (Owen 1976) and continues to rise. By 1981, half a million people were retiring from work each year (DHSS 1981). More recent projections for mid-1994 suggest that 10 642 000 people will have reached retirement age (60 years for women and 65 years for men) by 1995.

Ageing as a process has received considerable attention over time, and efforts made to halt its inevitability. There have been claims of elixirs of youth, while society spends considerable time and money to lessen the obvious effects of ageing by the use of anti-wrinkle creams, hair dyes and transplants, and surgical 'face lifts', for example. Although old age tends to be defined by chronological measures, biological ageing occurs at different rates in each individual, the only constant being that body cells will age in all individuals who live beyond maturity, and the effects of such ageing will be cumulative.

There is a number of theories about the ageing process. One is a developmental model of man in which life moves in stages from development in the uterus, through childhood, reproductive life and then old age. In this model, each stage is 'switched off' before the individual enters the next stage. Death is then seen as the final switching off. Although this model describes a process, it does not describe the mechanism behind the process, except to suggest that it is genetic.

Another theory is that of 'accumulation of random error', which is based on the idea of body tissue showing 'wear and tear' over time due to random errors in the transmission of information in the form of ribonucleic acid (RNA) from the genes to the cell body so that the activities of the parenchyma (active cells of an organ) will be impaired. This is seen as a cumulative process which will eventually affect the whole individual.

This latter theory explains the slower rate of cell division, growth and repair in the elderly which has implications if an individual sustains injury or becomes unwell due to disease. The slowed rate of cell production may be less than the rate of cell destruction, so that healing is delayed and disease processes are more difficult to reverse than in a younger age group.

As the ageing process progresses, morbidity rises, the elderly being prone to degenerative conditions. It could be argued that one of the costs of longevity is multiple disease when the body is least able to deal with it. De Beauvoir (1977), in discussing the relationship between old age and disease, suggested that 'old people are overtaken by chronic pathology'.

The major disabilities suffered by the elderly are vascular disease, especially heart disease and cerebrovascular accidents, chronic respiratory disease, musculoskeletal disorders, mental and nervous conditions and visual impairments. Other disabilities which may not necessarily bring an individual to hospital are incontinence and those conditions resulting from poor nutrition and environment.

The patients seen in hospital are generally showing the combined effects of normal physiological ageing and of disease processes. This may give an inaccurate and depressing view of old age where in fact many individuals, in spite of the ageing process, lead a full and rewarding life into extreme old age. There are increasing numbers of individuals living a relatively independent life well into their 80s and beyond.

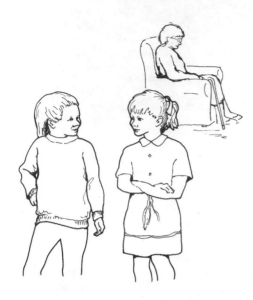

Psychological ageing

A slowing of regeneration of cells could be expected to bring a slowing in mental functioning to parallel the physiological changes. Difficulty in learning, remembering and adapting to change are areas where ageing is seen to have an effect, but often this effect is only illusory and related to observed behaviour rather than actual ability.

Much depends on the attitude of the individual. Those who remain mentally alert may have little difficulty in learning, and many elderly people take up new areas of interest when they retire. Self-image is important here, for if someone feels that he is 'useless' because he is no longer a working member of society, he may well become 'useless' by default. The 'generation gap' between old and young can have an effect in that the attitudes of others can reinforce feelings of 'being past it', so that the elderly person, instead of being encouraged to share his wisdom gained over the years, is relegated to a subordinate position in the home and in society.

Recent memory may suffer lapses in old age but often memory of the past is enhanced. This, too, varies from individual to individual. Memory lapses may result in the development of the habit of double-checking that actions have been taken (for example, locking the door or putting out milk bottles) or in accidents such as kettles being boiled dry or meals missed. In either situation, relatives may become irritated, worried and exasperated and this will have a severe effect on the individual's self-image.

An inability to adapt to change may be due not to mental changes but to physiological changes, such as failing vision, where the familiar situation can be handled but the new creates a challenge which may be resisted since it might mean admitting to deficits. Psychological ageing, then, may be largely produced by the attitudes of the elderly person, in terms of his concept of his own worth, by others' attitudes towards him which affect his self-image, or by physical deficits which he seeks to minimize by resisting change.

Social effects of ageing

It is not only by the immediate family that the self-image of an elderly person can be undermined, but by society in general. Expectations are laid down throughout life which set an individual's place in society and the way that individual is expected to behave. These expectations are largely tied to the work ethic. Young children are educated in preparation for employment, adults are expected to work, and those who do not are seen as a liability to society. The fact that all employees pay towards pensions, through their firm and/or the government, seems to have little effect on attitudes. Retirement could be seen as an earned opportunity for an easier life, yet all too often it is seen as something which is forced upon a person at a certain age and has to be borne along with possible financial hardship and a restricted lifestyle.

Such social factors will not only alter an individual's self-image but may also affect his physiological health if he is deprived of adequate nutrition, warmth and status. Many individuals choose their social companions from work. In old age, with no job, and peers and possibly a partner dying, loneliness may also be a social factor in ageing. Harper (1991) suggests that in order to enhance the quality of life and to encourage independent functioning in the elderly, it is important to take into account the interrelationship of physical, social and psychological factors.

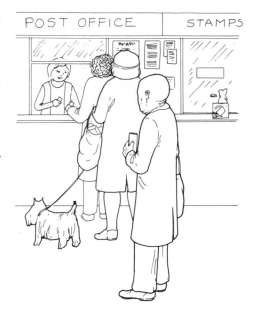

The needs of the elderly patient

Although care of the elderly is accepted as a separate area of both medical and nursing expertise, elderly patients are admitted to most hospital wards. They may be seen to have different needs from other patients because of the possibility of multiple diagnoses, which are exacerbated by the ageing process. Helping individuals to reach their potential while accepting that this may move in a negative direction requires imaginative care from all members of the health care team.

Assessment of the elderly patient needs particular care since methods of coping with deficits at home may prove difficult in hospital and give an inaccurate view of an individual's potential for self-care. For example, old age may be accompanied by sensory loss. In hospital this will be very apparent since visual deficits may lead to bumps and falls while auditory deficits will show up as the patient fails to respond to questions or directions.

Careful assessment may show that the layout of furniture at home is so well known that visual deficits do not impede mobility. Old people living alone often have the radio or television sound on very loud and have a family who know they have to raise their voices to be heard. In assessing normal coping mechanisms rather than the patient's performance in hospital, a more accurate picture may be built of the individual's potential for self-care, which hopefully will avoid over-dependence developing during a hospital stay. It is all too easy to allow an individual to become institutionalized in an environment with which he is not familiar (Denham 1990).

Mobility

Decreased mobility is a cause for concern on a number of counts, not least that it carries a risk of pressure sores which may take a long while to heal. Further, if an individual does not move, mental stimulation may be decreased, leading to apathy and possibly depression. Inability to get from place to place may cause problems of continence if the lavatory cannot be reached in time, and problems in maintaining adequate fluid intake and nutrition if it is an effort to get to the shops or indeed to the kitchen. There may also be problems of personal and environmental cleanliness leading to social isolation.

Individuals may be able to compensate for immobility at home. Many old people virtually live in the kitchen so it is only a few steps to the kettle and stove. They may have kindly neighbours who shop for them and provide stimulating company. They may have regular social services such as meals-on-wheels, a home-help or a regular visit from the district nurse or care assistant for personal hygiene.

Inability to reach the toilet in time may lead to the use of a plastic bucket kept conveniently by bed or chair. Problems often do not arise until either well-meaning relatives persuade the individual to come to live with them, or he is admitted to hospital because of physical deficits. The systems for coping which had been developed then become inappropriate so that the individual is seen to have multiple problems, one of which is incontinence.

Decreased mobility may occur for a number of reasons. Sensory loss, for example, may lead to an individual remaining at home where he feels safe. Physical illness leading to weakness or breathlessness, e.g. anaemia or chronic bronchitis, may lead to immobility and a reluctance to get up. Lack of mental stimulation, which may be linked to decreased mobility, may lead to complete immobility as the individual feels unable to make any effort. Physical pain may also lead to decreased mobility. This may be caused by disease, such as osteoarthritis or ischaemia, or by foot complaints, such as bunions or unattended toe nails.

When the patient is admitted to hospital many of the physical deficits may be treated. For example, a hearing aid may enhance auditory sensation and spectacles or an operation for removal of cataracts may improve vision. Chiropody may improve comfort of the feet, while treating the cause of physical deficits and relieving pain may help a patient towards increased mobility.

If the patient is nervous of the strange environment or depressed and apathetic, support will be needed to encourage him to move around. This aspect of care is easy to neglect on a general ward, particularly since it is time consuming. For example, it takes less time to bring a commode to the bedside than to help a patient walk to the toilet using a Zimmer aid.

Care should be aimed, where possible, towards rehabilitation, but this carries a risk, for when an unsteady patient is encouraged to become mobile he may fall. What tends to occur to counteract this is 'defensive nursing', in which the patient is over-protected to avoid accidents. The reality is that accidents will occasionally occur. What is important is that the patient is neither neglected nor over-protected.

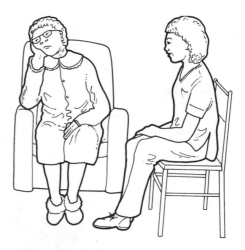

Incontinence

Incontinence may have physiological, psychological and sociological effects on the individual. Pressure sores are more likely to arise in incontinent than continent patients (Norton *et al.* 1975). There is also the problem of irritation caused by acid urine and the risk of infection following scratching of the sore skin. The incontinence may be both faecal and urinary, and cause the individual embarrassment. Vicious circles may arise, for, as immobility enhances the possibility of incontinence, incontinence itself may cause psychological and social embarrassment which reduces mobility, as the patient may not dare to move away from home and the handy bucket.

In the elderly, the bladder loses sensitivity to fullness, which may result in a lack of awareness of the need to micturate. When the bladder is full it will empty and this is described as sensory incontinence. Urge incontinence occurs when the feeling of a need to micturate has to be met immediately. This commonly occurs in urinary infection or in men where the prostate gland is enlarged. Incontinence may also be of the dribbling type, which may occur after prostatectomy or as a result of physical disease. Drugs, for example diuretics, may increase the possibility of urinary incontinence and stress may also have an effect, as may depression and apathy, where it is too much trouble to get out of the bed or chair to go to the toilet.

An individual may control his incontinence at home by strategically placed buckets, by the use of incontinence pads and pants (Figure 12.1) or more crudely by using pads of old sheeting to soak up the urine. He may deal with embarrassment about the condition and the smell by refusing social invitations and by keeping visitors at bay. If the individual lives with younger relatives, he may find himself in extreme disfavour if he dribbles onto carpets, good chairs and expensive mattresses. Relationships may disintegrate, leaving an individual feeling an outcast, useless and a disgrace to the family.

Mary Cotton suffered from occasional incontinence which she dealt with at home by having a plastic pail by her chair or bed, covered with a tea cloth. Unfortunately she had memory lapses which led to a small fire in her kitchen on one occasion, and the police taking her home from a shopping spree on another occasion. Her only daughter decided to take her into her home so that she would be safe.

Mrs Cotton had to take on the rules of her daughter's house, which did not allow pails or tea cloths in the living or bedrooms. She had to deal with the added stress of being treated as a naughty child when she ruined an electric kettle by putting it on the gas stove to heat, and put all the cutlery into the wrong drawer. Her incontinence increased, as did her mental aberration. She forgot that she was only allowed to sit on an old chair with a pad on it and, as a result, wetted an antique sofa. She awoke at nights and wet the floor while she looked for the non-existent pail.

The daughter was frantic and really believed that her mother was being deliberately naughty, when in fact Mrs Cotton was extremely distressed and miserable.

Fig. 12.1 Incontinence pads and pants. Reproduced with kind permission of Simcare Ltd.

Similar situations may occur if an individual is admitted to hospital. The change of environment will bring

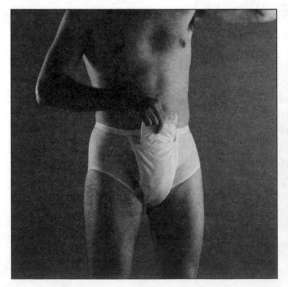

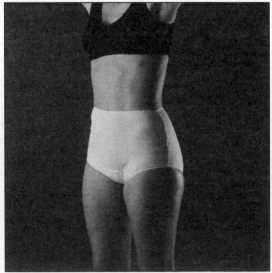

stress, as will the dependence on others for access to bedpan, commode or lavatory. The nurse may become impatient if she finds a wet bed when she brings a bedpan or if the patient urinates on the floor on his way to the toilet.

The situation may be eased for the patient if the nurse can gain an accurate assessment of the patient's problems and methods of coping. If, for example, the patient suffers from frequency, nursing care may include offering bedpans at hourly intervals. Similarly, if incontinence pads and pants, or something similar, are used at home, they should also be available in hospital. Such arrangements should reduce the patient's stress and help in maintaining maximum continence.

Individual feelings need to be appreciated. Incontinence can diminish any individual's self-image, especially those who have prided themselves on being clean. Admonishments and signs of disgust or intolerance on the part of the carers will do further harm, and make little contribution to rehabilitation.

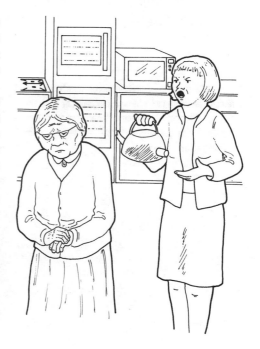

Urinary incontinence is a very common problem in the elderly, and faecal incontinence is not unusual, most often being due to chronic constipation. Diet may be a contributing factor. Hospital food is often low in fibre, or offers fibre in a form unacceptable to the patient. This, and reduced opportunities to exercise, may cause constipation in any patient. Faeces which are not passed at regular intervals tend to get hard and impacted as fluid is reabsorbed through the bowel wall. Faeces which are produced above the impacted mass, and which are unformed due to bacterial action, bypass the solid faeces and are passed as a loose offensive stool.

As with urinary incontinence, this may cause considerable stress and anxiety to the patient. Nursing care will include explaining to the individual why the problem has arisen and reassuring him that the impacted faeces will be removed and the cause dealt with where possible.

Enemas and suppositories, which may be used to clear an impacted bowel, are both potentially embarrassing procedures for a patient. Nursing care will include adequate explanation and reassurance that is strengthened by physical support, in that the patient will not be left without rapid access to bedpan, commode or toilet, and will be cleaned and freshened afterwards.

Whether incontinence is faecal, urinary or both, care should be taken to regularly clean and protect the patient's skin with barrier creams. Not only will this reduce the possibility of pressure sores or infections occurring,

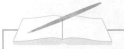

Look at the care plan for an elderly patient for whom you are responsible. Which problems are compounded by the ageing process? What goals have been set for handling two of these problems? Can you suggest further improvement to this patient's care?

but it will also reduce the offensive odour which arises from stale urine or faeces.

In rehabilitating an individual, incontinence cannot be considered in isolation. The patient's physical and psychological state may be affecting control, as may mobility, fluid intake and nutrition. Another important factor may be the clothes that are worn. Trousers with buttoning flies are often preferred by elderly men to the more quickly opened zip-fasteners of modern trousers. Underwear is often heavy and difficult to wash. If braces are worn, it can take a considerable time to prepare clothing so that a patient can have his bowels open.

Women have similar problems with corsets, voluminous knickers and several layers of clothes. There are clothes available for both men and women which aid rapid access for toilet purposes. In helping a patient towards self-care it is easy to forget discussion about suitable clothing when nightwear is being worn, as is usual on a general ward. Any discussion of clothes will need to take cognizance of the individual's beliefs about clothes and his financial state. It may be possible to adapt existing clothing in a way that is useful and acceptable to the elderly person.

Safety

Sensory loss, decreased mobility and incontinence may all affect an individual's safety. Bumps and falls may affect the integrity of the skin at best and the bones at worst, with fractures of the neck of the femur being common among the elderly. Poor mobility may affect safety, particularly if it is paired with urinating on the floor when the

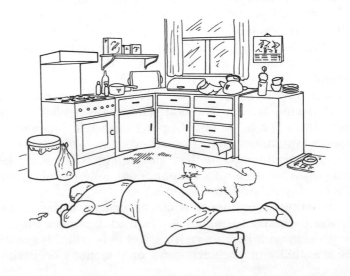

toilet cannot be reached in time. An elderly person, living alone, may be on the floor for hours after slipping on a puddle of urine.

Safety may also be affected by memory lapses. If a gas fire is turned on and not lit, fumes may overcome the individual. If meals are forgotten or the fire not lit, the body temperature may fall to a dangerous level. Other memory lapses may cause fires and the risk of burns, as in the case where a kettle boils dry and the individual picks it up by the overheated handle.

As the elderly person begins to suffer the deficits caused by ageing, a real problem arises for those who feel they are responsible for his safety. At first sight, taking the elderly person at risk into a loving family home may appear to be the perfect answer. However, problems may be similar to those of Mrs Cotton and her daughter, in that the daughter's home was simply not geared up for a forgetful, incontinent elderly woman. The result was, and is so often, misery on both sides.

One alternative is to leave the elderly person alone with adequate Social Services and neighbourhood support. One can argue that even if the individual has a smelly pail by the chair, and indulges in other unsavoury habits such as using a cup several times without washing it, or licking his spoons and forks and putting them away, he is not actually doing any harm to himself or others.

For the elderly, as for any individual, choices have to be made between the quality and quantity of life. In the main, if an individual is coping with living alone, albeit at an unacceptable level to his relatives, he should be left to be independent if that is what he chooses. If as a result he does fall or have an accident it should be seen as the cost of independence rather than the responsibility of his relatives.

When such a patient is admitted to hospital it may be tempting to view his condition as a case of neglect. It should be remembered that this is not necessarily the case. His damage on admission may be purely physical, whereas, in a strange place where his coping mechanisms are taken from him, his eventual damage may be both physical and psychological.

Of course there are elderly people who live with their families in harmony. This is easier in the extended rather than in the nuclear family, though here too, living with relatives may work well, especially if there is a 'granny flat' available which maintains privacy on both sides.

Defensive nursing has been mentioned in relation to mobility. What is required in hospital is preventive nurs-

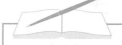

Think of an elderly person whom you know (preferably a family member). What is **your** attitude to his/her

1 intelligence
2 ability for self-care
3 general lifestyle?

Try to identify the factors affecting how you perceive the individual. If this elderly person were admitted to hospital, do you think that your colleagues' perception of him/her would be different from yours? In what ways would they differ?

Fig. 12.2 Zimmer aids.

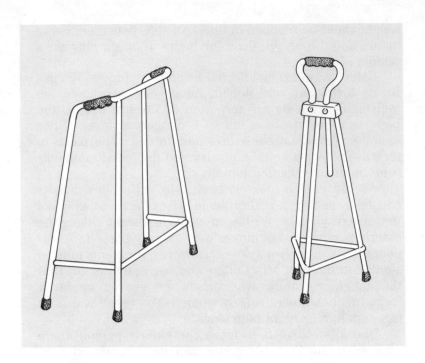

ing – the need to encourage mobility and prevent pressure sores and dependence being paramount in planning care. There are a number of aids to help an individual walk safely such as sticks and Zimmer aids (Figure 12.2). The physiotherapist may help an individual towards self-care while maintaining safety. The nurse will have a role in reinforcing and encouraging the patient so that his confidence is increased.

Dignity and identity

Too often, elderly individuals are treated as if they were irresponsible children rather than thinking adults who are dealing with the problems of ageing, loneliness and perhaps financial hardship. With failing faculties they may have to accept role reversal within the family and society as they grapple with decreased mobility, incontinence and other embarrassments.

This trend is often continued in hospital, where courtesies offered to other patients are frequently denied to anyone who is elderly. One example which has been mentioned in an earlier chapter is that of name. Being called 'Gran' can be seen to be both patronizing and offensive if it has not been established that the patient is happy with such a term. If asked, a patient may say, 'Oh, call me Granny Woodruffe – everyone does', while another may say, 'My name is Miss Bobbet'. Both deserve their title of choice.

Other areas which undermine an individual's dignity and identity are also associated with choice. Mobile patients may choose to sit by the bed, visit another patient or to go the day-room to watch television. The elderly immobile patient may be denied this choice by the nurse who puts him where she thinks he should be. Similarly sensory loss may lead a nurse to make meal choices rather than ask the patient. Even if hearing is affected and the individual is unable to read the menu, the nurse should attempt to discuss his preferences.

Dignity and identity will only be maintained by feedback from those with whom the patient comes into contact. Being treated as an individual of worth can help a patient to accept the deficits of ageing. The essence of a person does not change with an ageing body, and elderly people do not need the distress of being relegated to a 'geriatric' category.

Sexuality

Sexuality and sexual identity do not change as a part of the ageing process. Cormack (1985a) identifies the position of the elderly as often being given less attention than it should be because the youth-oriented society that many Western countries have developed places a further barrier in the way of fully considering the sexuality of all adult age groups. One of the problems here is in defining sexuality in terms of sexual activity. In fact, part of the sexuality of each individual is the need to be loved and to feel of worth. However, many elderly people do have an active sexual relationship and miss it considerably when they are hospitalized for any reason. It does not help an elderly patient if he feels that the young nurses who care for him ridicule any signs of sexuality in his behaviour.

A problem for the elderly is that they have to face the reality of their partner dying at a time when social contacts may be shrinking. Loneliness is part of the grief, but for many it is linked with sexual loss.

Mr McGregor had been married for almost 50 years when his wife died. When she had been dead for six months, Mr McGregor shocked his family by advertising for a companion.

The advertisement read 'Virile and active man of 76 years seeks female companion with a view to permanent relationship'. There were 20 replies, 19 from lonely widows wishing to remarry and one from a lonely homosexual. All the applicants were over 65 years old. Mr McGregor visited most of the women, taking them for drives, visits or meals. In the event he turned them all down, explaining to his son that he had hoped for a younger woman who would outlive him.

Many elderly male patients embarrass nurses by flirting with them and are subsequently dismissed as 'dirty old men'. In fact these patients may be suffering from sexual loneliness and simply enjoy the sight of young women around them. Each nurse will develop her own methods of dealing with male patients who attempt to flirt, and the elderly should be treated in the same way as the young. So often the elderly patient is admonished with reference to his age. The remark 'Oh, for heaven's sake – and you a grandfather?' diminishes a man's sexuality and the value of what might be a genuine compliment.

Similarly with female patients. It should not be assumed that elderly females do not retain sexuality.

Mrs Brown (a widow) was very insulted when the nurse who was assessing her ability to cope after mastectomy said, 'I usually ask a question about sexual adjustment but I guess you don't worry about that at your age'. Mrs Brown explained that her boyfriend lived in an adjoining flat and that the only reason they had not married was because it would reduce their pension.

Sexual activity may slow with age, but it does not necessarily cease. Similarly, sexual identity is an integral part of every human being throughout life.

Loneliness

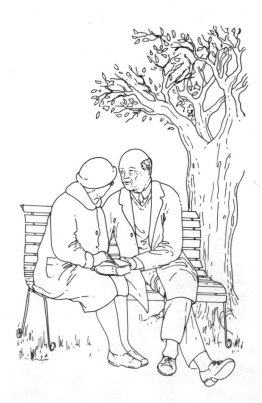

Some psychologists talk of 'disengagement' in the elderly, observing that interaction with society decreases with age. One theory is that this is a voluntary process in which isolation is chosen, while the other point of view is that society disengages from the old rather than the reverse.

What is undoubtedly true is that the elderly generally have fewer interactions than when they were young, and that, for many, loneliness is a real problem. Decreased mobility, embarrassment over incontinence, financial hardship and the increase in nuclear families are all factors which increase the risk of loneliness, as is age itself when peers may die or move away to live with relatives.

Over-60s clubs, SAGA holidays and day centres are examples of ways in which the elderly may meet and interact, but there remain many elderly people who are alone and lonely. When company is available for these people, they often talk endlessly as if to make up for the hours alone. This desire to talk – usually about the past – can be seen when an elderly lonely patient is admitted to hospital. He may talk to other patients or the nurse and may be nicknamed a 'chatterbox', yet the individual may go for whole days at home without talking to anyone.

In assessing elderly patients, loneliness should be considered as a potential problem. It may be that an individual is unaware of facilities in his area, or that relatives are unaware of how little interaction is available to the patient. Providing that the patient is unhappy about his isolation, it should be possible to improve this area of his life through social and voluntary services. Relatives may not be able or willing to visit regularly. This may be due to geographical location, work commitments or lifestyle, or simply that the family members are not close emotionally. The kindly elderly patient may also be a difficult elderly relative.

Confusion

Confusion may occur in the elderly due to physiological, psychological or social change. Physiological reasons include electrolyte and resulting fluid imbalance, infections, and diseases leading to a reduction in cerebral oxygenation. Psychological reasons include mental trauma such as bereavement, or upheaval such as occurs when an elderly person is moved into care. Social factors include a change of environment (Figure 12.3).

From the above, it can be seen that the ill, elderly patient admitted to hospital is very likely to be confused. The confusion is equally likely to be temporary in nature unless it is caused by physiological changes that cannot be reversed. It is important to make the situation clear to relatives who may be distressed by the manifestations of confusion.

Confusion may take many forms, the patient becoming abusive, failing to recognize friends and family, referring to past events as if they were happening at the moment, or becoming deluded about present people and surroundings. Alternatively the patient may become quiet and withdrawn, seeming to be unaware of place or time. It is dangerous to label people in such circumstances, since when a patient is labelled 'confused' this is often interpreted to mean that nothing said by the patient is to be taken seriously. The criteria for deeming an individual 'confused' must also be used with caution.

Fig. 12.3   Causes of confusion.

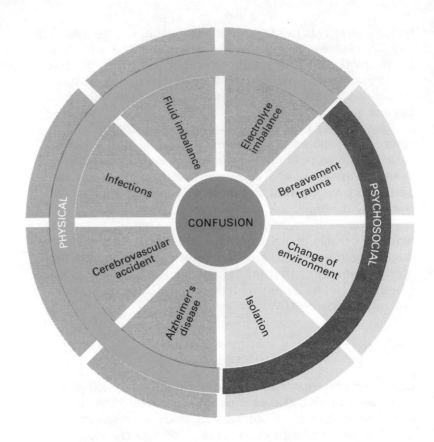

nnie Jones was admitted to hospital with a fractured neck of femur following a fall. She appeared confused after her operation and was later visited by a doctor who asked her a number of questions to ascertain her mental state. 'Who is the Prime Minister?', he asked. 'What day is it? and what month?' Mrs Jones knew the Prime Minister's name but could not recall the day of the week or the month. She burst into tears and was declared confused.

Later, Mrs Jones told a nurse that she had lost her watch which she described as silver with a white strap. The nurse told her not to worry. Several times during the day the patient asked about her watch and was told that she should not worry. The belief that the request for the watch was part of the patient's confusion was so strong that no one looked for it.

By evening, the patient was extremely agitated since the watch was of great sentimental value. Her agitation and aggression were seen as further signs of confusion until Night Sister, coming into the ward, stopped by Mrs Jones's bed. When asked for the watch, she looked in the locker, found the watch and gave it to the patient. The difference between Night Sister and the other nurses was that the Sister did not know the patient had been considered confused.

Confusion in hospital, due to the mental upset and social change associated with admission, may soon be resolved if the patient settles in well and learns to trust the staff. However, relatives may fear that this precludes the patient returning to safe self-care, especially if the confusion is linked with memory lapses. Careful assessment needs to be made of a patient's mental state. It may be that the temporary confusion of hospitalization will reappear for a while on discharge, since this will represent further upheaval. This can be monitored by community staff.

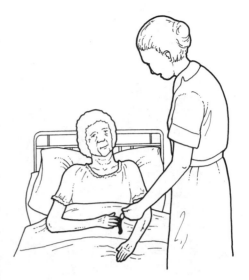

Permanent confusion is described as senile dementia or brain failure. Cormack (1985b) suggests that dementia is currently seen as the same as Alzheimer's disease and there is an increasing use of the term 'senile dementia of Alzheimer type'.

In this condition there is a slow and gradual onset of problems. The patient, before showing any signs of intellectual impairment, may be restless, agitated, irritable and particularly suspicious. This suspiciousness can be compounded by the effect on short-term memory and, in the later stages, on long-term memory, added to which there is a possibility of both hallucinations and delusions.

It can be seen that as the disease progresses, the individual's ability to make decisions or to live independently are severely affected. Relatives may be unwilling to take the patient into their home because of the many difficulties in the patient's behaviours and the physical danger that can be caused by confusion. Such patients usually require admission to a psychiatric ward for care.

Vi Stevenson lived alone in sheltered accommodation. She was a spry woman of 82 who was very proud of her home and her few possessions. Her relatives realized that she was getting confused when she appeared to forget recent events and spent a lot of time talking about the past. Because she was confused, she often mislaid things that she needed and this did not in the initial stages cause much problem. However, increasing suspiciousness and delusions caused Vi to come to believe that her possessions were being stolen by a neighbour. The Administrator of the sheltered accommodation decided that they could no longer have Vi in their care after she was found one rainy night standing outside a neighbour's window shouting, 'Christians don't steal'. Miss Stevenson had been looking for a particular hat, had not found it and become convinced that her neighbour had taken it from her.

As the dementia increases, the patient may need permanent care from others since they may be unable to remember to feed themselves, go to the toilet, wash themselves and other normal daily activities. What is important in nursing care is to distinguish between the normal forgetfulness of the elderly and senile dementia which, as has

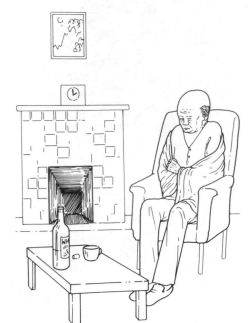

been seen, has more permanent and long-lasting effects.

Nutrition and warmth

Given the many problems that may be encountered by the elderly, it could be expected that any or all of them may be factors in reduced self-care, especially nutrition and warmth. Although the state pension in the UK is thought to be adequate for a healthy standard of living, and may be enhanced by supplementary benefits and rebates for the needy, there is nevertheless a considerable amount of poverty among the elderly.

Much of the poverty is secondary. That is, it is caused by the way the available money is spent rather than because the income is insufficient for survival. Much of the money which theoretically should buy goods to meet basic physiological needs, such as food and warmth, may be spent on meeting other needs. For example, the lonely person may find comfort in alcohol or attempt to buy company by providing refreshments or treats for visitors. That pensions do not usually provide enough money for more than basic needs is a social problem. The effects in terms of poor nutrition on the elderly may become a nursing problem when a patient comes into care.

Even if there is enough money for food and warmth, the elderly may still suffer from hypothermia and malnutrition because of other deficits. Poor mobility, sensory loss and memory lapses can all contribute, as may loneliness. It is not unusual for an elderly person to be admitted to hospital with a report stating that the individual's home has been found devoid of food, but that there was money in the house. In other instances, all that is found is empty alcohol bottles. One patient who was asked about this explained that 'whisky is warming, does not need cooking, relieves hunger pangs and provides cheer'.

Confusion may also lead to hypothermia and malnutrition in that the individual may lose his sense of time and place. Eating may occur on a haphazard basis but is unlikely to constitute a balanced diet, and it is probable that fires will not be lit. Some people may have automatic central heating, though many do not. Even here the confused person may suffer if he forgets to pay bills and the energy supplies are cut off.

In assessing a patient's nutritional needs it is important to understand his normal eating patterns and food preferences. Care should be planned not only to restore the individual's health but to ensure that his health does not deteriorate on discharge. This means organizing

Social Services for him such as meals-on-wheels, or perhaps arranging for new dentures if mastication is a problem.

In planning for the future the individual's co-operation must be sought. Meals-on-wheels may be dismissed as 'charity' which a person is too proud to accept. It may be that he does not understand that he will be able to pay for them. Exploring concerns will help to elicit the reasons for resistance to help. Similarly with dentures. If the patient does not accept the idea as useful, it is unlikely that he will wear the dentures.

The interrelated problems of the elderly which cause deficits that may lead to hospitalization are often put down to stubbornness on the part of the patient, along with resistance to change. Such stubbornness may in fact be a defence mechanism, for if an individual clings to the familiar, he can continue to cope, albeit uncomfortably and alone. The alternative may be unpalatable, as it often appears to involve giving up independence and becoming subordinate to family or institution. Each individual must have the right to choose unless he is a real hazard to himself or others.

Specific disease in the elderly

Elderly people may suffer from any disease but are very likely to suffer from those chronic diseases discussed in Chapter 10. Chronic bronchitis and congestive cardiac failure for example do not afflict the elderly as a group, but are usually the product of years of ill-health which are exacerbated by problems of ageing such as slowed cell regeneration, decreased mobility, and poor nutrition.

Some diseases, however, are more common in the elderly than in other age groups. Examples of some of those which are likely to be seen in elderly patients will be discussed, although it should be remembered that many elderly patients are suffering from a number of diseases, in addition to the normal ageing process.

Cerebrovascular accident (CVA)

THE DISEASE PROCESS

Of people with CVA, commonly called a 'stroke', 75% are over 65 years old. Strokes are caused by cerebral thrombosis, haemorrhage or occasionally by an embolism (Figure 12.4). Whatever the cause, the result is an inter-

Fig. 12.4 Cerebrovascular accidents.

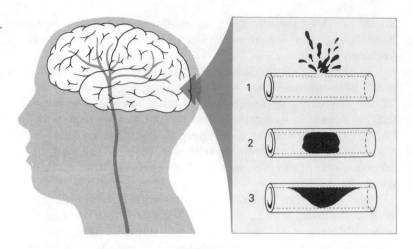

ruption of the blood supply to part of the brain. If the condition is due to thrombosis, this may be associated with atherosclerosis, a tumour causing pressure on cerebral blood vessels or any condition which is accompanied by a reduced intravascular pressure and stasis. If the thrombosis which forms does not become absorbed, necrosis of tissue in the surrounding area of the brain will occur and scar tissue will form.

Cerebral haemorrhage may also occur as a result of atherosclerosis where degenerative changes have weakened an artery. It may also occur as the result of weakness caused by an aneurysm which may be due to chronic inflammation or trauma. Hypertension can predispose to cerebral haemorrhage as pressure is exerted on weakened arterial walls. The resultant haematoma which forms causes pressure and a reduced blood supply to surrounding brain tissue, which is destroyed.

Emboli are a less frequent cause of CVA than thrombosis or haemorrhage. They may be formed from blood, fat, bacteria or tumour cells which are carried to the brain from other parts of the body via the circulation.

Physiological reactions

Physiological reactions will depend on the cause and severity of the CVA. If the cause is thrombosis, the reactions will be of gradual onset, whereas, in the case of haemorrhage or emboli, they will be sudden. Depending on the site and severity of the brain damage, the reactions may range from so slight as to go unnoticed, to relatively severe or so severe that the patient dies. About 50% of people die following CVA.

There are warning signs that give the alert to the possibility of CVA, especially if there is a history of atherosclerosis, hypertension or a recent fall with loss of consciousness. These include complaints of headaches, dizziness and blackouts, blurred vision, changes in speech, or stumbling movements. For the CVA of sudden onset, the individual may simply lose consciousness. In severe cases, coma may last several days and result in death. At the other end of the continuum, unconsciousness may be transient.

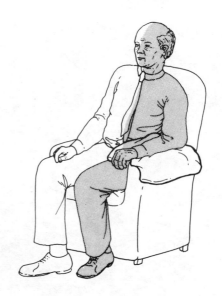

The conscious patient may have severe headaches as a reaction to intracranial pressure, and initial vomiting which is the result of stimulation of the vomiting centre in the medulla. Convulsive movements may also occur as neural pathways are affected by the damage to brain tissue.

Some level of paralysis will be likely to occur as the result of damage to brain tissue. Hemiplegia (paralysis to the side of the body opposite to the side of the brain lesion) is not uncommon. There will be loss of muscle tone and absence of normal reflexes on the affected side of the body. Babinski's reflex may be seen. This is the phenomenon of the big toe bending upwards instead of downwards when the sole of the affected foot is stroked.

If the brain damage is in the left cerebral hemisphere, aphasia may occur in right-handed people as a reaction to damage in the speech centre. Damage to the right cerebral hamisphere may affect the muscles used in speech and produce difficulties in articulation.

The individual's eyes may react to the brain damage. There may be papilloedema as a result of increased intracranial pressure (Figure 12.5) and the pupils may be constricted.

There is a wide range of reactions to brain damage but, in general, the nature and severity of the reactions will give an indication of the site and extent of the damage to brain tissue.

Psychological reactions

Intellectual capacity may be affected depending on the extent and site of the damage caused by the CVA. Psychological reactions to CVA are likely to be more severe in the individual who suddenly becomes unconscious and who later awakes to find himself in hospital with obvious disabilities. He may be shocked and anxious to find himself paralysed and unable to express himself. Fear may also be a reaction to such a situation.

If intellect is affected, the individual may show little reaction to his state. Relatives, however, are likely to react with anxiety and apprehension to the thought that the

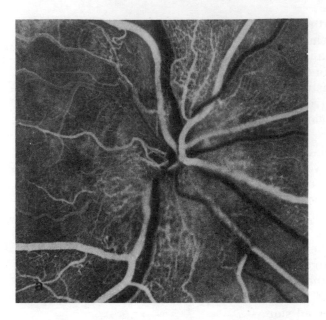
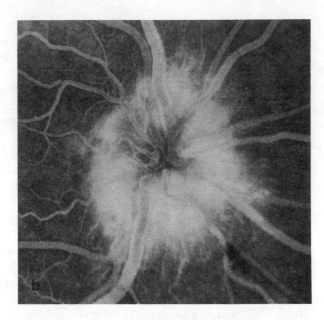

Fig. 12.5 Appearance of the retina in the early arterial phase (*left*) and late phase (*right*) of papilloedema. Reproduced from Swash and Mason (1984) with kind permission of the authors.

patient may become a 'cabbage'. Similarly, relatives are very likely to react with anxiety as a response to the patient's unconsciousness.

Social reactions

For the individual whose CVA was of gradual onset, hospitalization may be a relief as vague symptoms take on meaning. For those who suddenly become unconscious, social reactions will most likely occur within the family, whose members have to cope with the uncertainty of a serious diagnosis of doubtful outcome.

PLANNING NURSING CARE

Physical care

If the patient is unconscious, care will be planned as suggested earlier. For the conscious patient, the aim of care will be towards rehabilitation, given the constraints of any permanent disability. This will include the prevention of complications such as contractures, partial dislocation of joints (subluxation), pressure sores and respiratory difficulties.

The patient is likely to be nursed quietly in bed for the first few days of consciousness until it is established that bleeding, if present, has ceased. Depending on the severity of the CVA, a considerable amount of nursing care may be needed to maintain adequate breathing, nutrition and fluid intake. The skin of elderly patients is likely to be more vulnerable to pressure than that of younger patients, so especial care should be taken to retain its integrity.

Observations are important following a CVA. Blood pressure and recordings of temperature, pulse and respiration can indicate changes in response to the bleeding. A rise in blood pressure with a related slowing of respiration and pulse may mean that bleeding is continuing and causing increased intracranial pressure, while a weak pulse which is accompanied by a fall in blood pressure may mean a dangerous reduction in circulation due to blood loss from the system.

Fluid balance should be recorded. The patient may have intravenous fluids prescribed and, if unconscious or unable to control micturition, may be catheterized. If the patient has been unconscious, the swallowing reflex needs to be tested before a light nourishing diet is commenced. Medication may be prescribed for headaches but a balance must be maintained between relieving pain and masking neurological symptoms. For this reason aspirin is often the drug of choice. Other medication such as diuretics may be prescribed if symptoms suggest a need for them.

It is important for the nurse to report any changes in the patient's condition, whether improvement or deterioration, which may lead to a need for some modification of the care being given.

Communication is very important with patients, even when they appear to be unconscious, for it is known that hearing is the last faculty to disappear. The patient will need considerable reassurance as consciousness is regained for he may be very frightened about what has happened to him and what the possibilities are for the future.

As a patient becomes well enough to commence rehabilitation, other health professionals will be involved in his care. The physiotherapist and occupational therapist may be involved in physical rehabilitation if hemiplegia is present, while the speech therapist may be required for the aphasic patient. The nurse's role in rehabilitation is in co-ordination and support of the work of the specialist. For example, if an individual is learning to talk again following a CVA, the nurse should use every interaction with the patient as an opportunity to encourage speech and reinforce progress.

Psychological care

In order that a rehabilitation programme should have the maximum chance of success, the individual needs to be

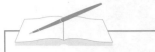

Taking account of the standard aspects of care following a CVA, design a critical pathway plan for a hypothetical patient. What variance would you expect if the patient were elderly?

motivated towards recovery. In the early days following CVA, major feelings may be so immersed in the horror of the present that the future does not register. The patient should be encouraged to express his feelings of fear, anger, guilt or anxiety if such feelings are present. If speech is affected, the patient may feel further trapped as he cannot verbalize his concerns. In this instance, writing may be a possible alternative for some patients.

Although it may be seen as 'natural' to react to disability, each individual will be different. It is important in planning care to assess levels of anxiety and depression and to refer to a counsellor or psychaiatrist if the patient appears unable to cope with his changed self- and body-image. It might be expected that any individual would automatically be motivated towards rehabilitation. Such an assumption cannot be made since each age has its own problems. The elderly person who has seen friends and family die may view his illness as the final straw. The resulting feelings of helplessness and hopelessness need working through with someone who is prepared to listen and understand, and possibly guide feelings into a more positive direction.

When rehabilitation starts, goals need to be carefully set. Knowledge of an individual, his interests and lifestyle can be an aid to setting meaningful goals which will attract the patient's interest. For example, if a patient's wife was going to have a birthday soon and the couple were close, there could be high motivation to learn to say 'Happy Birthday, darling' as a surprise on the day. Goals should be reachable, however, for failure could compound an individual's depression.

It is possible for many stroke patients to learn to speak and walk again and to care for themselves. Each patient requires a careful assessment of his potential for rehabilitation. Psychological support is required for the patient when planning a programme which will take time, effort and concentration on the part of the patient, his family and members of the health care team. This is a difficult area of patient teaching which will only succeed with the co-operation of the individual and his family.

Social care
In planning care, thought needs to be given to the patient's home circumstances. For the elderly patient living alone, a stroke may force him to decide to give up his home and accept the help of others. Such decisions should not be made lightly or while relatives are feeling noble rather than realistic. All avenues and possibilities should be ex-

plored and a decision made which is satisfactory for both the patient and his family.

For patients who can go home to a partner or friend, plans will need to be made so that rehabilitation which is commenced in hospital may continue into the community. This involves relatives since they will be the co-ordinators of the rehabilitation, with help from community services. The Social Services may be required if adaptation of the home is necessary, and can supply aids such as hand grips to fit to the wall near the lavatory and other items which help the patient in his efforts for self-care.

The strain of rehabilitation on an elderly person should not be overlooked. Relatives are as prone to feelings of depression and hopelessness as the patient. Further, they may get tired. Facilities for the family to have a rest should be available and considered as part of care, since if the family is able to cope, the individual may well spend the rest of his life in the community.

THE CARE PLAN

Priorities on the care plan will include protecting the patient from harm and further disability which could affect his chances for recovery. This includes basic nursing care in all areas where the patient is unable to look after himself.

After careful assessment, priority will be given to a realistic programme of rehabilitation. This will start when the patient has been helped to see the possibility of a worthwhile future which may be different from the past but no less rewarding.

The care plan should also include the relatives, who will need help in dealing with the crisis of a disabled individual, but who can be a potential source of help and encouragement to the patient.

Parkinson's disease (paralysis agitans)

THE DISEASE PROCESS

Parkinson's disease is relatively common in the elderly in that the usual onset is from 50 years upwards and 1% of the population over 60 years old suffers from the condition. Since it is a progressive and degenerative disease, many elderly patients with Parkinsonism may be seen on medical and geriatric wards.

The disease affects the functioning of the extra-pyramidal system of the brain, and is thought to be due to a reduction of dopamine, which is essential for normal functioning of the basal ganglia and for neurotran-

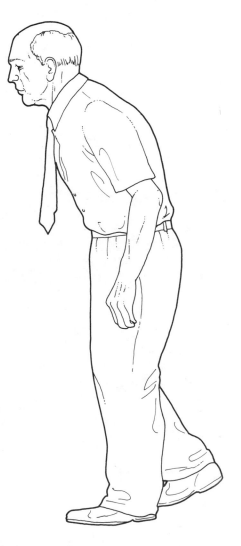

smission. Dopamine is produced by the substantia nigra and is excreted in urine (Tortora and Anagnostakos 1990). It has been found that patients with Parkinson's disease have low levels of urinary dopamine secretion, thus strengthening the theory of the link between the chemical and the disease.

The ageing process may in itself lead to a reduction of dopamine production and cause mild reactions similar to those of Parkinson's disease.

Physical reactions

The major physical reactions to the disease process are tremor, akinesia and muscular rigidity. These are thought to occur as a response to overactivity of neurones which are normally inhibited by dopamine (see Figure 12.6). These reactions develop slowly over time and may start with tremor of a hand when the individual is sitting quietly or resting, although it does not occur during sleep. Voluntary movement will stop the tremor, which will be more apparent when the individual is tired or stressed. As the disease progresses, other limbs may become involved. A typical reaction is that of a 'pill rolling' movement of finger and thumbs caused by tremor.

As the muscles become rigid, the individual may notice feelings of stiffness. There is tonic contraction of skeletal muscles which, as it increases, will lead to a slowing of voluntary movement and difficulties in mobility. Typically the patient will stand for some time before attempting to walk and, when he does, he will move with slow shuffling movements. Self-care may be affected since change of position may be difficult and manual dexterity may be affected.

The head and mouth may become involved as the disease progresses. The rigidity of muscles will affect facial expression, leaving the individual looking empty and expressionless. Speech will be slowed, slurred and expressionless. Eventually the patient may have problems in maintaining adequate nutrition as chewing and swallowing food becomes difficult. There may be over-secretion of saliva because autonomic nervous control is disturbed.

Since all muscles can become involved, problems may arise in breathing, particularly in coughing. The individual may complain of pain and of feeling generally unwell as a reaction to the increased ridigity of muscles and the malfunctioning of the autonomic nervous system.

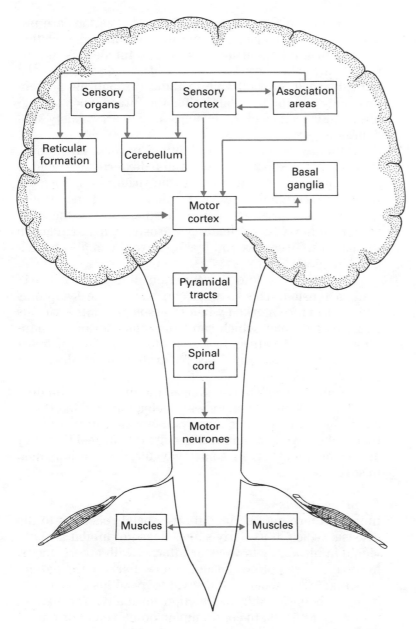

Fig. 12.6 Pathways in the control of voluntary movement.

Psychological reactions

Parkinson's disease progresses very slowly, often causing little difficulty until the condition is well advanced. Slight tremor may cause some psychological reactions but these may be no more than those of minor embarrassment and some concern about cause. Later, as muscle rigidity begins to affect normal lifestyle, concern may grow, so leading the individual to consult his doctor.

The diagnosis, particularly if the implications are understood, can cause considerable emotional reaction from both the patient and his family. Intellect is not affected until the very late stages of the disease, so the individual will be well able to think through his present problems and the possibilities for the future. Such a diagnosis may well lead to feelings of anger, anxiety and depression.

Difficulty in mobility and other normal functioning such as eating, speaking and manual dexterity may lead to acute embarrassment, as may the dribbling associated with over-secretion of saliva. Further, slowed speech and a mask-like expression may lead others to see the individual as slow-witted – leading to frustration and anger in the patient. Tiredness and feeling unwell can also have a psychological effect.

Relatives may find the situation difficult, which will lead to tension. This in turn can exacerbate symptoms which are more marked when stress is present. A vicious circle may develop which can cause considerable unhappiness, as the relatives feel guilty for their lack of tolerance, and the patient feels frustrated, miserable, and possibly depressed.

Spiritual beliefs may suffer as the individual wonders why he has been chosen to bear such an illness, but this is a variable reaction since many patients gain strength from their beliefs while others rail against fate or feel that they are being punished in some way for real or imagined misdeeds.

Social reactions

Initially, there may be few, if any, social reactions to the disease, which in its early stages does not inhibit an individual in his ability to work or interact with others. Later, however, as symptoms become more marked, the patient may react with social withdrawal to avoid his embarrassment in being unable to function normally. The patient may have difficulty in continuing in employment or pursuing active hobbies. Both will add to feelings of isolation. Social relations may also be affected since many individuals find difficulty in dealing with the obvious handicaps of others.

Sexual relationships may also suffer. The slow, expressionless, dribbling individual may bear little relationship to a former partner who was sexually attractive, and the individual himself may have problems with his social and sexual image. Further, muscle rigidity may make intercourse difficult for both partners since spontaneous movement is impeded. Many of the social reactions to

Parkinsonism may be sparked off by psychological tensions as much as by physical disability. This may be a problem for the whole family.

PLANNING NURSING CARE

Physical care

In planning physical care, the effects of chemotherapy will need to be monitored. The current drug of choice is levodopa, which is often prescribed in conjunction with an extracerebral dopa-decarboxylase inhibitor such as benserazide, which enables more of the drug to enter the brain. There are problems in the prescription of levodopa to patients with multiple pathology since there may be an effect on the action of other drugs. If the patient requires surgery, levodopa should be discontinued eight hours before the operation since its interaction with anaesthesia may cause cardiac arrhythmias.

The effect of levodopa is to replenish dopamine levels so that mobility is improved. There is less effect on tremor and, overall, the drug largely offers remission rather than cure. From a nursing view, monitoring is required of the side effects of the drug. These include anorexia, nausea, insomnia, postural hypotension, dizziness, tachycardia, arrhythmia and agitation. A dosage needs to be reached which improves mobility with the minimum of side effects. The benefits of levodopa are most obvious in the first few years of treatment. However, these benefits may decline and the adverse side effects become more severe. These may include abnormal involuntary movements. A classic sign is facial grimacing that is totally beyond the control of the patient and which can cause considerable distress.

By giving levodopa in combination with a decarboxylase inhibitor it is possible for a greater concentration of levodopa to reach the brain, with an accompanying decrease in peripheral side effects.

It is possible, because of the reactions to a diagnosis of Parkinson's disease, that the patient will need antidepressants as part of his drug regime.

In addition to chemotherapy, the individual will be encouraged to remain as mobile and independent as possible. The physiotherapist will organize a programme for the patient but the nurse has a role in encouraging the patient to carry out exercises and to remain as independent as possible. In any disabling illness this can be difficult since the patient may be experiencing emotions such as anger, despair or depression, which will affect motivation.

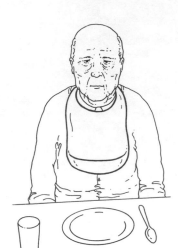

As the disease progresses, problems of self-care will increase and the patient may become incontinent. Basic nursing care will be required to deal with deficits while encouraging any possible self-care. There may be a temptation to do things for a patient because his own attempts are slow. It is important to allow time for the individual to complete tasks, rather than to foster dependence in the interests of efficiency. Elderly people may become anxious if they are hurried. For the patient with Parkinson's disease, anxiety will increase symptoms and feelings of helplessness.

In planning physical care, thought needs to be given to the possibility of discharge and any necessary help required by relatives. Involving family members in plans for the future may help them to understand the need to encourage self-care and to protect the individual's dignity. For example, the patient may dribble, and spill food if he feeds himself, yet he should be encouraged to remain independent in this area for as long as possible. Clothes that are easily washed and drip dry may be preferable to a large version of a child's bib for the patient's self-image.

Psychological care

Psychological care will be similar to that of any patient who is intellectually complete but has to face physical handicap. For the patient who has suffered a stroke there is at least the hope that physical ability will improve with a rehabilitation programme. For the patient with Parkinson's disease, the outlook may be very bleak, particularly when coupled with the ageing process and its limitations.

The individual must be allowed to express his feelings and it may be necessary to offer to refer him to another agency if talking alone does not result in his feeling more able to cope with his condition. If the patient is depressed he may need to see a psychiatrist, whereas if he is rejecting his faith, he may be helped by a minister. It is unrealistic to suppose that all patients will come to terms with their diagnosis but it is true that many will reach acceptance if they have a chance to consider and express their feelings about both the present and the future.

Relatives may also need to talk. If the patient lives alone, difficult decisions may need to be made about the future. If he lives with others, they will need to consider their role in his future. The patient must also be involved in such decisions, which may have psychological implications if the reality is painful and unpalatable.

Once the reality of the disease has been discussed, it is

essential that the individual is motivated towards the maximum mobility and self-care for as long as possible. Individuals will vary enormously in this respect. In some, anger may be channelled into determined independence while others may give up hope and become apathetic. It is a challenge to find motivators so that realistic goals may be set for continued self-care.

As the disease progresses, incontinence and increased dependence will be potential problems in that self-respect will suffer. The manner in which the nurse interacts with the patient can have an effect. If the patient is reprimanded for unsocial behaviour, his self-esteem will suffer a further loss. Positive action, however, such as regular offering of urinals, gentle cleansing of dribbling saliva, and care when feeding will help the individual to retain his identity in a difficult situation.

Social care

When a patient with Parkinson's disease is admitted to hospital, his illness will almost certainly have been with him for some time, although he may have been receiving medication from his General Practitioner. This means that social, and possibly sexual, problems may have been present for some time.

In planning care, when these problems have been assessed, it may be possible to suggest action which will help the patient and his family. There are many practical aids for the home such as strategically placed hand bars, raised toilets, and non-slip floor coverings, which will reduce dependence on others; and similarly with clothing. If button-up clothing is avoided and care given to ease of dressing, self-care may continue for longer than would be possible with conventional clothes. These practical measures will, in fostering independence, allow an individual to retain not only independence, but an acceptable self-image for the maximum time.

Problems with social relationships may take longer to resolve and expert help may be necessary. Involving both the patient and his family in discussions may prove useful since neither may be aware of the other's perspective. Increased understanding may decrease tension, although some partners may feel unable to cope with the change, especially if the patient's reactions to his disease appear to have affected his personality.

Sexual problems may need the help of a counsellor who is skilled in helping the disabled. Again, it must be remembered that there may be problems in terms of distaste for a disabled partner. Careful assessment is necessary in such situations, for many couples may not have

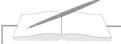

Mr Smith has Parkinson's disease. He lives with his (much younger) wife and is determined to remain independent on discharge from hospital. His problems include incontinence and difficulty with feeding and dressing. List the practical measures which might help the couple. Plan some open questions which will help you identify Mr Smith's reaction to his current situation.

problems and could be offended by inferences that difficulties exist. It is important to establish the nature of a relationship prior to identifying problems.

The Social Services may be able to assist with practical help so that a patient can remain in his own home. If this is not possible, the relatives' perspective needs to be understood so that individuals are not left feeling guilty because they cannot meet their relatives' or partners' needs.

THE CARE PLAN

The priorities for care will be concerned with enabling the patient to retain independence and self-respect for as long as possible. This will include monitoring medication and supporting the physiotherapy programme.

In the care plan, the individual should be assessed within the framework of his social situation, and his partner's and relatives' needs should be accepted.

Psychological care will include giving the patient the opportunity to express feelings in the hope that he will accept his diagnosis and become motivated to co-operate with the health care team.

Care will also be planned with the aim of returning the patient to society and with the best possible relationships, given the constraints of his disease.

Osteoarthritis

THE DISEASE PROCESS

Osteoarthritis is a chronic degenerative disease which is common in elderly patients, normally affecting one or more weight-bearing joints. The cartilage which normally protects the bones at their articulation point wears down over time until eventually the bone is exposed. Movement without protective cartilage produces thickening and irregularities of the bone surfaces with outgrowths (osteophytes), which may break off (Figure 12.7).

The exact cause of osteoarthritis is not known but the ageing process and overweight are thought to contribute to the condition. Trauma to the joint may also be a factor, although this has not been firmly established. The joints commonly affected are the hip, knee and spine. Joints of fingers and toes may also be affected by osteoarthritis.

Physical reactions

Reduced mobility and pain in the affected joint are reactions to the lack of a protective cartilage at articulation

Wear and tear causing thinning and cracking of articular cartilage

Loss of joint space

Osteophytes caused by bone overgrowth

Capsule contraction may deform joint

Exposed bone surface becoming thickened and polished

Fig. 12.7 Osteoarthritic damage to the hip.

points. The thickening of bones can be felt as enlarged joints which are irregular in shape. If osteophytes break off, there will be added pains as they impede the joints. Crepitus may be heard as the joint is moved.

Psychological reactions

The individual will be aware of the effect of the disease on his normal functioning and may well become frustrated as mobility is decreased. Pain may further reduce freedom of movement. There may be reactions of anger and misery if the condition is not treated. For the elderly person living alone, or with a partner who is also elderly, other problems affecting self-image may occur, such as incontinence and poor hygiene and self-care. If the patient is living with a younger relative, the decreased mobility may lead to early dependence, so affecting the balance of relationships.

Social reactions

Social reactions are those associated with reduced mobility and pain. There may be social isolation, a cessation of normal pursuits, and strain on personal relationships. Pain, if uncontrolled, may lead to outbursts of temper, so that the individual may be avoided by others.

PLANNING NURSING CARE

Physical care

The aim of physical care is to reduce pain, reduce the strain on the joint and maintain maximum mobility.

Pain may be relieved by analgesics, the most common of which is acetylsalicylic acid (aspirin). Patients on this drug need to be monitored for side effects such as intestinal bleeding. Sleeping on a firm mattress or with a board under the mattress may relieve pain at night since it will support the affected joint. Weight-bearing may be reduced by the use of a walking stick or Zimmer aid, and by curtailing unnecessary exercise. If the individual is overweight a reducing diet will be advised. Physiotherapy may be prescribed to maximize mobility while reducing strain on the affected joint.

The above measures are conservative in that the affected joints will not improve but continue to degenerate. Modern surgical procedures may be used either to immobilize the joint (arthrodesis) to relieve pain or for stability, or to replace part or all of the joint. Hip replacement operations are very successful and can return an individual to a fully mobile life (Figure 12.8). Unfortunately there are more individuals waiting for this operation than

Fig. 12.8 (a) Diagram and (b) X-ray of a hip prosthesis in place.

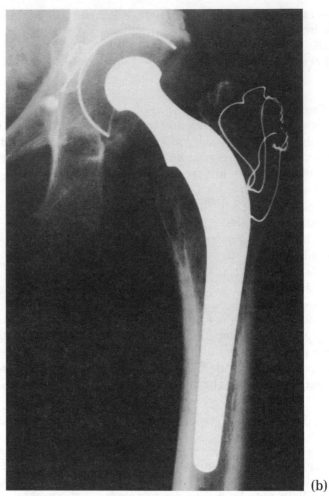

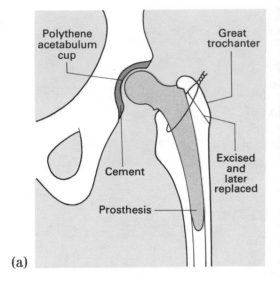

Polythene
acetabulum
cup

Great
trochanter

Cement

Excised
and
later
replaced

Prosthesis

(a)

(b)

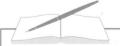

Make an appointment to be shown round your local hospital's physiotherapy department. Which aids are available to help patients with osteoarthritis to maintain independence? Try using two of these aids. Were they difficult to use? How did you feel when you were using them?

waiting lists will allow. This is reflected in the Patient's Charter which guarantees that admission for treatment by a specific date is no later than two years from the date when the Consultant put the patient on a waiting list. Elderly patients may be particularly frustrated by long waits when they feel that they already have limited time as active individuals. If the operation is performed and followed by physiotherapy, normal activities are usually resumed within three months, depending on the individuals's adaptation.

Psychological care

In planning psychological care, the individual's self-image should be taken into account. For example, weight-bearing may be reduced by use of a stick or aid but this may be unacceptable to the patient. There is an old saying that 'pride pinches'. In the context of osteoarthritis this means that many people would rather walk in pain without an aid than relieve weight at the cost of their self-image.

The promise of an operation may cause psychological problems if there is a long wait. The elderly person may feel that no one cares, and as a result become bitter about the health service. The nurse should be prepared to accept such feelings and, if appropriate, offer explanation of the way priorities are set. Although it may not help to know that most people wait for such an operation, it can take away the feeling of personal affront which may be present.

If dieting is necessary, the patient will need to be motivated. Realistic goals should be set and monitored so that pleasure may be taken in success. If hands are affected (Figure 12.9), boredom and frustration may need to be discussed and hobbies suggested which require less manual dexterity. The sight of affected hands which are gnarled with protrusions (Heberden's nodes) may cause distress which the nurse must accept. Elderly people do not necessarily stop caring about their appearance.

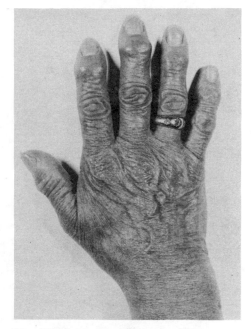

Fig. 12.9 Osteoarthritic damage to a hand. Reproduced from Swash and Mason (1984) with kind permission of the authors.

Social care

To help the individual maintain as normal a social life as possible, he should be assessed for aids which will help in the home and may be provided by the Social Services. A straight-backed firm chair is easier to get in and out of than a low soft one; the height of the lavatory can be raised along with other small adjustments to the home. Both the occupational therapist and the physiotherapist have an important role in assessing the individual's ability to live independently.

If an individual has a hip replacement he will need to learn to walk again without fear. Plans for care will include education on resuming normal pursuits which may have been discarded prior to operation. There is no set time for resumption of, say, driving, but a rule of thumb is that if it feels right, it is probably safe to go ahead. The consultant will advise the patient to lie on the unaffected side for at least two months to avoid pressure on the new hip joint. Apart from this constraint, there should be a gradual return to pain-free normality.

THE CARE PLAN

For the patient on conservative treatment, priorities will be given to pain relief and strategies to reduce weight bearing. Other priorities will include helping the patient

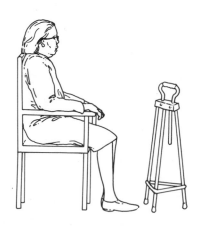

understand his disease so that his co-operation in care is assured.

The psychological implications for the patient and his family should be assessed and discussed. If the patient is awaiting surgery, plans should include helping the patient understand the concept of a waiting list.

For the post-operative patient, plans will be made to support the physiotherapist in a programme of rehabilitation and to think ahead to the needs of the patient and his family on discharge.

Summary

In this chapter, the ageing process has been described together with some of the problems and diseases which particularly affect the elderly. The list is not exhaustive since the elderly may suffer from any problem or disease which affects other age groups. What is particular to the elderly is the concept of multiple pathology.

The danger of labelling the elderly has been discussed in the hope that the members of this increasingly large group will continue to be treated as individuals, because inside their ageing bodies, they feel no different from any other human being.

References

Cormack, D. (1985a) *Geriatric nursing. A conceptual approach.* Ch. 3, Sexuality and ageing. Oxford: Blackwell Scientific Publications.

Cormack, D. (1985b) *Geriatric nursing. A conceptual approach.* Ch. 8, Diseases commonly experienced by the elderly. Oxford: Blackwell Scientific Publications.

De Beauvoir, S. (1977) *Old Age.* Harmondsworth, London: Penguin.

Denham, M. (1990) *Care of the long stay elderly patient.* London: Chapman and Hall.

DHSS (1981) *Growing older.* London: HMSO.

Harper, M. (1991) *Management and care of the elderly: psychosocial perspectives.* Sage Publications.

MacGuire, J. (1993) *Primary nursing in elderly care.* London: King's Fund.

Marshall, J. (1968) *The Old Poor Law 1795–1834. Studies in economic history.* London: Macmillan.

Norton, D., McLaren, R. & Exton-Smith, A. (1975) *Investigations of geriatric nursing problems in hospital.* Edinburgh: Churchill Livingstone.

O.P.C.S. (1995) PP2 No. 19. Mid 1992 based population projections. London: HMSO.

Owen, D. (1976) *In sickness and in health*. London: Quartet Books.

Shukla, R. (1994) *Care of the elderly*. London: HMSO Books.

Swash, M. & Mason, S. (1984) *Hutchison's clinical methods*, 18th edn. London: Baillière Tindall.

Tortora, G. & Anagnostakos, N. (1990) *Principles of anatomy and physiology*. London: Chapman & Hall.

Further reading

Bennett, C. (1992) *The essentials of health care of the elderly*. London: Edward Arnold.

Easterbrook, J. (Ed.) (1987) *Elderly care towards holistic nursing*. London: Edward Arnold.

Hollingham, P. (1990) *Care for the elderly*. London: Penguin Books.

Johnstone, M. (1982) *The stroke patient; principles of rehabilitation*. Edinburgh: Churchill Livingstone.

Solomon, E. P. & Davis, P. W. (1983) *Human anatomy and physiology*. Philadelphia: Saunders.

Tinker, A., McCready, C., Wright, F. & Selvage, A. (1994) *The care of frail, elderly people in the United Kingdom*. London: HMSO Books.

13

The Dying Patient

CHAPTER SUMMARY

The needs of the dying patient, 460
The need for knowledge, 461
Breaking bad news, 462
Hope, 466
The need for reassurance, 467
Emotional reactions, 467
Spiritual needs, 470
Cultural differences, 472
Social needs, 472
Physical needs, 474

Specific problems of the dying patient, 475
Anxiety, 475
Depression, 476
Fear, 477
Loss of dignity, 477
Loss of control, 478
Care when there can be no cure, 479

Focus of care, 479

The death of a patient, 480

The role of the relatives, 482
Collusion, 482
The relative as a visitor, 484

Meeting the needs of relatives, 485
Knowledge, 485
Reassurance, 486
Children, 487
Needs after death, 487
Reporting a death to a relative, 488
Practical needs, 488
Grief, 489

Summary, 491

References, 492

Further reading, 492

The needs of the dying patient

Almost every ward has patients who will not recover from illness. Sometimes they will be transferred to a hospice or they may be sent home to be cared for by relatives and friends with support from community services. Nevertheless, many will remain in hospital for the terminal stages of their illness to be cared for by the health care team. These patients require palliation rather than active treatment for their disease. It is only in recent years that palliative care has been accepted as a specialty. Prior to this, the dying patient was often seen in terms of failure on the part of medical and nursing staff who had learnt to believe that their role was to cure. As a result, the dying patient was often put in the bed nearest the door and given only minimal care.

Death is still a taboo subject in our society, and because of this dying patients may be avoided by the nurse or given inappropriate reassurance about their future. There has been a considerable amount of research in this area and it has been suggested that both doctors and nurses may not have accepted their own feelings about dying. This, in turn, may make it difficult to accept that a patient is dying and lead to a reluctance to interact with that patient.

In the Western world, we live in a relatively healthy society. Many nurses start their training not having seen a dead body. As a result, the nurse may feel worried or inadequate when caring for a dying patient and fail to identify the particular problems that the dying individual is facing in terms of his physical, social, psychological and indeed spiritual needs. In this area of nursing, as in any other, a sound knowledge is necessary plus insight into one's own feelings on issues that may trouble the patient. Accurate assessment is paramount so that actual deficits may be recognized, rather than generalized needs assumed which may not apply to a particular individual.

The need for knowledge

Some years ago there was considerable debate on whether a patient should be told that he is dying. Those suggesting that the patient should be told used the argument, among others, that the patient needs to have a chance to put his house in order and deal with unfinished business, while those against telling the patient argued largely on the basis that if a patient loses hope he may give up and die earlier. Thinking has changed considerably in recent years, and although there are still some health professionals who feel that information should be kept from the patient, the general feeling is that information should be given according to the needs of the individual concerned.

Giving information to a dying patient is a 'bad news' situation. In workshops on breaking bad news to patients (Faulkner *et al.* 1995), health professionals were quite open in admitting that they did not like to break bad news. Indeed, in Ancient Greece the bearers of bad tidings were killed. This links with health professionals' beliefs that they are somehow responsible for a patient's impending death. Major questions arise on who should break bad news, how it should be broken and where it should be broken, and who deals with the aftermath.

Nurses may feel that they are not responsible for telling a patient that he is dying, but if the paradigm is followed of giving information as the patient requests it, the patient may ask the person that he feels most comfortable with. This may be a nurse who will have to respond. Nurses too will be expected to deal with the aftermath of an individual having had his impending death confirmed. The classic work of Kubler-Ross (1970) describes the stages of adaptation to the knowledge that an individual cannot be cured. These are:

1 Denial and isolation
2 Anger
3 Bargaining
4 Depression
5 Acceptance

These stages produce a reasonable framework of what happens when a patient tries to come to grips with the notion that he will not get well and that his future is very foreshortened. However, all stages are not obvious in every patient, and some people may die without having truly accepted that this is their reality.

Breaking bad news

Because breaking bad news is not a pleasant task, there is a temptation to blurt it out bluntly and then back off. In fact it is very useful to check first on what the patient is making of the current situation. A common reaction to uncertainty is to look around for clues to what is happening and certainly a patient has to have thought of possibilities before he gets worried enough to go to his doctor. It may be that symptoms are similar to those of a friend or relative who was ill, and patients often make the link between their own symptoms and a correct diagnosis long before the doctor confirms that diagnosis. However, until the diagnosis is confirmed the patient may continue to hope that he is wrong in his expectation of bad news.

It is important to give patients bad news at a pace that suits them so that they may stop the professional at any

1 Assess patient's knowledge or suspicions
2 Give warning of reality
3 Break bad news at patient's pace
4 Allow space for news to be absorbed
5 Pick up pieces

Fig. 13.1 Strategy for breaking bad news.

time during this process. Figure 13.1 shows the strategy for breaking bad news in this way and shows that after the bad news the patient needs to have time to absorb the news and somebody there to pick up the pieces afterwards as they come to grips with a new reality.

Sonia had breast cancer. She had a mastectomy (Chapter 11) which was followed by chemotherapy. After a year, in spite of the treatment, Sonia had extensive secondaries. The doctor felt that he must tell Sonia that her chances of survival were very small.

Doctor I want to talk to you about your current situation
Sonia I'm not sure how I feel about that
Doctor I'm afraid the news is not good
Sonia You mean it's spread
Doctor I'm afraid so
Sonia Can you do anything doctor?
Doctor Well, we can certainly treat your symptoms and keep you comfortable
Sonia Are you telling me that you can't cure it?
Doctor Well, I'm sorry but that is what I have to tell you
Sonia I guessed that's how it was going to be
Doctor Do you need a little time now to think about this?
Sonia Well, I've thought about it and thought about it, but until just now I kept hoping that I was wrong
Doctor So you had thought that maybe this time . . . ?
Sonia My mother died of breast cancer at 37 and I'm 36. Have I got a year?

In the above rather painful sequence Sonia showed that she had thought that she might have reached a terminal stage but had hoped that the doctor would bring her better news. She needed some time to adapt to the knowledge, even though she had been afraid that it would be the case, and it was the nurse who spent time with her afterwards helping her to talk through her worries. By being given a warning and being allowed to set the pace, Sonia was able to absorb the news more readily than if it had been given in a blunt and uncaring way.

Some patients may raise the issue of their future before a health professional decides to tell them that they are not getting better. In such situations it is important that the nurse picks up the patient's cues that he is ready to talk about his current situation and future care.

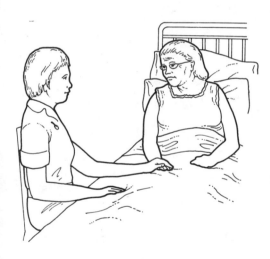

Patients' cues

Few patients in fact ask outright if they are dying. It is more common for a nurse to be asked obliquely, so the skill of picking up cues is all-important with these patients.

Vera, who was dying, said to her nurse, 'It is funny you know, my son is coming to see me from abroad for the first time in 17 years. Don't you think it is odd?' The nurse said, 'Well of course he would want to see you! Here, roll over so I can rub your bottom'. Her answer blocked Vera's enquiries. Later she tried again with another nurse who replied, 'Odd, I do not know your son. What do you think?', to which Vera replied, 'I think I must be dying – oh, it's not just Chris coming home, it's the fact that the treatment has stopped and I know I am not getting better'.

The second nurse allowed Vera to bring her own feelings out into the open without threat, since she was free to explore her problems with the nurse or to say something neutral if she was not yet ready to talk. However, turning the question around, to discover what the patient thought, could have posed a potential difficulty for the nurse, who might have had to accept the patient's problems and distress. Nurses may block questions in an attempt to protect themselves from patients' pain.

Vera was upset but seemed to enjoy the last week or two of her life as she mobilized her family into organizing the dispensing of her few precious items, and made clear her wishes for cremation. Other patients may not have reacted so positively, but as a general rule, if a nurse can assess a patient's readiness to discuss the future, talking will often bring eventual peace of mind to both the individual and his family.

If a patient is not ready for information, or if he is told in an insensitive way, he can become angry and hostile when told that he is dying.

Andrew was told that he was dying when the doctors decided that further treatment for his cancer would be of no avail. He became angry and denied that he was dying, accusing the doctors of incompetence. This was followed by feelings of guilt and depression which caused problems for his family. In such a situation, the nurse needs to remain calm and friendly until the patient is ready to talk.

Denial may be a strong coping mechanism for many people. If, during their life, they have dealt with difficulties by failing to believe that they exist, they are very likely to do the same if they are faced with a terminal diagnosis. If the patient remains in denial, this can cause problems for the family who cannot then discuss what the patient wants in the short future they have got, and one could argue that the denial should be broken and the patient made to face the truth. In fact, the patient may need his denial in order to manage his current situation. What the nurse can do is to check to see how solid the denial is. This is sometimes called 'looking for a window', and what it really means is asking the patient a checking question. The nurse might ask Andrew, for example: 'You say that the doctors are incompetent and that you aren't going to die. Is there ever any time, even momentarily, when you're not so sure about that?' This gives a patient the opportunity to share moments of concern which may show that the denial is partial only, or can also allow him to say, no, he never doubts for a moment that he'll get well. The latter statement means total denial, but even this may change over time as the events of each day add up and change Andrew's perception of what is happening to him.

Many patients, in fact, are very ambivalent about their diagnosis and prognosis. They may, on occasion, seem to accept perfectly that they are going to die and then at others, totally deny it. This ambivalence is usually followed by a readiness to accept impending death.

The above cases show the need to assess the patient's readiness to talk and to check for any cues he may give. If a patient says, 'I am dying, aren't I?' it is often useful to use a reflective technique to be sure he wants to know. It is possible that such a statement may be regretted immediately it is spoken, in which case the patient may well say, 'Oh, don't take any notice of me, I'm just feeling low today'. The nurse, however, will be alerted that the patient is thinking of discussing the future and should pick up further cues as they arise.

When patients face the fact of impending death, they often want to be given a time-scale. Such predictions are difficult to make with accuracy. The Consultant may be prepared to make a prediction for the patient in terms of weeks or months but, if not, it should not upset the patient if the nurse explains honestly the difficulty of giving more than an approximation (Faulkner and Maguire 1994). Many patients set goals for survival – to a daughter's wedding, their own birthday, or an anniversary – and seem to need hope from the nurse that the goal will be reached. Such goals appear to give purpose to the last few weeks of life, and should not be discouraged.

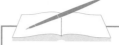

Work with a colleague. Compare two patients in your care – one who is recovering from disease and one who will not recover. How different are the problems on the care plan? Do you feel more comfortable with one of these patients than the other?

If yes, try to account for the difference. Discuss what you have learnt from this exercise with your colleague.

Consultants' directions versus patients' needs

The patient's need for knowledge is the business of every member of the health care team. There are some Consultants who continue to believe that patients should not know that they are dying, in the way that some believe that diagnoses such as cancer should not be divulged. This may be seen to cause difficulties for the nurse who finds herself talking to a patient who is ready for the truth. If the nurse picks up the patient's cues and assesses his current state of knowledge, she is often in a situation where, rather than breaking bad news, she is confirming the patient's tentative beliefs at a time when the patient has shown himself ready for such information. The nurse may, however, have to be a little assertive if the Consultant complains that information has been given that he did not feel was appropriate at the time.

There are benefits in having the knowledge that time is limited since it gives the patient a chance to complete unfinished business, to heal rifts, and to make plans.

A ndrew, when he had accepted the inevitability of death within three months, paid for his sister to come over from abroad for a holiday, sold his guns and transferred to his wife the deeds of their house. While his sister was with him he was determined to stay alive until his 50th birthday, which fell within a month. He actually lived until the day after his birthday, having requested particular music for the funeral service. Such an attitude is far from the feelings of hopelessness which some ascribe to the knowledge that one is dying.

If information at the appropriate time can be so positive, why should any health professional advise against it? In fact there is a belief that this knowledge may lead to depression and even suicide. A very few patients do react in this way but this is most likely because the patient is told his prognosis at an inappropriate time or in an inappropriate way. Some patients indeed may not move on from denial, and as a result may die without discussion. As long as individual needs are met, the nurse need not join the 'to tell or not to tell' debate.

Hope

The belief that if a patient is told he is dying he will give up hope is generally based on a very narrow view of hope, i.e. hope that the patient will recover. If hope is viewed in wider terms, it can in fact help the patient to manage his dying period better. It was seen above that Andrew, once he had accepted the inevitability of death, hoped not that he would get better but that he would live to his 50th birthday. Encouraging the setting of such short-term goals can give purpose to the period when a patient is dying and give considerable pleasure to both the patient and his family, because rather than simply waiting to die, the patient is actually living right up until the time he does die.

The need for reassurance

It is natural to want to be able to reassure patients when they are in distress. This is difficult with dying patients since the one thing they may wish to hear is impossible for a nurse to say. It may be a temptation to reassure with platitudes, but the problem here is that when the patient is ready to learn the truth, trust will go if the nurse has been making false promises. There are areas where reassurance can and should be given, but a nurse may face a dying patient who asks to be told that he will get well, and this reassurance cannot be given.

Emotional reactions

When individuals learn that they are unlikely to recover from their current illness and have to face the possibility of death, then there are three major emotional reactions. We saw that Andrew became very angry when he was told that he would not recover. Following on from anger are often emotions of guilt or blame. Few people wish to give up life and so being told that that is what is going to happen does generate a lot of anger for many people, and that anger is often directed at the health professionals who are caring for the patient. The anger is more likely to be diffused if it is acknowledged, made legitimate and then explored.

Mr Lodge had testicular cancer which was not diagnosed until he had secondaries in his liver. His anger was all directed at his General Practitioner, but when the nurse talked to him it became apparent that his anger was misdirected.

Mr Lodge	I told that GP six months ago and he wouldn't listen to me
Nurse	I can see how angry you are
Mr Lodge	Angry!
Nurse	Well, I guess in your situation I'd be pretty angry too, but I wonder if your anger really belongs with the General Practitioner
Mr Lodge	It's everywhere, it's everywhere. I suppose you're right. It isn't all with him. I've been a good sort of guy. I've always put myself out

for other people and now this has happened to me it makes me wonder just whether I'm a fool to believe that there's any sort of God who looks after us, and if there is, why the hell has he done this to me?

In the above exchange it will be seen that Mr Lodge was angry, not so much with the doctor who had failed to diagnose him, although there was some anger there, but primarily because his faith had been shaken. By exploring Mr Lodge's anger with him, it diffused and he then looked for logical reasons for why, at a reasonably young age, he had the sort of cancer from which he would not recover.

It is very common in these circumstances for the dying person to lay blame at someone's door or to manufacture guilt themselves. It may be, for example, that Mr Lodge could think of some things he had done that he was not too proud of and he might consider that his current situation was a punishment for these. In Mr Lodge's case he was blaming his God and the General Practitioner. Those feelings may change over time, but what is important for the nurse is to listen to the patient and to help him to work through the emotions that are generated by the reality of the fact that this person is going to die.

Mrs Brown had not been well for some time and was admitted to hospital with cancer of the lung and metastases in the stomach and liver. The Consultant thought she would live about a month but did not inform her of this diagnosis. Mrs Brown waited until a nurse was bathing her and asked, 'I will get over this won't I?' Such a question does not tell the nurse what the patient believes but appears to be a plea for reassurance. It would be easy to say, 'Of course you will! Now do cheer up' but such a reply may cause problems in the future. In this situation it is better to explore the question with the patient.

In Mrs Brown's case, the nurse asked her how she was feeling and the patient replied, 'That's the trouble, I feel so awful but no one has explained. It goes round and round in my head and I know I am not getting better'. The nurse was able to answer this by saying, 'I think you have to accept that you *are* very ill', to which came the astonishing reply, 'What a relief! I was afraid I was just being neurotic but couldn't manage to pull myself together'. It transpired that Mrs Brown had always been well and saw illness in terms of weakness on her part.

All patients are not like Mrs Brown, but nurses should avoid the trap of false reassurance. Alternatively, nurses should avoid being insensitive in their handling of impossible pleas for reassurance, since no one should deny the patient the right to hope. A statement in reply to a plea for reassurance of survival such as, 'Well, you know you are not at all well just now, but we will do our best for you' leaves the patient to hope, or maybe to begin accepting the truth without any lies being told. A blunt 'No, you won't get better, I'm afraid' could be quite devastating for the patient.

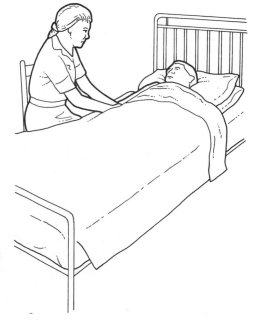

Pain

Patients may need reassurance that they will not die in pain. This can only be ascertained by careful assessment since there are strong cultural feelings about pain. The British idea of the 'stiff upper lip' may prevent many patients from admitting to pain. This may also be true of, for example, Moslem patients, who are taught to accept what is sent to them, in contrast to Continentals who feel free to show their emotions.

Of course this is a generalization, and pain thresholds do vary from individual to individual. There is, however, no reason why any nurse should not be able to reassure the patient that adequate pain control will be available. This will need co-operation from the patient in terms of honesty about pain levels. It is worth remembering that pain can be a more consuming problem than the actual thought of death.

Dying alone

A patient may worry that he will be left to die alone. This can be very important to him, even if he will slip into unconsciousness prior to death. From the nurse's point of view, it may seem impossible to reassure a patient that someone will be with him when he dies, given that wards are busy and staff overstretched. Yet dying is a lonely affair and, if possible, the patient's need should be met. What is often missed in hospital care is the knowledge that many patients appear to have foreknowledge of the time of their death. The following is one of many anecdotal accounts to support this view.

Mrs Brown went home to die. She was looked after by her two daughters, one of whom had moved in to be of help. Mrs Brown, although very ill, took a lively interest in day-to-day affairs and had decided that she would send her daughter to collect the several weeks' pension owed her on the following Monday. On Friday, she asked for the pension book. 'But Mother,' said her daughter, 'you were going to do this next Monday.' 'That would be too late,' replied Mrs Brown, and insisted that the pension be collected. Mrs Brown died the following afternoon.

Such stories, and there are many, could be dismissed as coincidence, but if they are true it is easy to understand a patient's need to know that he will not be alone when he dies. Such reassurance should be possible, and should be taken seriously by the nurse.

Relatives

Often, a patient will ask that a relative be summoned when his condition deteriorates. Again it should be possible to give reassurance on this point. A request of this sort may cause conflict for the nurse, especially if the patient deteriorates during the night. One can argue that it is pointless to disturb the relative's last peaceful night's sleep for some time to come, but promises made should be kept. Conflict can be avoided by being clear on what both patient and relative want, and whether the time of day (or night) makes a difference.

If a close relative is prepared to be with a dying patient, then nursing staff are relieved of the problem of the patient being alone. Thought must, however, be given to the relative, who may need support since death can be quite frightening and is compounded if the death means the loss of a loved one or close companion.

Other problems

Assessment of the dying patient will elicit other areas where reassurance is needed, some of them being highly individual. Everyone needs reassurance from time to time when circumstances make for feelings of insecurity. Some of the fears and worries elicited by illness and hospitalization have been discussed previously, where an individual may be dealing with the unknown. How much more frightening is death, where everything that is known and owned is left behind for the last time?

Spiritual needs

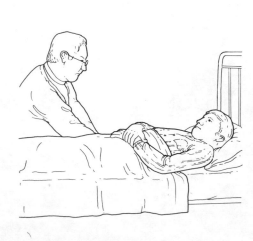

If death is a taboo subject, so too is the subject of one's spiritual beliefs. There is a common belief that spiritual = religious, and so the nurse's contribution to identifying spiritual needs may link with finding out what the patient's religion is and whether he would require a visit from his local religious leader. It could be argued that the clergy are the appropriate people to talk to patients about their spiritual needs, whether or not these include an element of religion. This, after all, is their area of expertise, and a nurse may not be able to answer all the patient's spiritual questions, may have a different religion from that of her patient, or, indeed, may not be a believer at all.

Yet in assessing a patient's deficits in terms of the whole person, such an argument will not hold and a distinction has to be drawn between ignoring a facet of an individual patient and accepting it, even if in the latter case the problem has to be referred elsewhere. What **is** important is that the nurse is prepared to assess the patient's problems, for being allowed to voice concerns may often help the patient considerably in sorting out thoughts and feelings.

Mrs Speke, knowing that she was dying, had the following conversation with her nurse:

Mrs Speke I wish I knew why I am stuck with this – I have always done my best I am sure
Nurse I am sure you have
Mrs Speke If only I could pray
Nurse Can't you?
Mrs Speke No, I just don't seem to believe any more. It's so frightening – maybe it all stops when I die
Nurse Look I can see you are worried, but I'm not sure I'm the best person to help you. Would you like to see the Chaplain?
Mrs Speke Oh, you do help, but yes – though I'm not sure what he will think of me
Nurse I'm sure he will try to understand and help you

Mrs Speke needed to air her concerns. The nurse felt that she could not really help but she did not block the patient. It is often difficult and embarrassing for a nurse to take part in such a conversation unless she does normally discuss religion socially, but this nurse, by listening, assessed a need and made an appropriate referral.

The nurse's beliefs

The nurse's personal beliefs should not get in the way of the patient concerned, even if those beliefs are different from the patient's. Each individual has a view of himself as a person and beliefs about what makes up that person. Religion may be an important part of an individual's spiritual beliefs but it may have a very small part to play. A nurse who has no religious beliefs may find it difficult to understand those of another individual. However, if a patient finds religion or other beliefs to be a support during illness and the dying period, to throw doubt on such beliefs is tantamount to removing hope. A nurse cannot offer proof that there is an afterlife and, indeed, the true believer does not need proof, but the belief that something happens after death has sustained many dying patients and will continue to do so.

Alternatively, the very religious nurse may be tempted

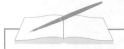

Read about one particular culture that you are not familiar with (Irish 1993). Compare the elements of that culture's beliefs about death and dying with your own. What are the major similarities? What are the differences?

to offer her beliefs to patients. Although it is true that crises in life can trigger forgotten faith, it is a very different thing, if angered by the events of life, to be told by someone to 'trust in the Lord'. Whether or not a nurse is a believer should not stop her listening to patients for long enough to assess their needs, and longer if she feels able to help them explore the deficits of faith caused by their illness.

Practical help

Depending on a patient's particular religion and the strength of his beliefs, there will be practical needs which the nurse can fulfil. The patient may request Communion at a time when the hospital does not have a service. The Chaplain can arrange this if it is thought that the need is great and the patient cannot wait until the next service.

Similarly a patient may express a need to confess. This most usually comes from Roman Catholic patients, who may be alarmed at the idea of dying without absolution. Patients may also request that a priest or minister is present at the time of death.

For a nurse to listen to such requests and deal with them seriously may be as important to the patient as physical care, especially when, from the patient's point of view, time is short.

Cultural differences

We live in a multiracial society where people have a variety of different religious backgrounds. People of different faiths require different actions in care of the dying and the nurse may need help in understanding the particular needs of people who have very different faiths from the standard Christian background common in the United Kingdom. Jews, for example, believe that when someone is dying this is such an important event that someone they love must be with them to rend and tear his or her clothes at the time of death. Neuberger (1994) considers those aspects of religious practice and ritual which may help people of ethnic minorities to die comfortably as they feel they are meant to. What is required from the nurse is the sensitive approach to areas which she may not have met before and which she may find difficult to understand.

Social needs

The dying patient may feel socially isolated for a number of reasons. There is much research to suggest that doctors and nurses avoid dying patients or those with fear-provoking diseases, so there is an immediate possibility of one source of interaction being reduced. Further, although patients in a ward will form a social community, they are likely to avoid contact with those patients who are seen to be very ill.

Friends and relatives may visit in profusion but they too may be upset or embarrassed at the thought of dying and may interact together round the bed, leaving the patient feeling sad and lonely. It is easy to criticize such apparent neglect of a patient's need to interact socially, but the reality is that most people are uncomfortable in the presence of the dying. It seems selfish to talk of personal concerns – so trivial in the face of death – or to discuss future plans with someone who has no future. To many, talking to the dying is a little like playing a game without knowing the rules. One is doubtful about making a move in case it brings penalties which may be painful.

Visitors

Visitors can be a useful social link for the patient but may need some support from the staff. The rule of two visitors only at each bed is probably useful for the dying patient, firstly because more might overtire him, and secondly because, with two, there is more chance of the interaction including the patient.

If the patient knows he is dying he may want to discuss practical matters with the family. They may find difficulty in talking openly of an impending death and may become upset. Nurses can help such visitors to cope with this situation by being supportive and by acting as role models. It may be that the patient wants to reach a certain goal – perhaps a birthday. He may get considerable pleasure from arranging a bedside party. Visitors can be encouraged to enter into his plans by realizing that such exercises buoy him up during what can be a very apprehensive time of life.

The patient who is denying the terminal nature of his illness may persist in talking about the future. He will be as distressed as any patient if he feels he is being avoided or his conversation blocked.

Nurses

Research has shown that nurses do not spend a great deal of time in social interaction with their patients. However, the dying patient should be assured of as much time from the nurses as are those patients who will recover. Facing up to mortality is difficult. Dying patients remind us of that mortality, yet it need not necessarily be a time of avoidance and sadness. Kubler-Ross (1975) sees death as 'the final stage of growth' and many religions look forward to heaven as a release from a sinful world.

Social interaction with the dying can be very rewarding. Patients are almost always interested in the nurse as a person and a little disclosure about future plans or current excitement may be diverting for a lonely dying patient. It is not so much what is said but that someone cares enough to take the trouble to say it which seems to count. The nurse's role in social interaction with a dying patient is to help that patient feel like a worthwhile individual, worthy of attention up to the moment of death.

Because most social interaction in a ward goes on between patients who are up and about, the patient confined to bed may well feel 'out of things'. Of course, if the patient is feeling very ill, solitude may be appreciated, but it is a fact of life that most people appreciate solitude more if it is chosen rather than imposed.

The nurse may be seen as a role model in that, if she ignores a patient, so may others. On the other hand, if she is seen to give a cheery word, or stop for a while with a patient, other patients will be more likely to stop to interact with him too. Patients may be worried by the dying patient because of inferences for their own recovery.

Mr Lacey, at 72, after his hip replacement, became quite friendly with the man in the next bed who had had a similar operation. This other patient also had a cardiac condition and became very ill and died. Mr Lacey was shaken, not just by the death but by the imagined implications for his own health.

It is not uncommon for dying patients to be put in a corner bed or in a side ward. Although there are good practical reasons for this, in that the patient may get more peace, will be more readily observed and more readily removed when dead, such placing can increase a patient's sense of social isolation.

Physical needs

Some researchers, e.g. Wilkes (1982), have listed those symptoms more likely to be experienced by the terminally ill patient. Although such a list may be useful in identifying the most common physical deficits which will be present in the dying patient, it is worth remembering that a physical assessment is necessary for all patients, whether or not a decision has been made about the likelihood of survival.

There is a certain danger in the labels 'dying patient' or 'terminally ill patient' in that misunderstandings are possible when it comes to the physical welfare of the patient. Is it necessary, for example, to worry about a balanced diet for someone who may be dead next week? Is there any point in working to prevent bedsores? In this respect, care should be no different from that given to any other patient. What is different is that there may be multiple needs which get more acute rather than showing improvement.

To assess the physical needs of the dying patient a knowledge will be necessary of the disease process(es) affecting him and of his ability to co-operate in his care. Some dying patients are bedfast and emaciated; others are reasonably nourished and out of bed up to their death. The label 'dying' says more about a patient's future than his present in physical terms and should not affect physical assessment.

Specific problems of the dying patient

If it is accepted that to label a patient as 'dying' or 'terminally ill' is simply to make a definite prediction about his future, then it should follow that such patients may have any psychological, social or physical problem experienced by the non-dying. They may also, however, have problems which are specific to the fact that they are not expected to recover from their current illness, problems which are related to the process of dying. Some of these problems are not exclusive to the dying patient, though the focus may be different for them. It is also worth remembering that each individual is different in his response to diagnosis and prognosis, so that these problems are not necessarily seen as standard to all patients.

Anxiety

A dying patient may not have been told his prognosis but yet may be suffering from anxiety. Perhaps what is happening to him does not make sense in terms of his ideas of recovery. Perhaps treatment is stopped without explanation or added symptoms appear as his condition worsens. It may be that a social trigger – perhaps a visit from relatives who live a long way away – will alert the patient

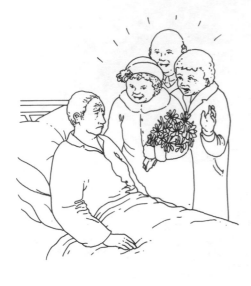

that all is not well. Anxiety will mount if a reasonable explanation of what is going on is not forthcoming.

Even a patient who knows his diagnosis may become anxious and unsure about the future, particularly if there is difficulty in finding someone who will share his concerns.

Such anxiety can grow as the full significance of what seems likely takes hold of the imagination. Diagnoses which cause anxiety because of their severity or implications have been discussed previously, but the reality of death can seem much worse in terms of its finality. Some dying patients, of course, are so ill that their levels of consciousness are impaired, but others may have weeks or months of lucid thinking time ahead of them. Without help, their anxiety may become severe.

Depression

Kubler-Ross cites depression as a stage which individuals go through between denying the reality of their impending death and its acceptance. This may lead to the assumption that it is natural to be depressed by the thought of dying, rather than seeing it as a problem. It was shown in Chapter 10 that depression may be severe enough to warrant psychiatric help when patients are coming to grips with a difficult diagnosis. The same is true when facing the thought of death. There will be degrees of depression which the nurse needs to identify so that appropriate action may be taken.

Certainly there is much for the patient to become depressed about, given that everything that is known will be left behind. Those with religious faith may be more philosophical but, again, there will be enormous variations between individuals.

Even if the diagnosis is not known to the patient, being ill for a long time can be very depressing, particularly if unpleasant physical effects, such as nausea, vomiting and pain, are present. More so, too, it there are no positive signs of recovery or indeed if there are signs of the condition worsening.

It is a common assumption that the elderly will be more ready to die than the younger patient, but this need not necessarily be true. Each will have his own reasons for wanting to live and his own particular concerns. The young mother may be depressed because she feels she is failing her children or because she will not see them grow up, whereas the elderly patient may be desperate to reach the age of 100 years and receive a telegram from the Queen. One can make value judgements on which of these is most important but this will not necessarily tally with the level of depression experienced.

Fear

Fear is an emotion commonly ascribed to dying patients but is often misinterpreted as a straight fear of death or of going into the unknown. If fear is identified as a specific problem for someone, it is important not to make assumptions about the causes, as these may be both multiple and surprising.

May, who knew she was dying, asked a lot of questions about what happened afterwards. The nurses could not understand this concern with details until May told them about a 'neighbour' who had apparently been buried, only to be discovered later in the mortuary. It appeared that two bodies had been confused and the wrong one taken away by the funeral directors. What May needed was reassurance on the hospital policy of labelling bodies after death since she was a Catholic and did not wish to lie in an alien cemetery.

Mr Armstrong, on the other hand, was afraid of dying in pain. He had accepted the reality of dying but was concerned with the 'how'.

The problem of fear is the same in both cases but the reasons, and therefore the possible solutions to the problems, are different. Unfortunately many people see being afraid as cowardly and for that reason alone may be loath to admit to such feelings. This is particularly so if the reason for the fear seems to be trivial. One can always find someone who is suffering more than oneself; this is often of no comfort whatsoever, but the knowledge of it may curb the disclosure of one's own fear.

Loss of dignity

Many symptoms experienced by dying patients may lead to loss of dignity, particularly as a patient weakens and is less able to take part in his own care. Such problems can include nausea, vomiting and incontinence, all of which can be very embarrassing to an individual. Confusion is also possible in the terminal stages of an illness. It may occur in bouts, with periods of lucidity in between, when the patient may become very distressed and perhaps feel that he has 'lost control'.

There are, of course, other situations where patients lose control and, with it, dignity. The dying patient is at maximum risk because matters will not improve, and because he may have several embarrassing symptoms.

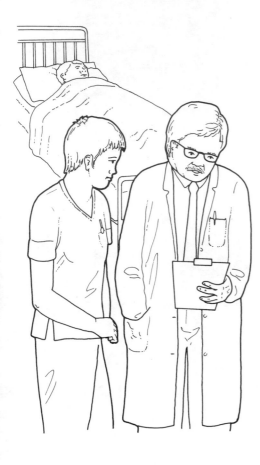

The situation becomes exacerbated if the patient ascribes the fact that he is largely ignored by doctors, nurses and perhaps family to his lack of control over his symptoms. Extreme misery can result.

Pain, which has been discussed in psychological terms, is a physical symptom common to many dying patients. It can become part of the problem of loss of dignity if the patient feels that he is being a nuisance by his inability to cope with it or by his constantly having to ask for analgesics. In the terminal stages of illness, analgesia should be given at regular intervals to control pain, and its effect carefully monitored. This allows for prescriptions to be changed promptly if necessary.

Loss of control

It has been seen that physical loss of control, whether through confusion or loss of bodily function, can cause distress. There is, however, also psychological or spiritual distress when the control over oneself as a person seems to be taken away. Mr Lodge in his terminal phase of illness seemed very unhappy, so that the nurse decided to talk to him.

Nurse   Mr Lodge, you look as if you've got lots of things on your mind. Do you want to talk?

Mr Lodge   I don't know. Do I get a choice?

Nurse   Do you get a choice?

Mr Lodge   Well, there doesn't seem to be anymore. I don't seem to be myself. Everybody else is making decisions for me. My wife couldn't handle me at home, so I'm here in the hospital. I can't make any decisions for myself anymore. I eat when you feed me, I get out when you get me out, I go back when you put me back. It would be lovely just to be me.

Mr Lodge felt that he had been totally taken over by the system and that he no longer had any control over any aspect of his life. His response was hostility and misery. In a hospital environment it is very difficult to meet individual needs in terms of the organization of the day, but by careful assessment it is possible to find out what the most important elements of control are for a patient and to allow the patient himself to make decisions about matters that are possible to alter within the constraints of the ward environment. Mr Lodge, when asked what he would like to do that would be different and would leave him feeling more that he had a say in the rest of his life, wanted to go home for weekends; he did appreciate that his wife could not manage to have him there all the time. By identifying this need and negotiating with Mrs Lodge and offering good community support, Mr Lodge was able to go home at weekends where he had his breakfast when he wanted it, got up when he wanted to, bathed or not as he wanted, and spent time with his family.

Care when there can be no cure

It will be seen that although there are specific problems commonly experienced by the dying, assessment may identify a number of problems no different from those of patients expected to get well. This raises the question of what is different in the care of the dying compared with that of other patients?

The decision that a patient is dying or terminally ill is usually made by a doctor, when active treatment is stopped because it will have no further effect on a progressing disease or condition. Such a prediction should not affect care but will affect the focus of such care.

When planning care for the dying patient it will no longer be focused on restoring that patient to his maximum state of wellness, but in maintaining his optimum level of social, psychological and physical well-being for the limited period left to him. This approach suggests the same positive and dynamic nursing care as is given to any patient. Assessment will need to be ongoing so that care may be planned on pertinent information. The eventual goal will be a peaceful and dignified death for the patient.

Focus of care

The focus of care will be on alleviating symptoms where possible and in minimizing other symptoms as they arise. In many instances, care plans will look little different from those of patients who are expected to get well. Any difference may be in goals, rather than care.

Taking mobility as an example, it can be seen that as a patient's condition deteriorates, he may be confined to bed. When a patient is expected to get well, plans may be made to improve mobility gradually. For the dying patient, the goals cannot move in this direction but each patient's plan for care can include that the patient is as mobile as possible and that he learns to accept the increasing limitations which will occur. In other words, mobility may be a concern but with a different focus for the dying patient.

Similarly with psychological problems. The need for information has already been discussed. In the patient who is expected to get better, information is required to help him towards maximizing his potential. For the dying patient, information may be required to help the patient accept the inevitability of his death and allow him to make the best use of the time he has left. In both cases the care includes the giving of information in response to deficits in knowledge. The difference lies in the focus of the care.

The dying patient, then, should have his care planned in the light of his symptoms and expressed needs. In many instances, problems identified may result in care plans which look for improvement. These may include the control of pain, alleviation of nausea and vomiting, and an improved psychological state. Positive results will help to maintain the dignity of the patient.

The reality of dying, however, may include symptoms which are difficult to control and distressing to the patient. In this area it is crucial that care is compassionate, and that the nurse is aware of the patient's distress so that she avoids making him feel guilty and uncomfortable about behaviour which is beyond his control.

Some patients may lose consciousness for a time before death occurs. Here, care will be the same as for any unconscious patient. Every patient has the right to be clean and comfortable for as long as he is alive, even if such care is time consuming and to no obvious avail. Continued respect for the patient is important for him, his relatives, and the health care team.

The death of a patient

Care does not cease on the death of a patient, but continues until the body has been removed from the ward. When a patient is thought to have died, he should be examined by a doctor and a death certificate issued. This is important since no funeral arrangements can be made until the relatives have the certificate, which will state the date, time and cause of death. A nurse is not generally authorized to sign the certificate.

What happens to the body after death will depend on a number of considerations. It is usual to bathe and tidy the body with the same respect given to the patient while he was alive, though relatives of some religious faiths, for example Jewish people, ask that the body is not touched by the nurses and will carry out these final acts themselves.

Hospital policy may vary on some points. It may be usual to pack cotton wool into orifices which may leak, such as the anus or vagina, or alternatively this may be carried out by the undertaker. Some hospitals provide shrouds, while others put the body into clean nightwear. Whatever the particular idiosyncrasies of the ward, the principle remains the same, i.e. that a patient, once dead, is clean and tidy to be taken to the mortuary and/or seen by his relatives.

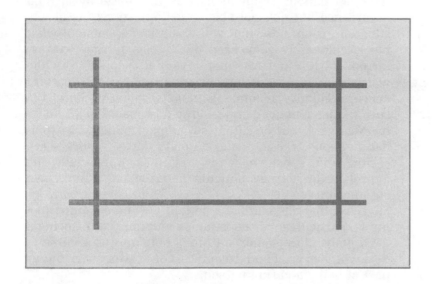

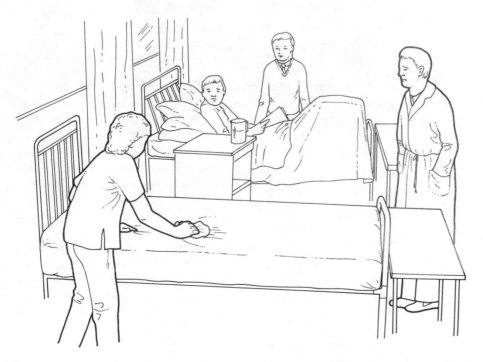

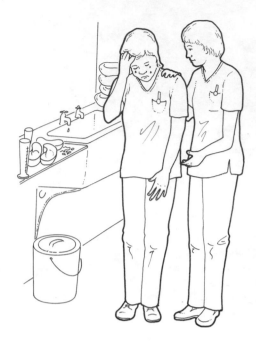

All bodies should be clearly labelled with the patient's name and hospital number. Some hospitals ask for a label on a wrist or ankle **and** one on the shroud.

When a body is removed from the ward, it is usual to close all curtains round other patients' beds while the porters bring in the mortuary trolley, and these are opened again when body and trolley have left.

It is often the case that the nurses will set about cleaning the empty bed and locker without explanation to the other patients. Patients may be very upset by such an occurrence but not feel able to ask questions. As in any situation, each individual will try to make sense of what has occurred. Is poor Fred dead? Has he been transferred? Is it usual to remove very ill people from the wards? Nurses need to be sensitive to the patients' natural concern and give a simple factual statement such as, 'I'm sure you have noticed how ill Fred has been. I'm afraid he has died now but he didn't suffer pain.' Such an explanation should reassure the patients that the nurses are caring and sensitive, and that they appreciate the apprehension felt by patients in the face of unknown circumstances.

Accepting the death of a patient may be upsetting to a nurse, particularly if she is junior and unused to seeing a dead body. More senior staff may help an upset nurse to deal with her grief and accept it – not as weakness, but as part of being a caring person.

The role of the relatives

The relatives of a dying patient often feel quite helpless when visiting the hospital. They may feel that their role is to be bright and cheerful when in fact they are frightened and concerned about the patient, the future and their role. Some may face the situation by denying the severity of the prognosis and setting themselves impossible goals for being positive about a future which will not occur.

Collusion

The possibility of some doctors withholding prognosis from a patient has been discussed. Such action may also be urged by relatives in the belief that it is in the best interest of the patient. The arguments may be powerful. For example, a man who has been married for 40 years may say he knows what is best for his wife and therefore asks that nurses and doctors withhold the truth. Certainly it will be true that this individual knows his wife much better than the nursing staff do, but this is not what collusion is really all about. It has been a common belief that relatives do not wish their loved ones to know that they are dying because they, the relatives, cannot cope with the resulting trauma. In reality, attempted collusion is primarily an act of love. No one wishes to hurt those that they love or indeed those that they feel responsible for, and so they hope that by remaining bright and cheerful and avoiding the issue of impending death then the loved one will have as much happiness as possible before they die.

For the nurse it is important to find out why a particular relative does not want his loved one to know and, more than that, what it is costing that person to hold the truth back from someone with whom they have had a very close relationship. Relatives will argue that they are happy to bear the cost of withholding the truth but if the nurse pursues this, it is very likely that the relative will admit that holding back the truth is causing problems.

Sandra Jones	I know what you're saying nurse. It is hard because sometimes there are things we can't say to each other because I'm so frightened that I'll let things out.
Nurse	How hard is that for you?
Sandra Jones	I'm prepared to bear it.
Nurse	Yes, but how hard is it?
Sandra Jones	(sigh) It's very hard.
Nurse	What do you think your husband is thinking?
Sandra Jones	That's the problem. We can't talk to each other, but I'm sure he couldn't bear it if he knew the truth.
Nurse	I wonder if you'll let me talk to him – not to tell him, to find out how he sees the current situation.

In the above exchange, the nurse identified the problem for the wife and that she was withholding the information because she cared so much about her husband, but by negotiating an opportunity to talk to the patient, she was able to find out that the husband knew perfectly well that he was dying but was himself trying to protect his wife. Such collusion is very common in times of crisis where each person knows the truth but is trying to protect the other. By breaking collusion, the couple can get together and move on in their relationship and in handling the particular trauma of the impending death. It is not always possible to break collusion. Many relatives are totally protective of their loved ones and many patients are in denial, but it is always worth the nurse attempting to break down the barriers that are caused by collusion (Faulkner 1992).

The relative as a visitor

The problem of being a visitor has been discussed in earlier chapters in terms of the strangeness of the situation and possible change in the role of the patient. When the patient is known to be dying, visiting can be difficult for both these and other reasons.

If the diagnosis and prognosis are known to all, there may be fewer constraints on conversation though relatives may be unsure how they should behave. The nurse can help and support the relatives if they find the situation distressing, and help them to understand the patient's need to talk through matters which might normally be seen as 'sick' or macabre.

Ellen Roberts was dying of cancer of the liver and realized that her time was limited. She was worried about how her husband would manage on his own but he was not prepared to discuss the future. Finally, Mrs Roberts persuaded her daughter-in-law to pack away the best china, give the linen tablecloths to friends and buy a number of drip dry items which could be managed by a man unused to fending for himself. Mrs Roberts' daughter-in-law coped quite well at visiting times as she fell in with her instructions. She finally broke down when Mrs Roberts wanted to discuss the catering for her funeral.

It can be seen that although Mrs Roberts was busy tying up 'loose ends', visiting was a strain for her relatives. A sensitive nurse can help to ease such burdens if only by being prepared to talk and listen.

Open visiting (which is normally allowed for the close relatives of dying patients) may cause problems if it is not discussed between nursing staff and visitors. It may be that if a relative is offered open visiting, he may feel obliged to spend more time at the hospital than he can reasonably manage. He will need to know that there are no such expectations of him.

Sometimes a relative does wish to stay at the bedside for long periods and is able to do so. In these instances the nurse should be aware of the length of time a relative has been sitting by the bed so that she can suggest a meal, a rest or a walk in the fresh air.

There is an aura around dying which may preclude

thoughts that the individual concerned may have been unpleasant to live with. A nurse may be shocked if relatives do not show care and concern for a dying relative. It is as well not to make judgements in such cases, since it may be that the individual who is dying has alienated those who had loved him and there is little feeling left when death is imminent.

Because visitors are individuals with commitments outside the hospital, there can be no expectations on how often they will come to see their relative or friend, or on how long they will stay. These visitors, however, will have expectations of the nursing staff, and special needs, which should be met.

Meeting the needs of relatives

Just as the needs of the dying patient may be identical to those of other patients, so it is with relatives. They have needs which are the same as those discussed in earlier chapters, but they also have special needs as they attempt to accept that the patient will not get better. This fact may pose both practical and psychological problems for a partner or family.

Knowledge

It is not unusual for doctors and nurses to leave relatives in ignorance of the severity of a patient's illness. This can cause problems all round if the patient is obviously deteriorating, since doubt can be cast on the competence of the nurses and doctors. It is understandable that there should be a desire to withhold bad news, but this would put the relative in a situation where he is trying to make sense of things which do not 'add up'.

Giving the diagnosis and prognosis to a close relative needs careful and sensitive handling, and must be considered in the light of what the patient understands about his illness. Brewin (1977) points out the difficulties for partners when one has knowledge that is withheld from the other.

It may be that the relative is the first to be told that the patient is dying. If so, it is at this point that collusion should be ruled out. One can expect denial and/or anger at such news and it may be that the information will not be accepted immediately. In many ways it is wise to adopt the same principles used for assessing a patient's readiness for information, but, whereas a patient may die without

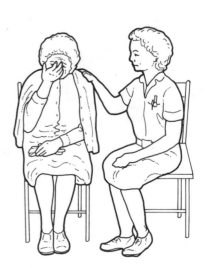

having discussed his impending death, a relative does need to be prepared in advance for the death.

When bad news is broken to a relative, time should be set aside so that questions may be asked, any possible reassurance given and care taken of what the relative will do next. If, for example, a wife is told that her husband will probably die in the next few weeks, she may be in no fit state to drive herself home immediately afterwards. She may feel calmer after a cup of tea or it may be necessary to telephone for another relative to take her home.

Once acceptance is reached, and this need not happen, many questions may arise such as when, how and where. Again, a sensitive approach is required, together with exploration of whether it is possible for the patient to die at home, or indeed if that is the wish of both patient and family.

If relatives at this time need to talk a lot after visiting or are constantly telephoning the ward, a busy nurse can lose patience. It is really important to remember how shattering the relative may have found the information and how difficult it is to deal with. His need for support from the ward staff is very real both in the early days and when death has occurred.

Reassurance

At first sight there seems little reassurance which can be given to the relative of a dying patient, but in fact there are many areas of concern where nursing staff can give reassurance and comfort.

One of the main feelings experienced by many relatives of dying patients is that of helplessness. They may need reassurance that their visits to the patient have value even if little is said. It may be that the patient will give feedback on how comforting a partner's presence can be, but many people are shy of disclosing their feelings directly, and the nurse may need to relay such messages.

Reassurance may be required that the hospital staff will not have expectations which the relative cannot meet in terms of visiting, helping in care, taking the patient home or being present at the death. Careful assessment is needed to discover to what degree the relative is able to be involved and reassurance should be given that the staff appreciate any difficulties of home commitments which may mean that the relative cannot, for example, leave children at night to be present at the time of death. Relatives may be frightened of death and indeed may not have seen or want to see a dead body. Reassurance may be needed that it is not obligatory to view the dead body.

On these and other matters it is important for the relative to feel safe enough with nursing staff to verbalize fears and worries without being made to feel selfish and uncaring. Concern may also be expressed on how the patient will die – will he be conscious? In pain? Will he look the same? Or make horrid noises? Explanations about death for the uninitiated can be reassuring as long as no false promises are made.

Children

Children are often excluded from the death of some grown-up or sibling who is very close to them. The arguments of their parents are very similar to those of collusion and the motivation is also similar. Parents will argue that their role in life is to keep their children free from harm and to look to their happiness, and arguments will be put forward that the children should be left happy as long as they can and, therefore, not be involved in the experience of dying. Relatives may discuss this with a nurse and make quite strong arguments for why their child is not being brought to see a dying relative.

For the nurse, this situation needs to be dealt with very similarly to that of collusion and it is often useful to ask a parent to think of reasons why perhaps the child should be involved as well as those which suggest that he should not. The important point here is this listing of pros and cons, which is called 'decision analysis'. The final decision on whether a child is involved or not is then made by the parent rather than imposed by the nurse.

If children are not involved and feel that they have somehow been isolated from the event of a loved one's death, they may be left feeling bitter and excluded and this can cause problems during the grieving process (Faulkner and Maguire 1994).

Needs after death

Death can occur in a number of ways. In this chapter the dying patient has been considered in terms of his failure to recover from disease. Such deaths may occur within a few weeks of diagnosis or may take months, but in either case, provided the relatives have been told the prognosis, there is an element of preparedness for what will happen.

Death may also occur suddenly as the result of a fatal accident, a physical phenomenon such as a massive heart attack, or murder or suicide. In these cases the relatives will be totally unprepared for the news of the death.

Reporting a death to a relative

If death has been expected after an illness of some duration, relatives will at least be expecting the news. Even so, the actual event may be extremely distressing and the nurse needs to be very sensitive in her approach, particularly if the message is being given over the telephone, when the relative may be alone and too shocked by the message to know what to do next.

If the death occurs in the night and the relative has asked to be informed, it is worth stressing that there is no expectation to come to the hospital immediately, but to come at a convenient time. Of course some relatives will want to be with the patient at the time of death, but, even here, they may not appreciate that death has actually occurred and it will be up to the nurse to point out gently that the patient is no longer breathing.

Should the death be sudden and unexpected, the news may be an enormous shock to relatives and it may be inadvisable to telephone in this event. It is possible that the police, the patient's GP or the local minister will be prepared to call personally at the house so that they can be as supportive as possible in what may be a very traumatic situation.

Practical needs

Because death is not an everyday occurrence in most families, many people have no idea of the practical implications. In the period immediately after death, the nurse can be both helpful and informative.

The doctor who certifies death will leave a certificate which the relatives are obliged by law to take to the Registrar of Births, Deaths and Marriages. If there is concern over the cause of death, a request may be made for a post-mortem examination, in which case the death certificate will be delayed.

Asking bereaved relatives to agree to a post-mortem or autopsy can cause distress. A tactful explanation of the need should be given rather than a blunt request. Relatives who object often feel that no useful purpose can be fulfilled now that death has occurred and are concerned at the possible mutilation of a much loved relative or partner. The nurse needs to be sensitive to these feelings while explaining why the request is being made.

Once the death is certified and registered, the funeral may take place. The nurse can show the relatives how to find an undertaker from the *Yellow Pages* and explain how a reputable one will be prepared to lift most of the organizational problems from them. Most undertakers are a tremendous help to a bereaved family and for that reason should be contacted early after the death. They will cover diverse matters such as explaining who is entitled to a death grant, dealing with flower orders and arranging times for the funeral service.

After death, the nurse's priorities are not always the same as the relatives'. The nurse needs to have the patient's belongings taken away so that the business of admitting new patients and caring for current ones may go on. The relative, on the other hand, may be coming to grips with what may be described as a life crisis and be temporarily unconcerned with mundane items such as the patient's clothes.

In this practical matter the nurse needs to show a sensitive approach when she has to ask a relative to check and sign for belongings which may trigger added grief. It may even be better if the relative is simply asked to collect the belongings 'within a few days' rather than upset a bereaved relative within hours of a death. It is not uncommon to see a crying individual carrying a suitcase along a hospital corridor. If relatives' needs are to be met an attempt should be made to avoid that sort of pain.

Not all relatives are upset by death.

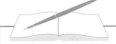

Look up the local standard for your area on informing a relative about the death of a loved one. Are the instructions clear and sensitive? Is advice offered, if required, on the practical steps to be taken after a death? How could the standards be improved?

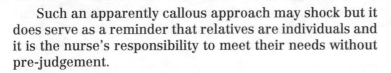

When Mrs Harris died, her friend was at the hospital within hours asking for the belongings and insisting on taking away flowers and pot plants which had been by the patient's bed.

Such an apparently callous approach may shock but it does serve as a reminder that relatives are individuals and it is the nurse's responsibility to meet their needs without pre-judgement.

Grief

Grief is a natural process which follows loss and can range in intensity from mild to severe, depending on how close the relationship had been between the individuals. Hospital nurses may not witness all the stages of grief but they may experience the early stage and need to be able to handle these emotions in the relatives.

The immediate reaction to the death of a loved one is one of shock and emotional numbing. Relatives may describe this period as 'walking in a dream', or 'being on automatic pilot'. In many ways, the planning and making arrangements for the funeral has a function in that it keeps the relatives occupied at a time when they are feeling 'switched off' from their emotions. The shock and numbness at a death may be followed by feelings almost of disbelief that the person is dead and there can be ambiguous behaviour in that the relative will be making plans for the funeral, sending out cards and feeling really upset, but at the same time looking for the dead person. This looking is called 'searching' and the nurse in hospital needs to understand that this is a natural part of the grieving process, because relatives of the dead patient may suddenly appear at the ward door for very trivial reasons, and what they are doing in fact is coming back to the last place where their loved one was alive.

In most individuals, this phase does not last very long but it can be quite upsetting to nurses who are unsure how to handle the situation. This is generally a very temporary phase. The nurse should accept the reason, however trivial, for the visit, be polite and then leave the relative to talk to other patients or simply to leave the building.

Working through grief can be seen in terms of tasks. Worden (1991) talks of four tasks for the bereaved person, the first of which is accepting that death has occurred and, secondly, feeling the pain of death. After this, the tasks are to accept life without the beloved person and fourthly, to be open to new relationships. The nurse on a ward where a patient has died may well be involved in helping a relative with these first two tasks of grieving. This generally means allowing that person to talk, to say how they feel, and to help them with the acceptance that the patient is not alive any more. Some relatives continue to visit the ward for some time after death, seeming to gain comfort from association with the last place where the patient was alive, and without necessarily demanding any input from the nurses.

Dealing with grief is painful. The old cliché 'laugh and the world laughs with you, cry and you cry alone' is often true. Yet the grieving relative may gain comfort from a nurse who will just **be there** and allow him to talk through his feelings. It is important that individuals do grieve and the nurse should be suspicious of the person who obviously cared for his relative but seems to be 'coping'. This individual may be denying grief an outlet. Such inhibited grief is known to lead to psychiatric problems, as in chronic grief, where the bereaved person often blames himself for what has happened.

The nurse's role is to be alert to the potential problems

of grieving relatives and she may feel that it is worthwhile to contact the district nurse or health visitor so that problems can be dealt with **before** psychiatric help is required. Many district and Macmillan nurses see 'bereavement visiting' as part of their role, and some hospitals have bereavement counsellors who visit relatives at intervals after a death has occurred. Even when death is accepted and the grieving process follows its natural course, there may be triggers to feelings of grief for some time to come such as anniversaries or special family occasions when the dead person is particularly missed.

Although nurses may find grief difficult to deal with, they may find a relative equally difficult if there is no sign of grief at all. Yet this does sometimes occur since all relationships are not happy. If rich Uncle Bill has sent his nephew £2 for Christmas every year and has been unpleasant as well, it should be possible to understand that the nephew's feelings on his uncle's death may be not grief but comfort from an inheritance.

Sometimes, too, relatives may seem relieved at their loved one's death, not because there is no sense of loss – which may come later – but because it has been painful to watch a prolonged and difficult illness.

W hen Ellen died after some months of discomfort, her husband stood at the end of the bed and said, 'Thank God for that'. He was not being callous, though it may have sounded so.

Summary

In this chapter the special problems of the dying patient and his relatives have been considered. It has been seen that these patients will not only have needs and problems in common with others, but will have specific problems associated with dying.

Care of the dying patient will be planned as for any other patient, but the focus of care and goals may be difficult.

Relatives, too, will have specific needs both while the patient is dying and after his death.

It is seen that the dying patient and his family require particularly sensitive care from the nursing staff.

References

Brewin, T. B. (1977) The cancer patient: communicator and morale. *British Medical Journal*, *2*, 1623–1627.

Faulkner, A. (1992) *Effective interaction with patients*. Edinburgh: Churchill Livingstone.

Faulkner, A., Argent, J., Jones, A. & O'Keeffe, C. (1995) Improving skills of doctors in imparting distressing information. *Medical Education*, *29*, 303–307.

Faulkner, A. & Maguire, P. (1994) *Talking to cancer patients and their relatives*. Oxford: Oxford University Press.

Irish, D. (Ed.) (1993) *Ethnic variations in dying, death and grief*. USA: Taylor and Francis.

Kubler-Ross, E. (1970) *On death and dying*. London: Tavistock Publications.

Kubler-Ross, E. (1975) *Death: the final stage of growth*. New York: Prentice-Hall.

Neuberger, J. (1994) *Caring for dying people of different faiths*. Mosby.

Simpson, M. A. (1975) Teaching about death and dying. In Raven, R. S. (Ed.) *The dying patient*. London: Pitman Medical.

Wilkes, E. (Ed.) (1982) *The dying patient*. Lancaster: MTP Press.

Worden, W. (1991) *Grief counselling and grief therapy*. London: Tavistock.

Further reading

Buckman, R. (1988) *I don't know what to say*. London: Macmillan.

Fallowfield, L. (1993) Giving sad and bad news. *Lancet*, *341*(8843), 476–478.

Faulkner, A., Maguire, P. & Regnard, C. (1994) Breaking bad news: a flow diagram. *Palliative Medicine*, *8*, 145–151.

Henley, A. (1988) *Good practice in hospital. Care for dying patients*. London: King's Fund Centre.

Hinton, J. (1979) *Dying*. Harmondsworth, London: Penguin.

Lammerton, R. (1990) *Care of the dying*. London: Penguin Books.

PART FIVE
EVALUATION AND DISCHARGE

14

Measuring Outcomes

CHAPTER SUMMARY

Outcomes in terms of patient satisfaction, 495
The patient as a judge of outcomes, 496
Satisfaction as a criterion, 497

Outcomes in terms of reduced dependence, 498
Physical outcomes, 498
Self-care, 500
Decision making, 500

Outcomes in terms of return to physical health, 501
Patients on a surgical ward, 501
Patients on a medical ward, 502

Elderly patients, 503
Measuring physical health, 503

Outcomes in terms of return to mental health, 504
Measuring mental health, 505

Outcomes in terms of patient potential, 508
Evaluating care of the chronically ill, 509
Evaluating care of the terminally ill, 509
Potential as a measure, 510

Summary, 511

References, 512

Further reading, 512

It was seen in Chapter 1 that by measuring outcomes it should be possible to evaluate care. There is, however, some difficulty in deciding, if care **can** be measured, how best to attempt such measurement. Should it depend on a patient's satisfaction, his ability to be independent, or on his improved health? If any or all of these, what are the criteria for success? If we maintain the concept of individuality, it will be seen that criteria for success can seldom be standard but will need to be set in the context of the particular circumstances of each patient.

Outcomes in terms of patient satisfaction

The number of patients who actually complain about the care they have received is relatively small. This may be less because they are satisfied than that the role of patient may be seen to preclude complaint. If complaints are made it is often after the patient is discharged, but as long ago as 1961 Maghee noted that the most common complaints made by patients were about lack of information and the quality of food; the annual Ombudsman's report continues to cite lack of information as a common complaint of patients.

If patients are involved in decisions about their care, it should be possible for nurse and patient to agree on expected outcomes. The individual should then be able to give an informed account of his satisfaction with particular aspects of his care.

The patient as a judge of outcomes

Since patients do not generally complain, it could be argued that using patient satisfaction to evaluate care has many difficulties, not least that patients may express satisfaction when in reality they may be disappointed in the results.

Many difficulties may be overcome by involving the patient at the point when problems are identified and care planned. If nurse and patient can agree on goals, then hopefully they will be able to discuss later whether the outcomes are as expected and whether the patient is satisfied with his progress. It may be that a patient's expectations are not realistic. This could lead to dissatisfaction, even if it is not expressed. An observant nurse may explore the cause for it and this may elicit the patient's frustrations and lay the groundwork for more realistic expectations of the outcome of care.

A patient's level of satisfaction is useful in measuring outcomes only if he understands what is possible. It was seen, for example, in Chapter 13 that the dying patient cannot expect to get well. He may, however, be satisfied that the care given affords him comfort and dignity. Similarly, the patient who has had a hip replacement may take considerable time and practice to walk normally. If this is not understood at the outset, there may be dissatisfaction with what is seen as 'slow progress'.

Pain control is another example where a patient needs to understand the problem. He can then appreciate that the initial goal may be to lessen pain while the appropriate drug and dosage are calculated. The longer term goal – of the individual being pain free – is reached as soon as possible after this. It is also important here that the individual is honest about his pain rather than stoic and uncomplaining because he does not want to make a fuss.

Communication skills are important in measuring patient satisfaction with outcomes. Consider the following conversation:

Nurse Well, Mr Lacey, you are feeling stronger today, aren't you?

Patient   Mm mm
Nurse   And walking easier
Patient   Well . . .
Nurse   You have nothing to worry about now

In fact this is a common, one-sided conversation in which the nurse tells the patient that he is feeling better. There is no measure of patient satisfaction with his walking. To gain information from the patient, a more open approach is needed, e.g.:

Nurse   Well Mr Lacey, how are you feeling today?
Patient   A little nervous still about walking
Nurse   About walking?
Patient   Yes, I am feeling able to walk further but it is still painful. I don't want to damage my leg
Nurse   You shouldn't damage your leg because it is held with a strong pin. I'll explain when we get you back to bed. I'll also get you something for the pain. How do you think we are doing in terms of our aims for you?
Patient   Well, I certainly reached Fred's bed on the target day. I am pleased about that and I know I need to be patient. It is tough though . . .

In the second conversation, the patient feels free to discuss nervousness and pain and his lack of patience. He appears satisfied that a stated goal has been reached but obviously wishes that more speedy progress could be made.

In using a patient's judgement of outcome, a distinction needs to be drawn between satisfaction that a planned outcome has been achieved and satisfaction with general progress to an outcome perceived by the patient as desirable, if not always possible.

Satisfaction as a criterion

For satisfaction to be used as a criterion for measuring outcomes, the satisfaction must be precisely defined. For example, Mr Lacey was able to say that he was satisfied that he had reached Fred's bed by the target date, and from this it can be assumed that the goal set, i.e. walking to Fred's bed by a certain date, was reached. But it can only be assumed that Mr Lacey was satisfied with the outcome if the criterion for success was simply walking a certain distance. If the quality of the walk was included in the expected outcome, it might be that Mr Lacey was not entirely satisfied.

The expected outcomes in Mr Lacey's case might be stated thus: (a) will walk from own bed to bed 9 by 4th

October, (b) walk will be pain-free, (c) patient will feel confident. Using patient satisfaction as a criterion it will be seen that outcome (a) has been reached but (b) and (c) need to be reassessed and new goals set.

Such precision is a reminder that, when goals are set, the expected outcomes should include some measure of quality. This is important because if, for example, Mr Lacey's progress is evaluated on physical performance alone, his pain may be missed. This could result in a setback after discharge when the patient may choose not to walk much in order to avoid the pain.

Satisfaction, then, can be seen as one criterion for evaluation if the terms of the satisfaction are clearly defined. A patient who is generally satisfied with the care received is rewarding to the nurses but will not necessarily provide feedback for evaluating the individual components of care. Finally, it must be remembered that 'satisfaction' is a value-laden word which will have different meanings for each individual. Precisely what a patient will express his satisfaction on may be stated, but it is more difficult to know what satisfaction means to that patient. Although one aim of nursing care should be that the patient is satisfied, it can be seen that other, more precise methods of evaluation are also necessary in order to judge if planned outcomes have been achieved.

Outcomes in terms of reduced dependence

An alternative method of evaluating care is by measuring a patient's move towards independence. This cannot, of course, apply to all nursing care since in some instances, e.g. terminal care, patients may be expected to increase their dependence on nursing staff. This is an important point, since if care is evaluated in terms of reduced dependence alone, it can be seen how dying patients might be labelled as failures. If care is to be evaluated in this way it is important that it should be applied only in those situations where reduced dependence can reasonably be expected.

Physical outcomes

If we think of Mr Lacey's problems with walking after operation, it can be seen that his ability to walk can be measured both in terms of his satisfaction with progress and in terms of his reduced dependence.

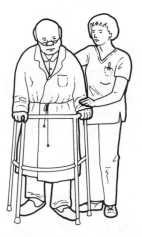
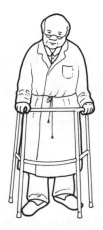
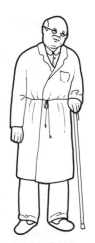

1 8th October   2 11th October   3 14th October

Initially, his walking may include a nurse and a Zimmer aid. If he is very apprehensive, two nurses may be required. If care is evaluated in terms of reduced dependence, the eventual goal may be that Mr Lacey can walk unaided (or with a stick) on discharge. Intermediate goals may be set by the physiotherapist and nurse to reduce his dependence in stages. If, for example, he reaches Fred's bed with two nurses and a Zimmer aid by 4th October, future goals might increase the daily distance covered while decreasing the physical support, first to one nurse and a Zimmer aid, then to the Zimmer aid alone, and from the Zimmer aid to a walking stick. Here, outcomes are measured in discrete stages that can be agreed by anyone observing Mr Lacey's progress. It can be seen that, if applicable, this method of evaluating care is more precise than patient satisfaction.

Outcomes may be measured in other areas of physical dependence as long as it is reasonable to expect the patient to become more independent. So often, goals are not reached because they are unrealistic.

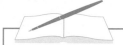

Choose a patient who is recovering well from his illness, and look at his case notes. By what criteria is his progress being measured? Is the patient satisfied with his progress? Suggest alternative ways of evaluating this patient's care.

Grace was an elderly patient who suffered from incontinence. Because she was worried about soiling, she constantly demanded to be taken to the lavatory. The nursing staff decided that Grace had a problem with bladder control and subsequently planned two-hourly visits to the lavatory. The aim was that the patient, by knowing when she could go to the toilet, would be less anxious. It was also expected that she would be continent.

In terms of outcomes, Grace was constantly asking nurses if it was time to go to the toilet, and was often distressed when she dribbled onto the floor. There was an increase in anxiety and in dependence, because the care planned was inappropriate for the patient and the goals set were unrealistic.

Self-care

Reduced dependence can also be seen in terms of a patient's ability to take on his own care. This is in line with Orem's (1971) concept of nursing, where progress is evaluated in terms of a patient's ability to undertake aspects of his care normally carried out by nurses. In fact, patients are normally only expected to carry out self-care that is expected to continue after discharge, and even then drugs are generally excluded, although there is a move towards self-medication trials in hospital by some Consultants. In all hospitals, the patient may have to learn to self-inject if this has been prescribed. Goals will be set in stages with evaluation of each set of outcomes being measured in terms of reduced dependence on nursing staff, as well as expertise in a particular task.

Reduced dependence through self-care may be in simple terms of learning to dress oneself and look after personal hygiene. The initial problems which caused dependence in these areas may be insoluble if the patient has a degenerative disorder such as rheumatoid arthritis. In this case solutions may be found in using clothes that are easy to put on and fasten and in aids to overcome physical disability. Outcomes will then be measured in terms of the patient's ability to put on the specially designed clothes. Goals which contained an expectation that the patient should manage normal clothes would be inappropriate and cause distress when followed by the inevitable failure.

Decision making

Reduced dependence should lead to a patient being able to make decisions about some aspects of his care. Sometimes an individual takes on the role of 'patient' to the extent that he will wait to be told before taking any actions, including getting out of bed or going for a bath.

Measuring outcomes of care should include an element of decision making. A patient may become more independent in terms of physical progress and self-care, but unless this includes an ability to make the decision to carry out an action, he is still dependent and may, on discharge, sit around all day, unsure of what he should be doing. Mr Lacey, for instance, might learn to walk unaided before discharge, but if he only gets out of bed when a nurse suggests he should, it can be seen that he is not making the decisions about his mobility.

Because of hospital routine, it is easy to control patients to the extent that they no longer contemplate inde-

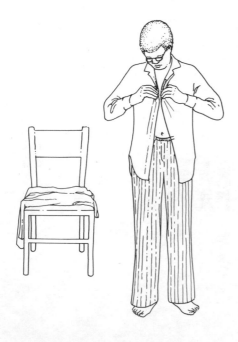

pendent action, yet prior to discharge it is crucial that a patient prepares to return to a situation in which he is, as far as possible, an independent decision maker. Evaluation of reduced dependence should take this into account.

A further difficulty for the patient in a return to independence is that goals that are set in hospital may not incorporate all aspects of life on discharge. These 'missing elements' may be areas that the patient finds difficult to talk about. This can lead to misunderstandings and to a patient being frightened of undertaking activities that were not discussed in hospital.

> Bill Jenkins recovered well from his myocardial infarct. While in hospital he followed a regime agreed with him by the nursing staff and took seriously the advice he was given about changes in his lifestyle. He was worried about translating the improvement while on the hospital ward into conditions at home and felt nervous about asking what might have seemed to be trivial questions about sexual activity and his jaunts to the pub and to football matches. As a result, on discharge, Mr Jenkins' activities were very similar to those on the ward in that he sat in the armchair quite a lot and felt unable to move on from the level of independence that he gained in hospital.

If Bill Jenkins had been helped to make independent decisions during his stay and rehabilitation, he would have been able to generalize much better back into the home environment.

Outcomes in terms of return to physical health

Much of nursing is geared to 'getting the patient better'. A patient comes in to hospital, is diagnosed, treated, recovers and is discharged. For cases who fit this pattern, evaluation of care in terms of return to physical health is quite logical. It must be remembered, however, that as with evaluating in terms of reduced dependence, it is only useful if there is a reasonable expectation that the patient **will** recover full health.

Patients on a surgical ward

Following surgery many patients fall into the category of people who will be expected to return to full physical health. Whether the operation is simple, e.g. appendicectomy, or more complex, e.g. hysterectomy, goals may be set which aim for a return to physical health. These will include physical healing, full mobility and a return to independence.

Goals set will be realistically staged and it may be that a return to full physical health may not occur until after the patient has been discharged. The patient who has had a simple appendicectomy, for example, may still feel the need for an afternoon rest after discharge, and the patient who has had a hysterectomy may not feel 100% fit for some months after discharge. This unexplained tiredness is often called 'post-surgical fatigue'.

In the hospital setting, evaluating care in terms of return to physical health may not mean that the patient is fully returned to health, rather that he is progressing towards full health at the expected rate. Although this expected rate may vary from individual to individual it is possible to predict normal recovery within certain limits.

Mrs Patel was admitted to hospital for tubal ligation to prevent further pregnancies. Post-operative care included the goal of early ambulation to prevent potential problems related to immobility. Since this is a relatively simple operation, it is expected that the patient will be out of bed the day after operation and fully able to look after her physical needs of hygiene and elimination within a few days.

Mrs Patel just wanted to sleep all day after the operation and barely managed to stay awake during visiting time. She resisted attempts to get her out of bed and needed help in walking to the toilet. This patient required reassessment by the nurse who initially felt that she was being lazy. When she realized that Mrs Patel really could not stay awake, a medical opinion was sought and the patient was found to have an underlying liver condition which had been exacerbated by anaesthesia. New goals had to be set for her return to physical health, which took into account both her operation and her liver condition.

Patients on a medical ward

Since many medical conditions are chronic it could be argued that it is not reasonable to set goals for the patient to return to full physical health because this will not be possible. The word 'chronic', however, needs to be used with caution since it can unnecessarily label a patient as unhealthy. One example of this is the patient with diabetes mellitus. It is true that the condition is chronic since the pancreas is unlikely ever to secrete enough insulin to maintain the individual's blood sugar at the correct level, but if treatment is effective, that is, if a proper balance is achieved between diet, exercise and insulin, goals could certainly be set for the patient to return to physical health.

When Molly Witherington was diagnosed as diabetic she was suffering from frequency of micturition, loss of weight and lethargy. After a medical decision had been made about treatment the nurses set goals for Mrs Witherington to return to full physical health.

By the time she was discharged the patient no longer suffered from frequency or lethargy and was putting on some weight. It is important when thinking of physical health not to exclude those patients whose health depends on replacement therapy and/or education.

Elderly patients

Because the elderly often have multiple diagnoses and degenerative diseases it is not always possible to evaluate care in terms of return to physical health. Each patient should be assessed as an individual and a decision made on the possibility of a return to as healthy a state as possible for that person.

The outcome of care of the patient admitted with hypothermia may well be a return to physical health, for example. In this instance, evaluation may also include an assessment of the patient's understanding of how to avoid getting too cold in the future and of the arrangements made to provide whatever help is necessary after discharge.

Measuring physical health

Measuring outcomes in terms of reduced dependence can be achieved simply by monitoring the amount of nursing intervention required. To measure physical health, many variables may need to be considered. It is usual to chart a number of observations for each patient on admission, such as temperature, pulse and respiration, blood pressure and urinalysis. These will give baseline data of the state of each individual on admission, as will a recording of weight and information about habits such as smoking, drinking and dietary intake. By continuing to monitor the patient and observe his behaviour, it is possible to measure change. The change may be in a negative direction if the patient is deteriorating, but positive change can be seen as a measure of a patient's return to physical health.

Since there is a range of normality in temperature, pulse and respiration, in other observations, and in metabolism and its effect on dietary needs, it would be ideal if data were available on each patient's normal healthy state. This may happen in the future with the increased

Fig. 14.1 Extensive pressure sores of the trochanters, sacrum and buttocks. Courtesy of Smith & Nephew Ltd.

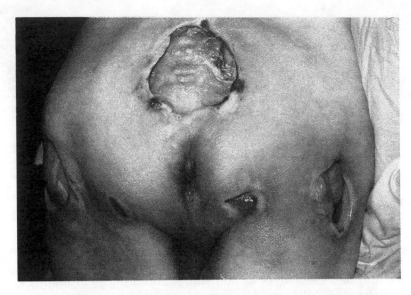

use of computers for the storage of information. Meanwhile, if a patient's measurements on admission are abnormal, measures of a return to physical health have to be monitored against an accepted norm.

In the case of trauma of any kind, a return to physical health may be measured in terms of healing. The progress of a pressure sore may be evaluated in terms of decreased depth and size (Figure 14.1), as may the varicose ulcers of the elderly. Wound healing may also be measured in terms of speed of healing and absence of infection.

Other, less precise, measures of a return to physical health may be by patient report. Again each individual differs in how much energy he normally expends and in the general pattern of his day. Only he will be able to say how his present state equates to what is normal for him.

Outcomes in terms of return to mental health

It was seen that illness and admission to hospital can cause stress to the patient. It is also recognized that stress may affect healing and recovery from illness. For these reasons, evaluation of care should not be simply in terms of physical recovery, if that is the expected outcome, but should also be concerned with mental recovery and the ability to cope with residual effects of disease.

Some conditions are well known to cause problems with mental health. There is a large literature on the psychological effects and psychiatric morbidity of cancer patients (Greer 1985; Thomas *et al*. 1987; Corney *et al*. 1992). Other diseases may also cause stress, particularly those where body image is changed or life in the future is going to be very different from how it was in the past. Before evaluation of psychological care can occur, each individual patient needs to be assessed and goals set, or referral made to an appropriate agency.

Measuring mental health

Measuring mental health is less simple than measuring, for example, a patient's temperature, pulse and respiration, although as in any measurement it is change which needs to be observed. As with physical health, knowledge of the patient's normal state would be useful, particularly when observing non-verbal behaviour. Just as there is a 'normal' body temperature with upper and lower limits, so there is a 'normal' range of mental behaviour with upper and lower limits. If it is not known what is normal for any one individual, it is difficult to make statements about mental state from observed behaviour.

If assessment of mental state gives a baseline of how the patient is coping on admission, goals may be set in stages for either the maintenance of mental health or, if there are problems on admission, a return to mental health.

Taking Mr Lacey as an example, it is reasonable to assume that his assessment on admission would have elicited that he was fearful of his forthcoming surgery. If pre-operative information was given, a goal could be set that, as a result of dealing with his questions, stress would be reduced. Measuring the effects of care in this instance could be by the patient reporting better understanding and a more tranquil approach to the forthcoming surgery.

Fear of walking following surgery may be reduced by offering information and by physical and psychological support. Evaluation of fear levels may be shown by Mr Lacey's attitude to walking. He may change from being apprehensive when asked to walk, to a state where his confidence increases from day to day. Such measurement may be said to be subjective, but, when feelings are concerned, concrete measurement is not possible.

Some patients may be so stressed by what is happening to them in hospital that their relatives comment on the change in their behaviour. After careful assessment by the nurse, it may be necessary to ask for a full psychiatric assessment where in-depth analysis may be made of the patient's current mental state and the effect of his illness on that state.

There are tools to measure the levels of psychiatric morbidity such as clinical anxiety and depression. However, these measuring tools are focused on a medical agenda and aim to quantify feelings. They do not explore the patient's reactions to his disease and there is an inherent danger in using psychopathology to look at the mental reactions of people who do not have psychiatric disease (Bowling 1992).

Patient report

For the patient to report his mental state, the nurse needs to be skilled in eliciting the patient's feelings. It should be possible to evaluate psychological care from a patient interview, though questions will need to be open and the patient will need to feel that he is safe in talking to the nurse.

Steve West had been told on the doctor's ward round that he had to have a colostomy. The nurse went to speak to him afterwards in an attempt to discover how he was coping with the idea of the impending operation. She started with an open question:

Nurse Well, Steve, how do you feel about the operation?
Steve (angrily) You don't expect me to be delighted I hope
Nurse Oh come on – it won't be so bad. I'll tell you what, why don't you talk to Mr Jones. He has had a colostomy for years
Steve I don't want to talk to bloody Mr Jones

The nurse was distressed at this interchange. She could see that Mr West had problems in coping but she was unable to identify them. Her mistake was in trying to reassure the patient without identifying his problems. She could not set goals for acceptance of the operation and evaluation could not take place. Better results might have been achieved if the nurse had explored the patient's anger in the following way:

Nurse Well, Steve, how do you feel about the operation?
Steve (angrily) You don't expect me to be delighted I hope
Nurse You seem very angry
Steve Yes – I am angry. The doctor tells me he is going to ruin my life and wanders off. It's all everyday to him
Nurse And to you?
Steve The end. I am engaged to be married – how can I expect Ruth to take on someone with a colostomy . . .

Here the nurse elicited one of Mr West's problems and goals were set which included talking to Ruth. It was later possible to evaluate whether the patient had moved towards acceptance of his operation. Other worries affecting his ability to cope were also elicited, goals set and Steve's return to mental health evaluated.

Behavioural measures

It is especially true that assessment is dynamic and continuous in the area of psychological well-being. A patient following mastectomy, for example, may have appeared to accept the operation on admission, but later shows that she is unable to cope by refusing to look at the scar. Goals will need to be set for looking at the scar and a time scale agreed between nurse and patient. Evaluation of outcomes will include measures of the observed change in attitude towards looking at the scar.

The above is an example of the need for both nurse and patient to be involved in making decisions. Compare the following:

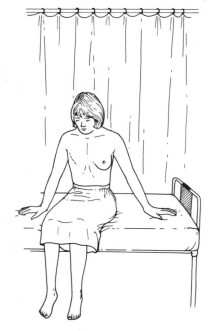

1

Joan Baker	Nurse, I'm very worried
Nurse	Well, there's no need to be worried. What are you worried about?
Joan Baker	I don't want to see myself when you take that dressing off
Nurse	Well, you've got to look at it sometime, you know. I get all my patients to look at their chest three days after the operation. Now, we'll leave that so you're going to look at it tomorrow.
Joan Baker	I'm not sure that I can.

2

Joan Baker	Nurse, I'm worried
Nurse	What are you worried about?
Joan Baker	I don't think I can bear to see the scar. I can't imagine myself without one of my breasts.
Nurse	Well, I think I can understand that but I wonder what we can do about it?
Joan Baker	I wish I never had to look again
Nurse	Perhaps we should make a plan so that you can build up to it
Joan Baker	You mean I could have a bit of space?
Nurse	But of course, if that would help
Joan Baker	I think it might be easier once it's healed
Nurse	Well, shall we set a plan so that you know what you're working to and maybe I could help by showing you some pictures when you are ready.
Joan Baker	Yeah, that might help, but I don't think I want to look today

Nurse	You don't have to look today, but what we will do is make a plan for building up to looking and since you'll be home by the time it's truly healed, we'll make sure that the Community Nurse takes over where I leave off in helping you with what I can see is quite a real problem.

In the first exchange, the nurse imposed a time limit for looking at the scar and left the patient feeling considerably worried and tense about the actual situation. In the second exchange the patient was left feeling more in control of the situation, though having agreed that goals would be set for a solution of the problem. Also the nurse had offered support in terms of allowing the patient to see photographs of other people prior to looking at herself. It is not uncommon for women, after mutilating surgery such as mastectomy, to be very concerned about body image. Very often they are offered photographs prior to the operation but this does not necessarily ease their concern for self image at the time when reality dawns.

It is relatively easy to forget that any illness can affect mental health by causing psychological problems. A patient's behaviour may alert the nurse to the possibility of problems. Some behaviour may be obvious, such as weeping or refusal of food. Less easy to assess is withdrawn or angry behaviour, especially if the nurse is not aware of the patient's normal behaviour. Evaluation can occur only if measurable goals have been set as the result of assessment. This assessment may also elicit psychological problems unrelated to the disease. It may be possible to set goals for improved mental health in this situation or it may be necessary, as with any psychological problem, to refer the patient to other agencies. In this case evaluation will take cognizance of outside help.

Outcomes in terms of patient potential

When Maslow (1969) put forward his theory of a hierarchy of needs for normal individuals, the ultimate goal was that the person would reach his potential when lower order needs were met. This model fits patient recovery well since it allows for potential to be reached on an individual level rather than being gauged against a perfect norm. If care is evaluated in terms of a patient reaching his potential, given that he may have long-term deficits, progress can be monitored at a realistic and possibly optimistic level.

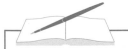

Look up both the national and local standards for evaluating patient care. Make comparisons of the two. What are the strengths of the local standards? How could they be improved?

Evaluating care of the chronically ill

Many patients suffer from diseases which are chronic, i.e. they have permanent deficits which cannot be rectified. One example of this is chronic bronchitis. The patient has deficits in breathing which may be alleviated but cannot be cured. To evaluate this patient's care in terms of a return to physical health would be inappropriate. Evaluation in terms of the patient reaching his potential can be a much more realistic measure of whether care has been effective or not, providing assessment had resulted in goals which were neither over- nor underoptimistic.

An elderly women was admitted to a geriatric ward stating that she was unable to walk. She was grossly overweight and had pain and stiffness in her legs. The medical diagnosis included osteoarthritis and drugs were prescribed to alleviate the pain.

Nursing assessment elicited the information that the woman preferred to be called Nancy rather than Mrs Griffiths, and that she was afraid to attempt walking. While at home her daughter had looked after her so that she had not needed to rise from her bed. It was agreed that Nancy was not reaching her potential as there was no reason why she should not walk with help. Because of the arthritis it was believed that a return to full health was not a reachable goal but that Nancy had the potential for self-care with limited mobility. Plans were made which included weight reduction, increased mobility and self-care. A time scale was agreed with the patient, who kept a diary of her weight, her time out of bed, and her success with efforts to walk.

Evaluation, in stages, to measure Nancy's progress led to reassessment and future goals being set. Nancy was not frustrated by the feeling that the impossible was being expected but was, rather, motivated to persevere as she became slimmer and more active.

This patient in fact more than reached the potential predicted by the nursing staff. Other patients may have a more limited potential than predicted because of unexpected factors. This is an example of the need for constant reassessment in the light of goals being achieved.

Evaluating care of the terminally ill

As with the chronically sick patient, the terminally ill will have deficits which cannot necessarily be reversed. Indeed, with these patients, deficits will be expected to increase rather than the reverse, and nurses may feel, as the patient deteriorates, that his potential is also decreasing.

Of course this is true, but just as goals may be set to achieve a higher potential for a patient who will get better, so goals may be reset for a lowered potential for the patient who is deteriorating. This should not be seen as failure; rather the result should be that each patient is gaining as much as possible from life in his present state. Evaluation should measure if this is being achieved. It depends on assessment which has resulted in plans for care with realistic goals. It may be that evaluation of a terminally ill patient's psychological state will show that the patient is despondent and sad. Reassessment may elicit information which can lead to plans to increase the patient's motivation to make the most of his time left. Re-evaluation may then measure changes in a positive direction which will show that the patient's potential for happiness, given his current deficits and limited future, is being met.

Potential as a measure

We have discussed the evaluation of individuals reaching their potential when a return to full health cannot be expected, but this does not mean that patients who are expected to return to full health may not also have their care evaluated in this way. In fact 'reaching potential' may be seen as a more ready measure than 'full health' since full recovery, if expected, may not always occur immediately or while the patient is in hospital.

It might be argued that to predict a patient's capabilities in the future is no more than guesswork, but it can be more than that since experience of a number of patients with similar conditions can give us a 'normal range' of recovery period or partial recovery rate. In assessing each individual, cognizance will need to be taken of those factors which may affect his recovery.

There is of course some guesswork attached to such predictions and this is a good reason why goals should be set in steps with the possibility of resetting if outcomes have been over- or underestimated. The patient's view is also important in decisions relating to reaching his full potential. In being involved, the patient's motivation to co-operate should increase and evaluation will be more likely to show that expected outcomes have been reached.

Quality assurance

It is not practical or feasible to evaluate every aspect of the quality of care (Redfern and Norman 1990; Koch 1992) but with changes in the NHS and the move to the purchaser/provider paradigm, there is a growing interest in measuring the overall care that is given in any particular unit. This activity of overall evaluation is sometimes called quality assurance and often called clinical audit. The aim is to measure the quality of care given and this involves devising tools that will actually measure the activities that make up total patient care. At present there is no general agreement on what should be measured and evaluated and how it should be measured, but audit and quality assurance exercises are in progress throughout the NHS (Ingleton and Faulkner 1994).

One of the big issues in audit is whether it should be carried out using external packages such as Qualpac, whether it should be carried out by an external body such as that offered by the Cancer Relief Macmillan Fund, or whether staff should devise their own measuring devices. Within these questions are the tensions caused by feeling that someone else is checking up on the nursing care given as opposed to nurses monitoring their own standards of care.

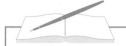

Choose two measures of audit that are commercially available. What are the stated aims of each package? What commitment is required from the staff to use each package, and what are the implications in terms of time, skills and costs? How would using each of these packages improve your standards of care? How does each package link with the local standards of care laid down for practice in your unit?

Summary

In this chapter it has been suggested that there are many ways to measure outcomes and so evaluate the nursing care of a patient.

These methods are not mutually exclusive but will depend very much on which aspects of care are being evaluated. For example, if outcomes are measured in terms of physical or mental health or in terms of a patient reaching his maximum potential, then such measures may be seen as global, giving a picture of the individual as a whole. A single measure for one aspect of care may also be used, such as reduced dependence – for example, Mr Lacey's ability to walk on his own.

Measuring care in subjective terms, i.e. patient satisfaction, may also be useful since one of the aims of nursing care is a satisfied patient. In this case there is the possibility that one measure, e.g. patient satisfaction, could conflict with another, e.g. reduced dependence, especially if nurse and patient have not agreed outcomes.

It has been seen that evaluation allows for reassessment and the setting of new goals based on progress to date.

Finally, the notion of quality assurance or audit has been introduced which aims to assess the current situation in a unit and ask questions about why care is delivered in the way it is and to look for improvements in the quality of care for a particular patient group.

References

Bowling, A. (1992) *Measuring health. A review of quality of life measurement scales*. Milton Keynes: Open University Press.

Corney, R., Everett, H., Howells, A. & Crowther, M. (1992) Psychosocial adjustment following major gynaecological surgery for carcinoma of the cervix and vulva. *Journal of Psychosomatic Research*, *36*, 561–568.

Greer, S. (1985) Cancer. Psychiatric aspects. In Granville Crossman (Ed.) *Recent advances in clinical psychiatry*, pp. 87–104. Edinburgh: Churchill Livingstone.

Ingleton, C. & Faulkner, A. (1994) *Quality assurance in palliative care: a review of the literature*, Occasional Paper No. 14. Sheffield: Trent Palliative Care Centre.

Koch, T. (1992) A review of nursing quality assurance. *Journal of Advanced Nursing*, *17*, 785–794.

Orem, D. E. (1971) *Nursing. Concepts and practice*. New York: McGraw-Hill.

Redfern, S. & Norman, I. (1990) Measuring the quality of nursing care: a consideration of different approaches. *Journal of Advanced Nursing*, *15*, 1260–1271.

Thomas, C., Madden, F. & Jehu, D. (1987) Psychological effects of stomas. *Journal of Psychosomatic Research*, *31*, 311–316.

Further reading

Benner, P. & Wrubel, J. (1989) *The primacy of caring. Stress and coping in health and illness*. Menlo Park, California: Addison Wellesley.

Harvey, G. (1988) The right tools for the job. *Nursing Times*, *84*(26), 47–49.

Marr, M. & Geibing, H. (1994) *Quality assurance in nursing: concepts, methods and case studies*. Edinburgh: Campion Press.

Parsley, K. & Corrigan, P. (1994) *Quality improvements in nursing and health care. A practical approach*. London: Chapman & Hall.

Rogers, S. (1991) Monitoring quality and standards. *Nursing Standard*, *6*(3), 17–19.

Schroeder, P. (1994) *Improving quality and performance. Concepts, programmes and techniques*. St Louis: Mosby Year Book.

Willis, L. D. & Linwood, M. E. (1984) *Measuring the quality of care. Recent Advances in Nursing, No. 10*. Edinburgh: Churchill Livingstone.

15

The Patient on Discharge

CHAPTER SUMMARY

Planning for discharge, 513
Discharge information, 515
Social conditions, 517

The need for patient education, 521
Understanding disease, 522
Understanding treatment, 523
Understanding precipitating factors, 523
Effective teaching, 524
Education for the recovery period, 528
Health promotion, 530

Self-image, 530
Mutilating surgery, 531
Patients on a medical ward, 531
Implications for discharge, 532

Practical considerations, 533
Notification of relatives, 533
Referral, 533
Transport, 534
Discharge against medical advice, 535
Discharge procedure, 536

The role of the relatives, 536
Physical care, 537
Emotional care, 537

Summary, 538

References, 539

Further reading, 540

Planning for discharge

Some patients are admitted to hospital with a clear idea of how long they will be in and what is likely to happen on discharge. Others may have only a hazy idea of their length of stay in hospital and little idea of the procedure for returning to their own environment. There is a move for much earlier return to the community for most patients and careful planning is required to make sure that when an individual returns to his own home, he has a clear idea of how to manage his life in relation to his recent illness or operation.

When a patient is in hospital, it is all too easy to concentrate on immediate problems and their solution or alleviation, without thinking ahead to the time of discharge. Even if the patient has been involved in his own care while in hospital, he seldom takes total responsibility for his welfare while he is undergoing treatment. In fact, although on admission a patient may have difficulty in adapting to his perceived loss of freedom, he may later become so accustomed to allowing others to take responsibility for his care that the idea of leaving the safe hospital environment can cause him concern.

Planning for discharge should start soon after admission so that the patient has time to absorb knowledge on his self-care for when he goes home, ask any questions which are troubling him and get used to the idea of the transition between hospital and home. The nurse will also need time to make any special arrangements which are necessary given the patient's individual circumstances.

Such pre-planning means that a careful assessment needs to be made of the patient's potential for self-care early on in his hospital stay. Preparation for discharge may then be linked to individual needs. Similarly, knowledge is necessary of the amount of support available from the patient's family so that care in the community can be arranged and community staff made aware of any problems.

Assumptions should not be made in planning a discharge since a nurse's previous experience may prevent account being taken of the unexpected. Many patients after surgery, for example, find difficulty in coping when they get home, yet technically they are no longer 'ill' in the accepted sense of the word. Faulkner and Maguire (1983) suggest that these patients do not necessarily get visited by community staff because they do not need the physical attention of the district nurse and may not be seen as a priority by the health visitor.

Ideally, the assessment document will have a section that covers the need or potential need for referral to the Social Services department (Figure 15.1). It should also have a section for discharge planning which should meet the local standards laid down in the Health Authority (Figure 15.2). If these sections of the assessment document are clearly laid out they will give the nurse a clear indication of the areas that she should cover on talking to a patient in the early stages of planning discharge.

In the absence of appropriate planning, problems may arise. The patient may be discharged without appropriate information or reassurance on his care at home. More importantly, the General Practitioner and relevant community service agencies may not know of the patient's potential discharge and needs. Similarly, if there has not been an adequate assessment prior to discharge, the facilities available to the patient at home may not be sufficient to enable him to cope there. Finally, the patient may

**TRIGGER FACTORS TO INDICATE NECESSITY FOR
REFERRAL TO SOCIAL SERVICES DEPARTMENT**

IF THE ANSWER TO QUESTIONS 6 + 7 IS **NO** OR **YES** TO QUESTION 8 A CORE
ASSESSMENT MUST BE CARRIED OUT BY THE NURSE.

		YES	NO
1.	Does the patient have a home to go to ?	☐	☐
2.	Has the patient got dependents at home who need care during Patients admission ?	☐	☐
3.	Does patient have a pet who needs care during admission ?	☐	☐
4.	Does patient need financial/legal advice ?	☐	☐
5.	Does patient have property that needs securing during admission ?	☐	☐
6.	Will patient be able to selfcare on discharge ?	☐	☐
7.	If the answer to question (6) is **NO**, is there a carer willing to care with/without support ?	☐	☐
8.	Will patient require more practical support from Social Services than that they were getting prior to admission ? (e.g. Home Care, Meal on Wheels, Day Centre).	☐	☐
9.	Does patient need opportunity to talk through anxieties re:	☐	☐
	Implications of illness	☐	☐
	Short term/long term future care	☐	☐
	Family/other issues	☐	☐

Answer **NO** to questions 1 & 6, answer **YES** to questions 2,3,4,5,7, & 8 and
refer to Social Worker.

Referring Nurse Signature: _____ Date: _____

Fig. 15.1 Example of assessment form to indicate necessity for referral to Social Services. Reproduced with kind permission of the Practice Development Unit, Seacroft Hospital, Leeds.

not actually be fit to leave hospital if planning and ongoing assessment has not occurred (DHSS 1988).

Discharge information

It is not unusual for patients to be given 'discharge information' on the actual day of discharge. Such information is unlikely to be retained for a number of reasons. Firstly, the patient is as likely to be under stress on discharge as when he was admitted. This may seem odd given that going home should be a joyous occasion, but in fact it is easily understood. Once again the patient is going into the unknown, not in terms of people or places but in terms of readjusting after a period of absence from home. He may wonder how he will cope, how his family will adapt to any

Fig. 15.2 Example of discharge planning form. Reproduced with kind permission of the Practice Development Unit, Seacroft Hospital, Leeds.

DISCHARGE PLANNING		
SERVICE	SIGNATURE	DATE
Discharge Date		
Patient Informed		
Family Informed		
TTO's		
Medication Explained to Patient		
Transport		
District Nurse		
G.P. Informed		
Any Other Services Arranged		
Outpatients Appointment		
Discharge Letter		
Specialist Nurse e.g. Macmillan, Stoma Nurse		

residual deficits of his illness and how he will manage his own care. He may be very apprehensive on the day of discharge and unlikely to remember information given to him.

Another reason against delaying discharge information until the actual day is that an individual can only remember a limited amount at a time. There has been considerable debate over the years on the noncompliance of patients with regard to medical advice. Ley and Spelman (1967) suggested that patients do not remember what they are told and, although this is an over-simplification of the reason for noncompliance, it could certainly be true if a patient is given considerable information all at once at a time of stress.

The vast body of research on health professionals'

abilities to interact effectively with their patients suggests that many patients simply do not receive adequate information based on their needs (Faulkner 1984; Faulkner and Maguire 1994; Sanson Fisher *et al*. 1991). Further, if discharge information is left until the last minute it could well be forgotten if a ward is busy or a nurse off sick who was responsible for a particular patient.

If local standards are observed and a formal documented structure is available for the discharge process (Bowling and Betts 1984), then potential problems should be avoided. In addition, it is useful to give the patient a discharge document which summarizes his move from the hospital back into the community (Figure 15. 3). Both patient and informal carers can then look at the document to make sure that they have understood the discharge information.

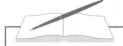

Choose a patient who will be discharged in the next two weeks. Who is the main carer? How much does the patient know about his discharge? What potential problems can you identify? Do you think the patient and carer are adequately prepared, to date, for discharge?

Social conditions

Occasionally there are problems with social conditions caused by a patient's deficits or discovered as a result of the patient's admission to hospital. Pre-planning is necessary in order that adjustments may be made in time for the patient's discharge. This can be a sensitive area if the conditions in which a patient has been living are poor, so any discussion needs to be handled with tact and understanding. Such matters are the concern of the health care team. There is little point, for example, in treating an elderly patient with hypothermia and then returning him to the same cold conditions which brought about the initial problems. The Social Services may be useful in this instance, although education of the patient may also be necessary.

Many individuals are totally unaware of the benefits available to them. Referral to a social worker will give the patient and family access to information which will help them to claim appropriate benefits. The Department of Social Security's leaflet FB31 (DSS 1994) lists the benefits available for those who are caring for someone, as do leaflets from the Carers National Association. There is also help available for those living alone who may need help with bills for fuel and other essential commodities, and some charities make grants to people. For example, the Cancer Relief Macmillan Fund makes grants to patients to help with the care of cancer patients at home.

The nurse, in assessing patients' needs on discharge from hospital, may have to deal with the pride of individuals who see such help as charity. What is important is that the patient is made as comfortable as possible on his

SEACROFT HOSPITAL : DISCHARGE PLAN

MEDICATION	DOSE	TIME	WHAT FOR

NUTRITIONAL SUPPLEMENTS:

DRESSINGS:

SPECIAL PRECAUTIONS:

COMPLIANCE AIDS PROVIDED:

If you have any queries regarding your drugs please contact:

SEACROFT PHARMACY HELPLINE

Dear

GP's Name:

Address:

Tel no:

Your discharge from .... ward has been arranged for

.... / .... /

You will be given a letter to take home to your GP which

will inform him or her of your care in hospital.

Diagnosis/treatment given ....

....

If you have any queries after you go home, please do not hesitate

to contact your Primary Nurse who is ....

or your Associate Nurse who is ....

on tel no: ....

Your District Nurse is .... tel no: ....

and will visit on ....

Your Homecare Manager is .... tel no: ....

and will visit on ....

Others:

Other information:

Fig. 15.3 Example of patient's discharge document. Reproduced with kind permission of the Practice Development Unit, Seacroft Hospital, Leeds.

DISCHARGE PLANNING CHECKLIST

SERVICE	SIGNATURE	DATE
DISCHARGE DATE		
PATIENT INFORMED		
FAMILY/CARER INFORMED		
THERAPISTS INFORMED		
PHYSIO		
OCC THERAPISTS		
DIETICIAN		
SPEECH THERAPIST		
TTOS/DRESSING		
MEDICATION EXPLAINED TO PATIENT/CARER		
DESTINATION ON DISCHARGE		
TRANSPORT/TYPE		
KEYS		
DISTRICT/ PRACTICE NURSE		
LIAISON NURSE		
HOMEHELP/WHICH DAYS		
MSW INFORMED		
OUTPATIENTS APPT/TRANSPORT REQUIRED		
GP LETTER		
INFORMATION SHEETS GIVEN		
COMPREHENSIVE ASSESSMENT		

Any special information/advice:

The following therapy/outpatients have been requested:

Date and type:

An outpatients appointment to see your Consultant is/is not required.

Details to be sent through the post.

Transport arranged Yes/No

May we take this opportunity to wish you all the very best and we

hope your stay with us at Seacroft has been a beneficial one.

Fig. 15.3 Continued.

return home and is helped to understand that appropriate help is every patient's right. It is also the aim to help patient and family cope.

Other help may be required which is more complex. For example, a patient may be discharged who can no longer manage stairs. It may be that arrangements can be made for him to have a room downstairs until more satisfactory arrangements can be made. Local councils are sympathetic to rehousing in these circumstances if the patient is not a home owner and/or is free to move. It is not a nurse's duty to make these arrangements but she should gather relevant information and refer the problem, with the patient's agreement, at the earliest possible opportunity.

One of the most difficult problems in planning discharge is that of the elderly patient who had previously lived alone but is no longer fit to do so. In this case it is crucial that the patient is involved in discussions about the problems of discharge.

Kate Mason had been admitted to hospital as an emergency, having fallen in her kitchen and been discovered by her daughter who visited some hours later. As Mrs Mason became well she was keen to go home and worried about her insurances falling behind if she was not there to pay the representative when he called. Until her admission, Mrs Mason had lived alone, having daily visits from her daughter. What she did not realize was that her daughter felt unable to continue care of her mother and had told both the Consultant and the Ward Sister that she wanted her mother 'put away'.

Mrs Mason first learned of her daughter's intentions when the Consultant told her she could no longer live alone and arrangements would be made to put her in a home. Kate was devastated and later that day knocked her lunch from the table and attempted to leave the hospital. A worried Sister, who did not understand Mrs Mason's behaviour, sent for a psychiatrist.

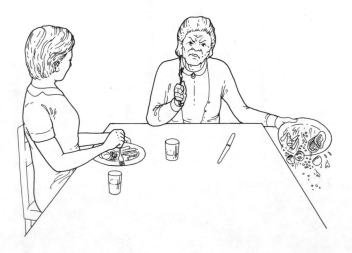

If discharge is going to mean dramatic change for the patient, it is essential to communicate openly with the patient and involve him in discussion of all the possibilities. Individuals have a right to choose (with a few exceptions such as the mentally ill) and may prefer to 'muddle along' in unsatisfactory conditions rather than submit to institutionalization. This may become a more contentious issue as health professionals become more litigation-conscious and argue for the 'best interests' of the patient. Health professionals in such situations need to make a careful assessment of the situation so that if the patient truly wants to return to an environment where all the evidence suggests that he may not cope well, or may come to harm, he may do so.

What is important here is that the **patient's** wishes are documented along with a record of family consultations. This should reflect that all avenues have been explored to help the patient cope in his chosen environment on discharge. If any patient feels that his wishes have been disregarded, he has the right to sue.

The importance of considering social conditions prior to discharge is that when a patient goes home he should have the best possible chance of maintaining his health at the maximum level. By carefully assessing need well in advance of discharge the necessary help can be obtained and known to be in place before the patient goes home. This may include referral to a social worker or to other services in the community. Such careful planning and documentation should ensure that the patient can remain at home and so lower the risk of readmission and of noncompliance with treatment regimens.

The need for patient education

For most nurses, the term 'patient education' usually brings to mind those patients who have to have obvious self-care on their return to the community: the patient with a stoma has to learn to deal with colostomy bags, the patient with diabetes to deal with insulin injections, and other patients with a variety of drugs or treatments.

Patient education is much more than this and may apply to practically all patients on discharge. Basically it should cover teaching the patient to understand his disease and treatment along with factors which may affect his future or have contributed to his present state. Health education was discussed in Chapter 2. To this the dimension of disease and treatment is being added so that the

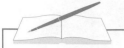

Choose a patient on your ward who is being prepared for discharge. Assess his knowledge of his disease. Assess his knowledge of his treatment. Is further help required for this patiet to understand his disease and treatment? If so, how can you help?

patient may return to optimum health given the constraints of his particular disease.

Research in the past has suggested that many patients are not taught to understand their disease and its treatment (Eardley *et al.* 1975; Faulkner 1980; Webb 1983; Faulkner and Maguire 1984). However, with the growth of specialist nurses with a remit to educate and support patients and their families this picture is changing. Examples are stoma care nurses, breast care nurses, cardiac rehabilitation nurses and nurses who work with patients who have a diagnosis of diabetes.

Understanding disease

An argument might be made that if a patient has been in hospital and has recovered from his disease or operation there is little point in worrying him with details before he goes home. If a patient has had a simple operation such as an appendicectomy this may be true, although it might comfort him to know that his appendix has no useful function. With many diseases, an understanding on the part of the patient may be a crucial factor in recovery.

The more a patient understands his disease and the need for particular treatments, the better he will cope with his current situation (Anderson 1987). This is particularly true for patients who are suffering from deficits which are permanent. For example, patients with diabetes need to have a clear understanding of the effect of their disease on the body so that they can understand the need for regular replacement of the deficit and the constraints which this imposes. Lowry (1995) suggests that patient information leaflets are useful to complement verbal information on both disease and its treatment.

When disease is linked with lifestyle, understanding is required to prevent recurrence. Patients who have had a myocardial infarction, for example, need to understand those situations which put undue strain upon the heart.

John Hughes had his first and second infarction when making love to his wife because he did not understand the link between exertion and its effect on his heart.

Traumatic surgery is also an area where patient understanding can be beneficial, and here especially, psychological factors need to be taken into account.

The patient with a stoma or following hysterectomy

or mastectomy are just three examples where lack of knowledge of the surgery and its effects can cause immense problems. People have to live with the effects of disease, maybe for a short while, maybe for a lifetime. No assumptions can be made that patients understand the implications of their disease without education from health professionals. Education should commence in hospital, considerably before discharge, and may need to be continued into the community. Increased knowledge should reduce not only recurrence and complications but should also reduce the psychological concerns of each patient.

Understanding treatment

If a patient understands his treatment regimen he is more likely to comply with the doctor's prescriptions. This understanding need not be highly technical but it should be linked with cause and effect. The patient who is prescribed diuretics should understand that her pills remove excess fluid from her body and that if she does not take them she may feel 'blown up'. That this link between her pills and her fluid balance is understood is more important than whether she talks of 'diuretics' or 'water pills'.

When treatment is unpleasant there is even more reason for the patient to be aware of its importance in relation to disease. Cytotoxic drugs, for example, may make a patient feel nauseous or actually produce vomiting. It is tempting to discontinue treatment on the grounds that 'the treatment is worse than the symptoms of the disease'. This can be a difficult area in patient education since there is seldom a guarantee that the drugs will be effective. Often there is a need for counselling and teaching in this situation. Sometimes treatment involves visits to out-patient departments. The patient is more likely to make the journey if there is a clear understanding of the reasons for the therapy. Otherwise resentment at the time and money spent for no apparent outcome can cause noncompliance.

Self-medication programmes may be useful in aiding compliance, since they educate the patient about his medication while he is in hospital and can substantially increase compliance on discharge (Sedgeworth *et al.* 1990; Johns 1990).

Understanding precipitating factors

It is not unusual for an individual to miss the link between lifestyle and disease. This may be due to a lack of knowledge or to denial of known facts. Patient education should aim to give insight into health-related factors and disease, though there may be some reluctance for a patient to accept knowledge which may require him to change the patterns of a lifetime.

It was seen in Chapter 2 that there are links between lifestyle and disease. For example, weight, smoking and alcohol consumption appear to be related to heart disease while smoking is also seen to be linked with many diseases, notably those affecting the respiratory system. Overweight is also thought to be linked with diabetes in older individuals. No assumptions can be made that any patient will have accepted these facts, yet, by the act of accepting this knowledge, a patient may decide to modify his behaviour and so have a positive attitude to his future health. In teaching patients this health educative aspect is often overlooked while emphasis is laid on the regimen required to maintain or improve the current condition.

Effective teaching

Teaching is a skill which all nurses need to learn if they are to help their patients. So often one hears a nurse or doctor exclaim, 'but I explained that to him!' when a patient seems unable to manage a simple task. It may be that an explanation **has** been given but for some reason it has not been understood by the patient.

Just as communication (Chapter 4) is a two-way interactive process, so is teaching. In fact communication skills can be seen as the basic bricks of teaching skills since, if there is no interaction, there will be no teaching or learning. The nurse may **tell** the patient what he needs to know but the message may be ignored, misunderstood or simply not heard.

In teaching a patient it is important to find out just how much he already understands and start from where he is in terms of knowledge or skills. If a concept is new to him it is important to start at the beginning. This is not such an obvious statement as it seems since when one is familiar with a particular skill or piece of knowledge, it is very difficult to avoid taking certain aspects for granted. There is a popular party game where individuals are asked to describe everyday procedures to an alien from another planet. One of the procedures is the tying of a knot. It is surprising how many people start with the knot itself and overlook the fact that the very beginning of the explanation should be a description of the string. To most individuals, string needs no explanation since it is part of everyday life.

Similarly it is common knowledge among medical and nursing staff that, for example, if a patient with diabetes is prescribed insulin, he is likely to have to take it for the whole of his lifetime. In teaching a patient to give his own injections, he needs first to understand the permanence of injections in his life in order to be motivated to learn.

Motivation

The idea of motivation is central to teaching. Psychologists have found that positive reinforcement, i.e. rewards, are the best motivators for learning. Punishment will also work but only if it is so severe as to be unethical in teaching humans. If patients are learning to manage their treatment prior to discharge the idea of positive reinforcement is very useful. As goals set for patient care should be reachable, similarly patient teaching should be planned in small steps.

Patients with a stoma, for example, need to learn to change their own bags, yet may find the whole idea of a stoma so repulsive that they avoid looking at it. The nurse's perception may be quite different – changing bags is an everyday procedure. To teach the patient to deal with his stoma requires careful assessment and plannning so that, by the time of discharge, the patient is competent to care for himself. The first step in teaching may be to help the patient look at his stoma. Forcing him to look at a prescribed time post-operatively is likely to cause stress, which will inhibit learning. Assessment, where the patient can verbalize his feelings, should help a nurse to plan this first step in self-care.

It will be seen that teaching is time consuming and requires considerable patience. Positive reinforcement means praising what is achieved in the correct manner and suggesting methods for rectifying mistakes. It is too easy to lose patience and say something negative such as, 'Oh, for heaven's sake, aren't you ever going to get it right?', rather than, 'Well, you have sealed the bag beautifully, but look, it's upside down – I expect it's because you see it from a different angle. Let's try again'. The first statement may cause the patient to feel a failure while the second should give him hope that he will eventually succeed.

Practice

If a patient needs to learn a skill such as changing a stoma bag, releasing a catheter or giving an injection, it will usually help to see the procedure carried out by the nurse. This gives a whole picture for the patient to remember

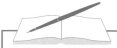

Borrow a copy of *Principles of Nutritional Assessment* by Gibson (1990). Arrange to work with a friend or colleague, and assess each other's standards of nutrition against the recommended standards. How did your feel about sharing this information? Will you make any changes to your own nutrition?

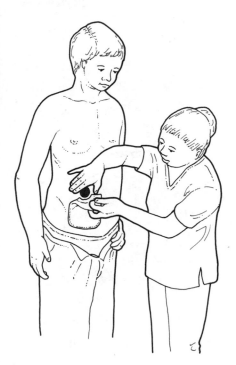

while he is learning the steps and thus he knows what he is aiming for in terms of the final skill.

If, for example, a patient with diabetes gets used to handling a syringe and insulin, understanding the need for cleanliness and the risks of infection, and working out his dose, it may be some time before he is ready actually to inject himself. During this time he can practise those steps which he has learned so that when he does actually inject he is confident that all other aspects of the procedure are correct. Similarly with the injection itself – this should be supervised by the nurse during a practice period until the patient has acquired the skill.

Allowing the patient to practise requires patience, especially on a busy ward where it would be easier for the nurse to carry out the procedure. Learning takes time but a patient who is competent in self-care is less likely to be readmitted to hospital.

Avoiding confusion

Some patients need to learn more than one skill prior to discharge. It is important not to confuse a patient if there are different procedures to be learned.

Miss Hope was diagnosed in an out-patient's clinic as having diabetes. She was 68 years old and the consultant decided that she could be stabilized at home with tolbutamide and a controlled diet. Before leaving the clinic Miss Hope was shown how to test her urine once and given her drugs with instructions on when to take them. The next day she was admitted as an emergency having swallowed her Clinitest tablets. Miss Hope had not learned the correct procedure for a number of reasons. Firstly, she was distressed to learn of her diagnosis. Secondly, she had not been allowed to practise testing her urine, nor yet to make a clear differentiation between the two bottles of tablets. Lastly, her eyesight was poor, a factor which had not been assessed.

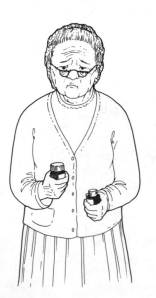

Incidents such as the one cited above can be avoided but adequate time is required. In a busy out-patients' department it may be necessary to involve a community nurse in visiting the patient's home to continue teaching and supervision should a specialist nurse not be available.

In teaching, confusion may be avoided by asking the patient to feed back his understanding at each stage of learning. Only in this way can the nurse be sure that the patient has gained understanding of a particular skill. Supervision of the actual procedure should continue until the individual is confident of his ability.

Written instructions

Many hospitals give written instructions to a patient prior to discharge to help him manage his treatment during the

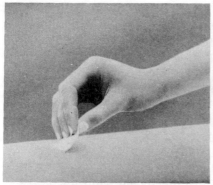

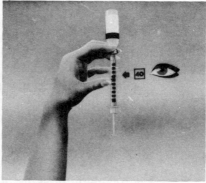

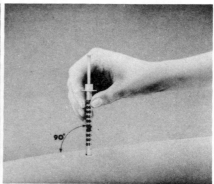

(a) Clean your injection site with an alcohol swab.

(b) Check the right dose. Remove the syringe from the bottle.

(c) With one quick motion, inject the needle into the skin straight in a 90 degrees angle.

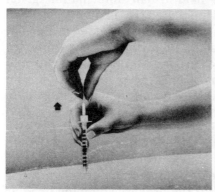

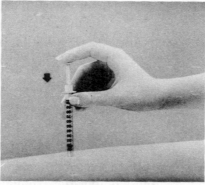

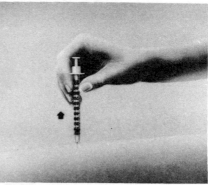

(d) While holding the barrel with one hand, pull up on the plunger about 2 to 4 units. Look for blood in the barrel. If there is blood, DO NOT INJECT THE INSULIN. The needle is in a vessel. Pull the needle out of the injection site, throw it away and start again, with a new syringe and a new injection site.

(e) If there is no blood, push the plunger down to inject the insulin.

(f) When the injection is finished pull the needle part of the way out, pausing for a moment.

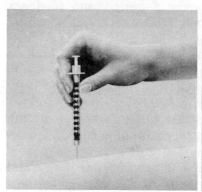

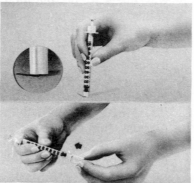

(g) Then, remove the needle completely from the skin.

(h) Bend the needle on a table and use the syringe cap to shield the needle. This prevents abuse of the syringe.

Fig. 15.4 How to inject insulin: an abstract of instructions to the patient. Courtesy of Becton Dickinson UK.

recovery period (Figure 15.3). These instructions will act as a useful *aide-mémoire* but do not replace the need for teaching. Such written instructions need to be discussed with the patient in order to ascertain that they are fully understood.

Some drug firms also issue written instructions for patients (e.g. Figure 15.4), but again these do not replace the need for patient teaching.

Education for the recovery period

The teaching of skills before discharge from hospital has been discussed. Equally important, but more neglected, is the need to give each patient information which will aid his recovery and future health. The information given should meet the needs of the patient (Faulkner 1984). Too often, information given to a patient is inaccurate and vague. For example, patients following hysterectomy are often told, 'Don't drive the car, don't lift heavy weights and don't have sex', rather than being given guidelines during which they adapt and recover so that they may indeed do all those things again. Similarly, advice to patients is often not linked to their lifestyle. For example, Faulkner (1980) found that nurses would tell patients who had had a mycardial infarct not to lift wardrobes, attend parties or work too hard. This leaves patients totally unable to work out whether they should lift the grocery shopping or their children.

Sometimes patients will ask questions about their care, their disease and their future. If this information is to be retained it should be given in clear language. Most people cannot remember more than six or seven pieces of information at a time. This means that teaching will need to be planned over a period and feedback gained from the patient to test that learning has occurred. Just as teaching a skill should build on previously learned units of the skill, so should knowledge be built up in steps.

There are some areas where patients may be loath to ask questions, notably on sexual matters. Faulkner and Maguire (1984) found that nurses were also loath to raise this subject, yet it is vitally important to many patients. A distinction may be drawn between sexual counselling and sexual advice. In teaching a patient about his after-care he needs definite knowledge on which to base his behaviour. If he also has problems he may need counselling so that he may work towards acceptance of a situation or towards solutions which are possible for him.

John Hughes had two infarctions while making love to his wife, and needed advice on love-making. If learning does not occur on how to manage this aspect of after-care the patient may be too scared to make love, which could damage his relationship with his wife, or lead to a further attack and the patient's possible death. Nurses may not have enough knowledge to teach on this aspect of care but should recognize from assessment when problems exist. Hopefully Mr Hughes will have been given advice on exercise. He will have been advised to walk rather than run and to gradually increase the amount of exercise taken. To understand this he needs to learn about the effect of exercise on the heart. If he can also understand how much energy is expended in making love, especially in the very common, so-called 'missionary position', where the male partner takes the dominant, most energetic role, he will also understand the need to take a more passive position when loving his wife.

It is in a situation like this when teaching and counselling may overlap. Mr Hughes may have rigid ideas about sexual behaviour and believe that only emasculated men allow their wives to take the 'dominant' position in love-making. He may not be open to suggestions for more gentle forms of sexual expression. If assessment of the patient reveals problems of this nature, it may be necessary to refer him to a trained sexual counsellor. The nurse will have met the individual's initial need to verbalize fears and will have taken appropriate action. The above example illustrates that an individual's personal beliefs will affect his willingness to accept information and advice. Teaching should not be attempted without prior assessment of the patient's knowledge and beliefs.

Teaching for recovery is concerned with maximizing potential. One would expect patients to be motivated to learn, albeit that learning to understand their disease and treatment may place restrictions on their lives. Occasionally a patient is not open to teaching because his perception of what life is about is different from that of the nurse.

Terry Ling was 46 when he had a cerebral haemorrhage. He made a good recovery with little impairment of function and understood well that in order to survive he had to lead a restricted life. Three weeks later he attended the wedding of the daughter of friends and at the reception asked the bride's mother to dance. As a nurse herself she asked him, 'Should you be doing this?' and he replied, 'Not if I want to survive, but I prefer to live'. He died a few weeks later having made an informed choice. It is often difficult for health professionals to accept the idea of informed choice, especially in the area of health promotion, perhaps the most difficult area of patient teaching.

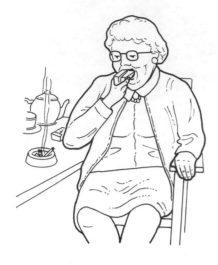

Health promotion

Patient teaching may require that an individual learns of the effects of his lifestyle on his current disease and future health. This is rather different in focus to the preventive health education discussed in Chapter 2. Ill-health may be seen as a lever to exert pressure on a patient to change his lifestyle, but this alone may not be enough. Some patients may link their 'heart attack' with smoking, for example, and give up in fright, but it is equally probable that many will rationalize matters such that they do not necessarily accept cause and effect.

If the nurse hopes to effect a change in behaviour such as in smoking, diet, alcohol, or mental health, she will have to accept that knowledge of the dangers of the present lifestyle may not be enough to break the habits of a lifetime. She will need to discover the patient's present level of knowledge and beliefs and find ways of motivating him to co-operate in a new regimen. Most people, for example, know that it is dangerous to smoke and over-eat. If disease calls for cessation of smoking or a modified diet it is essential that the patient understands the rationale for the change. Elliott *et al.* (1983) produced booklets giving hints on helping people give up smoking. Similar strategies may be used in other areas of health promotion.

Although a patient's disease may not be linked to unhealthy habits, the nurse may use his stay in hospital as an opportunity for preventive health promotion. The general public respects the opinion of health professionals and as long as the nurse is working towards informed choice rather than crusading, there should be no ethical dilemmas in attempting to achieve a more informed public. Planned teaching, based on a patient's needs, which have been carefully assessed, can be very rewarding. It should be integrated into all patient care so that the recovery and discharge period can be faced by the patient with the minimum of stress.

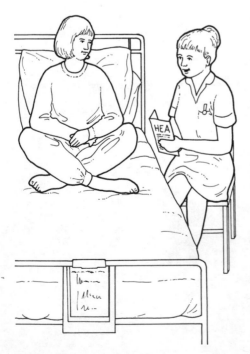

Self-image

Illness may affect an individual's self-image, and so add to any problems of discharge, since the individual going home does not feel the same person as the one who was admitted.

Mutilating surgery

Such feelings are true of almost every patient who has undergone mutilating surgery, whether it is major or minor and whether it is obvious to the outside world or not. Although the patient may worry while he is in hospital, his perceived deficiency is likely to be more important when he is discharged to the 'normal world'. The patient following mastectomy may feel a freak, or the amputee a figure of fun. If these patients are not assessed before and after discharge on their ability to cope in their normal environment, psychological problems may become severe to the extent that patients may refuse either to leave the house because they are 'ashamed', or to sleep with their partners because they feel 'unlovable'.

It was seen in Chapter 11 that other patients following surgery may have problems with their self-image which, if not faced while they are in hospital, may be exacerbated on discharge. Webb (1983) found that patients following hysterectomy are worried by the effect of their operation, some describing themselves as feeling 'neutered'. This could well have an effect on the patient's discharge, particularly in relationships with partners, so leading to psychological problems at a time when the emphasis needs to be on a return to health. Similarly with patients who have a stoma, where there is a change not only in body image but in body function. These patients may feel that other people are aware of offensive odour, that they are no longer 'normal' or that they are unacceptable to family and partner.

Some male patients may be temporarily impotent following surgery such as prostatectomy or the formation of a colostomy. This can have a traumatic effect on self-image in terms of virility and masculinity, especially if the patient is unaware of the temporary nature of the problem. Even if this problem arises while the patient is in hospital, it is unlikely that it will be verbalized because of the cultural taboos around talking about sexuality and the perceived inappropriateness of a male patient attempting to gain an erection while in hospital.

Patients on a medical ward

One could argue that medical patients' self-image need not be affected by their disease. Often, in fact, a patient may be affected by his diagnosis, or by his own (unexpected) reaction to that disease. It was seen in Chapter 4 that patients with carcinoma may feel there is a stigma

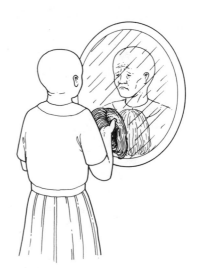

attached to their diagnosis and certainly it is well documented that such patients are avoided by hospital personnel. Since cancer may be equated with dying (Bond 1982) it would not be surprising if patients on discharge felt that they were treated differently by family and friends. Because self-image depends not only on the individual but on feedback from others, psychological stress may occur as the patient tries to fill his perceived role in society without the necessary feedback. The treatment for cancer may also affect self-image – loss of hair, libido and feelings of nausea will all bring changes to an individual's ideas about himself as a person.

Diagnoses which affect an individual's lifestyle may also affect self-image. If, for example, a patient needs to change employment as a result of his condition, his perception of self may change. If, alternatively, a disease is chronic, this 'label' may affect self-image, particularly in the case of diabetes, where the patient believes that he has to 'live by the clock'.

Any disease and its attendant deficits may affect self-image and hamper recovery, especially when individuals do not really understand what has happened or how to cope with what has occurred to them.

Implications for discharge

It is known that self-image may be affected by disease, treatment or surgery and this will have implications for the patient on discharge. Just as it is necessary to prepare the patient to cope physically, it is also crucial to assess his ability to cope psychologically with discharge and after-care.

Emotional after-care should warrant the same attention as physical after-care, in that those patients who may have problems in coping after discharge should be followed in the community so they can be quickly referred if their problems are not resolved. For this to happen there needs to be good liaison between ward and community staff, particularly if district nurses are involved who do not carry their own caseload (Chapter 17). The ward staff require the ability to assess the effect of illness on the patient's self image and the possible consequences if the patient seems unable to cope without further help.

It may be that the patient will show strong signs of distress prior to discharge, in which case referral to a counsellor or psychiatrist may be necessary before the patient is able to go home.

Practical considerations

When a date for discharge has been set, arrangements need to be made so that the return to the community is as free from stress as possible.

Notification of relatives

If a patient is given a date for discharge and is able to, he may well telephone relatives himself with the good news, or let them know at visiting time. Relatives may then see the Ward Sister/Manager and arrange a convenient time for taking the patient home.

It is not enough, however, simply to give a patient a discharge date and expect him to make the arrangements himself.

ilian had been admitted for minor surgery to remove a polyp from her face. She lived alone and travelled 50 miles on the bus to the hospital. When Lilian was told that she could go home she was too proud to tell the staff that her children lived too far away to fetch her or that she could not afford a taxi.

On the morning of discharge, a junior nurse, who was helping Lilian to pack, asked who was coming to collect her. When she realized that the patient planned to catch a bus, she reported the matter to the Ward Sister. Lilian was admonished for not being open with the staff and had to stay an extra day until hospital transport was available.

It is in fact the ward staff's duty to check that adequate arrangements are made for a patient's discharge. Lilian was discharged without anyone knowing that she was returning to a cold empty house. Patients are unlikely to proffer such information unless adequate assessment is made. If a patient does live alone, it may be that willing relatives will go and prepare the house, or take the patient to their home for a temporary period. No patient should be discharged until appropriate arrangements are made and confirmed.

Referral

When an individual is discharged, the hospital doctor sends a discharge letter to the patient's GP giving brief information about the patient's disease, treatment, present state and plans for follow-up. If the patient needs nursing care on discharge, the nursing staff will make contact with a community nurse (Figure 15.5). It is the

Fig. 15.5 Communications for referral prior to discharge.

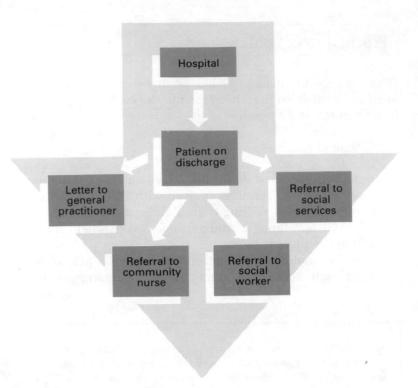

responsibility of either the Ward Manager or a liaison nurse who may be attached to the ward to make such referrals after consultation.

The letter to the GP may be given to the patient to deliver personally or may be sent through the post. Referral to a community nurse is often telephoned or faxed so that immediate attention is available at home, but this should always be followed by a written referral which gives adequate information about the patient's current state. Even if the GP and community nurse are notified of the patient's discharge in good time, it is usual to give the patient enough drugs and dressings to last for 48 hours, by which time a prescription for more may be obtained from the GP. It is essential that the patient understands when to take drugs, how many to take and how to apply treatments.

Transport

Hospital transport is available for all patients who need it. It is usually an ambulance or hospital car, though some authorities use volunteer car owners to transport patients, and some pay for taxis. Because such transport is expensive, those relatives who are prepared to collect patients by car are encouraged to do so. This may lead nurses to an expectation that every patient has such a relative. The danger of making this assumption is that individuals such as Lilian may find themselves travelling long distances by bus instead of in the relative comfort of hospital transport.

Each patient should be asked if transport is available to them. If not, transport should be arranged and relatives notified of the approximate time of the patient's arrival at home. An exact time cannot be promised since ambulances may be called to an emergency, so disrupting a planned schedule. If patients and relatives understand this there are less likely to be irate telephone calls or anxious patients.

A patient may have to attend the hospital after discharge as an out-patient. If so, the patient should have his appointment card before discharge if possible, and arrangements should be made for transport if necessary. Many patients do not know that they may be entitled to transport for out-patient treatment under certain circumstances. Miss Phipps, for instance, paid £6 per day for a taxi to take her to radiotherapy treatment until a nurse arranged transport for her.

Discharge against medical advice

Although discharge is accepted as a procedure arranged when a patient is ready to return to the community, occasionally a patient will decide that he wants to go home against the doctor's advice. He may be unhappy or angry or feeling that he is wasting his time. Apart from psychiatric patients who have been committed, being in hospital is a voluntary matter and every individual has the right to leave. However, if a patient does wish to leave it is important that a senior member of staff explores the reasons for the patient's decision and satisfies herself that the patient understands the implications of premature discharge.

Molly Witherington wanted to go home against medical advice. In this case, exploration of the reasons resulted in a compromise where the patient had two days out and then returned for treatment. Often, allowing a patient to talk through his feelings will result in a compromise or a change of heart. It is important for the nurse to remain cool in this situation. Opposing the patient is more likely to harden his resolve to go home than persuade him to stay.

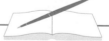

The next time a patient is discharged, keep a note of the following:

1 At what time was transport arranged?
2 Who helped the patient to pack?
3 When did transport arrive?
4 Where did the patient wait after he was dressed?

Do you think the discharge went smoothly? How could it have been improved?

A gypsy, Sam Bott, was in hospital in the terminal stage of cancer. One evening he became angry and demanded to go home. If Sister had said, 'Don't be silly, you have to stay here' she could have increased his anger. Instead she sat by the bed and said, 'Come on Sam, tell me about it'. Sam admitted to feeling imprisoned and 'hemmed in' since he was not used to sleeping indoors. He agreed to stay if his bed was wheeled outside in the daytime. This was achieved by covering it with plastic sheets if it rained. Sam remained in hospital until his death.

If a patient is determined to make his own discharge, he has to be seen by a doctor and sign a form which indicates that he is discharging himself against medical advice. This is a legal document which exonerates hospital staff from responsibility for that patient. It does not mean that the patient will be refused treatment in the future. Referral to a GP and community nurse should be made as necessary.

Discharge procedure

Whatever the circumstances of a patient's discharge, he should be asked to sign for any clothes or valuables which have been stored for him, and the nurse should ensure that all his belongings are safely packed.

There may be a wait between getting packed up and being collected which can be uncomfortable for the patient, especially if a zealous nurse has stripped his bed so there is nowhere to lie down. Any wait should be made as pleasant as possible. It may be that a comfortable chair in the day-room can be used if it is essential to get the bed ready for a waiting patient, but ideally he should feel that the territory of bed and locker will remain his until he leaves. Goodbyes should not be tinged with the feeling that the staff cannot wait to see the last of a patient.

The role of the relatives

It has been seen that relatives and friends have a part to play in the preparation of the patient's homecoming and perhaps in collecting him from the hospital. They can also play an important role in easing the transition between hospital and home, when the individual has to adapt from the role of patient to the role previously held in society with any additional adaptation required by the residual deficits of his disease.

Physical care

Relatives may need to be involved in physical care when a patient is discharged. It may be giving eye drops, monitoring drugs or producing a required diet. If this is envisaged, then they will need to learn what is required. As with patient education, time will be required and should be set aside so that, when a patient returns home, the relative feels confident that he can continue care of high quality.

Relatives will need to be assessed for willingness and ability to learn. Some may think that care at home should be given by community nurses while others will appreciate the chance to help the patient recover at home. Perhaps the most important point for relatives to learn before a patient's discharge is how much a patient may safely do for himself. It is possible to impede recovery by making a patient over-dependent with cossetting.

Sometimes it is useful for the patient and relative to learn together about after-care. This is particularly true in the sensitive area of relationships. Mr Hughes's need for information about the link between energy expended and its effect on the heart was discussed. His wife needed psychiatric treatment after his second infarction because she felt she was killing him. Her need for knowledge was as great as that of her husband.

Emotional care

Relatives may not realize the varying emotional effects of a changed self-image and may, without help, inadvertently fail a patient by not appreciating his problems. Perceptions may be different too. A husband may avoid

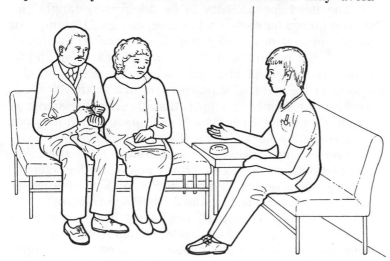

making loving advances to his wife after mastectomy or hysterectomy from consideration. She may interpret this as lack of interest because of her decreased attraction as a woman. If the couple do not talk, the resulting problems will increase tensions between husband and wife.

Similarly, the partner who will not allow the patient to resume a previous role will exacerbate problems of changed self-image. It may be that a mother will want to resume preparing her child for bed immediately. If the husband says, 'No, I'll do it, you can't carry her upstairs anyway', the mother feels excluded and useless. If, however, he says, 'OK, but let me carry her up until you are stronger', his wife will feel involved and wanted. If relatives can discuss these issues with health professionals **before** a patient's discharge, many problems could be avoided, as relatives can help patients to resume previous roles and avoid being overprotective.

Some patients are loath to give up the 'sick' role. This can be difficult for relatives if they do not understand how much a patient is able to do for himself on discharge. Preparation before discharge may prevent the perpetual invalid from developing and ruling a household.

Summary

In this chapter, the need for discharge planning to start as soon as possible after a patient's admission has been considered. It has been suggested that this should include adequate documentation of the potential need for social services and adequate documentation for the patient to take home.

The need for patients to be adequately taught the skills required for self-care has been discussed, along with the advantages of knowledge of disease and its treatment for both the patient and those who will care for him at home. The effect of changed body image has been discussed in the light of a patient's return to the 'normal' world and it has been shown that careful assessment is required to identify changes in self image which may not be obvious to others.

Practical considerations of discharge have been discussed along with the need for and procedure for referral, and the steps to be taken when a patient chooses to discharge himself against medical advice. Finally, albeit briefly, the role of relatives and carers has been considered in terms of smoothing the transition from hospital to home for the patient and avoiding unnecessary dependency, either because of relatives being overprotective or the patient being unable or unwilling to give up the 'sick' role.

References

Anderson, E. A. (1987) Pre-operative preparation for cardiac surgery facilitates recovery, reduces psychological distress and reduces the incidence of acute post-operative hypertension. *Journal of Consulting and Clinical Psychology, 55*(4), 513–520.

Bond, S. (1982) Communications in cancer nursing. In Cahoon, M. C. (Ed.) *Cancer Nursing. Recent Advances in Nursing, No. 3.* Edinburgh: Churchill Livingstone.

Bowling, A. & Betts, G. (1984) Communication: discharge. *Nursing Times, 80*(32), 31–33.

DHSS (1988) *Discharge of patients from hospital.* London: HMSO.

DSS (1994) *FB31. Caring for someone?* Heywood, Lancashire: Health Publications Unit.

Eardley, A., Davis, F. & Wakefield, J. (1975) Health education by chance. The unmet needs of patients in hospital and after. *International Journal of Health Education, 18*(1), 19–25.

Elliott, K., Faulkner, A., Randell, J. & Ward, L. (1983) 'Helping patients to give up smoking' leaflets. London: Health Education Council.

Faulkner, A. (1980) *The student nurse's role in giving information to patients.* Unpublished M.Litt. Thesis, Aberdeen University.

Faulkner, A. (1984) The consequence of ignorance: nurse/patient communication. In Brittain, J. (Ed.) *Consensus and penalties for ignorance in the medical sciences.* London: Taylor Graham.

Faulkner, A. & Maguire, P. (1983) Nursing is more than doing. *Journal of District Nursing, 1* (10), 9–13.

Faulkner, A. & Maguire, P. (1984) Teaching ward nurses to monitor mastectomy patients. *Clinical Oncology, 10,* 383–389.

Faulkner, A. & Maguire, P. (1994) *Talking to cancer patients and their relatives.* Oxford: Oxford University Press.

Gibson, R. (1990) *Principles of nutritional assessment.* Oxford: Oxford University Press.

Johns, C. (1990) Steps to self medication. *Nursing Times, 86*(11), 40–41.

Ley, P. & Spelman, M. S. (1967) *Communicating with the patient.* London: Staples Press.

Lowry, M. (1995) Knowledge that reduces anxiety. *Professional Nurse, 10*(5), 318–320.

Sanson Fisher, R., Redman, S., Walsh, R., Mitchell, K., Read, A. & Perkins, J. (1991) Training medical practitioners in information transfer skills: their new challenge. *Medical Education, 25,* 322–323.

Sedgeworth, C., Hudson, S., Jefferson, G. & Maclennan, W. (1990)

Pharmacist assessment of elderly patients' ability to self medicate. *The Pharmaceutical Journal, Feb 17*, 24–27.

Webb, C. (1983) Body image and recovery from hysterectomy. In Wilson-Barnett, J. & Fordham, M. (Eds.) *Recovery from illness*. Chichester: Wiley.

Further reading

Begg, D. (1993) How much should we tell our patients about drugs? *Prescriber*, *4*(10), 76–79.

Bird, C. & Cottrell, N. (1990) A prescription for self-help. *Nursing Times*, *86*(43), 52–57.

Dines, A. & Cribb, A. (1993) *Health promotion. Concepts and practice*. London: Blackwell Scientific Publications.

Ewles, L. & Simnett, I. (1992) *Promoting health. A practical guide*. Harrow: Scutari Press.

Farrow, S. (1993) Should we give them responsibility? Healthcare staffs' views on self-medication. *Professional Nurse*, *8*(5), 304–308.

Rankin, S. H. & Duffy, K. L. (1983) Patient education: issues, principles and guidelines. London and Philadelphia: J. B. Lippincott.

Wilson-Barnett, J. (Ed.) (1983) *Patient teaching. Recent Advances in Nursing, No. 6*. Edinburgh: Churchill Livingstone.

Wilson Barnett, J. & McCloud Clark, J. (1993) *Research in health promotion and nursing*. London: Macmillan.

Useful address

Carers National Association
20–25 Glasshouse Yard
London EC1A 4JS

PART SIX
CARE IN THE COMMUNITY

16

Life After Hospital

CHAPTER SUMMARY

Return to independence, 543
Out-patients' departments, 543
The specialist nurse, 546
Breaking the links, 547
Post-hospital depression, 547
Levels of activity, 549
Return to work, 549

Adjustment to reduced ability, 550
Changes in lifestyle, 550
Residual deficits, 551
Patients with poor prognosis, 552

The role of the family, 552
Emotional support, 553
Physical support, 555
Dying at home, 555

Summary, 556

References, 557

Further reading, 557

Return to independence

If a patient's discharge has been well planned, he will go home with enough understanding of his disease and treatment to continue his recovery without mishap. In some cases, the patient will be told to contact his GP if he has problems. In other cases, links may be maintained for some time with the hospital through the out-patients' department or via a specialist nurse.

Out-patients' departments

Many patients are followed up routinely after discharge from hospital by the Consultant at an out-patients' clinic. Ideally, an appointment card will be given to the patient before discharge. The alternative is for the appointment to be sent to the patient's home after discharge.

Appointments
A patient should know, before discharge, the approximate date of his first clinic appointment. If he does not subsequently hear from the hospital, he will know that an error has occurred and will be able to remind the Consultant through either the hospital or his GP.

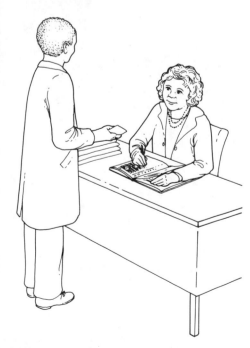

When Ingrid Olson was discharged from hospital after her mastectomy she knew only that she would be called to clinic to be fitted with a prosthesis. In fact her booking was overlooked and it was three months before she tentatively raised the matter with her district nurse. During that time she had not moved far from home, describing herself as a 'lop-sided freak'.

The clinic

Out-patients' clinics are run on an appointments system. Patients may be seen by their Consultant or one of the doctors on his team. Each patient has to take his appointment card to a clerk on arrival, who will then tell him where to sit until he is seen by the nurse or the doctor.

Clinics can be very frightening places. They are often large, open areas, and several Consultants may have a clinic on the same day. The patient may not realize that, once he has checked in, his notes will have been taken to the relevant nurse, and he may wonder how he will get his correct turn to be seen. It may be that the patient needs to be weighed and have urine tests, blood tests or observations taken before seeing the doctor. If so, these should be carried out with as much privacy and tact as possible to save embarrassment to the individual.

When Mrs Witherington went to the diabetic clinic for the first time, the nurse called her over to her desk to be weighed and have her urine tested. Mrs Witherington objected to her weight being shouted for all the clinic to hear and to being treated as a nuisance because she had not known she should have brought a specimen of urine with her.

To the nurse, the clinic will be an everyday occurrence, but to the patient it can be a bewildering and impersonal place. When Mrs Witherington was called in to see the Consultant, she had waited for an hour, miserably wondering if she was being punished for not knowing about the specimen. The Consultant's cheery, 'Well, you are doing fine – stay on the regimen and I will see you in two months', was over in a few moments and the patient was at the bus stop feeling foolish that she had not asked him any of the questions she had planned.

The nurse's role

The reality of out-patients' departments is that patients do have to wait. It may be that, because of an emergency, the doctor is late in arriving at the clinic. Alternatively, a new patient may take longer than the time allotted, or extra patients may be added to the list at the last moment. If the nurse explains any undue delay to the patients, they are less likely to feel that they are of little importance to the clinic staff. The Patient's Charter (revised 1995) sets standards for waiting periods, and the level of adherence

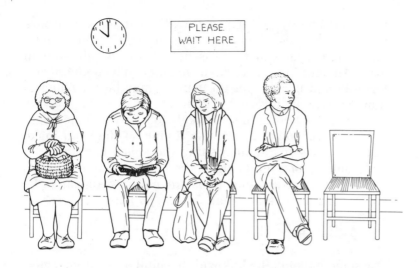

to these is one of the measures of the 'providing unit's' performance.

Similarly, a nurse can help a patient at the clinic by understanding that it may be difficult for him to raise matters with the doctor. If, when the patient is being weighed, the nurse asks an open question, e.g. 'Well, Mr Smith, how have things been since you went home?' she will give him the opportunity to express his concerns. If, for example, Mr Smith is concerned about pain in his leg at night, the nurse can forewarn the Consultant that this is a problem, and he in turn can raise the matter with the patient.

It may take some time for a patient to get to an out-patients' clinic. It may also be tiring if the patient has not fully recovered from his disease or operation. If, when he does arrive, he has the feeling that the long wait and short impersonal consultation are a waste of time, he may miss future appointments.

Follow-up clinics are important, however. Patients with cancer, for example, need follow-up appointments to ensure early detection of any spread after operation. For patients with diabetes it can mean better control and the early detection of complications; similarly for other conditions. Often, the nurse is the interface between patient and Consultant and can make a patient feel that the clinics are worthwhile even if there is sometimes a wait.

The nurse and the clinic environment

Strictly speaking, the clinical environment is not the responsibility of nursing staff. However, nurses can make a difference to the out-patient's department by making sure that it is as welcoming as possible. All too often the waiting

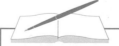

Visit your local out-patient department. What is the most recent magazine/journal? Is the refreshment area clearly signposted? How comfortable are the seats? How would you describe the overall environment? How could the area be improved?

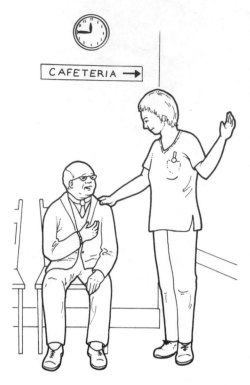

area is draughty and exposed with hard seats and bare walls. Magazines, if they are present, can be out of date and 'dog-eared' and there is not always a refreshment area. An hour in such an environment can be both uncomfortable and boring, yet the patient may be unwilling to move in case he misses his turn.

If a nurse knows there is likely to be a wait, she might give patients some idea of the timing so they can make realistic decisions about visiting the snack bar, taking a walk outside or even going to the toilet. From a patient's perspective, out-patients' departments may appear to be run for the staff rather than for the patients.

The specialist nurse

For some patients the link with hospital after discharge is the Specialist Nurse. Specialist nurses are increasingly used to fill the needs of certain groups of patients, being seen as experts in a particular area such as stoma care, diabetic care or mastectomy care (Figure 16.1). At present they tend to see all the patients in their area of specialization within a district, though Faulkner and Maguire (1983) suggested that they should be used as a resource by non-specialist nurses, seeing only those cases where special help is needed. With the 'new deal' for junior doctors, these nurses are expanding their role further, e.g. in haematology.

If a district employs specialist nurses, the patient will usually meet the nurse while he is still in hospital. A later visit can be a comforting link for the patient as he convalesces at home. Because the nurse is a specialist in her field she will be aware of the common problems facing the

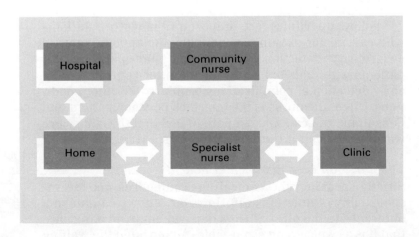

Fig. 16.1 The out-patient's contacts with the health care team.

patient and skilled enough to elicit the less common problems of each individual.

If, however, the role of the specialist nurse is as a resource for the community, the link between hospital and home may be made by a community nurse, who will know about the patient from the specialist nurse.

> **M**rs Witherington, for example, was seen in hospital by a diabetic nurse specialist. After discharge, the district nurse visited Mrs Witherington and established common ground by saying, 'I have been talking to Lesley, the diabetic nurse, about you and so I thought I would pop by to see how you are now that you are home.' Further links were made in the out-patients' clinic, when not only the doctor but the specialist nurse were in attendance.

The specialist nurse fills the role of practical nurse, teacher and adviser on physical care, and counsellor to patients. If she acts as a resource, her teaching role extends to other nurses. This co-operative role can be beneficial to both the specialist and non-specialist nurse, in that the specialist nurse will be able to maintain a balance between contact with patients, which can be emotionally draining, and her role as a resource to other health professionals.

Breaking the links

The return to independence means a gradual breaking of the links with hospital. For some patients this will be a simple matter, while others may take a considerable time to resume their normal activities.

Most patients have some time at home before returning to work. This time should be spent in gradually increasing activity so that, by the time work is resumed, no undue tiredness will be felt. An appendicectomy, which is seen by most people as a relatively simple operation, may leave a patient feeling tired for several weeks, while after a major operation, such as a hysterectomy, it may be two to three months before the patient feels really well again in all respects.

Post-hospital depression

Patients and their families need to understand post-hospital depression, which is quite a common occurrence once an individual has been home a short while. A patient after hysterectomy described it as follows:

It was all right while I was in hospital; we were all in the same boat. I did not have to worry about things there. Then I was so excited to be coming home, but it was different then. I'd had my stitches out and I suppose I felt that I should be better, but I was not. The children got me down and I did not want to be bothered with meals or the house — and I was so weepy.

These feelings of sadness and despair do not usually last long for, as the patient becomes stronger, he is more able to cope and his mood becomes more positive. Odd 'black' days may occur but these will be outnumbered by good days. Certainly the first week or so at home can be difficult. The visitors, flowers and cards usually cease, and expectations of a return to normal pursuits can seem overwhelming.

For some patients, the return home can be a sad time if they are seen to have recovered from their illness.

Madge Darnley lived alone and had a very quiet life. She did not mix much with colleagues at work and her closest contact was her mother with whom she had a rather ambivalent relationship. After a diagnosis of cancer and her admission to hospital for surgery, Madge's life changed overnight. Her mother became pleasant and co-operative, colleagues at work who had seemed aloof visited and brought flowers and presents, and other acquaintances took great care to offer support while she was ill. Soon after her return home, when she was seen to be coping well with her disease and its treatment, life started to return to its previous level where she spent much time on her own, her mother became difficult again and colleagues returned to the cool relationship that she had been used to. Madge missed the secondary gains of illness because it highlighted for her the value of other people to be caring and concerned for her.

Many groups of patients do not have links with the hospital after discharge and may be at a loss for someone to talk to. They may feel that they should 'pull themselves together' rather than worry their GP. If they do go to their GP they may not be treated with sympathy, for research such as that of Rosser and Maguire (1982) suggests that GPs are not so likely to respond to psychological distress as to organic disease. Indeed many GPs feel such responses to major surgery are 'natural' and do not, therefore, require special treatment.

It is of concern that some patients do not improve. For example, up to 25% of patients after mastectomy are known to suffer from clinical depression, which means that their depression becomes severe enough to warrant psychiatric help. Obviously such patients need to maintain their links with the hospital through specialist or community nurses so that those at risk can be identified early. Neglect of post-operative depression can lead to a patient becoming a suicide risk.

Any patient may suffer from psychological problems after his homecoming if he is unable to accept his diagnosis, prognosis, or changes in his normal functioning. Careful monitoring in the community will mean early identification of problems so that the patient can be helped to return to independence as soon as possible.

Levels of activity

There are many elements of ordinary daily living to which the patient needs to return. Some of these can cause concern if the patient is not sure what is permissible. Common examples are being out and about, shopping, lifting children, driving a car and resuming sexual activity.

Obviously each case must be treated individually, and if any activity is considered dangerous the patient should be informed. If not, a rule of thumb is to resume activities gradually and to stop if pain or discomfort is felt. Patients should feel free to discuss their return to normal health (for them) and no assumptions should be made about a patient's understanding. It is not uncommon, for example, for a patient after hysterectomy to believe that she should no longer make love. This sort of misunderstanding can strain relationships unnecessarily.

Return to work

When a patient who normally works is sick, he is allowed three days without certification. After that, the patient can sign his own sick note (SC2) for a period of four further days, making a week, after which he requires a sickness certificate (Med 3) from his doctor to send to his employer. Once certified 'sick' in this way, a return to work has to be approved by a doctor who will issue a 'final' certificate giving the date on which the patient may return to work.

There are accepted periods for people to stay away from work following different disorders. This will vary according to the type of treatment and how it has been performed. The move towards laser treatments and 'keyhole' surgery, for example, may mean that the patient returns to work earlier than if traditional surgery had been performed. However, in most situations, there will be a period of recovery before a return to work.

In a few patients there may be a reluctance to return to work, and this can be for a variety of reasons. After a long period at home, the patient may feel nervous about

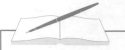

Find a colleague for this exercise. Each of you should think of a patient who has seemed reluctant to go home and another who was very anxious for discharge. What were the similarities between each pair of patients? What were the differences?

'fitting in' again at work. It is quite common to feel an outsider or to gain the impression that one has not been missed. It may be that work responsibilities have changed in the patient's absence and virtually a new job needs to be learned.

Some patients may find this a very difficult adjustment, giving rise to similar feelings as those experienced in adjusting from hospital to home. Anxiety about this final step in the return to independence may lead to sleeplessness and resultant tiredness, lack of interest in food, and mood swings. If the patient can be helped to understand his feelings, his return to healthy living will be eased.

Most patients make the transition from hospital to home and back to work relatively easily. Those who do not should continue to have help from the hospital and community so that they can deal with their problems. If those problems are psychiatric, prompt referral to a psychiatrist or social worker or other appropriate source should be made with the patient's agreement.

Adjustment to reduced ability

Not everyone who is discharged from hospital will return to total independence. Some may return to relative independence but have to accept changes in their lives, while others may never be independent again.

Changes in lifestyle

Some diseases, because of their nature, may lead a consultant to suggest a change of employment. Patients with coronary heart disease, for example, are known to be at risk of further infarctions. The Consultant in this case might recommend that the patient's employment should not put others at risk, so, for example, driving a bus or a taxi would be disallowed. Similarly, the patient himself should not be at risk, so being a steeplejack or a builder's labourer who stands on ladders and high buildings would similarly be discouraged.

It will be remembered that self-image depends on how we see ourselves and on how others see us. A change of work, or a period of unemployment because alternative work is not available, may have a serious effect on a self-image already affected by illness. The resulting unhappiness can delay recovery from illness and may cause depression. A positive approach to the patient is necessary in these circumstances along with a willingness to understand his discontent. Retraining may be possible, which will interest and motivate the individual to psychological adjustment.

Some patients may expect their disease to lead to changes in lifestyle. A patient newly diagnosed with diabetes may, for example, interpret instructions to lead a 'regular life' to mean that he can no longer work shifts. This is not necessarily true. A well-controlled patient with diabetes should be able to lead a normal life to the extent that colleagues will not necessarily know of his diagnosis. He may wish someone at work to know, but equally he may decide to live his life without fuss. What he **should** do, always, is carry a diabetic card (Figure 16.2) and have glucose available in order to avoid hypoglycaemic reactions.

There is of necessity a change in the patient's lifestyle in terms of diet, exercise and medication, which may cause problems in adjustment after discharge. However, with education, these individuals should be able to eat in restaurants or friends' homes, or go out for a drink without calling attention to their disability.

Residual deficits

Patients with both diabetes and with coronary heart disease are left with residual deficits. Although these may affect lifestyle, they will not necessarily mean reduced independence. Other patients have to accept on discharge that they will be less independent than formerly, either

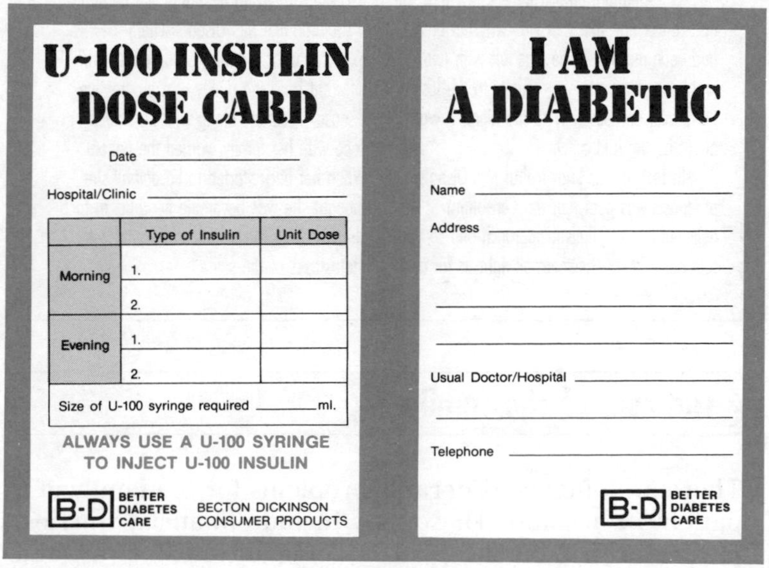

U~100 INSULIN DOSE CARD

Date ____________

Hospital/Clinic ____________

	Type of Insulin	Unit Dose
Morning	1.	
	2.	
Evening	1.	
	2.	

Size of U-100 syringe required ________ml.

ALWAYS USE A U-100 SYRINGE TO INJECT U-100 INSULIN

B-D BETTER DIABETES CARE BECTON DICKINSON CONSUMER PRODUCTS

I AM A DIABETIC

Name ____________

Address ____________

Usual Doctor/Hospital ____________

Telephone ____________

B-D BETTER DIABETES CARE

Fig. 16.2 The diabetic card.

because they are no longer strong enough to care for themselves or because some bodily function is impaired.

If, for example, a patient is newly paraplegic, the reality of never walking again may be confronted only after discharge, when the patient has to face adaptation to normal life within the confines of a wheelchair. Individuals vary enormously in their attitudes to such severe deficits, some appearing to cope well while others become bitter and angry. The acceptance of permanent deficits may be paralleled by bereavement. The patient is in fact grieving and may need considerable support in the process. Some individuals may be at risk of psychiatric morbidity if they cannot work through the grieving process.

Less dramatic, but equally inhibiting, are the deficits caused by chronic diseases. An example of this is the patient with chronic respiratory disease. After discharge, the patient may have to accept not only that life is restricted but that the condition is progressive. There may be problems in adjustment, both to the constraints of the disease and to an acceptance of the permanence of the disability.

Patients with poor prognosis

Some patients are discharged home without a proper understanding of their diagnosis or prognosis. This can lead to misconceptions about a return to independence.

To return to Ingrid Olson and her mastectomy operation as an example, the patient on discharge knew that she had cancer and that that was why her breast had been removed. She was left with two problems of adjustment – firstly to the loss of her breast and secondly to the niggling worry about having had cancer.

In fact, it was known that Mrs Olson's prognosis was poor, but the Consultant believed in an optimistic approach and so had told her that 'things seem all right as far as we can tell'. What bothered the patient was that she did not seem to be feeling better.

Adjustment on discharge can be difficult in a situation like Mrs Olson's where the expectation of a return to normal activities is different from the reality of a progressive disease. Tiredness along with an inability to cope with her family worried the patient. When her back started to be painful she thought she was becoming neurotic. In fact she was later readmitted to hospital with metastases of the spine.

The role of the family

There are often considerable problems for the family of a patient in hospital. These may include financial worries, particularly if the hospital is some distance away and visiting requires long journeys. There may also be problems of caring for children, continuing to work to capacity and even of finding time to cook and clean the house.

It is easy in any of these circumstances to start talking of how much better things will be when the patient comes home. The underlying assumption is that people in hospital are ill and that when they come home they are well. There may also be little understanding of convalescence or the needs of a patient to readjust to the home environment.

On the day that Ingrid Olsen came home from hospital she had been getting out of bed for probably two or three hours each day. She came home to a family whose members were looking forward to Mum's return and to the resumption of regular meals properly cooked, which Dad had not been able to provide. Within a few hours of homecoming, Ingrid was in tears, her husband was exasperated and the children were very puzzled by the tensions that they perceived. What Ingrid had required was to adjust gradually to being at home and to re-find her place in the home at her own pace. Her family, on the other hand, had been muddling through, desperate for the day when Mum and some sense of stability over the running of the home returned.

At the other end of the continuum are those relatives determined to care for the patient on discharge whether or not this is required.

Either approach can be detrimental to the patient's chances of adapting and reverting to his normal role in society. It was seen in Chapter 15 that relatives may need help from hospital staff **before** discharge in order to gain a clear picture of the patient's problems and abilities. This will give the family the best chance of understanding the reality of the period after discharge.

Emotional support

Emotional support is crucial to a patient's homecoming, no matter how minor or serious the reason for hospitalization. Generally, serious ill-health is not discussed socially, yet a common greeting is 'How are you?'.

Mrs Witherington met a friend in Woolworth's shortly after discharge who asked, 'How are you?'. The patient, still attempting to adapt to injections, urine tests, and a controlled diet, replied, 'Well, I am feeling all right in myself but I am not sure I will ever get used to the injections.' Her friend, who had expected the customary, 'Fine, how are you?', made a hasty retreat from something she could not deal with. This reticence to talk about how individuals really feel may lead to 'bottled up' emotions, which may suddenly erupt to the surprise of both patient and family.

The ideal role of the family in this situation is to provide an environment where the patient feels free to express his feelings. This can be difficult, especially if the prognosis is poor or a patient's deficits are permanent. Often, the preferred confidant is the patient's partner. It is easy for nurses to assume that a partner is prepared to take this role but the reality is often very different. Many couples do not talk together, especially about their sexual life, children, religious beliefs or finances. This lack of communication can cause severe problems unless nursing staff are aware and can offer a counselling and monitoring service.

Even if partners do talk, their perceptions may vary.

Bill found that he was impotent after his stoma operation. He talked to his wife about it, trying to show her how his whole self-image was affected. He also tried to explain that the stoma nurse had suggested that he masturbate as a recovery exercise. Bill had read some literature and tried to involve his wife in the masturbatory exercise, as suggested by the nurse. Bill's wife was disgusted and felt that Bill was using his illness to involve her in unnatural practices — further, she began to worry in case the operation had turned Bill into a permanent sexual pervert.

The problem here was that the stoma nurse had made suggestions without assessment of the relationship between husband and wife. Bill, desperate to return to normal, failed to see things from his wife's point of view, while she herself understood neither the problems nor that the suggestions about sexual behaviour came from the nurse. If relatives are to help a patient in adjustment after disease, they may first need insight into the nature of his post-operative concerns.

Emotional support is also required in the 'post-discharge blues' period. Although the patient may feel that everyone has unrealistic ideas about his ability to cope, relatives themselves may feel drained.

Mrs Witherington's husband, for example, had found life difficult while his wife was in hospital. He had taken time off work but did not find it easy to care for the children, cook and clean, and visit the hospital daily. Mrs Witherington, depressed at the thought of daily injections for life, thought her husband did not understand. On the first night he lost his temper and all his own frustrations came out — the endless washing, fretful children, miserable visiting. Finally he shouted, 'And I did not get a single card or bunch of flowers — you had **all** the sympathy.'

Such exchanges clear the air but do not happen between all couples. It is often the community or the specialist nurse who must help with emotional support for both the patient and the family.

If a patient is alone he is particularly at risk. In these circumstances neighbours or friends can be supportive and a specialist or community nurse may be invaluable in helping the patient to cope.

Physical support

Physical support was considered in Chapter 15. Certainly relatives need to discuss this with the nursing staff before the patient's discharge because there can be no assumptions about the support relatives can offer. The disabled or elderly patient may make the greatest demands on relatives.

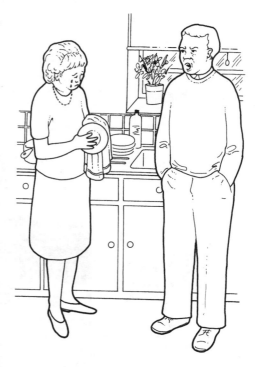

Often, in a rush of love when the patient is in hospital, a relative will make offers which in reality are unreasonable to expect. The aftermath of such offers can be severe. Renvoize (1978) talks of 'granny bashing' in situations where a family has taken in an elderly relative to live with them. Sympathy must go to any elderly person so treated, but understanding is also required of the severe strain put on a family that did not understand the full implications of the care they were offering.

Any disabled person can be demanding and querulous, and often the charming patient in hospital is very different at home. Of course there are reasons to rail against fate, and even to resent the family's freedom while feeling tired and inhibited oneself. However, even the most loving family can become worn down and divided if there is no acknowledgement and support of the care which they give.

Many hospital authorities recognize this problem and are prepared to take a dependant into care for periods of time to give the family a rest. This has been helped by recent legislation which has earmarked a proportion of social services funding for respite care. More co-operation of this kind could lead to a greater number of families being able to offer physical support to disabled relatives. This is equally necessary whether or not the individuals are able to live together harmoniously.

Dying at home

If relatives have a role in providing help and support after discharge for the patient who will either get better or survive, they also have an important role if the patient wishes to die at home. Approximately one in three of the population dies at home (Copperman 1983). With the NHS reforms and more emphasis on care in the community, this figure may increase, with a resultant expectation of support from informal carers.

Because the majority of deaths occur in hospital, the general public are relatively cushioned from knowledge of dying. If a relative wishes to die at home, the family will need to understand what is being undertaken and will need considerable support from community services. Many families are able to care for a dying relative at home if they know what to expect. It is the **unknown** which is so frightening.

L iz Francis was quite happy to care for her mother, who was dying of cancer. She had a smallholding and, although she had not met human death, her experiences with animals had given her a realistic approach to life.

One day her mother asked Liz to get her out of bed and fetch Liz's sister. She then insisted on sitting on the couch and asked the others to do the same. Obviously confused and angry, the mother shouted at Liz, 'It is not right. I wanted it to be as it was before'. Liz rushed out of the room frightened and upset. After her sister had put their mother back into bed, she comforted Liz and telephoned the doctor. Liz was unhappy about being alone with her mother after the incident and expressed relief at her death three days later.

Mr Mudd, on the other hand, nursed his wife alone at home with visits from the community nurses. He had seen his mother and sister die and knew what to expect. He told the nurses that he was happy to give his wife her last wish, that she should die at home. When she died, however, he told the nurse that he was glad. He was not being callous, but he was very tired.

In Chapter 13, we considered the needs of dying patients. These needs exist no matter where the individual is cared for, and if home is the place of choice, relatives may find themselves expected to meet many of the dying patient's needs. There are obviously many differences between a nurse and a relative looking after a patient. One of the crucial differences is that the nurse can go off duty. Relatives may give 24-hour care, especially if they are unaware of the support available to them. It is therefore important that, if a patient goes home to die, hospital nurses make sure that support in the community is available.

Summary

In this chapter, the transition from hospital to home has been considered from both the patient's and his family's viewpoint.

The need for links to exist between hospital and home has been discussed, along with the need for an eventual return to independence if this is possible.

Adjustment to reduced ability has been discussed in terms of both changes in lifestyle and the need for acceptance of chronic disability.

The role of the relatives has been discussed in giving emotional and physical support, and in the cost to the family members if they themselves are not supported.

Finally, consideration has been given to the patient who wishes to die at home, and the effect of this on his family.

References

Faulkner, A. & Maguire, P. (1983) Nursing is more than doing. *Journal of District Nursing*, *1*(10), 9–13.

Renvoize, J. (1978) *Web of violence. A study of family violence*, Harmondsworth, London: Penguin.

Rosser, J. & Maguire, P. (1982) Dilemmas in general practice: the care of the cancer patient. *Social Science and Medicine*, *16*, 315–322.

Further reading

Blyth, A. (1990) Audit of terminal care in general practice. *British Medical Journal*, *300*, 983–986.

Carey, J. (1994) *Older people and community care*. London: OPCS.

Copperman, H. (1983) *Dying at home*. Aylesbury: HM & M.

Department of Health (1993) *Caring for people*. London: Creese and Associates.

McKeehan, K. M. (1981) *Continuing care – a multidisciplinary approach to discharge planning*. London: C. V. Mosby.

Rosenthal, C. J., Marshall, V. S., Macpherson, A. & French, S. E. (1980) *Nurses, patients and families*. London: Croom Helm.

Smith, V. & Bass, T. (1982) *Communication for the health care team*. Adapted for the UK by Faulkner, A. London: Harper and Row.

Wilson-Barnett, J. & Fordham, M. (1982) *Recovery from illness*. Chichester: J. Wiley.

17
Community Services

CHAPTER SUMMARY

The district nurse, 559
Referrals, 559
The case load, 561
The health clinic, 561
The dying patient, 562
Bereavement visiting, 563
The nursing hierarchy, 564

The health visitor, 565
Referrals, 565
The case load, 566
The health clinic, 568
Health promoton, 568
Requirements of the preventive role, 569
The health visiting hierarchy, 570
The practice nurse, 570

The social worker, 571
Referrals, 572
The case load, 572

Support in the home, 573
The interrelated roles of nurses and social
   workers, 574
Home help, 574
Meals-on-wheels, 574

Alternative help in the community, 575
Good Neighbour Scheme, 575
Voluntary organizations, 575

Summary, 576

References, 577

Further reading, 578

Current policy on care in the community aims to build on the best of good practice which already exists. New reforms (DHSS 1990) aim to enable people to live an independent, dignified life at home or in the community for as long as they are able and wish to do so. This means that where, in the past, many people have stayed in hospital after operation or treatment for disease, they will be discharged into the community much sooner than before. Similarly, many patients, particularly the elderly, will be seen to be more appropriately cared for in the community than in a hospital. Key objectives of the Community Care Act, 1990 are:

- To promote the development of domiciliary, day and respite services to enable people to live in their own homes wherever feasible and sensible
- To ensure that service providers make practical support for carers a high priority
- To make proper assessment of need and good care management the cornerstone of high quality care
- To promote the development of a flourishing independent sector alongside good quality public services

■ To clarify the responsibilities of agencies and so make it easier to hold them to account for their performance

■ To secure better value for taxpayers' money by introducing a new funding structure for social care.

It can be seen from the above reforms that adjustment is necessary among the professionals offering care in the community. The work of social services is widening and the work of nurses and health visitors may also cover a wider range of responsibilities. An understanding of the role and function of health professionals and social services in the community will help hospital staff to make appropriate decisions to refer patients before discharge so that care and support can be continued into the community.

The district nurse

Traditionally, the district nurse has been seen as a practical nurse who gives physical care to those who need it. However, with the emphasis moving towards holistic patient care, the expectations are that district nurses will also undertake psychological care of those patients known to have difficulties in coping with their disease and treatment.

To become a district nurse, Registered Nurse (RN) or Enrolled Nurse (EN) qualifications are required. Since 1982 it has also been mandatory to undertake a course of training of at least six months in an institute of higher or further education.

The district nurse, once qualified, becomes part of the primary health care team (Figure 17.1) although she is not employed by the General Practitioner (GP). The team consists of GPs, midwives, district nurses, health visitors and practice nurses, the district nurse being attached to either a GP or a clinic. In either event, she does not select or identify her own case load, but depends on referrals from GPs, hospitals or other members of the community services.

Referrals

Dunnell and Dobbs (1982) suggested that approximately one-third of district nurses' time is spent on patients referred by the GP and over half on follow-up visits. This picture is rapidly changing as a result of the implementation of the Community Care Act (Forster and Laming 1992). There are, of necessity, closer links with social

Fig. 17.1 The structure of the primary health care team.

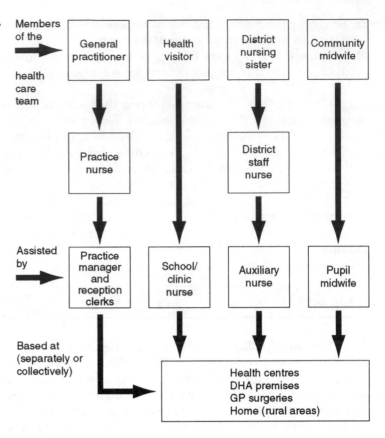

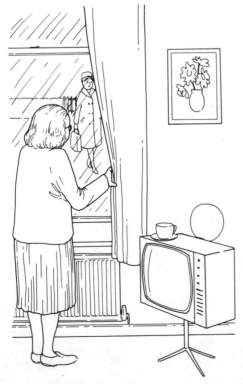

services as decisions are made on patients' needs for health care or social care. These changes, with their emphasis on community care, can have a considerable impact on the skills required by district nurses (Hugman and McCready 1993; Corbett *et al.* 1993) and on the way that they spend their time. Teams are becoming more diverse with varying responsibilities according to grade.

Research suggests that GPs are oriented to physical care. For example, in Chapter 16 it was shown that in interactions with cancer patients, GPs saw psychological problems as natural given the circumstances. Such attitudes will affect the type of problem referred to the district nurse and will underline her role in giving physical care. Similarly with referrals from hospital: most of these are of patients who require continuing physical care after discharge.

There is a growing concern about whether the existing skill mix in district nursing reflects the true needs in terms of workload (Department of Health 1992), with approximately 17% of time being spent on advice, counselling, reassurance or education. Faulkner's work (1984) suggests that the nurses would need further training in interactive skills before they could extend their role in this area.

The case load

The district nurse's case load will vary from one geographical area to another, but it is usually wide and varied, with many patients being visited in their own homes. Basic nursing care may constitute a considerable part of the district nurse's load. For example, a family may be able to nurse an elderly relative but need the help of a nurse for bathing and general hygiene of the patient. Other individuals, living alone, may manage with similar help. For the elderly patient, the nurse can be a cheerful addition to the day, which might otherwise be very lonely. She may be pressed to drink tea and provide company after her tasks are finished and this may cause problems for the nurse with a busy schedule.

The major difference between the district nurse and her hospital counterpart is that, in the community, the nurse is a visitor in the patient's home. This means that no matter what she is about to do for the patient, she is dependent on being invited into the house and on being allowed to carry out her tasks. Of necessity, this takes some of the formality from the nurse–patient relationship and depends on a considerable amount of trust from the patient. The district nurse may often have to remind herself that she is offering a service and can therefore ask that certain criteria are fulfilled. For example, the television may be blaring in a corner when the district nurse wishes to speak to a patient. She can ask that patient to turn the television off. It is advantageous for distict nurses to schedule their visits to these patients, with their agreement, so as to arrive at a time when other distractions are at a minimum. This helps the patient to plan accordingly, but also helps the district nurse to meet local standards for time-keeping and appointments.

The district nurse carries out many of the more sophisticated nursing tasks such as dressings, injections and removal of sutures, often in far from ideal circumstances. Introduction of CSSD (Central Sterile Supply Department) packs has reduced problems, but obviously the average home does not have the trays and trolleys which are taken for granted in hospital.

The health clinic

Those patients who are able to, may see the practice nurse at their local health clinic. District nurses may run their own clinics, e.g. well-women and family planning clinics, from the group practice or community health centre. Many GPs operate from a group practice and will have an office at a health centre which has a waiting room and clinical areas. The district nurse attached to a particular GP may be in attendance during surgery hours and will be available to give nursing care and advice to those patients referred to her.

The district nurse may also make decisions about which patients she will visit and which patients could attend at clinic. If a patient is discharged from hospital with sutures in, the nurse may encourage him to have them removed at the clinic to make sure he is beginning to get up and take short walks. Similarly with such tasks as dressings and injections. The nurse has autonomy in organizing her case load and in making decisions about her patients, although she will obviously work in close cooperation with the GP. Her aim at all times will be to deliver a high level of nursing care in the community.

The dying patient

One important area of the district nurse's work which can encompass total patient care is terminal care. About one-third of the population currently dies at home, cared for by relatives and friends, and often helped by the district nurse.

The majority of care in these circumstances is given by relatives and friends who are prepared to rearrange their lives so that the patient can remain at home. Feeding, washing and bed-making are usually managed by the family, as is sitting up with the patient at night when this is necessary. Often the bed is brought downstairs for ease of care. The nurse can offer expertise in bathing, dressings, and controlling pain by injection if necessary. She can also offer support to the family if they find difficulty in coping. For them to have the nurse's telephone number in an emergency may be a great comfort.

The district nurse may also facilitate day care for patients who are terminally ill. This is offered by many hospices throughout the country (Faulkner *et al.* 1992) and can be beneficial both to the patient, who can get out of the home on a regular basis into a supportive environment, and to the relative, who can get some space from the considerable burden of caring for a terminally ill patient. Further, many day care centres offer physical care that a relative may not be able to give on his own and so can lift the burden of the district nurse in terms of what is expected from her by the family and dying patient.

Dying patients may take a considerable amount of the nurse's time, especially if regular injections are required. By being prepared to give this time, an individual's right to die at home is maintained and relatives are given the chance to look after their own. When a patient dies at home, relatives will need help, just as they do when someone dies in hospital. If the death occurs in the night the relatives may not know what to do and may telephone the district nurse.

Death at home has to be certified by the GP, after which the undertaker will remove the body to the chapel of rest. Most undertakers provide a 24-hour service and can take a great deal of worry from the family in the organization of the funeral, just as they will if the patient dies in hospital (Chapter 13).

Some families may wish to keep the body at home until the funeral, where the coffin might be mounted on a table in the front room and left open for relatives to pay their last respects. This happens less often than formerly. Smaller houses and flats, with one living room, tend to preclude this practice.

The district nurse may be present at the death but more often it is the relatives who are with the patient. Unlike in hospital, a patient at home is not laid out by the nurse. This task is performed by the undertaker, although if the nurse is present she may straighten the body.

Bereavement visiting

If a patient dies at home, the district nurse may visit the family afterwards to see how they are coping with the loss. The nurse will need to understand the stages of grieving (Murray Parkes 1988; Faulkner 1995) so that she can counsel or refer in cases of abnormal grief or where the normal grieving process does not start.

In the absence of government policy on working with bereaved people (Faulkner 1993), the majority of work is carried out by volunteers. However, the district nurse has an important role in the early days after the death to call by and see how the grieving relatives are managing. It is not generally possible to tell how a relative will handle his grief until some weeks after the death, and whether the district nurse takes on the role of assessing a bereaved individual will vary considerably according to the philosophy of the health centre and the locality.

Even if the nurse does not visit in this way, the family may feel a need to keep in touch with the nurse who supported them during the weeks before the death. This may show in telephone calls about trivial matters. It is not unusual for a nurse to be asked to collect unused tablets even when the label clearly states that such drugs should be returned to the chemist. Similarly, the able relative, who could well return a Zimmer aid or commode, might ask the nurse to collect it.

The district nurse should be sensitive to these needs and many give of their own time to relatives who want to talk about their bereavement over a cup of tea. This concern with the family rather than the patient alone can make the district nurse's role very rewarding.

The nursing hierarchy

Although district nurses work with considerable autonomy, in close collaboration with GPs and practice nurses, and take the majority of referrals from the GP, they are in fact answerable to a nursing hierarchy, the members of which are in turn responsible for the efficient running of district nursing services (Figure 17.2). Although there are 18 000 or more nurses in the district nursing services, including auxiliaries (Department of Health 1992), the numbers are still seen to be below the ideal.

Constraints of staff numbers inevitably force management to reorder priorities, so district nurses may find themselves under pressure to give preference to certain aspects of care rather than others. The area most likely to

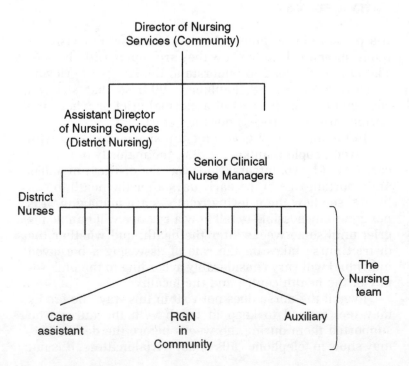

Fig. 17.2 An example of a district nursing hierarchy.

suffer is that of 'observational visits', i.e. those visits to patients where no physical care is needed. Such options may mean that certain groups of individuals, e.g. patients after mastectomy, hysterectomy and other surgical procedures, do not receive nursing visits even though it is accepted that they are at risk of social and emotional problems. Although specialist nurses may fill this gap, in effect this means that the district nurse's role is being eroded. The risk exists that she will return to the role of physical carer if resources do not let her fulfil the concept of holistic patient and family care.

Locate a patient on your ward who will shortly be discharged into the community, and who will require help from a district nurse.

What information do you consider is vital for the district nurse? How could the ward team best liaise with the district nurse to ease the patient's transition into the community?

The health visitor

The health visitor has a more preventive, educative role than the district nurse and is traditionally seen to be concerned mainly with the health of the pre-school child. However, her role also includes care and support for patients in the community and specifically includes emotional support.

To become a health visitor, RGN registration is essential with at least 12 weeks' experience in obstetrics or midwifery. There is a mandatory training for health visitors which takes place in institutes of higher and further education. These courses last for one academic year. After training, the health visitor becomes part of the primary health care team and, as with district nurses, she is either GP- or clinic-attached (Figure 17.1).

Referrals

The health visitor gives care to patients on the GP's list but carries her own case load. The GP may refer cases to her, as may the hospital sister or liaison nurse. She also has part of her case load from birth notifications, which will come to her direct, since she has a duty to visit all new babies on the GP's list at ten days old.

Other cases may derive from liaison with the district nurse, community midwife, social workers, schools and hospitals (Figure 17.3). As with the district nurse, follow-up visits will comprise a large part of her case load, the difference being that, whereas the district nurse primarily visits those who need physical care, the health visitor routinely visits normal families with pre-school children, to give advice and help on health and child care.

A growing area of concern for health visitors is in identifying child abuse. Because they work closely with

Fig. 17.3 The health visitor's
interactions with the health care team.

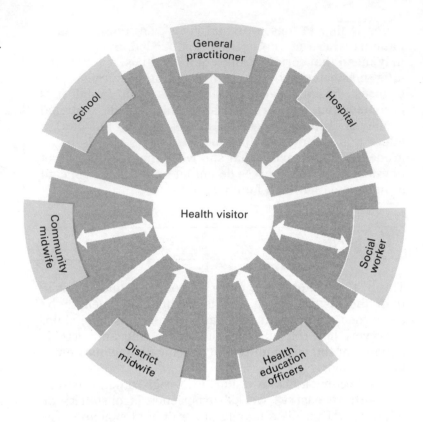

families both in their own homes and in the community,
they are seen to be ideally placed to observe early danger
signals of abuse and to provide support when this occurs
(Armstrong 1994).

The health visitor's case load may also include referrals of the elderly and the mentally ill, particularly where
the family needs help and support in order to cope. Part of
the training of health visitors is to recognize stress in
families so that support may be given before breakdown in
the family occurs.

The case load

Although theoretically the case load of the health visitor is
wide and varied, her major emphasis is usually on families
with children in the birth to five years age group. Orr
(1983) suggests that this is due to the large number of
reports stressing the need for disease prevention and child
health. The health visitor is certainly expected to visit all
families with children under five years old and to find
cases which need her help and advice. Much of her liaison
is with agencies concerned with sick children, child abuse
or non-accidental injury.

This liaison brings the health visitor into contact with social workers as well as hospital staff. This may involve multidisciplinary care of problem families, and occasional visits to court to report on a family's problems or ability to provide adequate care for their children. Some health visitors act as school nurses, but all liaise closely with schools and may continue to monitor problem families with older children. Although in family visiting the child appears central, the health visitor will monitor all individuals within that family (Luker 1992).

Although it is expected that all new babies will be visited and subsequently followed up, families are free to refuse the services offered. The family is the host with the right to refuse admission to a visitor. This can be difficult when those who refuse the services appear to be those who need them most. Health visitors often require patience and tact to gain the trust of a young mother who may see her as 'a spy from the welfare' rather than as a friendly adviser.

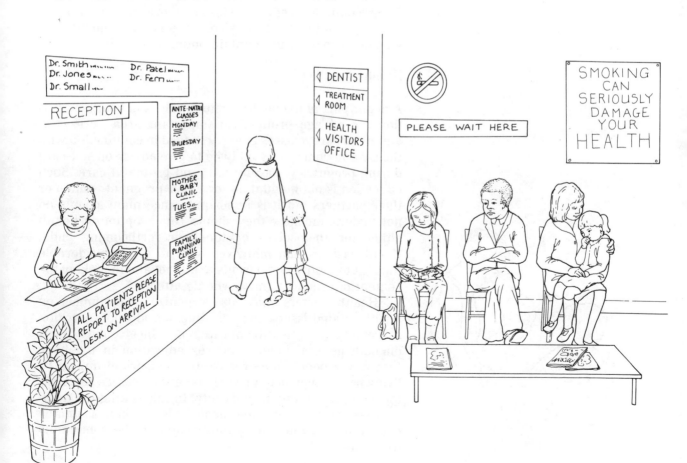

Care of the elderly is not generally seen as a high priority area for health visitors. However, their role in monitoring all members of a family can lead to early identification of problems in an elderly person or in family members who are trying to cope with different generations within the same home (McClymont 1991).

The health clinic

Since the health visitor deals largely with normal, healthy families, many of their needs may be met at the clinic, after the first post-birth visit has been made. Health centres will have regular clinics for mothers to attend with their children, where they will be advised about the prevention of disease by immunization and about the normal care and development of their children. Developmental screening will lead to early identification of problems so that appropriate action may be taken.

The health visitor may also be present with the practice nurse at the GP's surgery in a preventive capacity and for screening procedures. This collaborative aspect of the primary health care team's role is aimed at helping individuals to reach and maintain optimum health.

Health promotion

A major part of the health visitor's role is in health education for all age groups. An important area here is in antenatal care, classes being arranged in conjunction with the GP and community midwife to give advice on self-care during pregnancy, parentcraft, and postnatal care. Such education is not mandatory for either pregnant women or their partners but it is important, since many people do not understand how they should retain optimum health either for themselves or for their forthcoming child. Health visitors and midwives have to give considerable thought to motivating parents to attend, and to making the content pertinent to those who do attend.

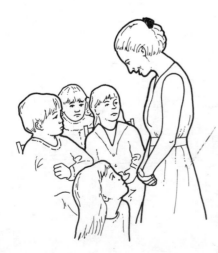

Health visitors may also organize programmes on health-related issues such as smoking, alcohol, nutrition and child abuse. Health education may be given in schools on both general health and sex education in the hope that young people may realize the dangers of unhealthy living before they take up such dangerous habits as smoking, drug abuse and promiscuity. In this setting the audience is captive and the health visitor has a unique opportunity to influence young people in the community (Drennan 1988).

Other health education advice may be given where groups of people meet, such as 'over 60s' clubs. The elderly may need advice and help on nutrition when finances are limited, on the necessity to keep warm in winter, or indeed on benefits to which they may be entitled. Such advice may be given on an individual basis in day-to-day visiting to those who do not attend clinics, groups or clubs, but it is always up to the individual to decide whether to heed the advice given. Health education may in this way offer informed choice to individuals in relation to their particular lifestyle and that of their families.

Requirements of the preventive role

It can be seen that the district nurse bases much of her care on the skills learned as a hospital nurse. The health visitor does not generally offer physical care but acts as an adviser, teacher and counsellor. It can be argued that every nurse requires these skills, but they are particularly required by the health visitor, who is offering a service to well people who may not see the need for involvement with a health professional.

Since much of her work revolves around the birth to five years age group, the health visitor needs in-depth knowledge of both normal and abnormal development so that she can help mothers to be realistic about their child's progress and offer support and referral when a child has problems.

Work with problem families requires health visitors to understand their clients and to build relationships which will facilitate the acceptance of help and advice. It is difficult to be non-judgemental of a parent who batters a child or indeed of an individual who batters an elderly relative. An ability to assess the circumstances of such behaviour can reveal the tremendous strain under which some families live, and lead to useful help being offered, rather than punishment.

The current emphasis in health visiting suggests that the role does not generally include many patients who have been discharged from hospital. This is an area which needs further exploration since such patients would benefit from monitoring in the community. A health visitor with well-developed assessment skills could offer useful support in the post-discharge period and fill a role in the early identification of problems. Faulkner and Maguire (1983) suggest that at present health visitors will only take on such a role if the patient has small children.

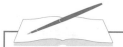

How could a health visitor contribute to patient care after discharge? How would you initiate the involvement of a health visitor as part of discharge planning?

The health visiting hierarchy

It can be seen that the health visitor enjoys considerable autonomy, while collaborating with many other health professionals. She is, however, answerable to a nursing hierarchy which, in the same way as district nursing managers, is responsible for a well-run service, given limited resources.

Managers, faced with these constraints, have to order priorities. Faulkner and Maguire (1983) found that several managers would not have health visitors involved in the aftercare of mastectomy patients because their stated priority was the birth to five years age group. As with district nursing, managers' policies may be seen to constrict the role of the health visitor. It may be that until increasing the number of community nurses is made a priority, many patients will not have their needs assessed or met after discharge. This can in turn lead to readmittance of patients who, with care, could have coped at home.

One way in which hospital staff can alert community managers to the wider needs of individuals after hospitalization is to refer those patients assessed to be at risk while in hospital to both district nurses and health visitors. Adoption of a more holistic approach to care in the community should also lead to a widening of the community nurses' role and to improved care for patients after discharge from hospital.

The practice nurse

The role of practice nurse was first established in the mid to late 1980s with a major role of screening, preventive care and support for patients. The practice nurse is employed directly by the GP. This can cause some problems in that there may be difficulties in accessing nursing support, leadership or clinical supervision within her general practice (RCN 1994). It can be seen that the role of the practice nurse can overlap with the roles of both district nurse and health visitor.

Because the practice nurse is based at the health care clinic, it is important that training and updating allows her both to deal with diagnostic and screening tests, health promotion and routine immunization, and to deal with emergency situations and common medical conditions (Hampson *et al.* 1994).

With good teamwork the practice nurse can be a useful interface between the GP, the health care centre and care in the community. Both the district nurse and health visitor can be aided by the role of the practice nurse and good liaison is essential for maximizing the potential for improved patient care.

The social worker

The primary health care team, i.e. GP, nurses and health visitors in the community, are part of the National Health Service and are concerned with the care and health of individuals in society. Care, both practical and financial, is also offered by the Social Services and an individual's needs for these services are assessed by a social worker. A social worker's training will depend on her background. If, for example, she has a first degree in a relevant subject, she can study for a postgraduate year in order to gain the certificate of social work training together with an MSc. Non-graduates may have to study for up to three years for the certificate alone.

Although social workers are occasionally attached to the primary health care team, they are more usually located in the Social Services area office. Wherever they are based, strong links may be expected with the primary health care team, since social workers assess the needs of their patients from Social Services and work with them in many situations.

Given the reforms in the NHS, there are now expected to be closer links between the GP, the Health Authority and the Social Services (DHSS 1990). For example, the decision to admit or discharge from hospital, although taken primarily on medical grounds, has now to take clear account of social and other factors. The Community Care Act states that wherever these social factors come into play there should be close consultation between Health Authorities and Social Service departments, it being seen to be most undesirable that anyone should be admitted to or remain in hospital when their care could be more appropriately provided elsewhere. As was seen in Chapter 12, there can be difficulties, particularly in care of the elderly, in determining the best place for a patient to be cared for. The *Oxford Times* (1995) highlights the problems of determining medical versus social problems, particularly since social workers are not trained in medical skills. The article summed up as follows:

We are reminded here of the social worker who called on Miss X, noticed a funny smell very like nail polish, and reported to her colleagues, 'I wonder what she's up to. Has she been secretly doing her nails hoping to get her claws into that old poppet of a pensioner living on his own opposite?'

The health visitor who called later that day about fitting a handrail in the loo also noticed the acetone like aroma and immediately and correctly diagnosed the onset of diabetes in Miss X, but that was all quite a time ago.

The social worker, in general, works closely with the health care team. Undoubtedly there are problems of what is medical and what is social, particularly in elderly people with multiple diagnosis, but in general the social worker's role is to work with the health care team towards the best decisions for patients in their care.

Referrals

The social worker's case load is diverse and comes from many sources. GPs, nurses and health visitors in the community may refer cases, as may hospital staff. Other referrals may come from schools, the police, Social Security offices or voluntary organizations such as the Citizens' Advice Bureau.

Social Services departments run a 24-hour service since a number of the cases referred need crisis intervention. Clients are free to refer themselves for help, or may be referred by friends or neighbours.

The case load

The social worker's case load encompasses all age groups, although children and the elderly are priorities along with the physically and mentally disabled. The poor and the homeless may also form part of the case load.

A large part of the social worker's time is spent in counselling clients and their families in an attempt to help them deal with their problems. Occasionally decisions have to be made to remove children from their parents because they are found to be at risk, emotionally or physically, and occasionally crisis intervention is necessary if families are unable to cope with life.

The activities of the social worker and the primary health care team may often be associated in patients on discharge from hospital since it is the Social Services which provides support in the home such as aids and home helps, and funds meals-on-wheels. Such support in the home may need to be arranged before discharge, particularly if changes are required in living accommodation. In this way, the hospital staff will link with the social worker to aid the patient's smooth return to society.

Social workers may also be involved in offering psycho-social support and counselling to some patients on discharge. However, if the social worker's case load is heavy with problem families, this aspect of after-care of hospital patients may take a low priority.

Other facets of the social worker's role which may affect patients on discharge are the provision of places in social centres for the physically disabled, holidays for the disabled (in collaboration with voluntary organizations) and short-stay care for a patient to provide relief for a family under the strain of coping. These services are arranged through the nurse or GP at the health centre.

Support in the home

An increasing number of patients, who would otherwise have to remain in hospital, can go home with support from the Social Services. Assessment may be made by the social worker or a rehabilitation adviser after nursing or medical staff have discussed the case. For patients who are left in physical deficit, the help required may be in the form of aids such as wheelchairs, commodes or specially designed cooking facilities. Occasionally, a home may need ramps or handrails to be added or doors widened for the patient to function properly, or the installation of a telephone to link him with outside support.

Some of these alterations and modifications may take time for the social worker or rehabilitation adviser to arrange. If, for any reason, the patient's home is not adaptable, rehousing may need to be arranged with the patient's permission. Elderly patients, particularly, are often loath to move, even from an inconvenient home. In such instances, it may be possible to offer to modify the ground floor so that the patient does not have to negotiate stairs.

If a patient has not been properly assessed prior to discharge, he may find that the cannot manage stairs or that he needs aids of some sort. In this case it will most likely be the district nurse who asks the social worker to arrange relevant aids or modifications for the home. Co-operation between the nurse and the social worker, whether in hospital or the community, can ensure that the patient is able to manage at home as soon as possible and with the minimum of fuss. A request for a commode, for instance, may only require the word of the nurse, while modification to the house will require careful assessment before work is approved.

The interrelated roles of nurses and social workers

At first sight, it may appear that there is a considerable overlap in the services offered by nurses and social workers, particularly in the case of health visitors. However, a major difference is that whereas the health visitor fulfils a largely preventive role, the social worker is responsible for enforcing legislation. This directly affects the relationship between professional and patient – or client – since the community nurse is a visitor in the home whereas the social worker has the right of entry. In fact, social workers and health visitors often work together with problem families (Sachs 1990) and use the case conference as a vehicle, not only to discuss plans of action, but to agree on the responsibility each professional will take in providing care and support.

The roles of the district nurse and the social worker are less likely to overlap; rather they are interdependent in that the district nurse depends on the social worker to assess and provide aid or support for patients, while the social worker depends on each member of the health care team for referrals. Understanding of each other's problems facilitates the best possible after-care for patients on discharge and those who need help to remain at home and retain their independence.

Home help

The Social Services provides a home help system for individuals who need physical assistance in running their homes. This service can ease the transition between hospital and home for those patients who cannot immediately resume their normal responsibilities. Home helps are not expected to do really heavy housework, but if for any reason an individual's home has become very dirty the Social Services will send in a team to clean it.

The home help service is financed by the Social Services and is often provided to individuals free of charge. However, there is no national policy on this service and in some areas there is a sliding scale for contributions based on the individual's income. This can cause problems in that many people, especially the elderly, are loath to discuss their income with strangers. Social workers, in their assessments, must learn to be very tactful when it is obvious that an individual needs help.

Meals-on-wheels

The meals-on-wheels service undertakes to provide the main meal of the day to individuals who are unable or

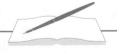

What experience do you have of Social Services? List four areas of support that can be provided by a social worker. When would it be most appropriate to contact Social Services for a patient in your care?

unlikely to prepare a proper meal for themselves. This service is aimed primarily at the physically disabled and the elderly. Although meals-on-wheels services are usually administered by the Women's Royal Voluntary Service (WRVS), they are financed by the Social Services. A small charge is made to the recipient of the meals, but this in no way reflects the actual cost of providing the service.

Meals-on-wheels are not generally available every day of the week, their frequency depending on the area and the number of helpers available, but the service does ensure nutritious meals for many individuals at minimal charge.

Alternative help in the community

The primary health care team, in collaboration with the social worker, can provide care and support for those who need it in the community. There is also other help available for those who do not actually require nursing services, or who require such services in addition to that available from the National Health Service.

Good Neighbour Scheme

In 1977 the then DHSS launched the Good Neighbour Scheme, which aims to involve individuals in monitoring those members of the community who are seen to be at risk, such as the elderly living alone.

Of course this already happens in many places, especially in small villages where the inhabitants all know each other. However, in many towns and cities, people may not even recognize their neighbours, let alone know whether they are alone or incapacitated. The Good Neighbour scheme makes a small payment to an individual in return for his taking an interest in his neighbour's welfare.

Voluntary organizations

There is a tremendous number of voluntary organizations offering help and support to those in need. Some, like the WRVS, work with the Social Services, while others work independently. District Health Authorities may give some financial help to such organizations but often the workforce makes no charge for its services and, as a result, runs on a very small budget.

Some voluntary services are specific, e.g. Alcoholics Anonymous, which helps individuals and Al-Anon who support their families, and the British Diabetic Association, which offers information and support to patients with diabetes. Other specific 'helping' agencies are CRUSE, for bereaved individuals, Victim Support, for those who have been victims of crime, and Relate, for those with relationship problems. Others, such as the Citizens' Advice Bureau, which provides information to anyone who requires it, or the Samaritans, which offers friendship to the lonely, sad or suicidal individual, are more general in their work.

Some organizations offer physical help to families that are coping with a relative at home and may need a break. The Marie Curie Foundation, for example, offers nurses to sit with patients at night, a service which most District Health Authorities, cannot afford to provide, while Macmillan nurses visit patients with cancer, although many Macmillan nurses are 'pump primed' by the charity and their salaries later paid by the Health Authority trust or the local hospice.

Voluntary organizations and associations can be seen to provide services not available through the NHS or the Social Services, and as such are invaluable in the community.

Summary

In this chapter, those services in the community that are available to help the patient and his family as he adjusts to a return to society have been considered.

District nurses are available to give physical and, ideally, emotional care to individuals, while the health visitor fulfils a preventive and counselling role. Because of constraints of time and finance, it has been seen that some groups of patients may not be included in the case load of either the district nurse or the health visitor.

Help is also available from the Social Services. This requires collaboration between community nurses and the social worker in order that aids, support and services may be promptly available for those in need.

Because the Social Services also operate under financial constraint, many voluntary organizations and associations have emerged to offer help, advice and support. Many of these organizations work closely with the Social Services departments.

The services described are important in the community since they mean that many individuals may remain in their own homes rather than having to be admitted to a hospital or other institution.

References

Armstrong, H. (1994) *Child protection for health visitors: a training resource*. London: HMSO.

Corbett, K, Meeham, L. & Sackey, V. (1993) A strategy to enhance skills. *Professional Nurse, October*, 60–63.

Department of Health (1992) *The nursing skill mix in the nursing service*. London: HMSO.

DHSS (1990) *Community care in the next decade and beyond*. London: HMSO.

Drennan, V. (1988) *Health visitors and goups: politics and practice*. London: Butterworth Heinemann.

Dunnell, K. & Dobbs, J. (1982) *Nurses working in the community*. Office of Population Censuses and Surveys, Social Survey Division. London: HMSO.

Faulkner, A. (1984) Teaching non-specialist nurses assessment skills in the aftercare of mastectomy patients. Unpublished Ph.D. Thesis, University of Manchester.

Faulkner, A. (1993) Developments in bereavement services. In Clark, D. (Ed.) *The future for palliative care*. London: Open University Press.

Faulkner, A. (1995) *Working with bereaved people*. Edinburgh: Churchill Livingstone.

Faulkner, A. & Maguire, P. (1983) Nursing is more than doing. *Journal of District Nursing*, *1*(10), 9–13.

Faulkner, A., Higginson, I., Egerton, H., Power, M., Sykes, N. & Wilkes, E. (1992) *Hospice day care. A qualitative study*. London: Help the Hospices.

Forster, A. & Laming, H. (1992) *Implementing caring for people*, (EL(92)65, CI(92)30). London: Department of Health.

Hampson, G., Bolde, N. & Takle, S. (1994) *Practice nurse handbook*. London: Blackwell Science.

Hugman, J. & McCready, S. (1993) Profiles make perfect practice. *Nursing Times*, *89*(27), 46–49.

Luker, K. (1992) *Health visiting. Towards community health nursing*. London: Blackwell Science.

McClymont, M. (1991) *Health visiting and elderly people. A health promotion challenge*. Edinburgh: Churchill Livingstone.

Murray Parkes, C. (1988) Bereavement as a psychosocial transition: processes of adaptation to change. *Journal of Social Issues*, *44*(3), 53–65.

Orr, J. (1983) Health visiting the UK. In Hockey, L. (Ed.) *Primary care nursing. Recent Advances in Nursing, No. 5*. Edinburgh: Churchill Livingstone.

Oxford Times, 6.1.95. That funny smell. Oxford.

Royal College of Nursing (1994) *Practice nurses' continuing education and professional development*. London: RCN.

Sachs, H. (1990) *A brave attempt – teamwork between health visitors and social workers on an inner city estate*. London: King's Fund.

Further reading

Baley, M. (1987) *District nursing*. London: Butterworth Heinemann.

Gaffin, J. (Ed.) (1981) *The nurse and the welfare state*. Aylesbury: H.M. and M.

Gordon, D. (1993) *Community social work. Older people and informal care: a romantic illusion?* London: Avebury Press.

Harrison, S. (1977) *Families in stress*. London: Rcn.

Hockey, L. (Ed.) (1983) *Primary care nursing. Recent Advances in Nursing, No. 5*. Edinburgh: Churchill Livingstone.

Jeffree, P. (1994) *The practice nurse*. London: Chapman & Hall.

Lahiff, M. (1981) *Hard to help families*. Aylesbury: H.M. and M.

Luft, S. (1994) *Nursing in general practice*. London: Chapman & Hall.

Meredith Davies, J. B. (1983) *Community health, preventive medicine and social services*. London: Baillière Tindall.

Robertson, C. (1991) *Health visiting in practice*. Edinburgh: Churchill Livingstone.

Sutton, C. (1994) *Social work, community work and psychology*. London: The British Psychological Society.

Tettersall, M. (1993) *Handbook of practice nursing*. Edinburgh: Churchill Livingstone.

18

The Changing Role of the Nurse

CHAPTER SUMMARY

Nurse–doctor relationships, 580
Problems in nurse–doctor relationships, 580
Responsibility for information, 583
Patient advocacy, 585

Research and the nurse, 587
Becoming a researcher, 588
Becoming research-minded, 589
Reading research reports, 591

The cost of nursing, 593
Physical costs, 593
Emotional costs, 594
The counselling role, 595
Burnout, 599

The need for support, 599
Peer support, 600
Managerial support, 600
Developing coping strategies, 601

Education, 603

Continuing education, 604
Reading, 605
In-service education, 605
Post-basic courses, 606
Graduate education, 606

Summary, 607

References, 607

Further reading, 609

The change from the traditional model of nursing to a more individualized approach to patient care has brought with it many changes to the role of the nurse. A major change can be seen in relationships with other health professionals, particularly with medical colleagues, in that the nurse will expect to be involved in decision making on patient care.

It was seen in Chapter 1 that the change in junior doctors' hours has led to an expansion of the nurse's role. The parameters of that changing role have still to be clearly defined, but in the meantime the nurse is increasingly involved in the planning and execution of patient care. The question of 'who does what' for the patient raises issues of the organization of care. Greene (1994) argues for patient-focused care which places the individuals with the most appropriate skills in the right position to undertake whatever task is at hand. This allows care to be built around the patient and his needs rather than around the organization. To implement such a system each job would need to be re-profiled to provide the appropriate mix of skills for particular care of a patient. Nurses' roles could change again in that housekeeping and domestic duties may be shed as they take nurses away from the patient and are not skilled activities, and some of the activities currently carried out by junior doctors would be taken on by the nurses. This theory, brought from the USA, fits in perfectly with the new deal for doctors (1991).

When care is based on patient's needs rather than on physical care alone, this brings about a change in the relationship with the patient. By taking an interactive and facilitative role with the patient, the nurse will be brought into close contact with the patient's emotional, physical and social reactions to disease and its treatment. The expanding role of the nurse will require that she has skills which allow her to assess the patient's needs, be able to act as a first level counsellor and know when to refer an individual to other available agencies. The nurse will also need to be an educator which requires that she understands theories of learning and motivation.

Expectations of nurses are also changing. The Briggs Report (1972) suggested that nursing should be research-based. This means that all nurses should be aware of the implications of research for their clinical practice, while some will perhaps carry out their own studies in patient care.

Change is not without trauma since, for many individuals, it means getting used to new concepts which may be uncomfortable. There is stress inherent in changed relationships and in having well-established practices questioned. The current approach to nursing is, in fact, not without personal cost to both nursing staff and their colleagues. Looking at the cost of nursing will in itself raise other issues such as the need for support and for continuing education so that practice and change may be managed without damage to the nurse as an individual.

Nurse–doctor relationships

Problems in nurse–doctor relationships

Traditionally, doctors have had considerable influence on nursing in that they have been involved in teaching, writing textbooks and choosing staff. Some would describe this influence as kindly paternalism, while a growing number of nurses see it as a wish to dominate. The problem is not new but has undoubtedly been exacerbated by the advent of the nursing process and the emerging role of the nurse as a thinking, accountable member of the health care team.

There are a number of theories to account for problems between medical and nursing staff. The feminist view is that inequality exists between the professions because most doctors are men and most nurses women. In this theory, nurses (i.e. women) are having to fight doctors (i.e. men) in order to shake off domination and become equal. A question arising from this theory relates to the meaning of 'equality'. Women who think medicine is a superior profession are free to train as doctors, and men may enter nursing. There is equality of opportunity in each profession. What is less assured is equality of status between the professions even though each is dependent upon the other for the provision of quality care to every patient.

As nurses take on responsibilities that had been held by junior doctors and as they shed some of their more mundane tasks which take them away from the patient, the difference in status is likely to be less obvious. The team approach to care also underlines the interdependence between individual members of the team, whether they be nurses, doctors or other health professionals.

Doctors might argue that there is inequality between the professions academically in that there is a vast difference between the entry requirements and length of training for the two professions. This is one viewpoint, although it loses sight of the more important issues to nurses of being responsible for their own profession and accountable for their own actions. Nursing, medicine and the paramedical professions all have differing demands in terms of entrance requirements and training but each produces professionals with distinct functions which are not interchangeable but which are interdependent.

The move to put nurse education into, or ally it with, higher education, and the growth of departments of nursing in many universities, is a move towards academic equality between the professions, especially since such nurses take up clinical posts after completing their degrees. When degrees were first set up for nurses, the department of nursing was usually either in a medical school or in the social sciences. Increasingly, nursing is a school within a university just as medicine is a school. The two schools may be linked but nevertheless nursing is no longer academically dependent on medicine. Doctors may sit on panels for nursing posts within the university and nurses will sit on selection panels for medical posts, and this reciprocity again underlines the interdependence of the professions.

Another theory to explain problems between the professions is that doctors are loath to lose the 'handmaiden' image of the nurse. Certainly doctors have been doubtful about the nursing process and the changing role of the nurse. Mitchell (1984), in making a case against the nursing process, mourns the growing independence of nursing and 'the progressive exclusion of doctors from nursing affairs'. This suggests that professional independence in nursing may be seen to be a threat to medical staff because it upsets the 'status quo'.

In giving up the handmaiden image, nurses must take responsibility for equable change. To blame doctors for 'clinging onto the past' suggests that nurses are still answerable to, and controlled by, the medical profession. Professional 'freedom' depends on the profession itself for, as Gilbran (1979) states in relation to freedom in general:

And what is it but fragments of your own self
you would discard that you may become free?
– For how can a tyrant rule the free and
the proud but for a tyranny in their own freedom
and a shame in their own pride?

Most nurses would consider it quite reasonable that doctors are not included in 'nursing affairs' and it seems equally reasonable to assume that most doctors would not consider involving nurses in 'medical affairs'. Nevertheless it is important that there should be close collaboration between the professions. For this to occur, each has to earn the respect of the other and each has to accept the unique role of the other. There can be professional sharing then, without threat to either group.

A differentiation used in this book has been that doctors diagnose and treat disease while nurses respond to a patient's reaction to his disease. If taken at its simplest level, the statement could be seen to infer that doctors do not need to concern themselves with individuals while nurses do not need to concern themselves with disease. Both statements are erroneous. Doctors **do** need to view each patient as an individual and Mitchell (1984) criticizes the nursing process approach to care because of its 'stereotype' of doctors as disease- rather than care-oriented. The unique function of the doctor is to diagnose and treat disease: this does not exclude him from caring. That nurses need to know about disease has been well stated in the text, but this does not make them medical diagnosticians, nor does it infer that they will necessarily prescribe medical treatment.

The concept of nurses and doctors becoming equal

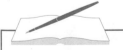

Jot down your major responsibilities as a nurse. How many of these can be carried out independently from other members of the team? Which responsibilities give **you** most satisfaction with your work?

partners in patient care is far from reality at present. For this reason, there are often divergent opinions on patient care which pose problems for the nurse. One such problem concerns the patient's level of information on disease, prognosis and treatment, while a more general problem is that of the nurse as the patient's advocate.

Responsibility for information

The team approach to care and the move towards patient-focused care should show that the responsibility for giving information to a patient or relatives is that of all team members. Difficulties may arise if the Consultant has very different views on the level of information to be given than do his nursing colleagues, and many Consultants still argue that, because they are legally responsible for the patient, they have the ultimate right to make a decision on how much information is given to a patient.

That a nurse is legally accountable for her actions is beyond dispute. What is important is the issue of how a nurse may meet her patients' needs if those needs are not similarly identified by the Consultant or indeed if they conflict with medical orders. This problem was dealt with briefly in Chapter 13 in respect of a patient's need to know his diagnosis and prognosis, but not in terms of the effect on nurse/doctor relationships.

Health professionals need to interact with each other and jointly make decisions which will affect patient care. If a Consultant feels strongly that a patient should not be told his diagnosis or prognosis, it is up to the nurse to negotiate ground rules for subsequent interactions with the patient. For example, many patients ask for information to confirm what they already suspect. In such situations the nurse can make a clear case to the Consultant that although she will not spell out a diagnosis or prognosis, she will in fact confirm what patients have already worked out and she will also answer questions honestly.

It may be that the Consultant has problems; he may wish to protect the patient from pain and himself from feelings of doubt and failure if the prognosis is poor. He may also have had a damaging experience with a patient who responded badly to the truth. Improvement in the ability to break bad news in a sensitive way (Faulkner *et al.* 1995) may, hopefully, overcome such problems.

Such negotiation allows the doctor and nurse to understand each other's point of view. This will have a positive effect on the whole team, given that the alternative is for the nurse to feel unrealistically controlled by the Consultant and subsequently to become hostile so that she attacks rather than negotiates. Any individual's reaction in such a situation is likely to be defensive and possibly autocratic, while the nurse will be left feeling frustrated and angry.

In any conflict, the best possible strategy for breaking deadlock is a cool, logical approach. It may be that a patient is ready to discuss her prognosis as follows:

Patient You know nurse, I can't see me getting out of here

Nurse Not getting out?

Patient Oh, you know, I'm going just the way our Mary went

Nurse How was that?

Patient Well she was sick, and lost weight – just like me – and then her skin went like mine. It wasn't long then before she died

Nurse Are you saying that you are dying?

Patient Yes. There isn't any other answer, is there? I'm not daft, yet no one wants to let me talk about it.

Nurse Would you like to talk now?

Patient Oh yes . . .

In the above example, the nurse felt that she had to allow the patient to talk. In so doing, she confirmed the patient's beliefs even though the Consultant had stipulated that this information should not be divulged. Afterwards the nurse met the Consultant, and told him that his patient had been told her prognosis. Because she expected a problem, she tried to protect herself by attacking the decision which she had overridden. The Consultant became furious and complained to Sister.

An approach which may work towards better understanding is a discussion that is not defensive. If the nurse had explained that the patient was ready to talk and had indeed asked to talk, the conversation might have proceeded along the following lines:

Nurse And so I was really confirming what she had worked out for herself, though I know you had thought we should not say anything.

Doctor (annoyed) I don't generally tell the patients – you know that. It takes away their hope.

Nurse Are you saying that I should have lied to her?

Doctor Well – not lied exactly

Nurse Well?

Doctor Well – how is she now?

Nurse She seems relieved to have it out in the open. You know, I really did check that she wanted to talk

> *Doctor* Hurumph. I suppose situations change – I'd like
> to look at Mrs Clark

In discussing the patient's needs, the nurse is describing a situation which required a certain action. The Consultant, unable to suggest an alternative, since few would advocate actual dishonesty, is likely to accept the reality, albeit unwillingly. Further, his original decision has not been questioned so that he can rationalize that changed situations required changed actions.

It is very important that differences between any two individuals do not deteriorate into a 'win–lose' situation, for, if each person feels the need to 'win', winning itself becomes more important than the cause of the conflict; losing is so often accompanied by a perceived loss of face and possible humiliation. This can be the reason for autocratic behaviour from doctors, who, rather than lose face, will use their perceived status in an attempt to control a difficult situation. While it is important that nurses treat doctors as colleagues, they should also attempt to see beyond the autocratic façade to the vulnerable human beneath.

The problem is complex and almost certainly some consultants will continue to control the amount of information given to patients, and react angrily if their wishes are not observed, no matter what the reason. As nurses are adapting to a changed role, their medical colleagues are having to give up firmly entrenched beliefs, which may not be easy. In proving herself, the nurse will need to show that she can be trusted. If, for example, a nurse accurately assesses a patient's need and readiness for information, the Consultant will, over time, learn to respect her judgement.

Just as each individual learns to interact with others, each nurse will need to learn how to interact effectively with colleagues, including doctors. Self-assurance arising from knowledge-based professionalism is a powerful tool, as is respect for colleagues as individuals. As health professionals learn to interact more effectively, both with their patients to identify needs and with their colleagues to understand each other's point of view, then patient care should become more a matter for the team rather than for any one individual (Faulkner 1992a).

Patient advocacy

There is concern that some of the decisions made for patients are not in their best interests and that the nurse has a role as the patient's advocate (Rich 1995). Unfortunately this may be interpreted as a collusion of nurse and patient against the medical professional, where it should be seen as the nurse performing a function for the patient that, for a number of reasons, he cannot perform for himself.

As patients become more articulate they may question medical decisions but feel unable to resist them. Alternatively, the nurse may question medical decisions on the basis of her own knowledge and experience. In either situation there is a potential for conflict between nursing and medical staff since the latter may feel that their professional expertise is being questioned. However, if the nurse is unhappy about prescribed treatment, it is her duty to raise the issue with the doctor in terms of her own professional accountability.

In the matter of mistakes in medical prescriptions, clearly it is possible to make an informed decision and ask for records to be corrected so that the correct drug or dosage may be given. What is more difficult is the situation where opinion is involved. This may include decisions on quality of life, the participation in drug trials or options concerning treatment. When the nurse involves herself with these decisions she becomes a potential advocate for the patient. This means that she must be able to put the patient's case to the Consultant cogently and without rancour.

'Advocate' means 'one who intercedes' or 'one who pleads the cause of another'. In other words, patient advocacy puts the nurse in the role of spokesman for, not protector of, the patient. If drugs are prescribed incorrectly, refusing to give them is a professional duty of the nurse in order to protect the patient. If the patient with carcinoma tells the nurse that he does not wish for chemotherapy and asks about alternative treatment, the nurse becomes the patient's advocate if she discusses the problem with the Consultant.

Difficulties arise if the Consultant does not wish to discuss his decision. He may say, 'I know best in this situation and I don't change my mind'. This will be very frustrating to a nurse who knows that there **are** alternative treatments. She is also likely to become angry that the concerns of her patient, or herself, are of so little importance to the doctor.

This situation is very similar to that of the divergence of opinion over giving a patient his prognosis, in that it can become a battle which the consultant will attempt to 'win' by tight control. It may be a temptation for the nurse to tell the Consultant that to refuse to change his mind or discuss the problem is a sign of weakness, not strength, and for her to advise the patient to refuse treatment. Both are

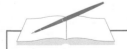

Imagine you are taking on the role of advocate for a patient in your care. How would you put your case to the Consultant? What strategies would you use to encourage co-operation?

likely to increase hostility between doctor and nurse, and undermine the patient's confidence in the health care team.

Approaching the Consultant for an equable discussion of the problem should lead to his discussing options with the patient, providing that he has not been made to feel defensive and inept. If this strategy is not successful, there is no reason why the nurse should not discuss options with the patient so that he has enough information to discuss his problem with the Consultant. The patient is then in the situation of making an informed choice.

When Molly Witherington did not wish to remain in hospital after her diagnosis of diabetes, it was to a nurse that she confided her worries about her small daughter. The nurse took on the role of patient advocate and, by fully explaining the situation to the Consultant, avoided the possibility of the patient taking her own discharge. That the registrar was not happy showed in his comment that the patient was uncooperative, but, in spite of that, the medical staff trusted the nurse's judgement.

It may seem that as medical and nursing staff are adapting to the changing role of the nurse, all the effort is being made by the nurses if they have to develop strategies with which to 'manage' their medical colleagues. Since doctors may not be motivated to change, this is the reality and is no different from any human interaction where it is known that diplomacy is almost always more effective than hostility and leads to improved relationships. If a nurse behaves as a colleague she cannot become a handmaiden, and if she avoids flattery as a means of managing her male colleagues she cannot fall into the trap of male domination.

Research and the nurse

Relatively, nursing research is still in its infancy in comparison with other disciplines. However, there is a growing body of knowledge arising from nursing research and a growing awareness in the profession of the implications of research findings. Research has been described by many as 'the systematic investigation towards increasing the sum of knowledge' and may be carried out in a small or large way. Whether a study is small or large scale, it has to be carried out with rigour if it is to be credible, which implies that the investigator needs some training in research methods.

A distinction needs to be made between a researcher

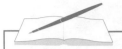

Choose an aspect of nursing that particularly interests you.

1 Find some references (your librarian will help you) on work in this area.
2 Choose two of the references and read them critically.
3 How has this exercise increased your knowledge of this area?
4 Can you see a need for further research? If so, how would you like to see it developed?

and a data gatherer. Medical staff often advertise in nursing journals for nursing staff to be involved in a research project. This very often involves the nurse in gathering medical data but does not necessarily teach her to be a researcher. A researcher is one who is involved in a project from conception to completion and who understands the methodological issues involved. The Briggs Report (1972) suggested that a few nurses need to be highly trained in this way and that all nurses needed to be 'research-minded'.

Becoming a researcher

Most nurses undertaking research are graduates, many of whom will register for a higher degree. There are, however, exceptions to this, since any nurse may become involved in a project in her own clinical setting provided that she can gain support in terms of time to undertake the work and finance if there are cost implications.

Many nursing posts have a research element within them. For example, teaching staff in university departments are expected to be actively involved in research as one of the facets of their work. Other posts are distinctly research posts. For example, at Trent Palliative Care Centre there are a number of research associates involved in various projects on aspects of palliative care. Within these posts there is an expectation that individual work will be written up for a higher degree. Courses can be taken while in post to improve knowledge of research methodology and of statistical and qualitative analysis. In this area there is increasing collaboration between health professionals to improve knowledge of patient care (Faulkner and Maguire 1994; Ingleton and Faulkner 1995).

Most undergraduate courses contain a research component which equips students to understand research and carry out a small study, the report of which contributes to their final examination mark. As a result, some individuals become interested in research as a potential career. Nurse graduates may have degrees in disciplines other than nursing, studying for a degree either before or after they have completed general nurse training. This means that nursing research is influenced by disciplines such as psychology, sociology and other sciences.

For a nurse to undertake research she will need finance which is available from a number of sources. The Department of Health and the Scottish Home and Health Department fund a number of research studentships each year for nurses to develop skills in research in an area of interest to them. The prerequisite to gaining these scholarships is often that the nurse must be acceptable to register for a course of study leading to a higher degree. It is also possible to apply for awards or bursaries which give partial support for a nurse to pursue a research project. Small charities such as Help the Hospices may be approached, as may larger organizations such as the Wellcome Trust, Cancer Research Campaign or the Medical Research Council.

Drug firms may also offer money for research, though they are largely concerned with drug trials and medical research. In addition, each NHS region has a research budget and they increasingly put out requests for protocols. For those nurses who are interested in becoming involved in research but who do not feel ready or able to write a protocol, then a post in a research unit will give a salary while the nurse is undertaking a study that has been designed by and funded to the Project Director.

Some research experience is required in order to produce a protocol and gain funding for research. For the nurse who wishes to undertake research but has little experience, it is possible to obtain help from an experienced researcher in a university department of nursing, for example. In looking for such help, someone with experience in the area to be studied should be found. The protocol will then be submitted in both names, the experienced researcher adopting a supervising role. This can be an advantage to the novice researcher in that funds are more readily available to researchers who have proved their ability with previous studies.

Becoming research-minded

The majority of nurses do not wish to become full-time academic researchers, but their contribution to nursing will be enhanced if they take an active interest in research and its relevance to their work. To be research-minded requires that each individual takes a questioning approach to practice rather than accept that nursing care is delivered in the only way possible. The following story illustrates this point:

A young man joined the Guards. One morning his sergeant gave him a pot of white paint and a brush, and told him to paint the white line on the parade ground. As the soldier started painting, he wondered what the line was for. His sergeant did not know but made enquiries. Finally it was discovered that the line was an aid to lining up horses for parade. Horses had not been kept in those barracks for 20 years.

It could be said that the soldier was research-minded

in that he questioned practice. Some nursing practice is a little like painting an obsolete white line. An enquiring mind may lead to improved practice and a higher standard of nursing care.

Being research-minded is more than questioning practice, however. It also requires that nurses take cognizance of research findings and their applicability to practice. This awareness is often confused with implementation of research findings, individuals writing to nursing journals, bemoaning the fact that little use is made of the research that is available.

In fact, much of the early nursing research was descriptive and on a small scale. This means that results are not generalizable, but they do give information on areas of patient care and may lead to further research which tests changes in practice. For example, in the early 1980s there were many descriptive studies about communication between nurses and their patients (Ashworth 1984; Faulkner 1980; Macleod Clark 1982). These studies and others showed without doubt that nurses did not have the necessary skills to communicate effectively with their patients, nor yet did they give priority to activities which were interactive and concerned with psychosocial care. Following these studies there has been an increased concern with teaching nurses to interact effectively with their patients and in developing courses to improve skills (Faulkner 1992b; Faulkner and Macleod Clark 1987; Faulkner and Maguire 1984, 1994). By providing, and evaluating, courses to improve the deficits in both nurses' and doctors' abilities to interact with their patients, it is hoped for an improvement in psychosocial care of patients. Further work will, hopefully, focus on whether improving nurses' skills to interact with their patients actually makes a difference to the patient's perception of the care that they receive.

Even if experimental work does not follow from descriptive work, much can be learned from descriptive research using a qualitative approach. For example, as long ago as 1972 Stockwell undertook a descriptive study into the popularity of patients. She was able to describe the behaviour of popular and unpopular patients and the nurses' attitudes to both groups. A research-minded nurse reading Stockwell's work and that of Roberts (1984), would become much more aware of the attitudes to patients in her own practice and of the influence of colleagues on her perceptions of others. This alone might result in a more understanding approach to the individuals in her care.

It can be seen that research can have an effect in several ways and at several levels. If the profession is research-minded, the findings of collaborative experimental studies will lead to a change in practice, while those of descriptive research will lead to heightened awareness, and possibly increased funding for experiments to show the direction in which change may be made.

One of the problems in nursing research is that of generalizability, since the smaller the study the less likelihood there is that the subjects being studied are representative of the whole population. It cannot be assumed that a few nurses will behave in the same way as all nurses. What can be assumed is that the more nurses there are in a sample, the more likely it is that they will begin to be representative of all nurses, particularly if they are chosen at random, i.e. by chance.

The idea of representativeness can be tested by tossing a coin. Since a coin has two sides and is unweighted it will be expected to fall on either one of its sides. If tossed a number of times it is reasonable to expect that it will land an equal number of times on each side – and may occasionally stand on its edge. In fact, if an unweighted coin is tossed ten times it may fall on one side eight times and the other only twice. If it is tossed 100 times it is more likely to fall an equal number of times on both sides. It can be seen that tossing the coin ten times gives a less representative picture of an unweighted coin than does the larger sample of 100.

This is an important concept for the research-minded nurse for, when she reads research reports, she should be aware of the size of the study. If the findings seem important but the study is small, it may be that replication is necessary on a large scale to test the generalizability of the findings before practice is changed. Given the above constraints, small-scale research remains important because it may give local awareness of local problems, and may lead to larger studies, which could lead to changes in practive and improved patient care.

Reading research reports

Research reports may be written at several levels. They may be in the form of a thesis which is submitted for a higher degree. A thesis should be written in such detail that the research could be replicated by other individuals, which often makes it tedious to read. Theses are held in the university library and may be borrowed on inter-library loan. The Royal College of Nursing, in an attempt to make nursing theses more available, has the Steinberg collection. This comprises copies of theses bought from the universities, with the permission of the authors, which are then kept in the Royal College of Nursing library in London.

Research reports may also be written as monographs or as 'research papers' which are published in journals. These are written in a more readable form than theses but contain less detail. The language may remain scientific or may be in a simpler style, depending on the journal and its readership.

Reading research reports can give useful information on current enquiry into nursing, but they should be read critically and with some knowledge of the process of research. Hawthorne (1983) produced a useful checklist for those wishing to understand the principles of research.

Briefly, a research report should contain the following:

1 *A clear statement of the problem*
This statement should set out the precise area which was studied, and any assumptions made about the problem.

2 *A referenced background to the study and/or literature review*
There are a number of methods of referencing literature pertinent to a topic. In this book, a modified Harvard system has been used (Lancaster 1974), that is, the author's surname has been used in the text, along with the year of publication. In this system, an alphabetical list of authors' names with the article title and journal or publisher is at the end of the document or, as in this book, at the end of each chapter.

If there are several authors of a book or paper, it would be clumsy to put them all in the text. The form then is that for more than three authors the text will contain up to the first three authors followed by '*et al.*'. This means 'and others'.

References in a report should be of 'key' works in the field, although lesser known work may be included. The idea of referencing is to acknowledge the work of others and to lead readers on to further reading. To use others' work or ideas without reference may be interpreted as plagiarism.

3 *The Research Method Used*
The report should outline the research method used and, ideally, the reasons for the choice. The sample size and characteristics should also be stated.

4 *Data Collection and Analysis*
Often there is a difference between the planned research and the data collection. The report should discuss any pilot work (that is, work to test methods or research instruments) and any problems encountered in data collection. Methods of analysis should be given.

5 *Results*

Results should be stated. It is often helpful if results are shown graphically. Pie charts, histograms or graphs give a more immediate sense of a result than written words.

6 *Discussion*

The discussion will normally portray the researcher's interpretation of results and may be followed by recommendation for further work or for a change in practice.

There is a move towards writing research reports in a way which highlights not only the results of the study but also the problems encountered during the research. It is necessary to appreciate that real research seldom follows the ideal textbook format.

To read reports and equate their findings to a nurse's own reality can add an extra dimension to the role of the nurse. Not only does research question practice and offer possibilities for change, it may also increase self-awareness in a nurse as she cares for her patients.

The cost of nursing

Individualized care which is based on research can be very demanding on the nurse. Her role includes that of carer, facilitator, educator, counsellor and confidante. She is also expected to relate constructively with other members of the health care team and keep up-to-date on developments within the profession. The costs can be counted in terms of physical, emotional and personal commitments to patients' care.

Physical costs

Few would dispute that nursing is hard physical work. This is demonstrated by the fact that nurses may retire earlier than those in other occupations. Acknowledging that the work is physically tiring leaves nurses with a responsibility to protect their health.

Throughout this book it has been seen that part of a nurse's role is to educate patients about their disease and its treatment and to help them optimize their physical health. It is therefore paradoxical that nurses often neglect their own health. For example, more nurses smoke than do those in other occupations and many use alcohol in order to relieve stress. Similarly, nurses are often above their ideal weight and this may be because of eating snacks and junk food rather than a proper meal while they are on duty. In workshops for health professionals in cancer and terminal care, it has emerged that many nurses and doctors use food and alcohol to handle the difficulties of their job (Faulkner and Maguire 1994). One nurse summed it up by saying, 'When the going gets rough, I buy myself chocolate and have a glass of wine'.

Unhealthy eating can make an individual vulnerable to infection and in nursing this is exacerbated by the very nature of the work. Some illnesses are considered as industrial injuries because of the risk factors in nursing. These include diseases such as tuberculosis and hepatitis type B. If a disease is accepted as being related to work, it carries special payment rights while the individual is unable to work.

Back injuries are not uncommon among nurses. These are often due to poor lifting technique, and can lead to prolonged time away from work and possible unemployment. All nurses should be taught to lift safely and effectively.

It can be seen that the physical costs of nursing can be high, especially if nurses do not put a value on maintaining their own physical health. Often problems are exacerbated by a perceived expectation that a nurse should not admit that she is unwell. This can lead to an individual continuing to work when she should be off sick.

It may appear that nurses are actually **careless** of their own health. Faulkner and Ward (1983) found that the only situation in which most nurses who smoked would give up cigarettes was if they themselves were pregnant. Their concern was for the new life rather than their own. In fact, this concern for others should be a motivation to a nurse to protect her health. If she has an unhealthy lifestyle this may well affect her level of performance on the ward, so affecting patient care.

Emotional costs

The physical costs of nursing cannot be divorced from the emotional costs. Nursing can be emotionally draining, especially in individualized care. Many patients have personal concerns which they may have been unable to share with others. The facilitative nurse, in her assessment of the patient, will allow him to talk through his problems. It is not unusual to hear a patient say, 'I know things have not changed, but I feel so much better now that I have told you about it'.

The patient may feel better but this can be at the nurse's expense. She may be upset by the nature of the

On page 118 you were asked to monitor your own food and fluid intake for 24 hours, with a few colleagues. How did your diet for the 24 hours compare with the standards set down in the (1991) *Health of the Nation* document? What, if any, changes did you make to your diet as a result of this exercise? How could monitoring your own diet help you in advising patients on diet?

problem, or feel frustrated because there is no solution. She may also identify with the patient and be unable to forget an incident. Another problem for the nurse is in being non-judgemental. Often she has to hear things from patients of which she does not approve, and this may lead to concerns that the patient interprets neutral behaviour as approval.

Giving emotionally to patients is not necessarily to deny feelings, but it is to deny censure. Empathetic responses to patients' feelings require that the nurse also 'feels'. It is this giving to a number of patients which can have an accumulative cost. Each nurse needs to know how much she can give and learn to be honest with herself and with others.

The classic work of Menzies (1970) suggested that nurses develop defences to protect themselves from becoming involved in patients' concerns. Task-allocated care helped this process since it tended to depersonalize individuals. Nursing as a process does not encourage such depersonalization. Rather it encourages the nurse to communicate with the patient. The most sophisticated communication and potentially the most emotionally draining is that of counselling.

The counselling role

If a nurse assesses a patient and identifies problems, it follows that solutions are sought. In physical problems, solutions may be reasonably clear-cut. For example, if pressure is a problem for the patient in bed, a regimen of pressure care can be instituted which the patient should readily understand and accept. Similarly, if a patient has problems in breathing when lying flat, nursing him in an upright sitting position may alleviate his distress. In both cases the nurse is being directive, basing her judgement on research, her own experience and known solutions to the problems. The patient may be involved in the decisions made but is likely to bow to 'superior' knowledge.

Dealing with emotional problems is very different, since the best solutions are those reached by the individual. Counselling is non-directive and its aim is to help an individual find acceptable solutions to soluble problems, or to learn to cope with insoluble ones. This may be very difficult for the nurse who, having assessed a problem, may see an 'obvious' solution. Unless the solution is acceptable to a patient, it will not relieve emotional distress.

Emotional problems may cover a wide spectrum, from those related to diagnosis and prognosis to more personal problems involving relationships and beliefs. A nurse will need knowledge and skills before she can take on a counselling role and will need to accept her own limitations. The process of counselling may be likened to the nursing process in that there are stages of assessment, planning, implementation and evaluation.

Assessment

Assessment, using the skills of communication described in Chapter 4, is required to identify the problem with which the patient cannot cope. If the problem is personal, it is particularly important that trust is established. It may be that the patient will require promises of confidentiality. This requires thought on the part of the nurse, for the problem may be one which, if shared, could help a patient's overall recovery. It is probably best to say something which will engender trust but leave room for negotiation, such as: 'I hope you feel you can trust me to be discreet but, if I can't help with your problem, I may need to refer you to someone else. Perhaps we can talk about that later.' What is important in building trust is that promises given should not be broken.

Active listening is important, as are facilitation, clarification and picking up cues. The patient may be ashamed of his problem, which may lead to hesitation, cues and ambiguous statements. Open questions, picking up cues and an unhurried facilitative approach should help the individual to verbalize his problem. The following extract gives an example of the skills of identifying a personal problem with which the patient (Mrs Springfield) could not cope.

Patient I am not sure about going home
Nurse Not sure? (reflecting)
Patient Well – it's so peaceful in here (cue)
Nurse But not at home? (picking up cue)
Patient No
Nurse How is it at home? (open question)
Patient I don't know how to tell you
Nurse Why don't you try? (facilitating)
Patient Well, it's John, my husband. He has become so rough lately
Nurse Rough – with you? (clarifying)
Patient Yes, over the last few months he has become very violent with me – and I can't get him to discuss it. If I hadn't had my work I would have gone crazy. But now the doctor has said I have to stay at home for three months because of the hysterectomy and I dread it

In the above extract, the nurse was able to identify a real problem. Without the appropriate skills she may have missed the problem by premature reassurance, blocking or missing cues, as follows:

Patient I am not sure about going home
Nurse Of course you are – you will be right as rain once you are there (premature reassurance)
Patient But it is so peaceful in here (cue)
Nurse (laughing) You must be joking! Come on, let's get you up (missed cue; blocking)

In this second extract, the patient may abandon her attempts to talk to the nurse. In fact, the nurse may not be able to handle a problem of this nature, but if she identifies it she can refer it on to someone who can.

Planning
In planning as a counsellor, skills are required to help the patient set goals or formulate strategies for coping with the problem. This can be a difficult stage for a counsellor who has to face her own feelings about the problem but resist giving advice on what to do. It may be obvious to the nurse, for example, that a battered wife should leave her husband. The patient, however, may have a very different perception of the situation. By allowing the patient to talk through the options, possible solutions may arise.

Before planning, more detail may be required of the exact problem. In Mrs Springfield's case, the nurse established that the violence only occurred when the couple were in the house alone together and appeared to be related to Mr Springfield's dissatisfaction with his employment. In assessing the problem the nurse established that Mrs Springfield had a coping strategy, i.e. throwing herself into her work, but that three months' convalescence had removed this. The patient's illness had in fact precipitated a situation where the patient, instead of accepting the problem, had to face it and find a solution. The nurse attempted to clarify the patient's attitude.

Nurse You say you would have gone crazy without your work. How did this help?
Patient Well, I am lucky, I have an absorbing job, so during the daytime I can just switch off – and I have been staying at the office quite late. And where before I would hurry home, I often stay with a friend overnight if I have to be somewhere early
Nurse Go on (prompting)
Patient Well, it doesn't change things but I can bear

what happens because I can get away – I don't mean that I don't mind – of course I do, but I have hoped he would get better – and I fill the house at weekends, the children or friends come over – oh – now I have to be at home I realize I just haven't faced things

Nurse And now? (prompting)

Patient Well, I can't escape any more

Nurse Is that what you want? (direct question)

Patient I sometimes think it's the only way. He won't go for treatment or to marriage guidance – in fact he says he only hits me because I like it. He isn't the man I loved anymore – but the thought of being on my own at my age is scary.

In the above extract, Mrs Springfield is beginning to consider her options. She will need to work through the possibilities open to her and perhaps agree to talk to someone expert in marital counselling who can help her. Her negative attitude to her husband may need to be explored, along with the possibility that he may be mentally ill and badly in need of help.

Implementation

When a patient has made decisions, implementation is in his hands. The counsellor may be supportive but if, for example, Mrs Springfield decides to leave her husband, only she can actually do the leaving. The nurse can, however, refer the patient to the Social Services if there are financial or housing problems.

Evaluation

More often than not, hospital nurses lose touch with patients after discharge. The nurse may never know, for example, if Mrs Springfield did leave her husband nor yet how the patient coped if she did leave. However, in some situations it is possible to evaluate the effects of counselling, particularly if the problems are concerned with coping with diagnosis and prognosis.

Summary

Although it can be rewarding to help a patient with her problems, it can also be emotionally expensive. The nurse who helped Mrs Springfield face the reality of her problem and the uncomfortable possibilities for dealing with it may have been appalled as she listened to the story. She may not have met a battered wife before or realized that it may not show on the outside. She may worry about her own parents or her boyfriend in addition to worrying about the patient. She may also feel that none of the solutions are palatable and that she has failed in some way. She may even disapprove of Mrs Springfield breaking up a marriage, no matter how violent the husband.

Burnout

If nurses do not consider their own needs in handling the emotions inherent in working with patients they may begin to show signs of strain. The Americans call this 'burnout' in that if the strain is neglected, eventually the nurse will have nothing left to give to her patients (Maslach 1981; Burnard 1991). Nurses may not notice the impending burnout in themselves because the signs are relatively subtle in their onset. However, other nurses may notice a change in colleagues and can then alert them in a sensitive way to the fact that they are no longer quite the cheerful and enthusiastic colleague they were before.

The major signs of burnout are loss of enthusiasm, loss of a positive attitude and the beginnings of a feeling that everything in life is awful and negative. This is generally followed by feeling unwell so that the nurse begins to take more time off sick than previously and spend more time at her General Practitioner (GP) with small ailments that previously would not have concerned her. Following on from tiredness, negative feelings and feelings of illness, a decrease in efficiency is noticed which is usually accompanied by a change in mood. This is followed by a loss of confidence and self-esteem, and if things do not improve for the individual, the nurse may become clinically depressed. At this point, the nurse will need professional help. The symptoms as described lead to the reality that a nurse can no longer use her own internal resources to deal with the everyday pressures of her career.

Burnout generally happens when a nurse is unsupported in her role so that the pressures and the emotional strain build up and have nowhere to go. There is considerably less risk of burnout in nurses who feel that they are supported in their role.

The need for support

It can be seen that nurses need both physical and emotional support if they are to give of their best to their patients and survive emotionally themselves. Most hospitals have health facilities for staff which can be used in addition to those offered by the GP. Some hospitals also hold clinics to help nurses give up smoking.

Emotional support is less well organized. In the UK, the Royal College of Nursing has a counselling service which any member may use by telephoning the counsellor. Some health authorities also provide counsellors for staff. What is less apparent is peer or managerial support for on-the-spot counselling, nor is there often help for learners to develop coping strategies.

Peer support

Peer support may be formal or informal. Formal support groups do exist in some hospitals. They give an opportunity for nurses to work through problems with their peers by talking about their feelings and the situations that they find most difficult to cope with. Much of the value of such groups is in the sharing of experiences and the discovery that other people also experience difficulties in their working lives. The feeling that others care enough to attend the group and listen to others' problems can be a valuable support mechanism even if problems are not solved.

Informal peer support may be available from a special colleague or friend who is prepared to listen and be supportive. This informal support is often reciprocal but not necessarily so. Informal support may also be available in groups, particularly of nurses who live together in a nurses' home and spend leisure time together. Individuals will choose those colleagues whom they can trust and who show a willingness to listen and be supportive.

Managerial support

Ideally, nurses should be able to turn to their managers for support. However, this is not always the case for a number of reasons. Rowden (1984) states that, 'A manager is one who gets his work done by getting others to do theirs. He must show an intelligent and humane understanding of the needs of the enterprise and of the people who work for him.'

Although these statements should be compatible they may be seen to be in conflict by some managers. If the manager is supportive to her staff – especially if the support requires that a nurse moves ward or has time off because she 'cannot cope' – work may be seen to suffer. An example may illustrate the point.

Nurse Shenton became very upset when a 45-year-old patient died after a coronary thrombosis. Sister reprimanded her, saying, 'If you are going to be a nurse, you will have to pull yourself together – other patients need attention'.

Sister was concerned with getting the work done rather than showing 'humane understanding' of her staff. In fact Nurse Shenton's father had died immediately before the nurse had started work on the medical ward three weeks earlier, and her upset was partially triggered by personal grief. Nurse Shenton discontinued her training, maintaining that she did not wish to belong to an 'uncaring profession'.

Had Sister given time to support Nurse Shenton and discover her problem, a nurse may not have been lost to the profession.

In fact, many managers have not been given help on how to support their staff and many see 'counselling' in terms of disciplinary action. Managers cannot be blamed for this, for without the skills they cannot provide the trust and facilitation required for counselling and supporting their staff.

Attitudes are as important as skills, for if a manager has a positive attitude towards staff she will, by definition, be supportive, even if she is unable to take the role of counsellor. Psychologists have known for many years that work improves with positive feedback, yet in many work situations the emphasis is on error. Giving the nurse praise for work well done can leave her feeling that progress is being made, while criticism of small errors can lead to frustration and eventually to lowered self-esteem.

The working environment can have a profound effect on a nurse's ability to cope with difficult situations, as can the knowledge that Sister is approachable and will understand if a nurse has problems. However, even if a manager is supportive, some nurses may fail to confide in her because they believe that they are meant to be able to cope. Admitting that some situations are difficult can be seen as admitting to weakness.

Each nurse has to make the decision on trusting a manager if she needs special support or the chance simply to talk. It may be that a particular tutor or a trained member of staff is helpful. The manager's role is to be available, to engender trust and to avoid censure.

Developing coping strategies

Often the most difficult situations to cope with are those that are new and unexpected. In a new situation, there may be no previous experience which helps to direct behaviour. If the situation is also unexpected, there is no time to plan action. Nursing offers many difficult situations, some of which are new and unexpected. In order to cope with these, knowledge is necessary of potentially difficult situations, skills are required to manage the situations, and self-awareness needs to be developed to explore feelings about the many issues involved.

Knowledge

Nurse education should prepare nurses for the realities of all areas of clinical practice. This knowledge should include preparation for facing death, dealing with fear-provoking diagnoses and prognoses, and considering potential problems which might be encountered. Many nurses have had little if any experience before training of death, violence or trauma, yet they are likely to meet all of these in some guise during their training. A nurse reacting badly to a battered baby on a paediatric ward said, 'If only I'd been prepared – I didn't know babies could be burned on purpose'. Lack of preparation can reduce a nurse's chances of coping.

Skills

If a nurse is skilled, she will feel more assured when delivering patient care, whether the care is physical or psychological. Such assurance should also help the nurse to be honest when she cannot deal with a situation so that she feels able to refer or ask for help without feeling a failure.

Self-awareness

Developing self-awareness can be painful but it can also help a nurse to cope with difficult situations as she explores her own feelings. For example, few people face their own mortality but, in nursing, meeting death is a reminder of that mortality, especially if the patient is of a similar age to the nurse. Understanding one's own feelings about death can help a nurse to cope not only with death itself but with the needs of the dying patient and his relatives.

In developing self-awareness, there is also a need to accept individual differences. The nurse who is herself fearful of dying may empathize with a patient who is frightened. She also needs to be able to help the patient who is stoic about death but has other pertinent concerns.

Self-awareness can make sense of reactions to specific situations if a nurse thinks through her actions. It may be that a nurse feels antipathy to a particular patient. In trying to understand the emotion a nurse may remember that someone whom she disliked in the past looked or sounded like the patient, or had the same name. Understanding may reduce the antipathy. If not, an honest 'I'm not the best person to care for Mr Tagholm' might be a solution.

There are numerous issues which a nurse will face which can be helped by self-knowledge. Attitudes and beliefs about abortion, euthanasia and life-support machines are just a few of these. In nursing, personal beliefs about abortion are allowed, as a nurse may refuse to help with the operation. In all other areas, the patient's needs are expected to override the nurse's personal views. This includes care of the patient before and after abortion.

It can be seen that nursing has stressful elements. Support can reduce this stress but the level of support required will vary from nurse to nurse. Each nurse needs to develop her own networks, which may include a partner, friend or relative who is not a nurse.

Education

There have been considerable changes in nurse education over recent years with a move from the nurse serving an apprenticeship in her training, which was service- rather than educationally-based, to true student status and emphasis on education for the expanding role of the nurse (Kendrick and Simpson 1992).

In 1986 the United Kingdom Central Council (UKCC) issued Project 2000, a new preparation for practice. The key proposals were:

1 That there would be a single level of registered practitioner
2 That there would be a specialized practitioner
3 That there would be a new helper grade
4 That learners would have a supernumerary status on the wards
5 That the training for enrolled nurses would be discontinued.

Within the document, the UKCC recommended true student status for learners as suggested by Briggs (1972).

In order to allow nurses to be supernumerary, a new grade of helper, called the health care assistant, was introduced to make up for the service contribution previously provided by student nurses. This change in nurse education brought a closer link with higher education in that first level registration and Diploma level qualification would be validated by the local university. All students would follow a common foundation programme and then select one of four specialist branches: adult nursing, children's nursing, mental health nursing or learning disabilities nursing. Salaries were replaced with a bursary.

The new training (P2K) was commenced in a number of districts in 1990 so that a number of courses have been completed and new ones started. Much of the criticism of P2K was in advance of its implementation and this reflects the fear that there would be a lack of information and, for the clinical staff who supervise the students, lack of ownership of the course because they were not involved in its planning. Tutors too could well feel threatened by having to teach at different levels and wondering whether their preparation for teaching is appropriate to the new style course.

Thompson (1989) interviewed some of the first students about their perception of the course. These learners had been attracted to nursing in general rather than to a new course but they did see that continuous assessment, which is a feature of P2K, was much fairer than examinations and they appreciated the set hours of working and holidays which mimicked the academic year. Initial supernumerary status was valued as was the cessation of the 'pair of hands' role. (Students are not rostered until after the Common Foundation Programme [CFP]).

One P2K student (Lancaster 1991) reports that the course helped her to take a more holistic view of care but was puzzled by the reluctance on the part of some clinical staff to absorb the changes.

What is important about the new learning status for nurses is that it will help them to be seen as practitioners and professionals in a way that was not possible before. In their expanding role (Chapter 1) they will be able to feel that they are colleagues of doctors rather than subservient to them. It is argued that this major change in relationships with other health professionals and the direction for the profession can only be achieved through the new educational programme (Henry and Pashley 1990).

Continuing education

No matter what the form of training, whether it be as a graduate nurse, a P2K nurse or a nurse who has undertaken traditional training, the point of registration is just the beginning of a professional career in the UK. All nurses need to continue their education through private study, and through attending courses, study days and conferences. These will not only serve the purpose of keeping up-to-date professionally, but also allow interaction with other health professionals and facilitate career development. Since 1990, all nurses who wish to continue practice have had to provide evidence of continuing education. The final content of PREP (Post-Registration Education and Practice) was agreed in March 1993 and came into force on 1 April 1995. All practitioners will have to comply with the statute by April 2001 in order to maintain an effective registration with the UKCC (Garbett 1995).

Choose one nursing journal. Where is the emphasis of its contents, e.g. clinical, research, management, or a mix? What do you see as a strength of the journal? How could it be improved?

Reading

There is a wide variety of nursing journals. Some are very general such as the *Nursing Times*, while others are more specific such as the *Journal of District Nursing* and *Journal of Cancer Care*. Some are specifically related to research. These include the *Journal of Advanced Nursing* and *Nursing Research*.

Choosing journals is a very personal matter, but as nursing becomes more research-based a point to note about a journal is whether its articles are referenced and use current research findings. Opinion is valuable but has more credibility if backed by research which is pertinent to the subject.

Most nursing libraries take a wide variety of journals. It is worth reading the journals of allied professions. The *British Medical Journal* and *The Lancet* often carry articles which are pertinent to nursing. Further, they help nurses to follow current medical thinking.

In-service education

Colleges of nursing provide in-service education for all grades of nursing staff. Newly qualified Staff Nurses may attend ENB accredited courses and study days while new staff are oriented to their new environment. A further function of in-service education is to help staff keep their knowledge base up-to-date and learn new skills.

Education may be in the form of study days, workshops or courses. The subjects covered reflect new advances in nursing and the expressed needs of staff. For example, when the nursing process was introduced, many in-service education tutors organized workshops and study days on 'implementing the process'. With the move towards trust status, trusts buy their training from colleges of nursing and health.

Staff can influence the content of in-service education programmes by stating clearly their perceived needs and by asking to attend courses. Outside speakers are often involved to give expert coverage of topics.

Post-basic courses

There is a wide variety of post-basic courses, some leading to further statutory nursing qualifications while others are certificated. There are courses leading to the qualifications of Health Visitor and District Nurse, both of which are taught in institutes of higher education. The health visitors' course lasts for one academic year, while the district nurses' course is for a minimum of six months plus a period of supervised practice. For both courses a period of clinical experience following registration as a nurse is required.

Nurses may also study for the Diploma in Nursing. Although the diploma is awarded from London University, the course is organized between colleges of nursing and an institute of higher education. The course is normally studied on a day-release basis over three years. An increasing selection of diplomas and higher degrees related to health studies are offered by a number of universities. A first degree is not always necessary for these providing that the candidate can show some signs of recent ability to study at the appropriate level.

Advanced Clinical Courses are available of varying duration which carry certificates from the relevant National Boards. In England and Wales, these were originally set up by the Joint Board of Clinical Nursing Studies, which has since been subsumed into the UKCC and its Boards. These courses are set up according to professional need and expertise which is available in an area. This means that nurses may have to travel some distance to undertake the course of their choice. The benefit is that, while on the course, the students should gain experience in a centre of excellence.

Other courses which do not carry a certificate are also available to nurses. In order to attend any course, whether or not it leads to qualifications or a certificate, a nurse may need to be seconded by her employing authority. In a time of financial cutbacks this may pose a problem and some nurses may be prepared to pay for their own education if they are allowed study leave. This raises the issue of whether continuing education is the responsibility of the nurse or the employer.

Graduate education

With the introduction of P2K and the need for colleges of nursing to ally themselves with higher education, there is an increasing number of degree courses offered in nursing. Some of these are basic undergraduate courses which lead to a degree and the registration of RGN. Others are for those nurses who are already registered who wish to work towards graduate status. Some of these courses may be studied on a day-release basis.

More nurses are studying for higher degrees. These may be in aspects of clinical nursing. For example, a Diploma in Community Care can be taken at Sheffield University and lead to the qualification of Master of Science. A similar Diploma with the option of leading to a Master of Science can be taken in Palliative Care. Usually the course is taught up to the level of Diploma and then the final year leading to the higher degree is often by research alone.

Continuing education, at whatever level, is important for both personal and professional growth and adds to the body of knowledge which makes nursing a profession in its own right.

Summary

In this chapter the diverse nature of nursing has been explored, showing that the nurse has a role which demands an effective working relationship with her medical colleagues and other members of the health care team.

Nursing itself demands a knowledge of research and a questioning approach to practice. It also requires that some nurses become researchers and share their findings with the profession.

The costs of nursing have been considered, along with the need for effective support networks. This includes peer support, managerial support and the development of self-awareness on the part of the nurse.

Finally, the considerable changes in nurse education have been briefly described and the need for continuing education has been discussed to facilitate both personal growth and the enhancement of the profession.

References

Ashworth, P. (1984) Communicating in an intensive care unit. In Faulkner, A. (Ed.) *Communication*, pp. 94–112. Edinburgh: Churchill Livingstone.

Briggs, A. (1972) *Report of the Committee on Nursing*. London: HMSO.

Burnard, P. (1991) Beyond burnout. *Nursing Standard, 5*(43), 46–48.

Faulkner, A. (1980) Communication and the nurse. *Nuring Times, 76*(21), 93–95.

Faulkner, A. (1992a) *Effective interaction with patients.* Edinburgh: Churchill Livingstone.

Faulkner, A (1992b) The evaluation of training programmes for communication skills in palliative care. *Journal of Cancer Care, 1,* 75–78.

Faulkner, A. & Macleod Clark, J. (1987) Communication skills teaching in nurse education. In Davis, B. (Ed.) *Nursing education research and developments,* pp. 189–205. London: Croom Helm.

Faulkner, A. & Maguire, P. (1984) Teaching ward nurses to monitor cancer patients. *Clinical Oncology, 10,* 383–389.

Faulkner, A. & Maguire, P. (1994) *Talking to cancer patients and their relatives.* Oxford: Oxford Medical Publications.

Faulkner, A. & Ward, L. (1983) The nurse's role as a health educator. *Nursing Times,* Occasional Paper, 79, 15.

Faulkner, A., Argent, J., Jones, A. & O'Keeffe, C. (1995) Improving skills of doctors in imparting distressing information. *Medical Education.*

Garbett, R. (1995) The Nursing Times guide to PREP. London: *Nursing Times.*

Gilbran, K. (1979) *The Prophet.* London: Heinemann.

Greene, A. (1994) Generic engineering. *Nursing Management, 1*(1), 26.

Hawthorn, P.J. (1983) Principles of research: a checklist. *Nursing Times, 79*(23), 41–43.

Henry, C. & Pashley, G. (1990) Carving out the nursing 90's. *Nursing Times, 86*(3), 45–46.

Ingleton, C. & Faulkner, A. (1995) *Quality assurance in palliative care: a review of the literature.* Occasional Paper No. 14. Sheffield: Trent Palliative Care Centre.

Kendrick, K. & Simpson, A. (1992) The nursing reformation. In Soothill, K., Henry, C. & Kendrick, K. (Eds.) *Themes and perspectives in nursing.* London: Chapman & Hall.

Lancaster, A. (1974) *Compiling references and bibliographies.* London: King's Fund Centre.

Lancaster, A. (1991) Project 2000: a nurse's view. *Nursing, 4*(32), 16.

Macleod Clark, J. (1982) Nurse/patient verbal interaction. Steinberg Collection. London: RCN.

Maslach, C. (1981) *Burnout: the cost of caring.* Englewood Cliffs, New Jersey: Prentice Hall.

Menzies, I. (1970) *Defence systems as control against anxiety.* London: Tavistock Press.

Mitchell, J. R. A. (1984) Is nursing any business of doctors? A simple guide to the 'nursing process'. *British Medical Journal, 288,* 216–221.

Rich, S. (1995) Meeting the challenges. *Nursing Times, 91*(4), 34–35.

Roberts, D. (1984) Non-verbal communication. Popular and

unpopular patients. In Faulkner, A. (Ed.) *Communication*, 3–28.

Rowden, R. (Ed.) (1984) *Managing nursing*. London: Baillière Tindall.

Stockwell, F. (1972) *The unpopular patient*. London: Royal College of Nursing.

Thompson, J. (1989) Starting with a bonus. *Nursing Times, 85*(37), 28–31.

Further reading

Abercrombie, M. L. J. (1979) *The anatomy of judgement*. Harmondsworth, London: Penguin.

Basford, L. & Slevin, O. (1995) Theory and practice of nursing. An integrated approach to nursing care for Project 2000. Edinburgh: Campion.

Burnard, P. (1990) *Nurse education, the way forward*. London: Scutari Press.

Calnan, J. (1984) *Coping with research*. London: Heinemann Medical.

Dolan, B. (1993) *Project 2000. Reflection and celebration*. London: Scutari Press.

Faulkner, A., Webb, P. & Maguire, P. (1991) Communication and counselling skills. Educating health professionals working in cancer and palliative care. *Patient Education and Counselling, 18*, 3–7.

Glover, J. (1982) *Causing death and saving lives*. Harmondsworth, London: Penguin.

Macleod Clark, J. & Hockey, L. (1989) *Further research for nursing. A new guide for the enquiring nurse*. London: Scutari Press.

Meichenbaum, D. (1983) *Coping with stress*. London: Century Publishing.

Reed, J. & Proctor, S. (Eds.) (1993) *Nurse education: a reflective approach*. London: Edward Arnold.

Robinson, J. & Gray, A. (1991) *Policy issues in nursing*. Milton Keynes: Open University Press.

Salvage, J. (1988) Professionalisation or struggle for survival. *Journal of Advanced Nursing, 13*, 515–519.

Stewart, W. (1983) *Counselling in nursing*. London: Harper and Row.

Watts, G. (1991) From vision to reality. *Nursing, 4*(32), 13–15.

Index

Page numbers appearing in **bold** refer to figures and page numbers appearing in *italic* refer to tables.

Abdominal pain 212, 218
Abdominal paracentesis 205, 295
Acetylsalicylic acid, *see* Aspirin
Acid–base balance 25, 40
Acidosis 299
Acquired immunodeficiency disease,
    see AIDS
Acupuncture 240
Acute medical conditions 245
Addison's disease *237*
Admission 67–82
  adjustment to ward
      environment 71–5, 79–80
  documentation 78–9
  information for patients 71, 77–8
  introductions 76
  notice of 69–70
  orientation to ward 76–7
  procedure 75–80
  stress on 70–1
  waiting for 76
Adrenal glands 35, *37*
Adrenaline 35, *37*, 46, 273
Adrenocorticotrophic hormone
    (ACTH) *37*
Ageing 424–7
  physiological 424–5
  psychological 426
  social effects on 426–7
AIDS 24, 347–50
  care plan 350
  disease process 347
  reaction to diagnosis 239–40
Airways maintenance **343**
Alcohol consumption 24, 524
  health education 23, 568
  in peptic ulcer 284
  restrictions 138
Alcoholics Anonymous 575
Alcoholism
  and cirrhosis of liver 291, 293
  and pneumonia 264
Aldosterone *37*, *234*, *237*
Alveoli
  in bronchitis 247
  in emphysema 252
Ambulance for transport of
    patient 534–5
Amylase *29*

Anaemia 257, 269, 323–30
  acquired 325
  aplastic *323*, 324, 326
  care plan 329–30
  in cirrhosis of liver 292
  diagnostic investigation 218
  disease process 323–7
  iron-deficiency *323*, 324
  pernicious 323, 324
  in renal failure 317, 320
  sickle cell 323, 324–5
  types 323
Anaesthetists 361
Anal canal 28
Analgesia 262, 368
Anatomical arrangement of body
    systems **42–4**
Aneurysms *214*, 442
Angina pectoris 276
Angiograms 224–5
Angiotensin *234*
Animal organs for
    transplantation 417
Ankylosis 335
Antibiotics 254, 267, 283, 287, 289,
    391
Antidiuretic hormone (ADH) *37*
Anuria 316
Anxiety
  and disease 115–16
  in dying patient 475–6
  see also Psychological problems;
    Stress
Aphasia 443
Aplastic anaemia *323*, 324, 326
Appendicectomy 398
  care plan 400
  laparoscopic 398
  the operation 398
  planning nursing care 399–400
Appendicitis **111**
Arteriograms 224–5
Arteriosclerosis 275
Arthrodesis 455
Ascites *205*, 238, 292
Aspirin 282, 337–8, 445, 455
Assessment 14–15
  and care plans 152
  in counselling 596–7

  diagnosis and 241
  of elderly patient 427–8
  forms 102, **515**
  of needs 83–104
Asthma 108, 110
  sputum in *205*
Atherosclerosis 275, 276, 309, 319,
    442
Atropine 215
Attitudes 48–9, 601
Autoimmune disorders 287, 291,
    313, *323*, 324
Azathiaprine 295

Babinski's reflex 443
Back injuries among nurses 594
Bacterial infections *207*
  sputum in *205*
Balanitis 299
Bandages 375
Barium enema *214*, 222, **223**
Barium meals 221–2
Barrier creams 431
Bedpans 290
Bedrest
  in acute renal failure 317
  in cardiac failure 271–2
  in cirrhosis of liver 295
  in myocardial infarction 277
  in peptic ulcer 284
  in rheumatoid arthritis 338
  in ulcerative colitis 289
Bedsores, *see* Pressure sores
Behaviour, assessment 507–8
Bereavement visiting 491,
    563–4
Bile ducts
  obstruction 404–5, **405**
  'T' tube for drainage 406
Bile pigments in faeces,
    absence 200–201, *201*
Bile salts *29*
Biliary colic 404
Biliary disorders *204*
Bilirubin in urine *204*
Biopsy *207*
  bone marrow 218–19
  breast 378
  gastrointestinal tract 212–14

Biopsy *contd*
  general factors 211
  liver 216–18
  needle for chest aspiration 204
  renal 215–16
  urinary tract 215
Bladder
  disease 113
  urethrogram 224
Blood
  in cerebrospinal fluid *207*
  clotting factors 293
  clotting time 217
  collection 217
  contaminated 348
  in faeces 200–201, *201*, 390
  loss 325
    see also Haemorrhage
  in sputum *205*
  in urine *204*
Blood gas in emphysema 252
Blood pressure (BP) 5, 127, 230–3
  in cardiac failure 270
  changes in *234*
  diastolic 231, *233*
  measurement 231–3, **232**
  and myocardial infarction 276
  normal limits *233*
  post-operative 363
  and shock 364–6
  systolic 231, *233*
Blood tests 196–7, **197**
  normal values *198*
Blood transfusion 287
  in anaemia 328
Blood vessels 31–2, **32**
Body image, *see* Self-image
Body systems 34–44
  anatomical arrangement **42–4**
  framework 41
  protective covering **40**, 41
Body tissue, investigations 206–19
Bone marrow
  biopsy 218–19
  depressed activity *323*, 324
  see also Aplastic anaemia
Bones **44**
Bowel movement 368–9
Bowel stoma formation, *see* Stoma
Brachial artery 231, **232**
Bradycardia 124
Brain 36
  disease, pulse rate in 124
  electroencephalogram (EEG) **229**,
    229–30
Breast cancer
  biopsy 207, 211, 218
  mammograms 220–1
  see also Mastectomy
Breast prosthesis 380–1, 383
Breathing
  Cheyne–Stokes 126
  difficulties (dyspnoea) 109–10, 126
    in bronchitis 247–8
    in cardiac failure 274
  exercises 406

sound of 126
in unconscious patient 342
see also Respiration
Breathlessness
  in anaemia 325
  in hyperthyroidism 310
Briggs Report 580, 603
Bristol Cancer Centre 240
British Diabetic Association 309,
  575–6
British Society for Digestive
  Endoscopy 209
Bronchiectasis *205*
Bronchitis 108, 110, 135, 150
  acute 246
  chronic 245–6, **246**
    and cardiac failure 269, 270
    and emphysema 251–2, 254
    gas exchange **255**
    sputum in *205*
  disease process 246–9
  in lung carcinoma 257
  social problems 251
Broncho-fibrescope 214
Bronchodilators 249, 254
Bronchopneumonia 265
Bronchoscopy 214–15
Bronchospasm 249
Bronchus, carcinoma **256**
Burns *204*, *234*, *237*, 339, 365

Caecostomy 390
Caecum **42**
Calcitonin *37*
Calcium 41
Cancer
  of bowel **111**, *214*, 222
  diagnosis, informing patient 137
  metastatic tumours 256–7
  see also Breast cancer; Lung
    cancer
Cancer Relief Macmillan Fund 511,
  517
Cancer Research Campaign 589
Capillaries 26–7, **27**
Carbimazole 311
Carbohydrates
  digestion *29*, 29–30
  intake in diabetes 301, 303–5
Carbon dioxide 254
Carboxypeptidase *29*
Carcinoma, *see* Cancer
Cardiac arrest 278, 280
Cardiac bed 272
Cardiac disease, *see* Heart
  disease
Cardiac failure *237*, 269–74
  care plan 274
  causes and effects **270**
  congestive *237*, 269
  disease process 269–71
  in emphysema 253
  oedema in *237*
  in renal failure 320
Cardiac massage 278
Cardiac output (CO) 230, *234*

Cardiovascular disease 108
Cardiovascular system 31–2, **32**
Care plans 16, 147–74, 269
  components 148–51
  critical pathways 154, **155–7**
  dynamic element 169–70, 173
  individualized 147, 158–9, 163
    format **153**, **155–7**, **159–62**
  multidisciplinary format **160–2**,
    171–2
  patient's role 163–4, 169
  standard 151–4
    limitations 152, 154
  see also under specific diseases
Carers National Association 517
Caring for People 22
CAT (computerized tomography)
  scans 225–6, **256**
Catheterization
  urinary tract
    after prostatectomy 412–13
    in incontinence 332
    for retention of urine 410, 412,
      413
Cell transport 30–1, **31**, 32
Central nervous system (CNS) 36
  control pathways **449**
Central Sterile Supply Department
  (CSSD) 561
  packs 371–2, **372**
Cerebral embolus 442
Cerebral haemorrhage 441–2
Cerebral injury 237
Cerebrospinal fluid (CFS) 205–6
Cerebrospinal fluid (CSF),
  abnormalities *207*
Cerebrovascular accident (CVA
  stroke) 320, 342, 441–7
  care plan 447
  disease process 441–4
  planning nursing care 444–7
Cervix, carcinoma 385
Charts 179–80, 183–4
  diabetes **183**
  fluid balance 180, **182**
  pain *263*
  urinalysis 180, **183**
Chemotherapy 258, 259–61,
  379
Chest, normal X-ray **220**
Cheyne–Stokes breathing 126
Child abuse 565–6, 568
Children, and dying patient 487
Chiropody 429
Cholangiogram 407
Cholecystectomy 404–9
  care plan 408–9
  laparoscopic 398
  the operation 404–6
  planning nursing care 406–8
Cholecystitis **111**, 406
Cholecystogram 224
Cholelithiasis **111**
Chronic disease 245, 245–6
  evaluating care 509
Chymotrypsin *29*

Circulatory system 31
  potential post-operative
    problems *364*, 366
Cirrhosis of liver 245, 291–2, **292**,
    293–8
  care plan 297–8
  disease process 291–3
  oedema in *237*
  planning nursing care 294–7
Citizens' Advice Bureau 576
Clean Air Acts 118
Clothes
  for disabled patient 452, 453
  disposal **373**
  and incontinence 432
Clubbing of fingers 253
Codeine 215
Cognitive dissonance 48
Colic 287
  biliary 404
Colleges of Nursing and Health
    605–7
Colon **28**
  carcinoma 390
Colonic washout, high 212
Colonoscopy 212–13
Colostomy 390
Coma
  after CVA 443
  dehydration in *237*
  diabetic 306, 309
  Glasgow coma scale **181**
  hepatic 292, 295
  hyperglycaemic 306
  hypoglycaemic 342
  see also Unconscious patient
Common cold 108, 110
Communication 50–2, 87–94,
    445
  need for 52
  non-verbal 90–4
    clothes 91
    eye contact 92
    observation 92–3
    posture 91–2
    touch 93–4
  surgeon and nurses 360
  verbal 51, 88–9
  see also Interviews
Community 57–60
  health risks 60
  social 59
  working 58–9
Community Care Act (1990) 558–9,
    571
Community nurse 526
  referral to 534
Community services 558–609
Complementary therapies 240–1
Confusion
  causes **438**
  in the elderly 437–40
Consent forms 361
Constipation 273, 368–9
  after barium 222
Contraceptives, oral *234*

Coronary thrombosis, *see* Myocardial
    infarction
Cortisol *37*
Cough 126
  in bronchitis 247–8, 250
  in cardiac failure 270
  in emphysema 253
  in lung cancer 257
  in pneumonia 268
Counselling 595–9
Creatinine 203
Cretinism 313
Crohn's disease **111**, *201*, 390
Cross-infection 356–8
CRUSE 576
Culture 60–2, 89
Cushing's disease *237*
CVA, *see* Cerebrovascular accident
Cyanosis 110
  in bronchitis 250
  in pneumonia 266, 267
Cystitis 113–14, 409, 413
Cystogram, micturating 224
Cystoscopy 215

Daily functioning, effect of illness
    on 116–17
Day centres 423
Day-rooms 72, 76
Death
  at home 562–3
  certificate 480, 488
  and organ transplantation 416–17
  see also Dying patient
Decision making by patient 500–1
Dehydration
  causes *237*
  as diagnosis *234*
Dentures, *see* Teeth, false
Department of Health 588
Depression 554
  in dying patient 476–7
  in lung cancer 262
  post-operative 547–9
Diabetes 106–7, 236, 245–6,
    298–310
  blood sugar analysis *198*, 199
  care plan 152, **164**, 309–10
  complications 309
  disease process 298–300
  fluid balance *237*, 299–300
    charts 180, **182**
  insulin dependent 302–3
  and ischaemic heart disease 275
  and lifestyle 551
  in mature people 299–300
  non-insulin dependent 301–2
  patient education 526, **527**
  physical reactions 306–7, *307*
  psychological problems 132
  and renal failure 319
  specialist nurse 546
  urinalysis 305
  in young people 299
Diabetes insipidus *237*
Diabetic card **551**

Diabetic coma 306, 309
Diagnosis 195–242
  cancer 137, 261–2
  co-ordination of information
    238–41
  investigations 196–242
  nurse's knowledge 150–1
  nurse's role 230–8
Dialysis, renal 318
Diarrhoea *237*
  in hyperthyroidism 310
  in ulcerative colitis 287–8
Diazepam 209, 215, 294
Diet
  in acute renal failure 318
  in anaemia 327
  before colonoscopy 212
  in biliary disorders 406
  in cirrhosis of liver 294
  in diabetes 303–5
  health education 24–5
  and ischaemic heart disease 275,
    280
  in peptic ulcer 283–4
  in radiotherapy 259
  and stoma 391, 394–5
  in ulcerative colitis 287–9
  see also Food intake; Nutrition
Digestive disorders 111–12
Digestive system 28, **28**
Digitalis 272
Diploma in Community Care 607
Diploma in Nursing 606
Diploma in Palliative Care 607
Diplopia 330
Disability, physical, adjustment
    to 551–2, 555
Discharge 513–40
  against medical advice 535–6
  implications 532
  information 515–17
  notification of relatives 533
  patient education 521–30
  plan form **518–19**
  planning for 513–15
  planning form **516**
  procedure 536
  psychological problems 549,
    554–5
  referral 533–4, **534**
  role of relatives 533, 537–8
  social problems 517, 520–1, 573
Disease
  deficits produced by 107–18
  physical signs 67–9
  process 105–30
  understanding 522–3
District nurse 559–65
  bereavement visiting 563–4
  case load 561
  local health clinic 561–2
  nursing hierarchy 564–5, **564**
  qualification course 606
  referral to 559–61
  terminal care 562–3
Diuretics 272, 294–5

Doctors
  in medical model of nursing 4–5
  see also Nurse–doctor relationship
Documentation, *see* Records
Dopamine 447–8
Drainage of wounds 376, 382, 407
Dressings 374–6
Drugs
  abuse 24
  administration in shock 366
  at discharge 534
  cytotoxic, *see* Chemotherapy
  for diabetes 301
  in hyperthyroidism 311
  and incontinence 429
  prescription sheets **177–8**
  records 176, 178–9
  in ulcerative colitis 289
Duodenum
  endoscopy 211–12
  ulcers 282
Dying patient 460–92
  anxiety 475–6
  depression 476–7
  dying alone 469–70
  emotional reactions 467–70
  evaluation of care 509–10
  fear 477
  home care 555–6
  hope 466–7
  information for **461**, 462–6
  knowledge needs 461–2
  loss of control 478–9
  loss of dignity 477–8
  pain 469
  physical needs 474–5
  planning nursing care 479–80
  reassurance 467
  relatives, *see* Relatives
  social needs 472–4
  spiritual needs 470–2
  visiting 473
  see also Death
Dysmenorrhoea 385
Dyspepsia *214*
Dysphagia 111, *214*, 330
Dyspnoea, *see* Breathing, difficulties
Dysuria 114

Elderly
  disease in 441–58
  meals-on-wheels 441
Elderly patient 422–59, 503
  assessment 427–8
  confusion 437–40
  dignity and identity 434–5
  discharge of 520–1
  incontinence 429–32
  loneliness 436–7
  mobility 428–9
  nutrition 440–1
  safety 432–4
  sexuality 435–6
  warmth 440–1
Electrocardiogram (ECG) **228–9**

Electroencephalogram (EEG) **229**,
    229–30
Embolism 441–2, **442**
  cerebral 442
  pulmonary *205*
Emergency admissions 397
Emotional costs of nursing 594–5
Emotional support from
    relatives 553–5
Emphysema 150, 251–6
  and chronic bronchitis 251–2,
    254
  disease process 251–3
  gas exchange **255**
  planning nursing care 254–6
Empyema of gallbladder 405
Encephalitis *207*
Endocrine hormones *37*
Endocrine system 34–5, **35**, 36
Endoscope **208**
  trolley **210**
Endoscopy 207–10
  gastrointestinal tract
    lower 212–14
    upper 211–12
  general factors 208–10
  indications and
    contraindications *214*
  respiratory tract
    (bronchoscopy) 214–15
  urinary tract (cystoscopy) 215
Enemas 212, 213, 431
  barium, *see* Barium enema
Enrolled Nurse (EN) 559
Epilepsy 230
Equipment, disposal **373**
Erythropoiesis, reduced *323*, 324
Evaluation of nursing care 17–18,
    169–70, **171–2**, 495–512
  in counselling 598
  mental health 504–8
  patient potential 508–11
  patient report 506–7
  patient satisfaction 495–501
  physical health 501–4
  reduced dependency 498–501
Exercise(s)
  breathing 406
  deficits associated with 116,
    322–3
  in diabetes 302, 305
  ECG 229
  in pneumonia 268
  post-operative 369, 383, 388
  in rheumatoid arthritis 338–9
Exophthalmia 310
Expression, facial 128
Extracorporeal shockwave lithotripsy
    (ESWL) 405
Extrasystole 125
Eyes
  in cerebrovascular accident 443
  in multiple sclerosis 330
Eysenck's introversion–extraversion
    scale 53

Facial expression 128
Faeces
  abnormalities *201*
  investigations 200–1, *201*
Family 56–7, 552–6
  extended **56**
  nuclear **56**
  in pneumonia 266
  see also Relatives
Fats
  in cirrhosis of liver 294
  digestion 30
Femoral hernia 401–2, **402**
Finger clubbing 253
Flatus tube **369**
Fluid balance 236–8
  in cardiac failure 270–1
  charts 180, **182**
  cirrhosis of liver 295
  disturbances 112–13, **113**, 114,
    117–18, *237*, 315
  maintaining 39–40
  in pneumonia 267
  in shock 366, 367
  in unconscious patient 343
  see also Dehydration; Oedema
Fluid intake
  after pyelogram 223
  after urethrogram 224
  in anaemia 327–8
  in colonoscopy 213
  in hyperthyroidism 311–12
  and radiotherapy 259
Folic acid 326, 327
  deficiency *324*
Follicle-stimulating hormone *37*
Food intake 26, 28–30
  deficits 110–12, 114, 117–18
  see also Diet; Nutrition
Fractures, bone 432.

Gallbladder 404–9
  cholecystogram 224
  empyema 405
  obstruction *201*
  see also Cholecystectomy
Gangrene in lower limbs 309
Gastric aspiration 399
Gastritis 245
General anaesthesia, and shock 365
General Nursing Council 3
General practitioners (GPs) 21
  action possibilities **68**, 68–9
  death certification 563
  notification of discharge 514, 534
  and practice nurse 570–1
Genito-urinary tract infections 358
Geriatric medicine 423
Glasgow coma scale **181**
Glomerulonephritis 319
Glossitis 325
Glucagon *37*
Glucose *29*, 235, 551
  blood 36, 299
  in cerebrospinal fluid *207*

Glucose *contd*
  meter 305–6, **306**
  reagent strip 305–6, **306**
  tolerance test 197, **199**, 199–200
  in urine 300
Glycerol trinitrate 277
Gonadotrophic hormones *37*
Gonads 34, **36**, 37
Good Neighbour Scheme 575
Guillain–Barré syndrome *207*

Haematemesis 212, 285
Haematoma, post-operative 374
Haematuria 215
Haemoglobin 217
Haemolysis
  acquired *323*
  hereditary *323*
Haemolytic anaemia 324–6
Haemolytic jaundice *201*
Haemoptysis *205*, 215, 257
Haemorrhage 217–18, *234*, *237*,
      285–6, 323
  cerebral 441–2
  external 376
  gastrointestinal 288
  oesophageal varices 292, 295
  post-biopsy 216, 217, 218
  post-operative 376–7
  primary 376
  secondary 376
  and shock 365
Haemorrhoids *201*, 212
Hair loss 260, 532
Hands
  osteoarthritis **457**
  washing 358
Head injury
  CSF after *207*
  dehydration in *237*
Headaches 295
Health
  concepts 20–1
  definition 20
  individual responsibility for 23–5
  measuring 503–4
  physiology 25–44
  sociological aspects 54–62
Health education 521–30, 568
Health Education Authority
      (HEA) 22–3, 281
Health Education Council (HEC)
      118
Health of the Nation 22
Health Promotion Unit 281
Health visitor 21, 514, 565–8
  case load 566–8
  health care team interaction **566**
  health clinics 568
  health education 568–9
  hierarchy 570
  preventive role 569
  qualification courses 606
  referrals 565–6
  and social workers 567

Hearing in unconscious patient 342,
      345
Heart 31
  electrocardiogram (ECG) 228–9
  transplantation 415
Heart disease
  ischaemic/coronary 163–4, 269,
      274–81
    care plan 163, **165–8**, 281
    disease process 274–7
    lifestyle 164, 550
    planning nursing care 277–81
  see also Cardiac failure
Heat treatment 339
Heberden's nodes 457
Heliobacter pylorus 282, 283
Help the Hospices 589
Hemiplegia 443
Hepatic coma 292, 295
Hepatitis 291
  B antigen *214*
  type B 594
Heredity
  blood defects 324–5
  and ischaemic heart disease 275
Hernia(s)
  irreducible 401
  reducible 401
  repair 400–4
    care plan 403–4
    the operation 400–1
    planning nursing care 401–3
  sites 401–2, **402**
  strangulation 401
Hiatus hernia **111**
Hip
  arthritis 135
  osteoarthritis **454**
  replacement 455–6, **456**
    social problems 138
HIV infection 24
HIV virus 347
Home helps 572, 574
Homeostasis
  diagram **39**
  maintenance 38–41
  and nervous system 36
Human growth hormone (HGH) *37*
Hydro-ureter 409
Hydronephrosis 409
Hygiene
  personal
    of nurses 356–7
    of patient 358
Hypercalcaemia 320
Hypercapnia 253
Hyperglycaemia *207*, 299, 302, 306,
      309
Hyperglycaemic coma 306
Hyperkalaemia 317
Hypertension
  in chronic renal failure 319
  portal 291
Hyperthyroidism
      (thyrotoxicosis) 269, 310–13

  care plan 313
  disease process 310–11
  planning nursing care 311–13
  pulse in 310
Hypervolaemia *234*
Hypoglycaemia 302, 306, 309
Hypoglycaemic coma 342
Hypothalamus 34–5, **35**, 38
Hypothermia 123–4, *124*, 440
Hypothyroidism (myxoedema) 245,
      313–15
  care plan 315
  disease process 313–14
  planning nursing care 314–15
Hypovolaemia *234*
Hypovolaemic shock *237*
Hypoxia 253, 323, 325
Hysterectomy 385–9
  care plan 389
  the operation 385–6
  planning nursing care 387–9
  psychological problems 386
  recovery after 386–7
  sexual activity after 387, 388, 549

Ileostomy 390
Immigrants 61–2
Immunosuppressants 289, 294,
      337–8
Impotence
  after stoma formation 392, 395
  and prostatectomy 410–11
Incontinence
  in elderly patient 429–32
  in multiple sclerosis 332
  pads and pants **430**
  in unconscious patient 343
  urinary 113
Independence, return to 543–50
Infection Control Nurse 356
Infections
  and anaemia *323*
  control 356–8
  of wounds 374
Influenza 346
Information
  co-ordination of 238–41
  for patients, at admission 71
  see also Patient education
Inguinal hernia 401–2, **402**
Insulin *37*, 298
  injections 302–3
  preparations 302–3
  treatment 302
Intensive therapy unit (ITU) 276
Interactions, *see* Social interactions
Interviews 94–102
  assessment forms 102
  clarification and encouraging
      precision 99
  closing 102
  control 100–101
  cues 97
  educated guesses 98–9
  questioning techniques 94–6

Interviews *contd*
  reassurance 100
  reflection 97–8
  silence 98
  summarizing 101–2
Intravenous fluids, post-
    operative 363, 367
Intravenous pyelogram
    (urogram) 222–4
Intrinsic factor 324
Investigations
  ascites 205
  blood 196–7, *198*, 198–200
  body tissue 206–19
  cerebrospinal fluid (CFS) 205–6,
    207
  diagnostic 196
  faeces 200–1
  sputum 203–4, *205*
  urine 201–3
  see also Urinalysis
Iodine 35
  deficiency 313
Iron-deficiency anaemia 324
Ischaemic heart disease, *see* Heart
    disease, ischaemic
Islets of Langerhans 35, **298**

Jaundice 112, 292, 293, 326
  cholestatic *201*
  haemolytic *201*
Joint Board of Clinical Nursing
    Studies 606

Ketones *204*, 235, 237, 299
Keyhole surgery 549
Kidneys
  biopsy 207, 215–16
  in diabetes 309
  disease 112–13, **113**, 223, 245
  failure, *see* Renal failure
  intravenous pyelogram 222–4
  transplantation 415
Koilonychia 325

Lactase *29*
Laparoscopic appendicectomy 398
Laparoscopic cholecystectomy 405
Laser 209
  treatment 549
Legal status of nursing records 187,
    189
Leukaemias 218
Leukocytes, polymorphonuclear, in
    CSF *207*
Levodopa 451
Life support procedures **279**
Lifestyle
  changes 132–3, 307–9, 550–1
  and disease 346
  health education 60, 523–4
Lipase *29*
Liver
  biopsy 207, 216–18
  cirrhosis, *see* Cirrhosis of liver

disease **111**, 112
  role in digestion 29–30
Local anaesthesia
  biopsy 216, 217
  endoscopy 209–11
London University: Diploma in
    Nursing 606
Loneliness in the elderly 427, 436–7
Luer Lok tap 204
Lumbar puncture 206
Lumpectomy 379
Lungs
  abscess, sputum in *205*
  carcinoma 108–9, **109**, 256–64
    care plan 264
    disease process 256–8
    planning nursing care 258–64
    pleural effusion in 204
    sputum in *205*
  in chronic bronchitis 246–7
  in emphysema 252–3
Lymphatic system 32
Lymphocytes in CSF *207*
Lymphoedema 379

Macmillan Cancer Service 576
Magnetic resonance imaging
    (MRI) 228
Malabsorption **111**, *201*
Malnutrition 440
Maltase *29*
Mammograms 220–1
Marie Curie Foundation 576
Maslow's theory of personality
    development **83**, 83–4
Mastectomy 378–85
  care plan 385
  modified radical 379
  the operation 378–80
  post-operative depression 548
  psychological problems 380,
    381–2, 383–4, 507–8
  social problems 380, 382, 384
  specialist nurse 546
Mastectomy Association 384
Meals-on-wheels 441, 572, 574–5
Medical Research Council 589
Medical ward 243–5
  patient in 502
  self-image of patients 531–2
  types 244–5
Melaena *201*, 285
Memory lapses 314, 426, 433
Meningitis 207
Mental health
  measuring 505–8
  outcomes 504–8
  personality 45–6
  see also Psychological problems;
    Stress
Metabolic activities **26**
Micturating cystogram
    (urethrogram) 224
Midwife, community 565
Minerals, digestion 30

Mobility
  in cardiac failure 271–2
  in elderly patient 428–9
  in multiple sclerosis 330
  observation of 129
  in osteoarthritis 454–5
  post-operative 369–70
  in rheumatoid arthritis 336, 337
  see also Exercise; Rest
Mouth care
  in acute renal failure 318
  in bronchitis 250
  in pneumonia 267
  in ulcerative colitis 289
Mucus in faeces 200–1, *201*
Multiple sclerosis *207*, 330–4
  care plan 334
  disease process 330–1
  planning nursing care 331–4
Muscles, in Parkinson's disease
    448–50
Muscular system **41**
Myocardial infarction 275, 276
  care plan 281
  planning nursing care 277–8
  psychological problems 280
  social care 280–1
Myxoedema, *see* Hypothyroidism

Nails 325
Nasogastric tube **286**
National Health Service (NHS) 21–2,
    571
Nausea 260, 532
Needs
  concept 83–8
  levels 84
  physiological 84–5
  psychological 86–7
  safety 85–6
Nephritis, acute *237*
Nervous system 36, 38
Noradrenaline *37*
Norton scale *135*
Nurse–doctor relationships 7–8, 261,
    579–83, 604
  problems in 580–3
  responsibility for information
    583–5
Nurse–patient interactions 11–12
  see also Communication
Nurse–social worker interaction 574
Nurses
  burnout 599
  continuing education 604–5
    in-service education 605–6
    post-basic courses 606
    reading 605
  counselling role 595–9
  and cross-infection 356–8
  and diagnosis 230–8
  education 603–4
  graduate 588
  graduate education 606–7
  in out-patients' departments 544–5

Nurses *contd*
  religious beliefs 471–2
  and research, *see* Research
  role 3–6, 579–609
    at admission 70–1
  support for 599–603
    by managers 600–1
    by peers 600
    development of coping
      strategies 601–3
  and task-oriented care 6–7
  uniforms 356
  see also District nurse; Enrolled
    nurse; Health visitor;
    Specialized nurse
Nursing
  costs of 593–603
    emotional 594–5
    physical 593–4
  defensive 429, 433
  focus 106
  medical model 3–5, *5*
  preventive 433
Nursing actions 15–16
Nursing care
  in acute renal failure 317–19
  aim evaluation 139–42
  in anaemia 327–9
  in bronchitis 249–51
  in cardiac failure 271–4
  in cerebrovascular accident 444–7
  in chronic renal failure 321–2
  in cirrhosis of liver 294–7
  in diabetes 301–9
  of dying patients 473–4
  in emphysema 254–6
  evaluation, *see* Evaluation of
    nursing care
  in haemorrhage 377
  in hyperthyroidism 311–13
  in hypothyroidism 314–15
  in ischaemic heart disease 277–81
  in lung carcinoma 258–64
  in multiple sclerosis 331–4
  in myocardial infarction 277–8,
    280
  osteoarthritis 455–7
  Parkinson's disease 451–4
  in peptic ulcer 283–5
  plans, *see* Care plans
  in pneumonia 267–9
  quality assurance 510–11
  in rheumatoid arthritis 337–40,
    342–5
  task-oriented 6–7
  in ulcerative colitis 288–91
  unconscious patient 342–5
  see also Post-operative care;
    Pre-operative care
Nursing history 14
Nursing journals 605
Nursing problems, *see* Problems
Nursing process 3, 12–18
  and counselling 596–9
  dynamic nature **13**

Nursing records, *see* Records
Nutrition 16
  in chronic bronchitis 250
  in cirrhosis of liver 294
  deficits 118, 281, 348
  in diabetes 303–5
  in the elderly 440–1
  health education 568
  in unconscious patient 342
  see also Diet; Food intake

Obesity 250, 299
Occupational therapist 445, 457
Oedema
  in acute renal failure 317
  in cardiac failure *237*, 269, 272
  causes *237*
  in chronic renal failure 320
  in cirrhosis of liver *237*, 292,
    293
  in lung carcinoma 257
  pitting 238
  pulmonary 238, 317
  in thrombosis *237*
Oesophagus
  disorders **111**
  endoscopy 211–12, *214*
  ulcers 282
  varices 292
Oestrogen *37*
Oliguria 237, 316
Organ Donation Register 417–18,
  418
Organ transplantation 414–19
  animal organs 417
  ethical problems 415–17
  physical problems 414–15
  psychological problems 417–19
Orthopnoea 377
Orthopnoeic position 272
Oscilloscope 228
Osteoarthritis 454–8
  care plan 457–8
  disease process 454–5
  planning nursing care 455–7
Osteodystrophy 319
Osteopathy Bill 240
Out-patients' departments 526,
  543–6
  appointments 543–4
  the clinic 544, 545–6
  nurse's role 544–5
Ovaries 35, *37*
  removal 385
Oxygen
  intake 25–6
    deficits 108–10, 114, 117–18,
      246–81, 347
  transport **31**
    in anaemia 323
Oxygen therapy
  in anaemia 327
  in bronchitis 249
  in cardiac failure 271
  in emphysema 254

  in myocardial infarction 277
  in pneumonia 267
Oxytocin *37*

Pain 116
  abdominal 212, 218
  angina pectoris 276
  chart **263**
  control 262, 496
  lung cancer 262, 264
  in myocardial infarction 276
  in osteoarthritis 454
  in peptic ulcer 282–3
  post-operative 136, 367–9
  in rheumatoid arthritis 336
Pancreas 35, 35–6, *37*
  in diabetes 298
  digestive enzymes 29
  microscopic structure **298**
Pancreatitis **111**
Papilloedema 443–4, **444**
Paracentesis, abdominal 205, 295
Paralysis, and cerebrovascular
  accident 443
Paralytic ileus 386
Paraplegia, adjustment to 552
Parasites, intestinal 111
Parathyroid glands **35**, *37*
Parathyroid hormone *37*
Parenteral therapy in ulcerative
  colitis 289
Parkinson's disease 447–54
  care plan 454
  disease process 447–51
  planning nursing care 451–4
  psychological problems 449–50,
    452–3
  social problems 450–1, 453–4
Pathology, understanding 106
Patient, potential, measuring 508–11
Patient advocacy 585–7
Patient education
  in anaemia 327–8
  in chronic bronchitis 249–50
  chronic renal failure 321
  cirrhosis of liver 294, 296–7
  in diabetes 307–9
  disease 522–3
  in emphysema 254–5
  in hip replacement 457
  in hyperthyroidism 312
  in ischaemic heart disease 278
  precipitating factors 523–4
  for recovery period 528–9
  for rheumatoid arthritis 338
  teaching methods 524–8
    avoiding confusion 526
    motivation 525
    practice 525–6
    written instructions 526, 528
  see also Health education;
    Information
Patients
  admission, *see* Admission
  counselling 595–9

Patients *contd*
  and cross-infection 358
  cultural differences 472
  documentation 175–84
  lifestyle 132–3
  as a person 8–12
  popular 11, 134
  problems 131–2
  prone position **216**
  roles 10–11
  satisfaction 495–501
  self-image, *see* Self-image
  in shock 366
  supine position **217**
  transfer sheet **188**, 190
  transport 534–5
  see also Nurse–patient interaction
Patient's Charter 22, 69, 147, 170,
    456, 544
Pensions, old age 423
Pepsin *29*
Peptic ulcer 282–7
  care plan 285
  complications 285
  disease process 282–3
  planning nursing care 283–5
Perception 47–8
Perforation, bowel 286–7, 288
Peripheral nervous system 36, 38
Peripheral resistance (PR) 231, *234*
Peristalsis 28
Peritonitis 398–400, 407
Pernicious anaemia *323*, 323–6
Personality 45–6
Physical activity, in bronchitis 247–8
Physiology of physical health 25–44
Physiotherapist 249, 445, 455, 457
Physiotherapy 332, 338
Picolax 212–13, **213**, 391
Pituitary gland 34–5, **35**
  anterior **36**, *37*
  posterior *37*
Placenta *37*
Platelet count 217
Pleural effusion 204–5
Pleurisy 266
Pneumonia 108–9, **109**, 245, 264–9
  care plan 269
  disease process 264–6
  in lung carcinoma 257
  lung sites **265**
  planning nursing care 267–9
  in renal failure 317
  sputum in *205*
Polydipsia 299
Polyneuritis, acute *207*
Polyuria 113, 116, 237, 320
Portal hypertension 292
Post-mortem 488
Post-operative care 363–71
  appendicectomy 400
  cholecystectomy 406–7
  hernia repair 403
  hysterectomy 388–9, *389*
  knowledge 370–1

mastectomy 382–4
  potential problems *364*
  prostatectomy 412–14
  and shock 364–6
  stoma formation 394–7
Post-operative depression 383, 386
Potassium 30
  and diuretics 272
Practice nurse 570–1
Pre-operative care 359–63
  appendicectomy 399
  avoiding complications 361–2
  cholecystectomy 406–7
  hernia repair 401–3
  hysterectomy 387
  mastectomy 381
  patient understanding of
    operation 359–61
  prostatectomy 410–12
  receiving the correct
    operation 362–3
  stoma formation 391–4
Pregnancy *214*
  bladder pressure 113, **115**
  ultrasound planning 228
Prejudice 48–9
Premedication, for endoscopy
    209–12, 215, 217
PREP (Post-Registration Education
    and Practice) 605
Prescription sheets **177–8**
Pressure areas, in ulcerative
    colitis 289
Pressure sores 259, 272, 284, **504**
  risk areas **135**
Primary health care team 571
  interaction with health visitor **566**
  out-patient's contacts with **546**
  roles **7**
  structure **560**
Problem family 569
Problems
  alleviation 141
  anticipation 135–9
    dangers 138–9
    physical problems 135–6
    psychological 136–7
    social 138
  class identification *139*
  definition 134
  goals 149–51
  identified 148–9
  insoluble 141–2
  nurse's 133–4
  patient's 131–2
  possible solutions 140–1
Progesterone *37*
Progress sheets **184–7**
Prolactin *37*
Propranolol 311
Prostate gland, enlargement 113–14,
    114
Prostatectomy 409–14
  the operation 409–10
  perineal 410

planning nursing care 410–14
  retropubic 410–11, **411**
  suprapubic **410**
  transurethral 410–11, **411**
Prostheses, breast 380–1, **381**, 383
Proteins
  in cerebrospinal fluid *207*
  digestion *29*
  in urine 320
Prothrombin time 217, 404
Pruritus 320
Psychiatrist, referral to 262, 290,
    328, 333, 340, 383, 532
Psychological individual 52–3
Psychological problems
  in acute renal failure 318–19
  after surgery 136–7; *see also*
    specific operations
  in AIDS 348, 349
  in anaemia 326, 328–9
  anticipation 136–7
  in bronchitis 248, 250–1
  in cardiac failure 271, 273–4
  cerebrovascular accident 443–4,
    445–6
  in chronic renal failure 320, 321
  in cirrhosis of liver 293, 296
  in diabetes 132, 300, 306–8
  discharge, *see* Discharge
  disease and 116–17
  in emphysema 253, 255
  in hyperthyroidism 310–11,
    312–13
  in hypothyroidism 314
  in lung carcinoma 257–8, 261–2
  in multiple sclerosis 331, 332–4
  in myocardial infarction 276–7,
    280
  in osteoarthritis 455, 456–7
  in Parkinson's disease 449–50,
    452–3
  in peptic ulcer 283, 284
  in pneumonia 266, 268
  in renal failure 316
  in rheumatoid arthritis 336,
    339–40, 344–5
  in ulcerative colitis 288, 289–90
  see also Anxiety; Depression;
    Self-image; Stress
Psychology of mental health 45–54
Pulmonary embolism *205*
Pulmonary hypertension 247
Pulmonary oedema 238, 270, 317
Pulmonary tuberculosis *205*
Pulse 124–5
  in anaemia 325
  in hyperthyroidism 310
  in myocardial infarction 276
  rate 124–5
  rhythm 125
  taking **124**
  volume 125
Pus
  in faeces 200
  in sputum *205*, 266

Pyelitis, acute 245
Pyelonephritis 319
Pyrexia 122–3, *124*, 224, 237

Qualpac 511
Questioning techniques 94–6
Questions
    closed 95
    leading 96
    open 95–6

Race Relations Act 61
Radionuclide imaging 227
Radiotherapy 258–9, 379
Reagent strips 234–5, **235**
Reassurance
    of patients 100
    of relatives 81, 486–7
Records 175–91
    changes 185
    drug 176, 178–9
    medical 175–6
    nursing
        and co-ordination 189–90
        as legal document 184–7,
            189–90
        progress sheets **184–7**
Rectum 28
Referral of problems 533–4
Registered General Nurse
        (RGN) 565, 607
Registered Nurse (RN) 559
Rehabilitation
    cerebrovascular accident 444–7
    wards 423
RELATE 576
Relatives 80–1
    and AIDS 348–9
    bereaved
        bereavement visiting 491
        grief 489–91
        needs after death 487
        practical needs 488–9
        reporting death to 488
    in cardiac failure 273–4
    in cerebrovascular accident 444,
        446–7
    in chronic bronchitis 250
    dying patient 470, 482–5
        children 487
        collusion 482–4
        knowledge 485–6
        reassurance 486–7
        visiting 484–5
    education of 328
    emotional care 537–8
    in emphysema 253–4, 255–6
    in lung cancer 259, 261–2
    in multiple sclerosis 331–4
    notification of discharge
        533
    in Parkinson's disease 452
    physical care by 537
    of unconscious patient 345
Religion, ministers of 262

Religious beliefs
    in chronic disease 333, 336, 340
    in dying patients 470
    of nurses 471–2
Renal biopsy 207, 215–16
Renal dialysis 318
Renal failure
    acute 316–19
        care plan 319
        dehydration *237*
        disease process 316–17
        planning nursing care 317–19
    chronic 319–22
        care plan 322
        disease process 319–21
        planning nursing care 321–2
Renin *234*
Research 587–93
    becoming research-minded
        589–91
    becoming a researcher 588–9
    reading research reports 591–3
Residual deficits 551–2
    see also Disability; Independence
Respiration 125–6
    cellular 25
    control 38–9
    rate 126
    rhythm 126
    sound 126
    see also Breathing; Oxygen intake
Respiratory acidosis 252
Respiratory disease, chronic,
        adjustment to 552
Respiratory system **27**
Rest
    in anaemia 327
    in cardiac failure 271–2
    deficits associated with 114–16,
        322–3
    and hysterectomy 389
    in pneumonia 267
Retinopathy, diabetic 309
Retirement 25, 422
Rheumatoid arthritis 334–41
    appearance and progression **335**
    care plan 340–1
    disease process 334–7
    planning nursing care 337–40
Rheumatoid factor 336
Rheumatoid nodules 336
Rogers' theory of personality
        development 45–6
Roles of individuals 10–11
Royal College of Nursing 591–2
Ryle's tube 399

Safety
    of the elderly 432–4
    in laser use 209
    patients' needs 85–6
Salpingo-oophorectomy,
        bilateral 385
Salt, dietary 272
Samaritans 576

Satisfaction, patient 495–501
Scanning 225–8
Scars 373
Scottish Health Education Group
        (SHEG) 23
Scottish Home and Health
        Department 588
Self-awareness of nurses 602–3
Self-care 339, 500
Self-image 9–10, 86–7
    and ageing 426
    at discharge 530, 532, 537–8
    in chronic bronchitis 250
    and employment 550–1
    surgery affecting 377–97, 531
        see also Hysterectomy;
            Mastectomy, Stoma
Sengstaken tube **297**
Sensation loss 342, 343
Sex education 568
Sexual advice 528
Sexual counselling 388, 528–9
Sexual problems
    after hysterectomy 387, 388
    after mastectomy 380, 383
    in Parkinson's disease 450, 453
    in rheumatoid arthritis 340
    and stoma 395–6
    see also Impotence
Sexuality 50
    of elderly patient 435–6
Shark's cartilage 241
Sheffield University: Master of
        Science 607
Shock
    anaphylactic 365
    cardiogenic 276, 364
    and haemorrhage 377
    hypovolaemic 365
    in peritonitis 399
    in pneumonia 267
    post-operative 364–6
Sickle cell anaemia *323*, 324–5, **325**
Sickle cell crisis 326, 327
Sickness certificate 549
Sigmoidoscopy 213–14
Skeletal system **40**, 41
Skin 128
    and radiotherapy 259
    in shock 365
    and stoma 394
Sleep disturbances 115–16
Smoking 24, 133
    and bronchitis 247, 249–50
    by nurses 594
    care plan 164, **165–8**
    in emphysema 254
    health education 23, 524, 568
    and ischaemic heart disease 275
    and lung carcinoma 257, 258, 264
    and myocardial infarction 280
    passive 257, 258
    and peptic ulcer 282, 284
    and pneumonia 264
Social class 54–5, *55*, 89

Social factors, and disease 117–18
Social interactions 49
  with dying patients 474
Social problems
  in acute renal failure 319
  after mastectomy 382
  in AIDS 348–50
  in anaemia 326–7, 329
  and appendicectomy 399–400
  bronchitis 248–9, 251
  in cardiac failure 271, 274
  cerebrovascular accident 444,
    446–7
  in chronic renal failure 321–2
  in cirrhosis of liver 293, 296–7
  in diabetes 300, 308–9
  in emphysema 253–4, 255
  hip replacement 138
  in hyperthyroidism 311, 313
  in hypothyroidism 314
  hysterectomy 386–7
  incontinence 138
  lung cancer 264
  in lung carcinoma 258
  in multiple sclerosis 331, 334
  in myocardial infarction 277,
    280–1
  in osteoarthritis 455, 457
  in Parkinson's disease 450–1,
    453–4
  in peptic ulcer 283, 284–5
  in pneumonia 264, 266, 268–9
  in rheumatoid arthritis 336–7,
    340
  in stoma formation 394, 396–7
  in ulcerative colitis 288, 290–1
Social services 22, 334, 340, 414,
    433, 447, 454, 571
  support in the home by 514–15,
    515
Social worker 567, 571–3
  care load 572–3
  discharge and 573
  and home helps 572
  referral to 572
Sociological aspects of health 54–62
Sodium 30
Specialist nurse 526, 546–7, 565
Speech, loss 257, 443
Speech therapist 445
Spider angioma 292
Spirituality 53–4
Splenectomy 329
Splints 338
Sputum
  abnormalities *205*
  collection 203–4
  in pneumonia 266
Staff on the wards 73–5
Status 55–6
Steatorrhoea *201*
Stercobilin *201*
Sterility 385
Sterilization of supplies and
    equipment 371–2

Sternal puncture 218
Steroids
  in rheumatoid arthritis 337–8
  in ulcerative colitis 289
Stoma 390–7
  bags 392, 394–5, **395**
  care plan 397
  impotence after 392, 395
  the operation 390–1
  patient education 394–7, 525
  planning nursing care 391–7
  psychological problems 392–4,
    395–6
  specialist nurse 396, 546
Stomach
  endoscopy 211–12
  obstruction 286
  ulcers 111, 282
Stomatitis **111**, 325
Streptokinase 277
Stress 46–7
  at admission 70–1, 136, 233
  in diabetes 306–7
  effects 12, 13
  in families 566
  and ischaemic heart disease 275,
    280
  in multiple sclerosis 333
  in nurses 603
  and outcomes 504
  in peptic ulcer 282
  in ulcerative colitis 288
  see also Psychological problems
Stroke, *see* Cerebrovascular accident
Subarachnoid haemorrhage *207*
Sucrase *29*
Suicide 316, 318
  and depression 549
Suppositories 213, 223, 273, 431
Surgery 5–6
  and cirrhosis of liver 294
  'cold' 355
  exploratory 355
  post-operative care, *see*
    Post-operative care
  pre-operative care, *see*
    Pre-operative care
  psychological problems after
    136–7
  replacement 414–19
  see also specific operations
Surgical ward 353–5
  cleaning 357–8
  infection control 356–8
  patient care 359–71, 501–2
  types 354–5
Sutures 374
Sweat 34
Synovial membrane 334–5

'T' tube in bile duct 406–8
Tachycardia 124
Teeth
  diseased 111
  false 211, 214, 343

Temperature 118–19, 121–4
  anal (rectal) site 122
  axillary site **122**
  intervals for 119, 121
  maintenance 38
  observations 122
  oral site **121**, 121–2
  pulse and respiration (TPR) 5,
    125, 230
    chart **120**
    charts 179–80, 233, 235
    post-operative 363
  role in recognizing disease 127
  taking 119
Testes **35**, *37*
Testosterone *37*
Thalassaemia *323*, 325, 326
Thermometers 119, **121**
Thrombosis *237*
  cerebral 441–2
  coronary, *see* Myocardial
    infarction
  oedema in *237*
Thyroid gland *37*
Thyroid hormones 35
Thyroid-stimulating hormone
    (TSH) 34, *37*
Thyroidectomy 311, 313
Thyrotoxicosis, *see* Hyperthyroidism
Thyroxine (T_4) *37*, 310, 314
Tiredness 257
  in anaemia 327
  in hyperthyroidism 310
Tomograms 220–1, **221**
Tonsillitis **111**
Tranquillizers 294, 312
  for biopsy 216, 217
Transport of patients 534–5
Trent Palliative Care Centre 588
Tri-iodothyronine (T_3) *37*, 310
Trypsin *29*
Tuberculosis 594
  pulmonary *205*
  tomogram **221**
Tumours, biopsy 218

Ulcerative colitis **111**, *214*, 222,
    287–91, 390
  care plan 291
  disease process 287–8
  faecal abnormalities *201*
  planning nursing care 288–91
Ultrasound scanning 227–8
Umbilical hernia 401–2, **402**
Unconscious patient 317, 323, 341–6
  care plan 345–6
  planning nursing care 324–5
  see also Coma
Uniforms, nurses' 356
United Kingdom Central Council
    (UKCC) 603, 605
Uraemia
  and prostate gland
    enlargement 409
  in renal failure 316, 317, 320

Urethrogram 224
Urinalysis 5, 127, 201–3, *204*,
    233–6
  charts 180, **183**
  in diabetes 305
Urinary tract
  catheterization, *see*
    Catheterization, urinary tract
  endoscopy/biopsy 215
  infection 409
  investigation 224
  obstruction 409
Urine
  abnormalities *204*, 234–6
  collection 202
    24-hour specimen 202–3
    'clean' specimen 202
    early morning specimen 202
  excretion, disturbances 113–14,
    367, 409
  glucose in 236–7
  incontinence, *see* Incontinence
  investigations 201–3
  normal characteristics *234*
  in renal failure 316
  see also Micturition
Urobilinogen 235
Urogram 222–4
Urokinase 277
Uterus, carcinoma 385

Vagina, surgery 388
Vaginitis 299
Varicose ulcers 504
Vasoconstriction 266, 316, 325
Veins **31–2**
Venous thrombosis 268, 272, 284
Vesico-ureteric reflux 224

Victim Support 576
Viral infections 265
Visiting 473, 484–5
Visual deficits 426
Visual display unit (VDU) 226
Vitamin A 30
Vitamin B$_{12}$ 294, 327
  deficiency (pernicious
    anaemia) *323*, 323–6
Vitamin B 30
Vitamin C 30
  deficiency 324, 326
Vitamin D 30, 319
Vitamin E 30
Vitamin K 404, 406
Vitamins 294
  digestion 30
Vomiting *237*, 276
  in peptic ulcer 283, 285

Waiting, lists for admission 397
Walking, difficulties with 141, 336,
    455
Walking sticks 455
Wards
  for the elderly 423
  environment of, patient
    adjustment 71–5
  mixed-sex 244
  noise and smell 72–3
  personnel 73–4
  structure 71–2
  see also Medical wards; Surgical
    wards
Warmth
  in the elderly 440–1
  in shock 365
Waste product elimination 32–4

Water
  body 31
  elimination 33–4
Weight 524
  change 127
  gain 314
  loss 112, 257, 311
  see also Obesity
Wellcome Trust 589
Wheelchairs 340, 552
Wigs 260
Women's Royal Voluntary Service
    (WRVS) 575
Work, return to 549–50
Working for Patients 22
World Health Organization
    (WHO) 20
Wounds 373–7
  asepsis 373
  and cross-infection 356–8
  CSSD packs 371–2, **372**
  drainage 376
  dressings 374–6
  haemorrhage 376–7
  healing 372–4, 504
    'secondary intention' 373–4,
    374

X-rays 216, 219–28
  barium meal 221–2
  CAT scanning 225
  contrast studies 221
  mammogram 220–1
  straight 219–20
  tomogram 220
  types 219

Zimmer aid 429, **434**, 455, 499